Nurse Practitioner
Certification Examination and Practice Preparation

FOURTH EDITION

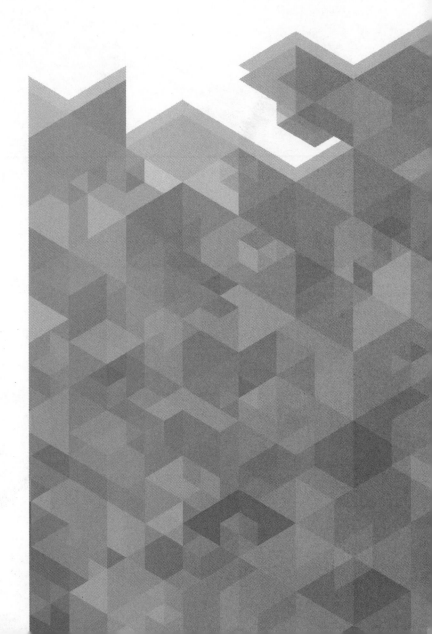

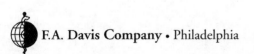

Nurse Practitioner
Certification Examination and Practice Preparation

FOURTH EDITION

Margaret A. Fitzgerald,
DNP, FNP-BC, NP-C, FAANP, CSP, FAAN, DCC
President, Fitzgerald Health Education
*   Associates, Inc.*
North Andover, Massachusetts
Family Nurse Practitioner
Greater Lawrence Family Health Center
Lawrence, Massachusetts

F.A. Davis Company • Philadelphia

F. A. Davis Company
1915 Arch Street
Philadelphia, PA 19103
www.fadavis.com

Printed in the United States of America

Last digit indicates print number: 10 9 8 7 6 5 4

Publisher, Nursing: Joanne Patzek DaCunha, RN, MSN
Director of Content Development: Darlene D. Pedersen, MSN, APRN, BC
Content Project Manager: Echo Gerhart
Design & Illustration Manager: Carolyn O'Brien
Electronic Project Editor: Sandra Glennie

As new scientific information becomes available through basic and clinical research, recommended treatments and drug therapies undergo changes. The author(s) and publisher have done everything possible to make this book accurate, up to date, and in accord with accepted standards at the time of publication. The author(s), editors, and publisher are not responsible for errors or omissions or for consequences from application of the book, and make no warranty, expressed or implied, in regard to the contents of the book. Any practice described in this book should be applied by the reader in accordance with professional standards of care used in regard to the unique circumstances that may apply in each situation. The reader is advised always to check product information (package inserts) for changes and new information regarding dose and contraindications before administering any drug. Caution is especially urged when using new or infrequently ordered drugs.

Library of Congress Cataloging-in-Publication Data

Fitzgerald, Margaret A., author.
  Nurse practitioner certification examination and practice preparation / Margaret A. Fitzgerald. — Fourth edition.
    p. ; cm.
  Includes bibliographical references and index.
  ISBN 978-0-8036-4074-0 (alk. paper)
  I. Title.
  [DNLM: 1. Nursing Care—methods—Examination Questions. 2. Certification—Examination Questions. 3. Nurse Practitioners—Examination Questions. WY 18.2]

RT120.F34
610.73076—dc23

                                                        2014008482

Dedication

To my dear brother, Jack (John Edward Fitzgerald, Jr.), and amazing sister-in-law, KT (Kathleen Thomas), two of the bravest people I know, with much love and admiration.

Contributors

Kara L. Ashley, M.Ed.
Northeast Association of Learning Specialists

Victor Czerkasij, MA, MS, FNP-BC, NP-C
Associate Lecturer
Fitzgerald Health Education Associates, Inc.
Clinical Practice, Skin Cancer and Cosmetic
    Dermatology, PC
Cleveland, Tennessee
Adult and Pediatric Dermatology
Dalton, Georgia

Carolyn Buppert, NP, JD
The Law Offices of Carolyn Buppert
Boulder, Colorado

Kahlil Ahmadi Demonbreun, DNP, RNC-OB, WHNP-BC, ANP-BC
Instructor
College of Nursing
Medical University of South Carolina
Clinical Practice, Women's Health Nurse Practitioner
Palmetto Primary Care Physicians
Charleston, South Carolina

Susan Feeney, MS, NP-C, FNP-BC
Senior Lecturer
Fitzgerald Health Education Associates, Inc.
Clinical Practice, Wright and Associates Family Healthcare
Amherst, New Hampshire
Assistant Professor
Director of Graduate Nursing Education
Rivier University
Nashua, New Hampshire

Jordan Hopchik, MSN, RN, FNP-BC, CGRN
Gastroenterology Nurse Practitioner
Philadelphia VA Medical Center
SGNA Scholar, DNP Student
La Salle University
Philadelphia, Pennsylvania

Scharmaine Lawson-Baker, DNP, FNP-BC, FAANP
Advanced Clinical Consultants
New Orleans, Louisiana

Louise McDevitt, MS, ACNP-BC, ANP-BC, FNP-BC, FAANP
Senior Lecturer
Fitzgerald Health Education Associates, Inc.
Clinical Practice, Grace Cottage Family Practice
Townshend, Vermont
Assistant Clinical Instructor
University of Vermont Medical School and
Graduate School of Nursing Family Nurse Practitioner
    Program
Burlington, Vermont

Sally K. Miller, PhD, AGACNP-BC, AGPCNP-BC, FNP-BC, FAANP
Senior Lecturer
Fitzgerald Health Education Associates, Inc.
Clinical Practice, Nevada Health Center
Las Vegas, Nevada
Clinical Professor
Drexel University College of Nursing and Health Professions
Philadelphia, Pennsylvania

Monica N. Tombasco, MS, MSNA, FNP-BC, CRNA
Senior Lecturer
Fitzgerald Health Education Associates, Inc.
Clinical Practice, CRNA, Catholic Medical Center
Manchester, New Hampshire
Nurse Practitioner, Emergency Medicine
Central New Hampshire Emergency Physicians
Huggins Hospital
Wolfeboro, New Hampshire

Christy M. Yates, MS, FNP-BC, NP-C, AE-C
Senior Lecturer
Fitzgerald Health Education Associates, Inc.
Clinical Practice, Family Allergy and Asthma
Louisville, Kentucky

Acknowledgments

This book represents a sum of the efforts of many people.

I thank my family, especially my husband, and business partner, Marc Comstock, for their support and patience as they lived through this experience.

I thank the staff of Fitzgerald Health Education Associates, Inc. for sharing me with this project for many months. To the contributing authors, your insight has helped increase the value and helpfulness of this publication.

I thank the patients and staff of the Greater Lawrence (MA) Family Health Center, where I have practiced for more than 25 years, as they continue to serve as a source of inspiration as I developed this book. Gracias.

I thank Joanne DaCunha, Echo Gerhart, and the F.A. Davis staff for their ongoing encouragement.

Last but not least, I thank the thousands of nurse practitioners who, over the years, have participated in the Fitzgerald Health Education Associates, Inc. Nurse Practitioner Certification courses. Your eagerness to learn, thirst for knowledge, dedication to success, and commitment to excellence in healthcare provision continue to inspire me. I am privileged to be part of your professional development.

Introduction

The scope of practice of the nurse practitioner is wide, encompassing the care of the young, the old, the sick, and the well. This book has been developed to help the nurse practitioner develop the knowledge and skills to successfully enter nurse practitioner (NP) practice and earn certification, an important landmark in professional achievement.

This book represents a perspective on learning and practice developed during my years of practice at the Greater Lawrence (MA) Family Health Center and as an NP and professional speaker. In addition, my experiences through the years of helping thousands of NPs achieve professional success through conducting Fitzgerald Health Education Associates, Inc. NP Certification and Advance Practice Update Courses influenced the development and presentation of the information held within.

This book is not intended to be a comprehensive clinical text; rather, it is meant to be a source to reinforce learning and a guide for the development of the information base and critical thinking skills needed for safe, entry-level NP practice. The reader is encouraged to answer the questions given in each section and then check on the accuracy of the response. The discussion section is intended to enhance learning through highlighting the essentials of primary care NP practice. The numerous tables can serve as a quick-look resource not only as the NP prepares for entry to practice and certification but also in the delivery of ongoing care.

—MARGARET A. FITZGERALD, DNP, FNP-BC, NP-C,
    FAANP, CSP, FAAN, DCC
    President
    Fitzgerald Health Education Associates, Inc.
    North Andover, Massachusetts
    Family Nurse Practitioner
    Greater Lawrence (MA) Family Health Center
    Lawrence, Massachusetts

Contents

Health Promotion and Disease Prevention

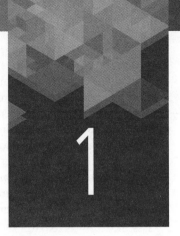

1

Primary Prevention Measures

1. An example of a primary prevention measure for a 78-year-old man with chronic obstructive pulmonary disease is:
   A. reviewing the use of prescribed medications.
   B. conducting a home survey to minimize fall risk.
   C. checking FEV1 (force expired volume at 1 second) to FVC (forced vital capacity) ratio.
   D. ordering fecal occult blood test (FOBT).

2. Which of the following is an example of a primary prevention activity in a 76-year-old woman with osteoporosis?
   A. bisphosphonate therapy
   B. calcium supplementation
   C. ensuring adequate illumination in the home
   D. use of a back brace

3. Secondary prevention measures for a 78-year-old man with chronic obstructive pulmonary disease include:
   A. screening for mood disorders.
   B. administering influenza vaccine.
   C. obtaining a serum theophylline level.
   D. advising about appropriate use of car passenger restraints.

4. Tertiary prevention measures for a 69-year-old woman with heart failure include:
   A. administering antipneumococcal vaccine.
   B. adjusting therapy to minimize dyspnea.
   C. surveying skin for precancerous lesions.
   D. reviewing safe handling of food.

5. Which of the following products provides passive immunity?
   A. hepatitis B immune globulin (HBIG)
   B. measles, mumps, and rubella (MMR) vaccine
   C. pneumococcal conjugate vaccine
   D. live attenuated influenza vaccine (LAIV)

6. Active immunity is defined as:
   A. resistance developed in response to an antigen.
   B. immunity conferred by an antibody produced in another host.
   C. the resistance of a group to an infectious agent.
   D. defense against disease acquired naturally by the infant from the mother.

7. Which of the following is usually viewed as the most cost-effective form of healthcare?
   A. primary prevention
   B. secondary prevention
   C. tertiary prevention
   D. cancer-reduction measures

8. An 18-year-old woman with allergic rhinitis presents for primary care. She is sexually active with a male partner and is 1 year post-coitarche; during this time she had had two sex partners. An example of a primary prevention activity for this patient is:
   A. screening for sexually transmitted infection.
   B. counseling about safer sexual practices.
   C. prescribing therapies for minimizing allergy.
   D. obtaining a liquid-based Papanicolaou (Pap) test.

9. When a critical portion of a community is immunized against a contagious disease, most members of the community, even the unimmunized, are protected against that disease because there is little opportunity for an outbreak. This is known as _____ immunity.
   A. passive
   B. humoral
   C. epidemiologic
   D. community

Answers

1. B.	4. B.	7. A.
2. C.	5. A.	8. B.
3. A.	6. A.	9. D.

Primary prevention measures include activities provided to individuals to prevent the onset or acquisition of a given disease. The goal of primary prevention measures is to spare individuals the suffering, burden, and cost associated with the clinical condition and is the first level of healthcare. An example is health-protecting education and counseling, such as encouraging the use of car restraints and bicycle helmets, counseling about safer sexual practices, and providing information on accident and fall prevention. Given its focus on preventing illness or injury, primary prevention is usually viewed as the most effective form of healthcare.

Immunizations and chemoprophylaxis are also examples of primary prevention measures. Active immunization through the use of vaccines provides long-term protection from disease. In herd or community immunity, a significant portion of a given population has immunity against an infectious agent; the likelihood that the susceptible portion of the group would become infected is minimized (Fig. 1–1). Passive immunity is provided when a person receives select antibodies, usually via the administration of immune globulin (IG), after exposure to an infective agent. This immunity is temporary and requires the patient to present post-exposure; the protection provided by IG usually starts within hours of receiving the doses and lasts a number of months. The use of vaccines to produce lasting disease protection is preferred to passive immunization through the use of IG. Another example of passive immunity is the acquisition of disease protection provided from mother to unborn child via the placenta. Secondary prevention measures include activities provided to identify and treat asymptomatic persons who have risk factors for a given disease or in preclinical disease. Examples include screening examinations for preclinical evidence of cancer, such as mammography and cervical examination with a Papanicolaou test. Other examples of secondary prevention activities include screening for clinical conditions with a protracted asymptomatic period, such as a blood pressure measurement to detect hypertension and a lipid profile to detect hyperlipidemia (Table 1–1).

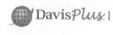 **See full color images of this topic on DavisPlus at http://davisplus.fadavis.com | Keyword: Fitzgerald**

Tertiary prevention measures are part of the management of an established disease. The goal is to minimize disease-associated complications and the negative health effects of the conditions to the patient. Examples include medications and lifestyle modification to normalize blood glucose levels in individuals with diabetes mellitus and in conjunction with the treatment of heart failure, aimed at improving or minimizing disease-related symptoms.

DISCUSSION SOURCES

http://www.cdc.gov/excite/skincancer/mod13.htm, Centers for Disease Control and Prevention: Levels of Prevention

http://www.niaid.nih.gov/topics/pages/communityimmunity.aspx, National Institute of Allergy and Infectious Disease: Community Immunity

Influenza Immunization

10. When advising a patient about injectable influenza immunization, the nurse practitioner (NP) considers the following about the use of this vaccine:
    A. Its use is not recommended in sickle cell anemia.
    B. Its use is limited to children older than 2 years.
    C. Its use is limited due to containing live virus.
    D. Its use is recommended for virtually all members of the population.

11. A middle-aged man with chronic obstructive pulmonary disease who is about to receive injectable influenza vaccine should be advised that:
    A. it is more than 90% effective in preventing influenza.
    B. its use is contraindicated in the presence of psoriasis vulgaris.
    C. localized reactions such as soreness and redness at the site of the immunization are fairly common.
    D. a short, intense, flulike syndrome typically occurs after immunization.

12. A 44-year-old woman with asthma presents asking for a "flu shot." She is seen today for an urgent care visit, is diagnosed with a lower urinary tract infection, and is prescribed trimethoprim-sulfamethoxazole. She is without fever or gastrointestinal upset with stable respiratory status. You inform her that she:
    A. should return for the immunization after completing her antibiotic therapy.
    B. would likely develop a significant reaction if immunized today.
    C. can receive the immunization today.
    D. is not a candidate for any form of influenza vaccine.

13. Which of the following statements best describes amantadine or rimantadine use in the care of patients with or at risk for influenza?
    A. Significant resistance to select strains of influenza limits the usefulness of these medications.
    B. The primary action of these therapies is in preventing influenza A during outbreaks.
    C. These therapies are active against influenza A and B.
    D. The use of these products is an acceptable alternative to influenza vaccine.

14. Which of the following statements best describes zanamivir (Relenza) or oseltamivir (Tamiflu) use in the care of patients with or at risk for influenza?
    A. Initiation of therapy early in acute influenza illness can help minimize the severity of disease when the illness is caused by a nonresistant viral strain.
    B. The primary indication is in preventing influenza A during outbreaks.
    C. The drugs are active only against influenza B.
    D. The use of these medications is an acceptable alternative to influenza vaccine.

Section 1: Preventive Services Recommended by the USPSTF

The U.S. Preventive Services Task Force (USPSTF) recommends that clinicians discuss these preventive services with eligible patients and offer them as a priority. All these services have been given "A" or a "B" (recommended) grade from the Task Force.

Recommendation	Adults		Special Populations	
	Men	Women	Pregnant Women	Children
Abdominal Aortic Aneurysm, Screening	✓			
Alcohol Misuse Screening and Behavioral Counseling Interventions	✓	✓	✓	
Asymptomatic Bacteriuria in Adults, Screening			✓	
Breast and Ovarian Cancer Susceptibility, Genetic Risk Assessment and BRCA Mutation Testing		✓		
Breast Cancer, Screening		✓		
Breastfeeding, Primary Care Interventions to Promote		✓	✓	
Cervical Cancer, Screening		✓		
Chlamydial Infection, Screening		✓	✓	
Colorectal Cancer, Screening	✓	✓		
Congenital Hypothyroidism, Screening				✓
Depression in Adults, Screening	✓	✓		
Diabetes Mellitus (Type 2) in Adults, Screening	✓	✓		
Folic Acid to Prevent Neural Tube Defects		✓	✓	
Gonococcal Ophthalmia Neonatorum, Preventive Medication				✓

Figure 1-1 Preventive services recommended by the U.S. Preventive Services Task Force (USPSTF). Available at http://www.ahrq.gov/clinic/pocketgd2012/gcp12s1.htm.

Continued

Section 1: Preventive Services Recommended by the USPSTF *(continued)*

Recommendation	Adults		Special Populations	
	Men	Women	Pregnant Women	Children
Gonorrhea, Screening		✓	✓	
Hearing Loss in Newborns, Screening				✓
Hepatitis B Virus in Pregnant Women, Screening			✓	
High Blood Pressure (Adults), Screening	✓	✓		
HIV, Screening	✓	✓	✓	✓
Iron Deficiency Anemia, Prevention				✓
Iron Deficiency Anemia, Screening			✓	
Lipid Disorders in Adults, Screening	✓	✓		
Major Depressive Disorder in Children, Screening				✓
Obesity in Children and Adolescents, Screening				✓
Osteoporosis, Screening		✓		
Phenylketonuria, Screening				✓
Rh (D) Incompatibility, Screening			✓	
Sexually Transmitted Infections, Counseling	✓	✓		
Sickle Cell Disease, Screening				✓
Syphilis Infection, Screening	✓	✓		
Syphilis Infection in Pregnancy, Screening			✓	
Tobacco Use in Adults and Pregnant Women, Counseling	✓	✓	✓	
Visual Impairment in Children Ages 1 to 5, Screening				✓

Figure 1-1—cont'd

TABLE 1-1
Secondary Prevention Principles

Principle	Comment
Prevalence is sufficient to justify screening.	Routine mammography is appropriate in women but not men.
Health problem has significant effect on quality or quantity of life.	Target diseases for secondary prevention include hypertension, type 2 diabetes mellitus, dyslipidemia, and certain cancers.
The target disease has a long asymptomatic period. The natural history of the disease, or how the disease unfolds without intervention, is known.	Treatment is available for the target disease. Providing treatment alters the disease's natural history.
A population-acceptable screening test is available.	The test should be safe, should be available at a reasonable cost, and have reasonable sensitivity and specificity.

Source: http://www.clevelandclinicmeded.com/medicalpubs/diseasemanagement/preventive-medicine/principles-of-screening/, Principles of Screening

15. When advising a patient about the influenza nasal spray vaccine, the NP considers the following:
    A. Its use is acceptable during pregnancy.
    B. Its use is limited to children younger than 6 years.
    C. It contains live, attenuated virus.
    D. This is the preferred method of influenza protection in the presence of airway disease.

16. Approximately _____ of healthcare providers receive influenza immunization annually.
    A. one-quarter
    B. one-half
    C. two-thirds
    D. three-quarters or more

17. The most common mode of influenza virus transmission is via:
    A. contact with a contaminated surface.
    B. respiratory droplet.
    C. saliva contact.
    D. skin-to-skin contact.

18. In an immunocompetent adult, the length of incubation for the influenza virus is on average:
    A. less than 24 hours.
    B. 1 to 4 days.
    C. 4 to 7 days.
    D. more than 1 week.

19. Influenza protection options for a 62-year-old man with hypertension, dyslipidemia, and type 2 diabetes mellitus include receiving:
    A. live attenuated influenza vaccine via nasal spray.
    B. high-dose trivalent inactivated vaccine (TIV) via intramuscular injection
    C. trivalent inactivated vaccine (TIV) in standard dose via intramuscular injection.
    D. appropriate antiviral medication as the initial onset of influenza-like illness.

20. Which of the following should not receive vaccination against influenza?
    A. a 19 year-old with a history of hive-form reaction to eating eggs
    B. a 24-year-old woman who is 8 weeks pregnant
    C. a 4-month-old infant who was born at 32 weeks of gestation
    D. a 28-year-old woman who is breastfeeding a 2 week old.

21. A healthy 6-year-old girl presents for care. Her parents request that she receive vaccination for influenza and report that she has not received this vaccine in the past. How many doses of influenza vaccine should she receive this flu season?
    A. 1
    B. 2
    C. 3
    D. 4

Answers

10. D.	14. A.	18. B.
11. C.	15. C.	19. C.
12. C.	16. D.	20. C.
13. A.	17. B.	21. B.

An individual who presents with an abrupt onset of signs and symptoms including fever, myalgia, headache, malaise, nonproductive cough, sore throat, and rhinitis typically has uncomplicated influenza illness, more commonly known as "the flu." Children with influenza commonly have acute otitis media, nausea, and vomiting in addition to the aforementioned signs and symptoms. Although the worst symptoms in most uncomplicated cases resolve in about 1 week, the cough and malaise often persist for 2 or more weeks. Individuals with ongoing health problems such as pulmonary or cardiac disease, young children, and pregnant women also have increased risk of influenza-related complications including pneumonia. Rarely, influenza virus infection also has been associated with encephalopathy, transverse myelitis, myositis, myocarditis, pericarditis, and Reye syndrome.

Influenza viruses spread from person to person largely via respiratory droplet from an infected person, primarily through a cough or sneeze. In an immunocompetent adult, the influenza virus has a short incubation period, with a range of 1 to 4 days (average of 2 days). Adults pass the illness on 1 day before the onset of symptoms and continue to remain infectious for approximately 5 days after the onset of the illness. Children remain infectious for 10 or more days after the onset of symptoms and can shed the virus before the onset of symptoms. People who are immunocompromised can remain infectious for up to 3 weeks.

Historically, the risks for complications, hospitalizations, and deaths from influenza are higher among adults older than age 65 years, young children, and individuals of any age with certain underlying health conditions than among healthy older children and younger adults. In children younger than 5 years, hospitalization rates for influenza-related illness have ranged from approximately 500/100,000 for children with high-risk medical conditions to 100/100,000 for children without high-risk medical conditions. Hospitalization rates for influenza-related illness among children younger than 24 months are comparable to rates reported among adults older than 65 years. Influenza strains such as H1N1, an influenza A virus also known as swine flu, and H5N1, an influenza A virus also known as avian flu, appear to cause a greater disease burden in younger adults.

Considering these factors, influenza, regardless of the viral strain, is not just a bad cold, but rather a potentially serious illness with significant morbidity and mortality risk across the life span. Even in the absence of complications, this viral illness typically causes many days of incapacitation and suffering and the risk of death. The influenza vaccines are about 70% to 80% effective in preventing influenza or reducing the severity of the disease. The injectable vaccine does not contain live virus and is not shed; there is no risk of transmitting an infectious agent to household contacts. Mild to moderate illness or current antimicrobial therapy is not a contraindication to any immunization, including the administration of the influenza vaccine.

Immunization rates against influenza for individuals with chronic illness are typically the highest, although there is considerable room for improvement. Certain groups have very low immunization rates and should be targeted for improvement. These include persons who live with or care for persons at high risk for influenza-related mortality and morbidity. Persons who provide essential community services should be considered for vaccination to minimize disruption of essential activities during influenza outbreaks. Students and other persons in institutional or other group-living situations should be encouraged to receive vaccine to minimize the risk of an outbreak in a relatively closed community. According to the recommendation of the Centers for Disease Prevention and Control (CDC), all members of the population age 6 months and older should receive annual immunization against seasonal influenza. If supply of influenza vaccines is limited, certain groups at highest risk of influenza complication or transmission should be prioritized for immunization. (Table 1–2).

TABLE 1-2
Advisory Committee on Immunization Practices (ACIP) Recommendations on Influenza Immunization

Routine influenza vaccination is recommended for all persons aged 6 months and older. While everyone should get a flu vaccine each flu season, certain patient populations are at high risk of having serious flu-related complications or live with or care for people at high risk for developing flu-related complications. Populations include:

- All children aged 6 through 59 months.
- Adults and children who have chronic pulmonary (including asthma) or cardiovascular (except isolated hypertension), renal, hepatic, neurological, hematologic, or metabolic disorders (including diabetes mellitus). Individuals age 50 years of age and older.
- Persons who have immunosuppression (including immunosuppression caused by medications or by HIV infection).
- Women who are or will be pregnant during the influenza season.
- Children and adolescents (aged 6 months – 18 years) who are receiving long-term aspirin therapy and who might be at risk for experiencing Reye's syndrome after influenza virus infection.
- Residents of nursing homes and other long-term care facilities.
- American Indians/Alaska Natives.
- Persons who are morbidly obese (BMI ≥40) kg/m^2.
- People who live with or care for those at high risk for complications from flu, including:
  - Healthcare workers.
  - Household contacts of persons with medical conditions that put them at high risk for complications from the flu.
  - Household contacts and out of home caregivers of children aged ≤59 months and adults aged ≥50 years, with particular emphasis on vaccinating contacts of children less than 6 months of age. (These children are too young to be vaccinated.)

TABLE 1-2

Advisory Committee on Immunization Practices (ACIP) Recommendations on Influenza Immunization—cont'd

All children aged 6 months to 8 years who receive a seasonal influenza vaccine for the first time should receive 2 doses spaced ≥4 weeks apart.

There are a variety of vaccines to protect against influenza currently available.

- Trivalent inactivated vaccine (TIV) in standard dose administered intramuscularly approved for all ages ≥6 months who have no other contraindications. This is the typical "flu shot." A quadrivalent inactivated vaccine is also available.
- Intradermal TIV in a lower dose when compared to standard flu vaccine administered IM (9 mcg rather than 15 mcg of each strain per dose) in a smaller volume (0.1 mL rather than 0.5 mL) approved for use in adults 18 to 64 years of age, with a preferred injection site over the deltoid.
- Inactivated TIV containing a greater dose of antigen when compared to standard flu vaccine (60 mcg rather than 15 mcg per dose) approved for use in adults age ≥65 years
- Live, attenuated influenza vaccine (LAIV) via nasal spray: A flu vaccine made with live, weakened flu viruses that is given as a nasal spray. The viruses in the nasal spray vaccine do not cause the flu. LAIV (trivalent or quadrivalent) is approved for use in healthy individuals, excluding pregnant women, ages 2 through 49 years.
- A trivalent cell culture-based inactivated influenza vaccine, which is indicated for persons aged 18 through 49 years.
- A recombinant hemagglutinin (HA) vaccine, which is indicated for persons aged 18 through 49 years.

The following recommendations apply when considering influenza vaccination of persons who have or report a history of egg allergy.

1. Persons who have experienced only hives following exposure to egg should receive influenza vaccine. Because little data are available for use of LAIV in this setting, IIV (inactivated influenza vaccine) or RIV (recombinant influenza vaccine) should be used. RIV is egg-free and indicated for persons 18–49 years of age. IIV (egg- or cell-culture-based) can also be used with the following additional safety measures:
   - Vaccine should be administered by a healthcare provider who is familiar with the potential manifestations of egg allergy.
   - Vaccine recipients should be observed for at least 30 minutes for signs of a reaction following administration of each vaccine dose.
2. Persons who report having had reactions to egg involving angioedema, respiratory distress, lightheadedness, or recurrent emesis, or persons who required epinephrine or other emergency medical intervention may receive RIV3, if aged 18–49 years and there are no other contraindications. If RIV3 is not available or the recipient is not within the indicated age range, such persons should be referred to a physician with expertise in the management of allergic conditions for further risk assessment before receipt of the vaccine.
3. All vaccines should be administered in settings in which personnel and equipment for rapid recognition and treatment of anaphylaxis are available.
4. Some persons who report allergy to egg might not be egg allergic. Those who are able to eat lightly cooked egg (scrambled eggs) without reaction are unlikely to be allergic. Conversely, egg-allergic persons might tolerate egg in baked products (bread, cake other bakery products); tolerance to egg-containing foods does not exclude the possibility of egg allergy. Egg allergy can be confirmed by a consistent medical history of adverse reactions to eggs and egg-containing foods, plus skin and/or blood testing for immunoglobulin E antibodies to egg proteins.
5. For individuals who have no known history of exposure to egg, but who are suspected of being egg-allergic on the basis of previously performed allergy testing, consultation with a physician with expertise in the management of allergic conditions should be obtained prior to vaccination. Alternatively, RIV3 may be administered if the recipient is aged 18–49 years.
6. A previous severe allergic reaction to influenza vaccine, regardless of the component suspected to be responsible for the reaction, is a contraindication to receipt of influenza vaccine.

Source: http://www.cdc.gov/flu/professionals/acip/2013-summary-recommendations.htm

The Advisory Committee on Immunization Practices (ACIP), sponsored by the CDC, recommends that healthcare administrators consider the level of vaccination coverage among healthcare personnel (HCP) to be one measure of patient safety quality programs; keeping HCP well and on the job is particularly important, given the increased patient volume and work burden to the healthcare system during flu season. At least three-quarters of all HCP report having had an influenza vaccination during a recent influenza season. This rate of immunization marks a significant improvement from rates in prior decades but falls far short of universal immunization for this important target population. Highest rates are found in acute care facilities where influenza vaccination is mandatory, whereas lowest rates are noted in long-term care facilities. Injectable trivalent influenza vaccine (TIV), more commonly called the "flu shot," is available in a variety of forms. (See Table 1–2 for details on candidates for each vaccine).

The nasal spray flu vaccine, also known as live attenuated influenza vaccine (LAIV) (FluMist), differs from the injectable influenza vaccine. Administered via a well-tolerated nasal mist, LAIV offers an easily administered, noninjection method of influenza immunization. LAIV contains influenza viruses that are sufficiently weakened as to be incapable of causing disease but with enough strength to stimulate a protective immune response. The viruses in the LAIV are cold-adapted and temperature-sensitive. As a result, the viruses can grow in the nose and throat but not in the lower respiratory tract, where the temperature is higher. LAIV is approved for use in healthy people ages 2 to 49 years old. Individuals who should not receive LAIV include children younger than 2 years; adults older than 49 years; patients with a health condition that places them at high risk for complications from influenza, including chronic heart disease, chronic lung disease such as asthma or reactive airways disease, diabetes or kidney failure, and immunosuppression; children or adolescents receiving long-term high-dose aspirin therapy; people with a history of Guillain-Barré syndrome; pregnant women; and people with a history of allergy to any of the components of LAIV. Adverse effects of LAIV include nasal irritation and discharge, muscle aches, sore throat, and fever.

Two special influenza immunization situations bear mention. Children younger than 9 years who are receiving initial influenza immunization need two doses of vaccine separated by 4 or more weeks. Pregnant women should be immunized against influenza; the vaccine can be given regardless of pregnancy trimester. Because of the change in the respiratory and immune system normally present during pregnancy, influenza is five times more likely to cause serious disease in a pregnant woman when compared with a nonpregnant woman. In addition, women who are immunized against influenza during pregnancy are able to pass a portion of this protection on to the unborn child, providing important protection during the first 6 months of life. Flu vaccine is also safe to give during lactation. Children younger than 9 years who are receiving initial influenza immunization need two doses of vaccine separated by 4 or more weeks.

Until recently, egg allergy was considered a contraindication to receiving all forms of influenza vaccine. Current recommendations advise that most individuals who are allergic to eggs can safely receive influenza vaccine (Table 1–2).

In the Northern Hemisphere, the optimal time to receive any influenza vaccine is usually in fall months, at least 1 month prior to the anticipated onset of the flu season; this timing is reversed in the Southern Hemisphere. The vaccine is given annually and its contents are reflective of the viruses anticipated to cause influenza for the upcoming flu season. In the United States, four antiviral drugs are approved by the Food and Drug Administration (FDA) for use against influenza: amantadine (Symmetrel), rimantadine (Flumadine), zanamivir (Relenza), and oseltamivir (Tamiflu). The adamantane derivatives (amantadine and rimantadine) are approved only for treatment and prevention of influenza A, whereas the neuraminidase inhibitor drugs (zanamivir and oseltamivir) are approved for use in influenza A and influenza B. Ongoing CDC viral surveillance has shown high levels of resistance of influenza A viruses to amantadine and similar medications. Because of this significant level of resistance, amantadine and rimantadine are no longer recommended by the CDC for the treatment of influenza. Relatively little resistance to the antiviral drugs oseltamivir and zanamivir has been noted in North America, but higher levels have been noted in Asia and other parts of the world. The healthcare provider should keep well informed of these developments.

Zanamivir and oseltamivir are used to treat influenza A and B infections caused by susceptible viral strains; if treatment with either of these drugs is started during the first 2 days of illness, the time a person feels ill is shortened by approximately 1 day. Zanamivir is inhaled and can cause bronchospasm, especially in patients with asthma or other chronic lung disease. The adverse effects of oseltamivir are largely gastrointestinal; the risk of nausea and vomiting is significantly reduced if the medication is taken with food.

Although many antiviral medications carry indications for the post-exposure prevention of influenza, all have a less favorable adverse reaction profile than influenza vaccine; these products are also significantly more expensive. Active immunization against influenza A and B is the preferred method of disease prevention.

DISCUSSION SOURCES

Centers for Disease Control and Prevention, http://www.cdc.gov/flu/index.htm, Seasonal Influenza

Centers for Disease Control and Prevention, http://www.cdc.gov/flu/healthcareworkers.htm, Influenza Vaccination Information for Healthcare Workers / Influenza Vaccination

Centers for Disease Control and Prevention, http://www.cdc.gov/flu/professionals/antivirals/index.htm, Antiviral Drugs

Measles, Mumps, and Rubella Immunization

22. When considering an adult's risk for measles, mumps, and rubella (MMR), the NP considers the following:
   A. Patients born before 1957 have a high likelihood of immunity against these diseases because of a history of natural infection.
   B. Considerable mortality and morbidity occur with all three diseases.
   C. Most cases in the United States occur in infants.
   D. The use of the MMR vaccine is often associated with protracted arthralgia.

23. Which of the following is true about the MMR vaccine?
   A. It contains inactivated virus.
   B. Its use is contraindicated in patients with a history of egg allergy.
   C. Revaccination of an immune person is associated with risk of significant systemic allergic reaction.
   D. Two doses at least 1 month apart are recommended for young adults who have not been previously immunized.

24. A 22-year-old man is starting a job in a college health center and needs proof of German measles, measles, and mumps immunity. He received childhood immunizations and supplies documentation of MMR vaccination at age 1.5 years. Your best response is to:
   A. obtain rubella, measles (rubeola), and mumps titers.
   B. give MMR immunization now.
   C. advise him to obtain IG if he has been exposed to measles or rubella.
   D. advise him to avoid individuals with skin rashes.

25. Concerning the MMR vaccine, which of the following is true?
   A. The link between use of MMR vaccine and childhood autism has been firmly established.
   B. There is no credible scientific evidence that MMR use increases the risk of autism.
   C. The use of the combined vaccine is associated with increased autism risk, but giving the vaccine's three components as separate vaccines minimizes this risk.
   D. The vaccine contains thimerosal, a mercury derivative.

26. Which of the following is not recommended to receive the MMR vaccination?
   A. A 1-year-old boy with a history of hive-form reaction egg ingestion
   B. A 24-year-old woman who is 20 weeks pregnant
   C. A 4-year-old girl who was born at 32 weeks of gestation
   D. A 32-year-old woman who is breastfeeding a 2 week old.

■) Answers

22. A.	24. B.	26. B.
23. D.	25. B.	

The MMR vaccine contains live but weakened (attenuated) virus. Two immunizations 1 month apart are recommended for adults born after 1957 because adults born before then are considered immune as a result of having had these diseases (native or wild infection); vaccine against these three formerly common illnesses was unavailable until the 1960s. As with all vaccines, giving additional doses to patients with an unclear immunization history is safe. (See Figure 1–2 for adult immunization schedules.) A quadrivalent vaccine, protecting against measles, mumps, rubella, and varicella (chickenpox), is also available and usually used to immunize younger children.

Rubella typically causes a relatively mild, 3- to 5-day illness with little risk of complication to the person infected. When rubella is contracted during pregnancy, however, the effects on the fetus can be devastating. Immunizing the entire population against rubella exploits herd or community immunity and protects pregnant women from contracting rubella and therefore eliminating the risk of congenital rubella syndrome in the unborn. Measles can cause severe illness with serious sequelae, including encephalitis and pneumonia; sequelae of mumps include orchitis and possible decreased male fertility.

In the past, a history of egg allergy was considered a contraindication to receiving MMR vaccine. The vaccine now is deemed safe in people with egg allergy. However, patients with a history of anaphylactic reaction to neomycin or gelatin should not receive MMR. The MMR vaccine is safe to use during lactation, but its use during pregnancy is discouraged because of the theoretical but unproven risk of congenital rubella syndrome from the live virus contained in the vaccine. MMR vaccine is well tolerated; there have been rare reports of mild, transient adverse reactions such as rash and sore throat.

At the request of the CDC and the National Institutes of Health (NIH), the Institute of Medicine and National Academy of Sciences conducted a review of all the evidence related to the MMR vaccine and autism. This independent panel examined completed studies, ongoing studies, published medical and scientific articles, and expert testimony to assess whether or not there was a link between autism and the MMR vaccine. The groups concluded that the evidence reviewed did not support an association between autism and the MMR vaccine. Although the preservative thimerosal, a mercury derivative, has been mentioned as a possible autism contributor, the MMR vaccine licensed for use in the United States does not contain this preservative.

DISCUSSION SOURCES

Centers for Disease Control and Prevention, http://www.cdc.gov/vaccines/default.htm, Vaccines and Immunizations

Centers for Disease Control and Prevention, http://www.cdc.gov/vaccines/vpd-vac/measles/default.htm#clinical, Measles

Centers for Disease Control and Prevention, http://www.cdc.gov/vaccines/vpd-vac/rubella/default.htm, Rubella (German measles)

Centers for Disease Control and Prevention, http://www.cdc.gov/vaccines/vpd-vac/mumps/default.htm, Mumps

Recommended Adult Immunization Schedule—United States - 2014

Note: These recommendations must be read with the footnotes that follow
containing number of doses, intervals between doses, and other important information.

Figure 1. Recommended adult immunization schedule, by vaccine and age group[1]

VACCINE ▼ AGE GROUP ►	19-21 years	22-26 years	27-49 years	50-59 years	60-64 years	≥ 65 years
Influenza [2,*]	1 dose annually					
Tetanus, diphtheria, pertussis (Td/Tdap) [3,*]	Substitute 1-time dose of Tdap for Td booster; then boost with Td every 10 yrs					
Varicella [4,*]	2 doses					
Human papillomavirus (HPV) Female [5,*]	3 doses					
Human papillomavirus (HPV) Male [5,*]	3 doses					
Zoster [6]					1 dose	
Measles, mumps, rubella (MMR) [7,*]	1 or 2 doses					
Pneumococcal 13-valent conjugate (PCV13) [8,*]	1 dose					
Pneumococcal polysaccharide (PPSV23) [9,10]	1 or 2 doses					1 dose
Meningococcal [11,*]	1 or more doses					
Hepatitis A [12,*]	2 doses					
Hepatitis B [13,*]	3 doses					
Haemophilus influenzae type b (Hib) [14,*]	1 or 3 doses					

*Covered by the Vaccine Injury Compensation Program

For all persons in this category who meet the age requirements and who lack documentation of vaccination or have no evidence of previous infection; zoster vaccine recommended regardless of prior episode of zoster

Recommended if some other risk factor is present (e.g., on the basis of medical, occupational, lifestyle, or other indication)

No recommendation

Report all clinically significant postvaccination reactions to the Vaccine Adverse Event Reporting System (VAERS). Reporting forms and instructions on filing a VAERS report are available at www.vaers.hhs.gov or by telephone, 800-822-7967.

Information on how to file a Vaccine Injury Compensation Program claim is available at www.hrsa.gov/vaccinecompensation or by telephone, 800-338-2382. To file a claim for vaccine injury, contact the U.S. Court of Federal Claims, 717 Madison Place, N.W., Washington, D.C. 20005; telephone, 202-357-6400.

Additional information about the vaccines in this schedule, extent of available data, and contraindications for vaccination is also available at www.cdc.gov/vaccines or from the CDC-INFO Contact Center at 800-CDC-INFO (800-232-4636) in English and Spanish, 8:00 a.m. - 8:00 p.m. Eastern Time, Monday - Friday, excluding holidays.

Use of trade names and commercial sources is for identification only and does not imply endorsement by the U.S. Department of Health and Human Services.

The recommendations in this schedule were approved by the Centers for Disease Control and Prevention's (CDC) Advisory Committee on Immunization Practices (ACIP), the American Academy of Family Physicians (AAFP), the American College of Physicians (ACP), American College of Obstetricians and Gynecologists (ACOG) and American College of Nurse-Midwives (ACNM).

Figure 2. Vaccines that might be indicated for adults based on medical and other indications[1]

VACCINE ▼ INDICATION ►	Pregnancy	Immuno-compromising conditions (excluding human immunodeficiency virus [HIV])[4,6,7,8,15]	HIV infection CD4+ T lymphocyte count [4,6,7,8,15] < 200 cells/μL	HIV infection CD4+ T lymphocyte count ≥ 200 cells/μL	Men who have sex with men (MSM)	Kidney failure, end-stage renal disease, receipt of hemodialysis	Heart disease, chronic lung disease, chronic alcoholism	Asplenia (including elective splenectomy and persistent complement component deficiencies)[8,14]	Chronic liver disease	Diabetes	Healthcare personnel
Influenza [2,*]	1 dose IIV annually		1 dose IIV or LAIV annually		1 dose IIV annually						1 dose IIV or LAIV annually
Tetanus, diphtheria, pertussis (Td/Tdap) [3,*]	1 dose Tdap each pregnancy	Substitute 1-time dose of Tdap for Td booster; then boost with Td every 10 yrs									
Varicella [4,*]	Contraindicated			2 doses							
Human papillomavirus (HPV) Female [5,*]	3 doses through age 26 yrs			3 doses through age 26 yrs							
Human papillomavirus (HPV) Male [5,*]	3 doses through age 26 yrs			3 doses through age 21 yrs							
Zoster [6]	Contraindicated			1 dose							
Measles, mumps, rubella (MMR) [7,*]	Contraindicated			1 or 2 doses							
Pneumococcal 13-valent conjugate (PCV13) [8,*]	1 dose										
Pneumococcal polysaccharide (PPSV23) [9,10]	1 or 2 doses										
Meningococcal [11,*]	1 or more doses										
Hepatitis A [12,*]	2 doses										
Hepatitis B [13,*]	3 doses										
Haemophilus influenzae type b (Hib) [14,*]	post-HSCT recipients only	1 or 3 doses									

*Covered by the Vaccine Injury Compensation Program

For all persons in this category who meet the age requirements and who lack documentation of vaccination or have no evidence of previous infection; zoster vaccine recommended regardless of prior episode of zoster

Recommended if some other risk factor is present (e.g., on the basis of medical, occupational, lifestyle, or other indications)

No recommendation

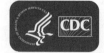

U.S. Department of Health and Human Services
Centers for Disease Control and Prevention

These schedules indicate the recommended age groups and medical indications for which administration of currently licensed vaccines is commonly indicated for adults ages 19 years and older, as of February 1, 2014. For all vaccines being recommended on the Adult Immunization Schedule: a vaccine series does not need to be restarted, regardless of the time that has elapsed between doses. Licensed combination vaccines may be used whenever any components of the combination are indicated and when the vaccine's other components are not contraindicated. For detailed recommendations on all vaccines, including those used primarily for travelers or that are issued during the year, consult the manufacturers' package inserts and the complete statements from the Advisory Committee on Immunization Practices (www.cdc.gov/vaccines/hcp/acip-recs/index.html). Use of trade names and commercial sources is for identification only and does not imply endorsement by the U.S. Department of Health and Human Services.

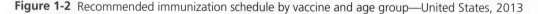

Figure 1-2 Recommended immunization schedule by vaccine and age group—United States, 2013

Footnotes
Recommended Immunization Schedule for Adults Aged 19 Years or Older: United States, 2014

1. **Additional information**
   - Additional guidance for the use of the vaccines described in this supplement is available at www.cdc.gov/vaccines/hcp/acip-recs/index.html.
   - Information on vaccination recommendations when vaccination status is unknown and other general immunization information can be found in the General Recommendations on Immunization at www.cdc.gov/mmwr/preview/mmwrhtml/rr6002a1.htm.
   - Information on travel vaccine requirements and recommendations (e.g., for hepatitis A and B, meningococcal, and other vaccines) is available at http://wwwnc.cdc.gov/travel/destinations/list.
   - Additional information and resources regarding vaccination of pregnant women can be found at http://www.cdc.gov/vaccines/adults/rec-vac/pregnant.html.

2. **Influenza vaccination**
   - Annual vaccination against influenza is recommended for all persons aged 6 months or older.
   - Persons aged 6 months or older, including pregnant women and persons with hives-only allergy to eggs, can receive the inactivated influenza vaccine (IIV). An age-appropriate IIV formulation should be used.
   - Adults aged 18 to 49 years can receive the recombinant influenza vaccine (RIV) (FluBlok). RIV does not contain any egg protein.
   - Healthy, nonpregnant persons aged 2 to 49 years without high-risk medical conditions can receive either intranasally administered live, attenuated influenza vaccine (LAIV) (FluMist), or IIV. Health care personnel who care for severely immunocompromised persons (i.e., those who require care in a protected environment) should receive IIV or RIV rather than LAIV.
   - The intramuscularly or intradermally administered IIV are options for adults aged 18 to 64 years.
   - Adults aged 65 years or older can receive the standard-dose IIV or the high-dose IIV (Fluzone High-Dose).

3. **Tetanus, diphtheria, and acellular pertussis (Td/Tdap) vaccination**
   - Administer 1 dose of Tdap vaccine to pregnant women during each pregnancy (preferred during 27 to 36 weeks' gestation) regardless of interval since prior Td or Tdap vaccination.
   - Persons aged 11 years or older who have not received Tdap vaccine or for whom vaccine status is unknown should receive a dose of Tdap followed by tetanus and diphtheria toxoids (Td) booster doses every 10 years thereafter. Tdap can be administered regardless of interval since the most recent tetanus or diphtheria-toxoid containing vaccine.
   - Adults with an unknown or incomplete history of completing a 3-dose primary vaccination series with Td-containing vaccines should begin or complete a primary vaccination series including a Tdap dose.
   - For unvaccinated adults, administer the first 2 doses at least 4 weeks apart and the third dose 6 to 12 months after the second.
   - For incompletely vaccinated (i.e., less than 3 doses) adults, administer remaining doses.
   - Refer to the ACIP statement for recommendations for administering Td/Tdap as prophylaxis in wound management (see footnote 1).

4. **Varicella vaccination**
   - All adults without evidence of immunity to varicella (as defined below) should receive 2 doses of single-antigen varicella vaccine or a second dose if they have received only 1 dose.
   - Vaccination should be emphasized for those who have close contact with persons at high risk for severe disease (e.g., health care personnel and family contacts of persons with immunocompromising conditions) or are at high risk for exposure or transmission (e.g., teachers; child care employees; residents and staff members of institutional settings, including correctional institutions; college students; military personnel; adolescents and adults living in households with children; nonpregnant women of childbearing age; and international travelers).
   - Pregnant women should be assessed for evidence of varicella immunity. Women who do not have evidence of immunity should receive the first dose of varicella vaccine upon completion or termination of pregnancy and before discharge from the health care facility. The second dose should be administered 4 to 8 weeks after the first dose.
   - Evidence of immunity to varicella in adults includes any of the following:
     — documentation of 2 doses of varicella vaccine at least 4 weeks apart;
     — U.S.-born before 1980, except health care personnel and pregnant women;
     — history of varicella based on diagnosis or verification of varicella disease by a health care provider;
     — history of herpes zoster based on diagnosis or verification of herpes zoster disease by a health care provider; or
     — laboratory evidence of immunity or laboratory confirmation of disease.

5. **Human papillomavirus (HPV) vaccination**
   - Two vaccines are licensed for use in females, bivalent HPV vaccine (HPV2) and quadrivalent HPV vaccine (HPV4), and one HPV vaccine for use in males (HPV4).
   - For females, either HPV4 or HPV2 is recommended in a 3-dose series for routine vaccination at age 11 or 12 years and for those aged 13 through 26 years, if not previously vaccinated.
   - For males, HPV4 is recommended in a 3-dose series for routine vaccination at age 11 or 12 years and for those aged 13 through 21 years, if not previously vaccinated. Males aged 22 through 26 years may be vaccinated.

5. **Human papillomavirus (HPV) vaccination (cont'd)**
   - HPV4 is recommended for men who have sex with men through age 26 years for those who did not get any or all doses when they were younger.
   - Vaccination is recommended for immunocompromised persons (including those with HIV infection) through age 26 years for those who did not get any or all doses when they were younger.
   - A complete series for either HPV4 or HPV2 consists of 3 doses. The second dose should be administered 4 to 8 weeks (minimum interval of 4 weeks) after the first dose; the third dose should be administered 24 weeks after the first dose and 16 weeks after the second dose (minimum interval of at least 12 weeks).
   - HPV vaccines are not recommended for use in pregnant women. However, pregnancy testing is not needed before vaccination. If a woman is found to be pregnant after initiating the vaccination series, no intervention is needed; the remainder of the 3-dose series should be delayed until completion of pregnancy.

6. **Zoster vaccination**
   - A single dose of zoster vaccine is recommended for adults aged 60 years or older regardless of whether they report a prior episode of herpes zoster. Although the vaccine is licensed by the U.S. Food and Drug Administration for use among and can be administered to persons aged 50 years or older, ACIP recommends that vaccination begin at age 60 years.
   - Persons aged 60 years or older with chronic medical conditions may be vaccinated unless their condition constitutes a contraindication, such as pregnancy or severe immunodeficiency.

7. **Measles, mumps, rubella (MMR) vaccination**
   - Adults born before 1957 are generally considered immune to measles and mumps. All adults born in 1957 or later should have documentation of 1 or more doses of MMR vaccine unless they have a medical contraindication to the vaccine or laboratory evidence of immunity to each of the three diseases. Documentation of provider-diagnosed disease is not considered acceptable evidence of immunity for measles, mumps, or rubella.
   Measles component:
   - A routine second dose of MMR vaccine, administered a minimum of 28 days after the first dose, is recommended for adults who:
     — are students in postsecondary educational institutions;
     — work in a health care facility; or
     — plan to travel internationally.
   - Persons who received inactivated (killed) measles vaccine or measles vaccine of unknown type during 1963–1967 should be revaccinated with 2 doses of MMR vaccine.
   Mumps component:
   - A routine second dose of MMR vaccine, administered a minimum of 28 days after the first dose, is recommended for adults who:
     — are students in a postsecondary educational institution;
     — work in a health care facility; or
     — plan to travel internationally.
   - Persons vaccinated before 1979 with either killed mumps vaccine or mumps vaccine of unknown type who are at high risk for mumps infection (e.g., persons who are working in a health care facility) should be considered for revaccination with 2 doses of MMR vaccine.
   Rubella component:
   - For women of childbearing age, regardless of birth year, rubella immunity should be determined. If there is no evidence of immunity, women who are not pregnant should be vaccinated. Pregnant women who do not have evidence of immunity should receive MMR vaccine upon completion or termination of pregnancy and before discharge from the health care facility.
   Health care personnel born before 1957:
   - For unvaccinated health care personnel born before 1957 who lack laboratory evidence of measles, mumps, and/or rubella immunity or laboratory confirmation of disease, health care facilities should consider vaccinating personnel with 2 doses of MMR vaccine at the appropriate interval for measles and mumps or 1 dose of MMR vaccine for rubella.

8. **Pneumococcal conjugate (PCV13) vaccination**
   - Adults aged 19 years or older with immunocompromising conditions (including chronic renal failure and nephrotic syndrome), functional or anatomic asplenia, cerebrospinal fluid leaks, or cochlear implants who have not previously received PCV13 or PPSV23 should receive a single dose of PCV13 followed by a dose of PPSV23 at least 8 weeks later.
   - Adults aged 19 years or older with the aforementioned conditions who have previously received 1 or more doses of PPSV23 should receive a dose of PCV13 one or more years after the last PPSV23 dose was received. For adults who require additional doses of PPSV23, the first such dose should be given no sooner than 8 weeks after PCV13 and at least 5 years after the most recent dose of PPSV23.
   - When indicated, PCV13 should be administered to patients who are uncertain of their vaccination status history and have no record of previous vaccination.
   - Although PCV13 is licensed by the U.S. Food and Drug Administration for use among and can be administered to persons aged 50 years or older, ACIP recommends PCV13 for adults aged 19 years or older with the specific medical conditions noted above.

Figure 1-2—cont'd

9. Pneumococcal polysaccharide (PPSV23) vaccination
- When PCV13 is also indicated, PCV13 should be given first (see footnote 8).
- Vaccinate all persons with the following indications:
  - all adults aged 65 years or older;
  - adults younger than 65 years with chronic lung disease (including chronic obstructive pulmonary disease, emphysema, and asthma), chronic cardiovascular diseases, diabetes mellitus, chronic renal failure, nephrotic syndrome, chronic liver disease (including cirrhosis), alcoholism, cochlear implants, cerebrospinal fluid leaks, immunocompromising conditions, and functional or anatomic asplenia (e.g., sickle cell disease and other hemoglobinopathies, congenital or acquired asplenia, splenic dysfunction, or splenectomy [if elective splenectomy is planned, vaccinate at least 2 weeks before surgery]);
  - residents of nursing homes or long-term care facilities; and
  - adults who smoke cigarettes.
- Persons with immunocompromising conditions and other selected conditions are recommended to receive PCV13 and PPSV23 vaccines. See footnote 8 for information on timing of PCV13 and PPSV23 vaccinations.
- Persons with asymptomatic or symptomatic HIV infection should be vaccinated as soon as possible after their diagnosis.
- When cancer chemotherapy or other immunosuppressive therapy is being considered, the interval between vaccination and initiation of immunosuppressive therapy should be at least 2 weeks. Vaccination during chemotherapy or radiation therapy should be avoided.
- Routine use of PPSV23 vaccine is not recommended for American Indians/Alaska Natives or other persons younger than 65 years unless they have underlying medical conditions that are PPSV23 indications. However, public health authorities may consider recommending PPSV23 for American Indians/Alaska Natives who are living in areas where the risk for invasive pneumococcal disease is increased.
- When indicated, PPSV23 vaccine should be administered to patients who are uncertain of their vaccination status and have no record of vaccination.

10. Revaccination with PPSV23
- One-time revaccination 5 years after the first dose of PPSV23 is recommended for persons aged 19 through 64 years with chronic renal failure or nephrotic syndrome, functional or anatomic asplenia (e.g., sickle cell disease or splenectomy), or immunocompromising conditions.
- Persons who received 1 or 2 doses of PPSV23 before age 65 years for any indication should receive another dose of the vaccine at age 65 years or later if at least 5 years have passed since their previous dose.
- No further doses of PPSV23 are needed for persons vaccinated with PPSV23 at or after age 65 years.

11. Meningococcal vaccination
- Administer 2 doses of quadrivalent meningococcal conjugate vaccine (MenACWY [Menactra, Menveo]) at least 2 months apart to adults of all ages with functional asplenia or persistent complement component deficiencies. HIV infection is not an indication for routine vaccination with MenACWY. If an HIV-infected person of any age is vaccinated, 2 doses of MenACWY should be administered at least 2 months apart.
- Administer a single dose of meningococcal vaccine to microbiologists routinely exposed to isolates of *Neisseria meningitidis*, military recruits, persons at risk during an outbreak attributable to a vaccine serogroup, and persons who travel to or live in countries in which meningococcal disease is hyperendemic or epidemic.
- First-year college students up through age 21 years who are living in residence halls should be vaccinated if they have not received a dose on or after their 16th birthday.
- MenACWY is preferred for adults with any of the preceding indications who are aged 55 years or younger as well as for adults aged 56 years or older who a) were vaccinated previously with MenACWY and are recommended for revaccination, or b) for whom multiple doses are anticipated. Meningococcal polysaccharide vaccine (MPSV4 [Menomune]) is preferred for adults aged 56 years or older who have not received MenACWY previously and who require a single dose only (e.g., travelers).
- Revaccination with MenACWY every 5 years is recommended for adults previously vaccinated with MenACWY or MPSV4 who remain at increased risk for infection (e.g., adults with anatomic or functional asplenia, persistent complement component deficiencies, or microbiologists).

12. Hepatitis A vaccination
- Vaccinate any person seeking protection from hepatitis A virus (HAV) infection and persons with any of the following indications:
  - men who have sex with men and persons who use injection or non-injection illicit drugs;
  - persons working with HAV-infected primates or with HAV in a research laboratory setting;
  - persons with chronic liver disease and persons who receive clotting factor concentrates;
  - persons traveling to or working in countries that have high or intermediate endemicity of hepatitis A; and

12. Hepatitis A vaccination (cont'd)
  - unvaccinated persons who anticipate close personal contact (e.g., household or regular babysitting) with an international adoptee during the first 60 days after arrival in the United States from a country with high or intermediate endemicity. (See footnote 1 for more information on travel recommendations.) The first dose of the 2-dose hepatitis A vaccine series should be administered as soon as adoption is planned, ideally 2 or more weeks before the arrival of the adoptee.
- Single-antigen vaccine formulations should be administered in a 2-dose schedule at either 0 and 6 to 12 months (Havrix), or 0 and 6 to 18 months (Vaqta). If the combined hepatitis A and hepatitis B vaccine (Twinrix) is used, administer 3 doses at 0, 1, and 6 months; alternatively, a 4-dose schedule may be used, administered on days 0, 7, and 21 to 30 followed by a booster dose at month 12.

13. Hepatitis B vaccination
- Vaccinate persons with any of the following indications and any person seeking protection from hepatitis B virus (HBV) infection:
  - sexually active persons who are not in a long-term, mutually monogamous relationship (e.g., persons with more than 1 sex partner during the previous 6 months); persons seeking evaluation or treatment for a sexually transmitted disease (STD); current or recent injection drug users; and men who have sex with men;
  - health care personnel and public safety workers who are potentially exposed to blood or other infectious body fluids;
  - persons with diabetes who are younger than age 60 years as soon as feasible after diagnosis; persons with diabetes who are age 60 years or older at the discretion of the treating clinician based on the likelihood of acquiring HBV infection, including the risk posed by an increased need for assisted blood glucose monitoring in long-term care facilities, the likelihood of experiencing chronic sequelae if infected with HBV, and the likelihood of immune response to vaccination;
  - persons with end-stage renal disease, including patients receiving hemodialysis, persons with HIV infection, and persons with chronic liver disease;
  - household contacts and sex partners of hepatitis B surface antigen–positive persons, clients and staff members of institutions for persons with developmental disabilities, and international travelers to countries with high or intermediate prevalence of chronic HBV infection; and
  - all adults in the following settings: STD treatment facilities, HIV testing and treatment facilities, facilities providing drug abuse treatment and prevention services, health care settings targeting services to injection drug users or men who have sex with men, correctional facilities, end-stage renal disease programs and facilities for chronic hemodialysis patients, and institutions and nonresidential day care facilities for persons with developmental disabilities.
- Administer missing doses to complete a 3-dose series of hepatitis B vaccine to those persons not vaccinated or not completely vaccinated. The second dose should be administered 1 month after the first dose; the third dose should be given at least 2 months after the second dose (and at least 4 months after the first dose). If the combined hepatitis A and hepatitis B vaccine (Twinrix) is used, give 3 doses at 0, 1, and 6 months; alternatively, a 4-dose Twinrix schedule, administered on days 0, 7, and 21 to 30 followed by a booster dose at month 12 may be used.
- Adult patients receiving hemodialysis or with other immunocompromising conditions should receive 1 dose of 40 mcg/mL (Recombivax HB) administered on a 3-dose schedule at 0, 1, and 6 months or 2 doses of 20 mcg/mL (Engerix-B) administered simultaneously on a 4-dose schedule at 0, 1, 2, and 6 months.

14. *Haemophilus influenzae type b* (Hib) vaccination
- One dose of Hib vaccine should be administered to persons who have functional or anatomic asplenia or sickle cell disease or are undergoing elective splenectomy if they have not previously received Hib vaccine. Hib vaccination 14 or more days before splenectomy is suggested.
- Recipients of a hematopoietic stem cell transplant should be vaccinated with a 3-dose regimen 6 to 12 months after a successful transplant, regardless of vaccination history; at least 4 weeks should separate doses.
- Hib vaccine is not recommended for adults with HIV infection since their risk for Hib infection is low.

15. Immunocompromising conditions
- Inactivated vaccines generally are acceptable (e.g., pneumococcal, meningococcal, and inactivated influenza vaccine) and live vaccines generally are avoided in persons with immune deficiencies or immunocompromising conditions. Information on specific conditions is available at http://www.cdc.gov/vaccines/hcp/acip-recs/index.html.

Figure 1-2—cont'd

Pneumococcal Immunization

27. When advising an adult patient about pneumococcal immunization, the NP considers the following about the vaccine:
    A. The vaccine contains inactivated bacteria.
    B. Its use is contraindicated in individuals with asthma.
    C. It protects against community-acquired pneumonia caused by atypical pathogens.
    D. Its use is seldom associated with significant adverse reactions.

28. Of the following, who is at greatest risk for invasive pneumococcal infection?
    A. a 68-year-old man with chronic obstructive pulmonary disease
    B. a 34-year-old woman who underwent splenectomy after a motor vehicle accident
    C. a 50-year-old man with a 15-year history of type 2 diabetes
    D. a 75-year-old woman with decreased mobility as a result of severe osteoporosis

29. All of the following patients received pneumococcal vaccine 5 years ago. Who is a candidate for receiving a second dose of antipneumococcal immunization at this time?
    A. a 45-year-old man who is a cigarette smoker
    B. a 66-year-old woman with COPD
    C. a 35-year-old man with moderate persistent asthma
    D. a 72-year-old woman with no chronic health problems

30. Identify whether the item has the characteristics of 23-valent pneumococcal polysaccharide vaccine (PPSV23) or 13-valent pneumococcal conjugate vaccine (PCV13).
    A. Routinely used in early childhood _____
    B. Use is associated with greater immunogenicity _____
    C. Routinely used in all well adults age 65 years or older _____
    D. Not licensed for use in children younger than 2 years of age _____

Answers

27. D.
28. B.
29. B.
30. A = PCV13, B = PCV13, C = PPSV23, D = PPSV23

Pneumococcal disease, caused by the gram-positive diplococcus *Streptococcus pneumoniae,* results in significant mortality and morbidity. The pneumococcal polysaccharide vaccine (Pneumovax PPSV23) contains purified polysaccharide from 23 of the most common *S. pneumoniae* serotypes.

Pneumococcal conjugate vaccine (Prevnar, PCV13) contains purified capsular polysaccharide from 13 serotypes of pneumococcus and is used in select adult populations, particularly the immunocompromised. Use of PCV13 is associated with greater immunogenicity when compared with PPSV23, but it does not provide protection against as many pneumococcal serotypes, and is routinely used in childhood. PPSV23 is not licensed for use in children younger than age 2 years.

Whatever the form used, the pneumococcal vaccine primarily protects against invasive disease such as meningitis and septicemia associated with pneumonia and disease caused by *S. pneumoniae*; this organism is the leading cause of death from community-acquired pneumonia (CAP) in the United States. The polysaccharide form protects from approximately 90% of the bacteremic disease associated with the pathogen, whereas the conjugate form is protective from approximately 70%. These immunizations are ineffective, however, against pneumonia and invasive disease caused by other infectious agents, including *Mycoplasma pneumoniae*; *Chlamydophila* (formerly *Chlamydia*) *pneumoniae*; *Legionella* species; and select gram-negative respiratory pathogens such as *Haemophilus influenzae, Moraxella catarrhalis,* and *Klebsiella pneumoniae.*

Indications for adults to receive pneumococcal vaccine include a variety of chronic health problems such as chronic lung disease (including asthma), chronic cardiovascular diseases, diabetes mellitus, chronic liver disease including cirrhosis, chronic alcohol abuse, cigarette smokers age 19 years or older, malignancy, chronic renal failure or nephrotic syndrome, functional or anatomic asplenia (e.g., sickle cell disease or splenectomy [if elective splenectomy is planned, vaccinate at least 2 weeks before surgery]), immunocompromising conditions or recipient of immunosuppressing medications, select organ transplant, cochlear implants, and cerebrospinal fluid leak. Other individuals for whom vaccination is indicated include residents of nursing homes or other long-term care facilities, and all adults 65 years or older regardless of health status. Consideration should also be given to recommending PPSV23 for Alaska Natives and American Indians ages 50 through 64 years who are living in areas in which the risk of invasive pneumococcal disease is increased.

Protection from invasive pneumococcal disease in a person with HIV warrants special mention; the risk of pneumococcal infection is up to 100 times greater in people with HIV infection than in other adults of similar age. Once the diagnosis of HIV infection is made, the patient should receive both PCV13 and PPSV23 vaccines as soon as possible; PCV13 is given first followed by PPSV23 8 weeks later. A second dose of PPSV23 should be administered at least 5 years after the initial dose, and a third dose should be administered at age 65 years if the person was younger than age 65 years at the time of HIV diagnosis. Updated recommendations for all adults age 65 years and above require use of both vaccines.

Revaccination after 5 years after the first PPSV23 dose is recommended for individuals older than age 2 years but younger than age 65 years who are at highest risk of pneumococcal infection or are at greatest risk of having a rapid decline in antibody levels, including sickle cell disease, splenectomy, chronic renal failure, nephrotic syndrome, immunocompromise, generalized malignancy, or on immunosuppressing medications. If initial PPSV23 vaccine was received at age 65 years or older, a repeat dose is not required. This immunization, with initial and repeat vaccination, is generally well tolerated (Table 1–3).

DISCUSSION SOURCES

Centers for Disease Control and Prevention, http://www.cdc.gov/vaccines/vpd-vac/pneumo/vac-PCV13-adults.htm, PCV13 (Pneumococcal Conjugate) Vaccine

Centers for Disease Control and Prevention, http://www.immunize.org/askexperts/experts_pneumococcal_vaccines.asp, Pneumococcal Vaccines (PCV13 and PPSV23)

▪ Hepatitis B Vaccination

31. Concerning hepatitis B virus (HBV) vaccine, which of the following is true?
A. The vaccine contains live, whole HBV.
B. Adults should routinely have anti-hepatitis B surface antibody titers measured after three doses of vaccine.
C. The vaccine should be offered during treatment for sexually transmitted diseases in unimmunized adults.
D. Serologic testing for hepatitis B surface antigen (HBsAg) should be done before hepatitis B vaccination is initiated in adults.

TABLE 1-3

Pneumococcal Vaccine Adverse Reactions

Local Reactions Including Pain, Redness	30%–50%
Fever, myalgia	Polysaccharide (Pneumovax 23-valent polysaccharide vaccine) = Uncommon, <1% Conjugate (Prevnar 13-valent conjugate vaccine) = 11%–40% in children, significantly less in adults with adverse reaction profile similar to 23-valent polysaccharide vaccine
Severe, potentially life-threatening	Rare

Source: www.cdc.gov/mmwr/preview/mmwrhtml/mm5934a3.htm

32. In which of the following groups is routine HBsAg screening recommended?
A. hospital laboratory workers
B. recipients of hepatitis B vaccine series
C. pregnant women
D. college students

33. You see a woman who has been sexually active with a man newly diagnosed with acute hepatitis B. She has not received hepatitis B vaccine in the past. You advise her that she should:
A. start a hepatitis B immunization series.
B. limit the number of sexual partners she has.
C. be tested for hepatitis B surface antibody (HBsAb).
D. receive hepatitis B immune globulin (HBIG) and hepatitis B immunization series.

34. Hepatitis B vaccine should not be given to a person with a history of anaphylactic reaction to:
A. egg.
B. baker's yeast.
C. neomycin.
D. streptomycin.

35. Risks associated with chronic hepatitis B include all of the following except:
A. hepatocellular carcinoma.
B. cirrhosis.
C. continued infectivity.
D. systemic hypertension.

36. Jason is a healthy 18-year-old who presents for primary care. According to his immunization record, he received two dose of HBV vaccine 1 month apart at age 14 years. Which of the following best describes his HBV vaccination needs?
A. He should receive a single dose of HBV vaccine now.
B. A three-dose HBV vaccine series should be started during today's visit.
C. He has completed the recommended HBV vaccine series.
D. He should be tested for HBsAb and further immunization recommendations should be made according to the test results.

37. All of the following individuals have not received vaccination against HBV. The vaccine should not be given in which of the following patients?
A. a 35-year-old man with multiple sclerosis
B. a 25-year-old woman with a past history of Guillain-Barré syndrome
C. a 48-year-old woman with systemic lupus erythematosus
D. a 28-year-old man who is acutely ill with bacterial meningitis

38. In the United States, universal childhood HBV began in what year?
   A. 1962
   B. 1972
   C. 1982
   D. 1992

39. You see Harold, a 25-year-old man who recently had multiple sexual encounters without condom use with a male partner who has chronic hepatitis B. Harold provides documentation of receiving a properly timed hepatitis B immunization series. In addition to counseling about safer sexual practices, you also advise that Harold:
   A. needs to repeat his hepatitis B immunization series.
   B. receive a single dose of HBV vaccine.
   C. be tested for hepatitis B surface antibody (HBsAb).
   D. should receive hepatitis B immune globulin (HBIG) and a single dose of the hepatitis B immunization series.

Answers

31.	C.	34.	B.	37.	D.
32.	C.	35.	D.	38.	C.
33.	D.	36.	A.	39.	B.

Hepatitis B infection is caused by the small double-stranded DNA hepatitis B virus (HBV) that contains an inner core protein of hepatitis B core antigen (HBcAg) and an outer surface of HBsAg. The virus is usually transmitted through an exchange of blood and body fluids, including semen, vaginal secretions, and saliva, via percutaneous and mucosal exposure. Groups at particular risk for HBV acquisition include sex partners of people with HBV infection; sexually active persons who are not in a long-term, mutually monogamous relationship (>1 sex partner during the previous 6 months); men who have sex with men; injection drug users; household contacts of persons with chronic HBV infection; patients receiving hemodialysis; residents and staff of facilities for people with developmental disabilities; and travelers to countries with intermediate or high prevalence of HBV infection. Additional at-risk groups include healthcare and public safety workers at risk for occupational exposure to blood or blood-contaminated body fluids. Infants born to mothers with HBV infection are at particular risk for HBV acquisition.

Hepatitis B infection can be prevented by limiting percutaneous and mucosal exposure to blood and body fluids and through immunization. Recombinant hepatitis B vaccine, which does not contain live virus, is well tolerated but is contraindicated in those who have a history of anaphylactic reaction to baker's yeast (Table 1–4). As with all vaccines, immunization against HBV should be delayed in the face of

TABLE 1-4

Personal Immunization Contraindications

Anaphylactic Reaction History	IZ to Avoid
Neomycin	IPV, MMR, varicella
Streptomycin, polymyxin B, neomycin	IPV, vaccinia (smallpox)
Baker's yeast	Hepatitis B
Gelatin, neomycin	Varicella zoster
Gelatin	MMR

Source: www.cdc.gov/vaccines/recs/vac-admin/contraindications.htm

serious or life-threatening illness. The vaccine is generally well tolerated and is administered in a three-injection series. If the vaccine series was interrupted after the first dose, the second dose should be administered as soon as possible. The second and third doses should be separated by an interval of at least 8 weeks. If only the third dose is delayed, it should be administered as soon as possible; the entire three doses series does not need to be repeated. Universal childhood vaccination against HBV started in 1982; as a result, one major at-risk group is adults born before that date who have not been offered the vaccine. Healthcare and public safety workers are recommended to be HBV immunized; receiving this vaccine is often a requirement of employment. Additional groups who should be offered HBV vaccine include persons with chronic liver disease and HIV infection. Because of increased risk of developing chronic HBV, unvaccinated adults with diabetes mellitus who are aged 19 through 59 years should also be encouraged to receive HBV vaccine. All other persons seeking protection from HBV infection, whether acknowledging specific HBV risk, are candidates for immunization.

Acute hepatitis B is a serious illness that can lead to acute hepatic failure, particularly in patients with underlying liver disease. Approximately 5% of adults with hepatitis B infection develop chronic hepatitis B; chronic hepatitis B is a potent risk factor for the development of hematoma or primary hepatocellular carcinoma and hepatic cirrhosis. Although usually appearing clinically well, a person with chronic hepatitis B continues to be able to transmit the virus.

Without intervention, approximately 40% of infants born to mothers with HBV will develop chronic hepatitis B and approximately one-fourth of the infected infants will go on to die from chronic liver disease. As a result, all pregnant women should be screened for HBsAg at the first prenatal visit, regardless of HBV vaccine history. The HBV vaccine is not 100% effective; in addition, woman could have carried HBV before becoming pregnant. Women at particularly high risk for new HBV acquisition during pregnancy should be retested for HBsAg in later pregnancy. In cases in which maternal HBsAg status is unknown, a situation common in children who have been adopted internationally, consideration should be given to testing the child for evidence of perinatal acquisition of HBV infection.

About 90% to 95% of individuals who receive the HBV vaccine develop HBsAb (anti-HBs) after three doses, implying protection from the virus. As a result, routine testing for the presence of HBsAb after immunization is not recommended. HBsAb testing should be considered, however, to confirm the development of HBV protection in individuals with high risk for infection (e.g., select healthcare workers with anticipated high levels of blood and body fluid exposure, injection drug users, sex workers) and individuals at risk for poor immune response (e.g., dialysis patients, immunosuppressed patients). Booster doses of HBV vaccine are recommended only in certain circumstances. For patients receiving hemodialysis, the need for booster doses should be assessed by annual testing for antibody to HBsAg (anti-HBs or HBsAb). A booster dose should be administered when anti-HBs levels decline to less than 10 mIU/mL. For other immunocompromised persons (e.g., people with HIV, hematopoietic stem-cell transplant recipients, and persons receiving chemotherapy), the need for booster doses has not been determined. When anti-HBs levels decline to less than 10 mIU/mL, annual anti-HBs testing and booster doses should be considered for individuals with an ongoing risk for exposure. Ongoing serologic surveillance in the immunocompetent population is not recommended.

Post-exposure prophylaxis is effective in preventing HBV infection. In a person who has written documentation of a complete HBV vaccine series and who did not receive post-vaccination testing, a single vaccine booster dose should be given with a nonoccupational known HBsAg-positive exposure source. A person who is in the process of being vaccinated but who has not completed the vaccine series should receive the appropriate dose of HBIG and should complete the vaccine series. Unvaccinated persons should receive HBIG and hepatitis B vaccine as soon as possible after exposure, preferably within 24 hours of the at-risk exposure. Testing for HIV, hepatitis A, and hepatitis C should also be offered; where applicable, post-exposure prophylaxis should be offered. Owing to the complexity of care, intervention for the person with occupational exposure should be done in consultation with experts in the area.

DISCUSSION SOURCES

Centers for Disease Control and Prevention, http://www.cdc.gov/mmwr/preview/mmwrhtml/rr5516a1.htm?s_cid=rr5516a1_e, A comprehensive immunization strategy to eliminate transmission of hepatitis B virus infection in the United States: recommendations of the Advisory Committee on Immunization Practices. Part II

Centers for Disease Control and Prevention, http://www.cdc.gov/hepatitis/hbv/hbvfaq.htm,Hepatitis B FAQs for Health Professionals

Smallpox Immunization

40. Which of the following best describes how the variola virus that causes smallpox is transmitted?
    A. direct deposit of infective droplets
    B. surface contact
    C. blood and body fluids
    D. vertical transmission

41. Smallpox disease includes which of the following characteristics?
    A. usually mild disease
    B. lesions that erupt over several days
    C. loss of contagiousness when vesicles form
    D. lesions all at the same stage during the eruptive phase of the illness

42. Smallpox vaccine contains:
    A. live vaccinia virus.
    B. a virus fragment.
    C. dead smallpox virus.
    D. an antigenic protein.

Answers

40. A.   **41. D.**   **42. A.**

Smallpox is a serious, contagious, and sometimes fatal infectious disease caused by the variola virus. There are a variety of clinical forms, of which variola major is the most common and severe form, carrying a fatality rate of around 30%. Smallpox in its naturally occurring form was globally eradicated after a successful worldwide vaccination program; the last U.S. case of smallpox was in 1949, and the last naturally occurring case in the world was in the late 1970s. As a result, routine vaccination for the general public was discontinued in the United States in 1972. Laboratory stockpiles of the variola virus do exist, however, and could be used as a bioterrorism agent.

Smallpox is typically spread from person to person via direct deposit of infective droplets onto the nasal, oral, or pharyngeal mucosal membrane or in the alveoli of the lungs; direct and fairly prolonged face-to-face contact is required. Smallpox is sometimes contagious during the onset of fever (prodrome phase), but it is most contagious with the onset of rash. At this stage, the infected person is usually very sick and not able to move around in the community. The infected person is contagious until the last smallpox scab falls off. Less commonly, smallpox can be spread through direct contact with infected bodily fluids or contaminated objects such as bedding or clothing. Rarely, smallpox has been spread by virus carried in the air in enclosed settings such as buildings, buses, and trains. Smallpox cannot be transmitted to humans by insects or animals, and animals cannot become ill with the disease.

Exposure to the virus is followed by an incubation period of about 7 to 17 days, during which the individual does not have any symptoms and the disease is not contagious. The prodromal stage lasts 2 to 4 days, during which the individual has a temperature of 101°F to 104°F (38.3°C to 40°C), malaise, headache, body aches, and sometimes vomiting. The individual is likely contagious at this time but is typically too sick to carry on normal activities. In the next stage, the rash appears first as small red spots on the tongue and in the mouth that develop into open sores that spread large amounts of the virus into the mouth and throat. The individual becomes most contagious at this time. The rash appears on the skin, starting on the face and spreading first to the arms and legs and then to the hands and feet. Usually the rash spreads to all parts of the body within 24 hours, and the temperature typically decreases. By day 3 of the rash, the skin lesions become raised, and by day 4, the lesions fill with a thick, opaque fluid and become umbilicated. The temperature often increases again until the lesions crust over, in about another 5 days. About 1 week later, the crusts begin to fall off, usually leaving a pitted scar. The individual remains contagious until all of the crusts have fallen off.

Although smallpox and varicella cause vesicular lesions, the clinical presentation of smallpox differs considerably from that of varicella (chickenpox). In varicella, the lesions typically erupt over days and are at various stages; some are vesicular, whereas some older lesions may be starting to crust over. In smallpox, all the skin lesions are usually at the same stage.

Smallpox treatment is largely supportive; no smallpox-specific therapy is currently available. An individual with suspected smallpox must be swiftly isolated. The NP should be aware of which local experts and governmental authorities need to be notified for a suspected case of smallpox.

In anticipation of possible exposure via bioterrorism, smallpox vaccination has been offered to or required of selected health and defense personnel, such as first responders, emergency healthcare providers, and members of the military. Vaccination within 3 days of smallpox exposure prevents or significantly reduces the severity of smallpox symptoms in most people, whereas vaccination 4 to 7 days after exposure likely offers some protection from disease or may modify the severity of disease. The U.S. government has stockpiled enough vaccine to vaccinate every person in the United States in the event of a smallpox emergency.

Made from a live smallpox-related virus called vaccinia, the vaccine is given through a unique immunization method: A two-pronged needle is dipped into the vaccine solution. When removed, the needle retains a droplet of the vaccine. The needle is then used to prick the skin numerous times in a few seconds, producing a few drops of blood and some local discomfort. A red, itchy bump develops at the vaccine site in 3 to 4 days; this progresses to a large draining pustule over the next few days. During the second week, the blister begins to dry up, and a scab forms. The scab falls off in the third week, leaving a small scar. Until the scab falls off, the vaccine recipient can shed the vaccinia virus. Although this is not the smallpox virus, infection with vaccinia virus can result in serious cutaneous illnesses including generalized vaccinia and eczema vaccinatum. As a result, the vaccination site must be cared for to prevent the vaccinia virus from spreading. As with most vaccines, mild reactions include a few days of arm soreness and body aches. Fever is occasionally reported. The NP needs to be aware of current recommendations for smallpox vaccine candidates and vaccine contraindications.

DISCUSSION SOURCE

Centers for Disease Control and Prevention, http://www.bt.cdc.gov/agent/smallpox/clinicians.asp, Smallpox Overview for Clinicians

Varicella-Zoster Virus Vaccination

43. Which of the following statements is correct about the varicella vaccine?
    A. It contains killed varicella-zoster virus.
    B. The use of the vaccine is associated with an increase in reported cases of shingles.
    C. Varicella vaccine should be offered to adults who were U.S. born prior to 1980 and report a childhood history of chickenpox.
    D. Although highly protective against invasive varicella disease, mild cases of chickenpox have been reported in immunized individuals.

44. For which of the following patients should an NP order varicella antibody titers?
    A. a 14 year old with an uncertain immunization history
    B. a healthcare worker who reports having had varicella as a child
    C. a 22-year-old woman who received two varicella immunizations 6 weeks apart
    D. a 72 year old with shingles

45. A woman who has been advised to receive varicella-zoster immune globulin (VZIG) asks about its risks. You respond that IG is a:
    A. synthetic product that is well tolerated.
    B. pooled blood product that often transmits infectious disease.
    C. blood product obtained from a single donor.
    D. pooled blood product with an excellent safety profile.

46. Maria is a 28-year-old healthy woman who is 6 weeks pregnant. Her routine prenatal laboratory testing reveals she is not immune to varicella. She voices her intent to breastfeed her infant for at least 6 months. Which of the following represents the best advice for Maria?
    A. She should receive VZV vaccine once she is in her second trimester of pregnancy.
    B. Maria should be advised to receive two doses of VZV vaccine after giving birth.
    C. Once Maria is no longer breastfeeding, she should receive one dose of VZV vaccine.
    D. A dose of VZIG should be administered now.

47. How is the varicella virus most commonly transmitted?
   A. droplet transmission
   B. contact with inanimate reservoirs
   C. contact transmission
   D. water-borne transmission

Answers

43. D.	45. D.	47. A.
44. B.	46. B.	

Varicella-zoster virus (VZV) causes the highly contagious, systemic disease commonly known as chickenpox; VZV infection typically presents with 300 to 500 vesicular lesions, fever, itch, and fatigue. The virus is transmitted via respiratory droplet and contact with open lesions. Chickenpox can be serious, especially in infants, adults, and individuals of all ages who are immunocompromised. A history of naturally occurring or wild varicella infection usually confers lifetime immunity. Reinfection is, on rare occasion, seen in immunocompromised patients, however. More often, reexposure causes an increase in antibody titers without causing disease. Although most cases are seen in children younger than 18 years, the greatest rate of mortality from varicella is in adults 30 to 49 years old. Prior to the availability of the VZV vaccine, chickenpox was a prevalent childhood illness.

Evidence of immunity to varicella includes documentation of age-appropriate vaccination with VZV vaccine, laboratory evidence of immunity or laboratory confirmation of disease, birth in the United States before 1980, or the diagnosis or verification of a history of varicella disease or herpes zoster by a healthcare provider. Among adults born before 1980 with an unclear or negative varicella history, most are also seropositive. Confirming varicella immunity through varicella titers, even in the presence of a history of varicella infection, should be done in healthcare workers because of their risk of exposure and potential transmission of the disease.

The varicella vaccine is administered to children after their first birthday with a repeat dose usually given between ages 4 and 6 years. Older children and adults with no history of varicella infection or previous immunization should receive two immunizations 4 to 8 weeks apart. In particular, healthcare workers, family contacts of immunocompromised patients, and daycare workers should be targeted for varicella vaccine, as should adults who are in environments with high risk of varicella transmission, such as college dormitories, military barracks, and long-term-care facilities. Pregnant women should be assessed for evidence of varicella immunity. Women who do not have evidence of immunity should receive the first dose of varicella vaccine on completion or termination of pregnancy and before discharge from the healthcare facility. The second dose should be administered 4 to 8 weeks after the first dose. The vaccine is highly protective against severe, invasive varicella. Mild cases of chickenpox may be reported after immunization, however. Because this is a live, attenuated virus vaccine, it should be used with caution in certain clinical situations (Table 1–5).

For healthy children and adults without evidence of immunity, vaccination within 3 to 5 days of exposure to varicella is beneficial in preventing or modifying the disease. Studies have shown that vaccination administered within 3 days of exposure to rash is at least 90% effective in preventing varicella, whereas vaccination within 5 days of exposure to rash is approximately 70% effective in preventing varicella and 100% effective in modifying severe disease. For individuals without evidence of immunity who have contraindications for vaccination but are at risk for severe disease and complications, use of VZIG is recommended for post-exposure prophylaxis. VZIG, as with all forms of IG, provides temporary, passive immunity to infection. IG is a pooled blood product with an excellent safety profile.

TABLE 1-5
Live, Attenuated Virus Vaccines

Vaccine prepared from live microorganisms or viruses cultured under adverse conditions leading to loss of virulence but retention of their ability to induce protective immunity.

Live Attenuated Virus Vaccine Examples	Precautions For Use in Special Populations
MMR (Measles, mumps, rubella) Varicella (Chickenpox)	Pregnancy because of theoretical risk of passing virus to unborn child
Intranasal influenza virus vaccine (FluMist) Zoster (Zostavax)	Immune suppression, with the exception of HIV infection, because of potential risk of becoming ill with virus
	With HIV infection, live virus vaccines usually are not given with CD4 T lymphocyte cell counts <200 cell/uL. See adult immunization guidelines for further information.
Rotavirus vaccine (oral vaccine only given to young infants)	Use contraindicated in infants diagnosed with severe combined immunodeficiency (SCID)

Source: www.cdc.gov/vaccines/pubs/acip-list.htm

The NP should check current recommendation about post-exposure prophylaxis.

The VZV can lie dormant in sensory nerve ganglia. Later reactivation causes shingles, a painful, vesicular-form rash in a dermatomal pattern. About 15% of individuals who have had chickenpox develop shingles during their lifetime. Shingles rates are markedly reduced in individuals who have received varicella vaccine compared with individuals who have had wild or native VZV disease. The virus is present in the vesicles seen in shingles. If an individual without varicella immunity comes in contact with shingles skin lesions, that individual could contract chickenpox. An individual with shingles cannot transmit shingles to another person.

DISCUSSION SOURCE

Centers for Disease Prevention and Control, http://www.cdc.gov/vaccines/vpd-vac/varicella/default-hcp.htm, - Varicella Vaccination: Information for Healthcare Providers

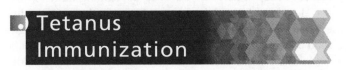

Tetanus Immunization

48. An 18-year-old man has no primary tetanus immunization series documented. Which of the following represents the immunization needed?
    A. three doses of diphtheria, tetanus, and acellular pertussis (DTaP) vaccine 2 months apart
    B. tetanus IG now and two doses of tetanus-diphtheria (Td) vaccine 1 month apart
    C. tetanus, diphtheria, and acellular pertussis (Tdap) vaccine now with a dose of Td vaccine in 1 and 6 months
    D. Td vaccine as a single dose

49. Which wound presents the greatest risk for tetanus infection?
    A. a puncture wound obtained while gardening
    B. a laceration obtained while trimming beef
    C. a human bite
    D. an abrasion obtained by falling on a sidewalk

50. A 50-year-old man with hypertension and dyslipidemia presents for a primary care visit. He states, "It has been at least 10 years since my last tetanus shot." He should be immunized with:
    A. Td.
    B. Tetanus IG.
    C. Tdap.
    D. None of the above, owing to his concomitant health problems.

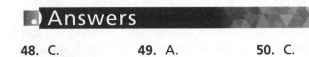

Answers

48. C.   49. A.   50. C.

Tetanus infection is caused by *Clostridium tetani,* an anaerobic, gram-positive, spore-forming rod. This organism is found in soil, particularly if it contains manure. The organism enters the body through a contaminated wound, causing a life-threatening systemic disease characterized by painful muscle weakness and spasm (lockjaw) with at least a 10% mortality rate. Diphtheria, caused by *Corynebacterium diphtheriae,* a gram-negative bacillus, is typically transmitted from person-to-person contact via respiratory droplets or cutaneous lesion. This organism causes a severe illness involving the respiratory tract, including the appearance of pseudomembranous pharyngitis and possible airway obstruction. Owing to high immunization rates, a confirmed case of diphtheria has not been reported in the United States for more than a decade.

In the developed world, tetanus and diphtheria are uncommon infections because of widespread immunization. Because protective titers wane over time, and adults are frequently lacking in up-to-date immunization, most cases of tetanus occur in adults older than 50 years.

A primary series of three tetanus vaccine injections sets the stage for long-term immunity. A booster tetanus dose every 10 years is recommended, but protection is probably present for 20 to 30 years after a primary series. Using Td vaccine rather than tetanus toxoid for primary series and booster doses in adulthood also assists in keeping diphtheria immunity (Fig. 1–2). Early childhood tetanus and diphtheria immunizations also include acellular pertussis vaccine, providing protection for this highly contagious cough-transmitted illness. A single dose of Tdap during adulthood provides additional protection from pertussis. For adults receiving initial immunization, a series of three vaccine doses is needed. Two of the three can be Td, and one should be Tdap. Rarely have cases of tetanus occurred in persons with a documented primary tetanus series.

The use of tetanus and diphtheria with or without acellular pertussis immunizations is well tolerated and produces few adverse reactions. A short-term, localized area of redness and warmth is quite common and is not predictive of future problems with tetanus immunization.

When a patient presents with a clean minor wound and an unclear tetanus immunization history or inadequate tetanus immunization (0–2 doses), a dose of tetanus vaccine should be provided. In the presence of all other wounds and an unclear or inadequate tetanus immunization history (0–2 doses), a dose of tetanus vaccine with tetanus immunoglobulin (TIG), an example of passive immunization, is advised. With TIG use, temporary immunity is provided.

DISCUSSION SOURCES

Centers for Disease Control and Prevention, http://www.cdc.gov/ncidod/dbmd/diseaseinfo/diptheria_t.htm, Vaccine preventable disease: Diphtheria

Centers for Disease Control and Prevention, http://www.cdc.gov/vaccines/pubs/pinkbook/tetanus.html, Vaccine preventable disease: Tetanus

Centers for Disease Control and Prevention, http://www.immunize.org/askexperts/experts_per.asp, Ask the Experts: Diphtheria, tetanus, pertussis

Hepatitis A Vaccination

51. Of the following, the most common route of hepatitis A virus (HAV) transmission is:
    A. needle sharing.
    B. raw shellfish ingestion.
    C. ingestion of contaminated food or water.
    D. exposure to blood and body fluids.

52. When answering questions about HAV vaccine, the NP considers that it:
    A. contains live virus.
    B. should be offered to adults who frequently travel to developing countries.
    C. is contraindicated for use in children younger than age 6 years.
    D. usually confers lifelong protection after a single injection.

53. Usual treatment for an adult with acute hepatitis A includes:
    A. interferon-alfa therapy.
    B. high-dose ribavirin.
    C. parenteral acyclovir.
    D. supportive care.

54. Peak infectivity of persons with hepatitis A usually occurs:
    A. before onset of jaundice.
    B. at the time of maximum elevation of liver enzymes.
    C. during the recovery period.
    D. at the time of maximum disease-associated symptoms.

55. In the United States, what proportion of all reported hepatitis A cases have no specific risk factor identified?
    A. Approximately 25%
    B. Approximately 50%
    C. Approximately 75%
    D. Nearly 100%

56. Which of the following represents the food or beverage that is least likely to be contaminated with the hepatitis A virus?
    A. a lettuce salad
    B. a bowl of hot soup
    C. a plate of peeled mango
    D. a glass of ice tea

Answers

51. C.	53. D.	55. B.
52. B.	54. A.	56. B.

Hepatitis A infection is caused by HAV, a small RNA virus. Transmission through the fecal–oral route is the primary means of HAV transmission in the United States. Often, a member of a household or someone who lives in close contact with others introduces the infection into the group. In developing countries with limited pure water, most children contract this disease by age 5 years. In the United States, nearly half of all reported hepatitis A cases have no specific risk factor identified. Among adults with identified risk factors, the majority of cases are among men who have sex with other men, persons who use illegal drugs, and international travelers.

HAV replicates in the liver, is excreted in bile, and is shed in stool. Peak infectivity in acute hepatitis A occurs during the 2-week period before onset of jaundice or elevation of liver enzymes, when concentration of virus in stool is highest. Once jaundice occurs, the amount of HAV in the stool diminishes. Effective methods to inactivate HAV include heating or cooking foods to temperatures >185°F (>85°C) for 1 minute or disinfecting surfaces with a 1:100 dilution of sodium hypochlorite, the active component of household bleach, in tap water. For travel to developing nations, the traveler should be advised to avoid foods that are usually eaten raw, including fruits and many vegetables. Thorough food cooking largely eliminates this risk.

Additional candidates for HAV immunization include men who have sex with men, individuals who reside in or travel to areas where the disease is endemic, food handlers, sewage workers, persons working with HAV-infected primates or with HAV in a research laboratory setting, day-care workers, long-term-care residents and workers, and military and laboratory personnel. Injection drug users also benefit from the vaccine. HAV is rarely transmitted sexually or from needle sharing; rather, injection drug users often live in conditions that facilitate HAV transmission.

In the majority, hepatitis A typically causes a self-limiting infection with a very low mortality rate. However, coinfection with hepatitis A and C, with hepatitis A and B, or acute hepatitis A in addition to a chronic liver disease can lead to a rapid deterioration in hepatic function. Individuals with chronic hepatitis B or C or any chronic liver disease should be immunized against HAV. Individuals who have clotting-factor disorders and are receiving clotting-factor concentrates who have not had hepatitis A should also be immunized. Any person anticipating close personal contact, such as a household member or caregiver, with an international adoptee during the first 60 days after arrival in the United States from a country with high or intermediate endemicity is also encouraged to be immunized; the HAV vaccine should be given at least 2 weeks prior to the arrival of the adoptee if possible. All children and anyone who requests HAV protection should receive HAV vaccine.

HAV vaccine, which does not contain live virus, is usually well tolerated without systemic reaction. Single-antigen vaccine formulations should be administered in a two-dose schedule at either 0 and 6–12 months (Havrix), or 0 and 6–18 months (Vaqta). If the combined hepatitis A and hepatitis B vaccine (Twinrix) is used, administer three doses at 0, 1, and 6 months; alternatively, a four-dose schedule can be used, administered on days 0, 7, and 21–30 followed by a booster dose at month 12. Optimally, HAV vaccine should be given 4 to 6 weeks prior to travel to an area where the disease is endemic. With HAV exposure, immune globulin or HAV vaccine can be given with 2 weeks to minimize the risk of hepatitis A infection.

Treatment for HAV is largely supportive. There is no chronic form of the infection.

DISCUSSION SOURCES

Centers for Disease Control and Prevention, http://www.cdc.gov/hepatitis/hav/index.htm, Hepatitis A Information for Healthcare Professionals
(See also Figures 2–1 and 2–2.)

Poliovirus Vaccination

57. Which of the following statements is true about poliovirus infection?
    A. It is transmitted via the fecal–oral route.
    B. Rates of infection among household contacts are about 30%.
    C. Sporadic outbreaks continue to occur in North America.
    D. It is transmitted via aerosol and droplets.

58. A 30-year-old man with HIV lives with his two preschool-aged children. Which of the following statements best represents advice you should give him about immunizing his children?
    A. Immunizations should take place without regard for his health status.
    B. The children should not receive influenza vaccine.
    C. MMR vaccine should not be given.
    D. The children should not receive poliovirus immunization.

Answers

57. A.   **58.** A.

Polioviruses are highly contagious and capable of causing paralytic, life-threatening infection. The infection is transmitted by the fecal–oral route. Rates of infection among household contacts can be as high as 96%. Since 1994, North and South America have been declared free of indigenous poliomyelitis, largely because of the efficacy of the poliovirus immunization. The vaccine is available in two forms: a live-virus vaccine that is given orally (oral polio vaccine [OPV]) and an injectable vaccine that contains inactivated poliovirus (IPV). When OPV is used, a small amount of weakened virus is shed via the stool. This shedding presents household members with possible exposure

to poliovirus, resulting in a rare risk of vaccine-associated paralytic poliomyelitis (VAPP). Because of VAPP risk, OPV is no longer used in the United States, but it is used in other countries. Use of IPV, containing inactivated virus, poses no such risk.

DISCUSSION SOURCE

Centers for Disease Control and Prevention, http://www.cdc.gov/vaccines/vpd-vac/polio/default.htm, Polio Vaccine

Preventing Disease

59. When working with a middle-aged man with a body mass index of 33 kg/m² on weight reduction, an NP considers that one of the first actions should be to:
    A. add an exercise program while minimizing the need for dietary changes.
    B. ask the patient about what he believes contributes to his weight issues.
    C. refer the patient to a nutritionist for diet counseling.
    D. ask for a commitment to lose weight.

60. A sedentary, obese 52-year-old woman is diagnosed with hypertension and states, "It is going to be too hard to diet, exercise, and take these pills." What is the least helpful response to her statement?
    A. "Try taking your medication when you brush your teeth."
    B. "You really need to try to improve your health."
    C. "Tell me what you feel will get in your way of improving your health."
    D. "Could you start with reducing the amount of salty foods in your diet?"

61. During an office visit, a 38-year-old woman states, "I drink way too much but do not know what to do to stop." According to the Stages of Change Transtheorectical Model, her statement is most consistent with a person at the stage of:
    A. precontemplation.
    B. contemplation.
    C. preparation.
    D. action.

62. During an office visit, a 48-year-old man who smokes two packs of cigarettes per day states, "My kids are begging me to quit. My dad smoked and died when he was 80. I am not sure what all the fuss is about." According to the Stages of Change Transtheoretical Model, his statement is most consistent with a person at the stage of:
    A. precontemplation.
    B. contemplation.
    C. preparation.
    D. action.

63. Linda is a 52-year-old woman who presents for a follow-up visit for hypertension, type 2 diabetes mellitus, and dyslipidemia. She has a 50-pack year cigarette smoking history, quit smoking 6 months ago, and now reports smoking about 10 cigarettes per day for the past 2 weeks while being particularly stressed during her 78-year-old mother's recent serious illness. Linda states, "I give up. I guess I cannot quit." Which of the following is the most appropriate response to Linda's statement?

A. Do you think your mother's illness was a trigger for your smoking?

B. Can we work on a plan to help you to get back to being smoking-free?

C. Once your mom is well again, you should try quitting again.

D. You sound really discouraged about this.

Answers

59. B.	61. B.	63. B.
60. B.	62. A.	

Possessing information about methods for preventing disease and maintaining health is an important part of patient education. Knowledge alone does not ensure a change in behavior, however. NPs need to consider many factors in patient counseling and education (Box 1–1).

In providing primary care, the NP should maintain an attitude that the patient is capable of changing and achieving improved health. Change occurs dynamically and often unpredictably. A commonly used change framework is based on the work of Prochaska and DiClemente and is known as the Stages of Change Model/Transtheoretical Model (TTM). In this model, five stages of preparation for change are reported.

- Precontemplation: The patient is not interested in change and might be unaware that the problem exists or minimizes the problem's impact.
- Contemplation: The patient is considering change and looking at its positive and negative aspects. The person often reports feeling "stuck" with the problem, unable to figure out how to change to solve or minimize the health issue.
- Preparation: The patient exhibits some change behaviors or thoughts and often reports feeling that he or she does not have the tools to proceed.
- Action: The patient is ready to go forth with change, often takes concrete steps to change, but is often inconsistent with carrying through.
- Maintenance/relapse: The patient learns to continue the change and has adopted and embraced the healthy habit. Relapse can occur, however, and the person learns to deal with backsliding.

As health counselor, the NP provides a valuable role in continually "tapping" the patient with a message of concern about health and safety, helping to move the person in the precontemplation stage to the contemplation stage. After the patient is at this stage, presenting treatment options and support for change is a critical part of the NP's role. During action and maintenance stages, the NP needs to be positive

---

BOX 1-1
Orderly Approach to Patient Education and Counseling

■ Assess the patient's knowledge base about factors contributing to the problem.
■ Evaluate the contribution of the patient's belief system to the problem.
■ Ask the patient about perceived barriers to action and supporting factors.
■ Match teaching to the patient's perception of the problem.
■ Inform the patient about the purpose and benefit of an intervention.
■ Give the patient an anticipated time of onset of effect of a therapy.
■ Suggest small rather than large changes in behavior.
■ Give accurate, specific information.
■ Consider adding new positive behaviors, rather than attempting to discontinue established behaviors.
■ Link desired behavior with established behavior.
■ Give a strong, personalized message about the seriousness of health risk.
■ Ask for a commitment from the patient.
■ Use a combination of teaching strategies, such as visual, oral, and written methods.
■ Strive for an interdisciplinary approach to patient education and counseling, with all members of the team giving the same message.
■ Maintain frequent contact with the patient to monitor progress.
■ Expect gains and periodic setbacks.

Source: Freda MC: http://www.medscape.com/viewarticle/478283_3, Issues in Patient Education

and encouraging, even with the occasional relapse. With relapse, an important message to convey to the patient is that he or she was successfully able to make the change once and can do it again and that the patient is continuing to learn how to change behavior. Using statements that begin with "we" convey the message that the NP is there to help facilitate success.

DISCUSSION SOURCE

Substance Abuse and Mental Health Services Administration, http://www.samhsa.gov/co-occurring/topics/training/change. aspx, Motivational Interviewing and the Stages of Change

Cancer Screening

64. Which of the following women should have screening for cervical cancer?
    A. An 18-year-old who has a history of genital warts
    B. A 17-year-old with coitarche 3 years ago and four male sexual partners
    C. An 80-year-old with heart failure and a remote history of normal Pap test results
    D. A 21-year-old who has had one male sexual partner and consistent condom use

65. Which of the following is a recommended method of annual colorectal cancer screening for a 62-year-old man?
    A. digital rectal examination
    B. in-office fecal occult blood test (FOBT)
    C. at-home FOBT
    D. sigmoidoscopy

66. Which of the following types of cancer screening is not routinely recommended in a 55-year-old woman?
    A. breast
    B. skin
    C. endometrial
    D. colorectal

Answers

64. D.   **66.** C.   **66.** C.

Cancer screening is an important part of providing comprehensive primary healthcare. Adherence to current, nationally recognized guidelines is an important part of effective clinical practice. At the same time, different organizations can have slightly different guidelines. When this occurs, rather than be concerned about the minor difference, focus on the commonalities. At the same time, all guidelines advocate for a 50-year-old woman to have a mammogram. All organizations are in agreement that a Pap test should not be done prior to age 21 years, nor continue to be conducted in elderly women with anticipated short

life spans. Please see additional information on cancer screening in other chapters of this book.

DISCUSSION SOURCES

American Cancer Society, http://www.cancer.org/healthy/find-cancerearly/cancerscreeningguidelines/american-cancer-society-guidelines-for-the-early-detection-of-cancer, American Cancer Society Guidelines for the Early Detection of Cancer

United States Preventive Services Task Force, http://www.uspreventiveservicestaskforce.org/adultrec.htm#cancer, cancer screening

Tobacco Use

67. The components of brief intervention for treating tobacco use include:
    A. Ask, Advise, Assess, Assist, Arrange.
    B. Advise, Intervene, Counsel, Follow up, Prescribe.
    C. Document, Counsel, Caution, Describe, Demonstrate.
    D. Advise, Describe, Confer, Prescribe, Document.

68. Brief intervention that provides motivation to quit tobacco use should be:
    A. used at every clinical visit that the tobacco user has, regardless of reason for the visit.
    B. offered when the tobacco user voices concern about the health effects of smoking.
    C. applied primarily during visits for conditions that are clearly related to or exacerbated by tobacco use, such as respiratory tract disease.
    D. when the clinician is conducting a comprehensive health assessment, such as with the annual physical examination.

69. The use of FDA-approved pharmacologic intervention in tobacco use:
    A. makes little difference in smoking cessation rates.
    B. reliably increases long-term smoking abstinence rates.
    C. is helpful but generally poorly tolerated.
    D. poses a greater risk to health than continued tobacco use.

70. You see a 48-year-old patient who started taking varenicline (Chantix) 4 weeks ago to aid in smoking cessation. Which of the following is the most important question to ask during today's visit?
    A. "How many cigarettes a day are you currently smoking?"
    B. "On a scale of 0 to 10, how strong is your desire to smoke?"
    C. "Have you noticed any changes in your mood?"
    D. "Are you having any trouble sleeping?"

Answers

67. A.   **68.** A.   **69.** B.   **70.** C.

Tobacco use poses a tremendous health hazard; tobacco-related diseases result in a significant burden to public health and healthcare costs. Tobacco dependence is a chronic disease that often requires repeated intervention and multiple attempts to quit. Effective treatments exist, however, that can significantly increase rates of long-term abstinence. Treating tobacco use and dependence guidelines from the Agency for Healthcare Research and Quality (AHRQ) offer the following recommendations for smoking cessation.

Clinicians and healthcare delivery systems must consistently identify and document tobacco use status and treat every tobacco user seen in a healthcare setting. Brief tobacco dependence treatment is effective. Clinicians should offer every patient who uses tobacco at least the brief treatments shown to be effective. An example of a brief intervention includes the "5 As": Ask, Advise, Assess, Assist, Arrange (Table 1–6). This strategy should be used with all tobacco users, including individuals with no current desire to quit because this can serve as a motivating factor in future attempts to discontinue tobacco use.

Individual, group, and telephone counseling are helpful, and their effectiveness increases with treatment intensity. Two components of counseling—practical counseling (problem solving/skills training) and social support—are especially effective, and clinicians should use these when counseling patients making a quit attempt. Telephone quit line counseling has been shown to be effective with diverse populations and has broad reach. Clinicians and healthcare delivery systems should ensure patient access to quit lines and promote quit line use.

Tobacco-dependence treatments are effective across a broad range of populations. Clinicians should encourage every patient willing to make a quit attempt to use the counseling treatments and appropriate medications. Numerous effective medications are available for tobacco dependence, and clinicians should encourage their use by all patients attempting to quit smoking—except when medically contraindicated or with specific populations for which there is less evidence of effectiveness (i.e., pregnant women, smokeless tobacco users, light smokers, and adolescents). These medications include nicotine replacement therapy (NRT) (e.g., patch, gum, inhaler, nasal spray, and lozenge) and medications to reduce the desire to smoke (bupropion [Zyban, Wellbutrin] and varenicline [Chantix]).

The use of these medications reliably increases long-term smoking abstinence rates. Generally, the risk associated with the use of these medications is less than that associated with continued tobacco use. Adverse effects occasionally attributed to the use of smoking cessation medications are sometimes actually a result of nicotine withdrawal. The FDA added a warning, however, regarding the use of varenicline. Specifically, depressed mood, agitation, changes in behavior, suicidal ideation, and suicide have been reported in patients attempting to quit smoking while using varenicline. Patients should tell their healthcare provider about any history of psychiatric illness before starting this medication; clinicians should also ask about mental health history before starting this medication. Close monitoring for changes in mood and behavior should follow.

Counseling and medication are effective when used by clinicians as solo interventions for treating tobacco dependence. The combination of counseling and medication is more effective, however, than either alone. Clinicians should encourage all individuals making a quit attempt to use both counseling and medication. For an individual who is not interested in quitting, motivational intervention is often helpful and should be provided at every clinical visit.

Treatments for tobacco dependence are clinically effective and highly cost-effective relative to interventions for other

---

TABLE 1-6
Five As

Ask about tobacco use	Identify and document tobacco use status for every patient at every visit.
Advise to quit	In a clear, strong, and personalized manner, urge every tobacco user to quit.
Assess willingness to make a quit attempt	Is the tobacco user willing to make a quit attempt at this time?
Assist in quit attempt	For the patient willing to make a quit attempt, offer medication and provide or refer for counseling or additional treatment to help the patient quit.
	For patients unwilling to quit at the time, provide interventions designed to increase future quit attempts.
Arrange follow-up	For the patient willing to make a quit attempt, arrange for follow-up contacts, beginning within the first week after the quit date.
	For patients unwilling to make a quit attempt at the time, address tobacco dependence and willingness to quit at next clinic visit.

Source: http://www.ncbi.nlm.nih.gov/books/bv.fcgi?rid=hstat2.section.29645#29648, AHQR supported clinical practice guidelines: Treating tobacco use and dependence

clinical disorders. Providing insurance coverage for these treatments increases quit rates. Insurers and purchasers should ensure that all insurance plans include the counseling and medication identified as effective in the AHRQ guidelines as covered benefits.

DISCUSSION SOURCE

Tobacco Use and Dependence Guideline Panel, Treating Tobacco Use and Dependence: 2008 Update. Rockville (MD): US Department of Health and Human Services; 2008 May. Available from: http://www.ncbi.nlm.nih.gov/books/NBK63952

Neurological Disorders

2

Cranial Nerves

1. Assessing vision and visual fields involves testing cranial nerve (CN):
   A. I.
   B. II.
   C. III.
   D. IV.

2. You perform an extraocular movement test on a middle-aged patient. He is unable to move his eyes upward and inward. This indicates a possibility of paralysis of CN:
   A. II.
   B. III.
   C. V.
   D. VI.

3. Loss of corneal reflex is in part seen in dysfunction of CN:
   A. III.
   B. IV.
   C. V.
   D. VI.

4 to 6. Match the CN with the appropriate function or test.

4. CN I	A.	Tongue and throat, swallowing
5. CN VII	B.	Sense of smell
6. CN IX	C.	Facial asymmetry, drop of mouth (Bell's palsy)

Answers

1. B.	**3.** C.	**5.** C.
2. B.	**4.** B.	**6.** A.

Knowledge of the cranial nerves (CNs) is critical for performing an accurate neurological assessment. Because these are paired nerves arising largely from the brainstem, a unilateral CN dysfunction is common, often reflecting a problem in the ipsilateral cerebral hemisphere.

Cranial Nerve Mnemonic

A commonly used mnemonic for identifying and remembering the cranial nerves is: *On Old Olympus Towering Tops, A Finn And German Viewed Some Hops.* The details of the cranial nerves are as follows:

- CN I—Olfactory: You have one nose, where CN I resides. Its function contributes to the sense of smell.
- CN II—Optic: You have two eyes, where you will find CN II. Function of this CN is vital to vision and visual fields and, in conjunction with CN III, pupillary reaction.
- CN III—Oculomotor: CN III, the eye (*oculo-*) movement (*motor*) nerve, works with CNs III, IV, and VI (*abducens*, which helps the eyeball abduct or move). The actions of these CNs are largely responsible for the movement of the eyeball and eyelid.
- CN IV—Trochlear: This nerve innervates the superior oblique muscle of the eye.
- CN V—Trigeminal: Three (*tri*) types of sensation (temperature, pain, and tactile) come from this three-branched nerve that covers three territories of the face. For normal corneal reflexes to be present, the afferent limb of the first division of CN V and the effect limb of CN VII need to be intact.
- CN VI—Abducens
- CN VII—Facial: Dysfunction of this nerve gives the characteristic findings of Bell's palsy (facial asymmetry, droop of mouth, absent nasolabial fold, impaired eyelid movement).
- CN VIII—Auditory or vestibulocochlear: When this nerve does not function properly, hearing (auditory) or balance is impaired (vestibulocochlear). Rinne's test is part of the evaluation of this CN.
- CN IX—Glossopharyngeal: The name of this CN provides a clue that its function affects the tongue (*glosso*) and throat (*pharynx*). Along with CN X, the function of this nerve is critical to swallowing, palate elevation, and gustation.

- CN X—Vagus: This CN is involved in parasympathetic regulation of multiple organs, including sensing aortic pressure and regulating blood pressure, slowing heart rate, and regulating taste and digestive rate.
- CN XI—Accessory or spinal root of the accessory: Function of this CN can be tested by evaluating shoulder shrug and lateral neck rotation.
- CN XII—Hypoglossal: Function of this CN is tested by noting movement and protrusion of the tongue.

DISCUSSION SOURCE

http://www.med.yale.edu/caim/cnerves/, Cranial nerves, accessed 9/20/13.

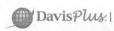 See full color images of this topic on DavisPlus at **http://davisplus.fadavis.com | Keyword: Fitzgerald**

Bell's Palsy

7. You examine a 29-year-old woman who has a sudden onset of right-sided facial asymmetry. She is unable to close her right eyelid tightly, frown, or smile on the affected side. Her examination is otherwise unremarkable. This presentation likely represents paralysis of CN:
   A. III.
   B. IV.
   C. VII.
   D. VIII.

8. Which represents the most appropriate diagnostic test for the patient in the previous question?
   A. complete blood cell count with white blood cell (WBC) differential
   B. Lyme disease antibody titer
   C. computed tomography (CT) scan of the head with contrast medium
   D. blood urea nitrogen and creatinine levels

9. In prescribing prednisone for a patient with Bell's palsy, the nurse practitioner (NP) considers that its use:
   A. has not been shown to be helpful in improving outcomes in this condition.
   B. should be initiated as soon as possible after the onset of facial paralysis.
   C. is likely to help minimize ocular symptoms.
   D. may prolong the course of the disease.

Answers

7. C.   8. B.   9. B.

Bell's palsy is an acute paralysis of CN VII (in the absence of brain dysfunction) that is seen without other signs and symptoms. Though the exact cause is unknown, the condition is believed to result from inflammation of the cranial nerve within the temporal bone, presumably related to mechanical compression. Bell's palsy is often linked to viral infections, including herpes simplex virus, herpes zoster, Epstein-Barr, cytomegalovirus, adenovirus, rubella, and mumps virus. Other conditions can mimic facial muscle weakness observed with Bell's palsy, including stroke, infection, Lyme disease, and tumors. Diagnostic approaches that can be used to determine the cause of the symptoms include electromyography (to measure electrical activity of the facial muscle in response to stimulation); imaging scans to rule out tumor or skull fracture are typically only ordered when there is uncertainty with the diagnosis and are not routinely ordered. Appropriate antibody testing for Lyme disease should be obtained in a patient presenting with signs of Bell's palsy; Bell's palsy is a rare finding during secondary stage of Lyme disease.

For most people, Bell's palsy is temporary and symptoms usually start to improve within a few weeks with complete recovery by 6 months. A small percentage of people will have permanent symptoms. Updated guidelines from the American Academy of Neurology (AAN) recommend the use of corticosteroids to treat Bell's palsy. Current evidence demonstrates little benefit on the use of antivirals as part of Bell's palsy therapy. With ocular involvement, such as impaired eye closure and abnormal tear flow, consultation with an eye care professional should be obtained. The use of tear substitutes, lubricants, and eye protection may be needed to reduce the risk of corneal drying and foreign-body exposure to the eye.

DISCUSSION SOURCES

Anderson, P. AAN Guideline on Bell's Palsy. http://www.medscape.com/viewarticle/774056/

Lo, B. http://emedicine.medscape.com/article/2018337-overview. eMedicine: Bell's palsy

Gronseth GS, Paduga R; American Academy of Neurology. Evidence-based guideline update: Steroids and antivirals for Bell palsy: Report of the Guideline Development Subcommittee of the American Academy of Neurology. *Neurology* 79:2209–2213, 2012.

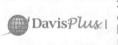 See full color images of this topic on DavisPlus at **http://davisplus.fadavis.com | Keyword: Fitzgerald**

Headache

10. A 40-year-old man presents with a 5-week history of recurrent headaches that awaken him during the night. The pain is severe, lasts about 1 hour, and is located behind his left eye. Additional symptoms include lacrimation and nasal discharge. His physical examination is within normal limits. This clinical presentation is most consistent with:
    A. migraine without aura.
    B. migraine with aura.
    C. cluster headache.
    D. increased intracranial pressure (ICP).

11. A 22-year-old woman presents with a 3-year history of recurrent, unilateral, pulsating headaches with vomiting and photophobia. The headaches, which generally last 3 hours, can be aborted by resting in a dark room. She can usually tell that she is going to get a headache. She explains, "I see little 'squiggles' before my eyes for about 15 minutes." Her physical examination is unremarkable. This presentation is most consistent with:
    A. tension-type headache.
    B. migraine without aura.
    C. migraine with aura.
    D. cluster headache.

12. Indicators that a headache can be the presenting symptom of a serious illness and may require neuroimaging include all of the following except:
    A. headaches that occur periodically in clusters.
    B. increasing frequency and severity of headaches.
    C. headache causing confusion, dizziness, and/or lack of coordination.
    D. headache causing awakening from sleep.

13. Prophylactic treatment for migraine headaches includes the use of:
    A. amitriptyline.
    B. ergot derivative.
    C. naproxen sodium.
    D. clonidine.

14. Among the following beta blockers, which is the least effective in preventing migraine headache?
    A. acebutolol
    B. metoprolol
    C. atenolol
    D. propranolol

15. Antiepileptic drugs useful for preventing migraine headaches include all of the following except:
    A. divalproex.
    B. valproate.
    C. lamotrigine.
    D. topiramate.

16. Evidence supports the use of all of the following vitamins and supplements for migraine prevention except:
    A. butterbur.
    B. riboflavin.
    C. feverfew.
    D. ginkgo biloba.

17. You are examining a 65-year-old man who has a history of acute coronary syndrome and migraine. Which of the following agents represents the best choice of acute headache (abortive) therapy for this patient?
    A. verapamil
    B. ergotamine
    C. timolol
    D. sumatriptan

18. A 45-year-old man experiences rapidly progressing migraine headaches that are accompanied by significant GI upset. Appropriate acute headache (abortive) treatment includes all of the following except:
    A. injectable sumatriptan.
    B. dihydroergotamine nasal spray.
    C. oral naproxen sodium.
    D. zolmitriptan nasal spray.

19. With migraine, which of the following statements is true?
    A. Migraine with aura is the most common form.
    B. Most migraineurs are in ongoing healthcare for the condition.
    C. The condition is equally common in men and women.
    D. The pain is typically described as pulsating.

20. In tension-type headache, which of the following is true?
    A. Photophobia is seldom reported.
    B. The pain is typically described as "pressing" in quality.
    C. The headache is usually unilateral.
    D. Physical activity usually makes the discomfort worse.

21. Risk factors for cluster headaches include all of the following except:
    A. over 65 years of age.
    B. heavy alcohol use.
    C. heavy tobacco use.
    D. male gender.

22. Treatment options in cluster headache include the use of:
    A. nonsteroidal anti-inflammatory drugs (NSAIDs).
    B. oxygen.
    C. the triptans.
    D. all of the above therapies.

23. Which of the following oral agents has the most rapid analgesic onset?
    A. naproxen (Naprosyn)
    B. liquid ibuprofen (Motrin, Advil)
    C. diclofenac (Voltaren)
    D. enteric-coated naproxen (Naproxen EC)

24. The mechanism of action of triptans is as a(n):
    A. selective serotonin receptor agonist.
    B. dopamine antagonist.
    C. vasoconstrictor.
    D. inhibitor of leukotriene synthesis.

25. Limitations of use of butalbital with acetaminophen and caffeine (Fioricet) include its:
    A. energizing effect.
    B. gastrointestinal (GI) upset profile.
    C. high rate of rebound headache if used frequently.
    D. excessive cost.

26. The use of neuroleptics such as prochlorperazine (Compazine) and promethazine (Phenergan) in migraine therapy should be limited to less than three times per week because of their:
    A. addictive potential.
    B. extrapyramidal movement risk.
    C. ability to cause rebound headache.
    D. sedative effect.

27. Which of the following statements about ergotamines is false?
    A. are effective for tension-type headaches
    B. act as 5-HT1A and 5-HT1D receptor agonists
    C. have potential vasoconstrictor effect
    D. should be avoided in the presence of coronary artery disease

28. With appropriately prescribed headache prophylactic therapy, the patient should be informed to expect:
    A. virtual resolution of headaches.
    B. no fewer but less severe headaches.
    C. approximately 50% reduction in the number of headaches.
    D. that lifelong therapy is advised.

29. A 48-year-old woman presents with a monthly 4-day premenstrual migraine headache, poorly responsive to triptans and analgesics, and accompanied by vasomotor symptoms (hot flashes). The clinician considers prescribing all of the following except:
    A. continuous monophasic oral contraceptive.
    B. phasic combined oral contraceptive with a 7-day-per-month withdrawal period.
    C. low-dose estrogen patch use during the premenstrual week.
    D. triptan prophylaxis.

30. A first-line prophylactic treatment option for the prevention of tension-type headache is:
    A. nortriptyline.
    B. verapamil.
    C. carbamazepine.
    D. valproate.

31. A 47-year-old woman experiences occasional migraine with aura and reports partial relief with zolmitriptan. You decide to add which of the following to augment the pain control by the triptan?
    A. lamotrigine
    B. gabapentin
    C. naproxen sodium
    D. magnesium

32. A 68-year-old man presents with new onset of headaches. He describes the pain as bilateral frontal to occipital and most severe when he arises in the morning and when coughing. He feels much better by mid-afternoon. The history is most consistent with headache caused by:
    A. vascular compromise.
    B. increased intracranial pressure (ICP).

    C. brain tumor.
    D. tension-type with atypical geriatric presentation.

33. Systemic corticosteroid therapy would be most appropriate in treating:
    A. tension-type headache.
    B. migraines occurring on a weekly basis.
    C. intractable or severe migraines and cluster headaches.
    D. migraines occurring during pregnancy.

34. When evaluating a patient with acute headache, all of the following observations would indicate the absence of a more serious underlying condition except:
    A. onset of headache with exertion, coughing, or sneezing.
    B. history of previous identical headache.
    C. supple neck.
    D. normal neurological examination results.

35. Common secondary headache causes include all of the following except:
    A. brain tumor.
    B. intracranial bleeding.
    C. intracranial inflammation.
    D. cluster headache.

36 to 38. Match the female:male ratio for each type of primary headache listed:
    36. Tension-type headache   A. 1:3 to 1:8
    37. Migraine without aura   B. 3:1
    38. Cluster headache   C. 5:4

39 to 43. Indicate the appropriate course of action (head CT scan, head MRI, or neither) for each of the following patients:

39. A 45-year-old man who presents with a sudden, abrupt headache. Upon questioning, he appears somewhat confused with decreased alertness to his surroundings.

40. A 48-year-old woman with a history of breast cancer who presents with 3 month history of progressively severe headache, and bulging optic disk.

41. A 24-year-old man who presents in the ED following a motor vehicle accident. He exhibits confusion and falls in and out of consciousness.

42. A 57-year-old woman with a prior history of a brain tumor that was removed 8 years ago. She complains of headaches that have been increasing in frequency and intensity over the past month.

43. A 37-year-old man diagnosed with cluster-type headache that is alleviated with high-dose NSAIDs.

44. In counseling a patient who experience migraines, you recommend all of the following lifestyle changes to minimize the risk of triggering a headache except:
    A. avoiding eating within 1-2 hours of AM awakening.
    B. limiting exposure to cigarette smoke.
    C. avoiding trigger physical activities.
    D. implementing strategies to reduce stress.

45. A 37-year-old woman complains of migraine headaches that typically occur after eating out in restaurants. Potential triggers that can influence the onset and severity of migraine symptoms include all of the following except:
A. **cheese** pizza.
B. pickled or fermented foods.
C. freshly baked yeast products.
D. baked whitefish.

The primary headaches, including migraine, tension-type, and cluster headache, are the most common chronic pain syndromes seen in primary care practice (Table 2–1). Development of the appropriate diagnosis is critical to caring for patients with headache (Table 2–2). Despite the existence of

Answers

10. C.	22. D.	34. A.
11. C.	23. B.	35. D.
12. A.	24. A.	36. C.
13. A.	25. C.	37. B.
14. A.	26. B.	38. A.
15. C.	27. A.	39. CT scan
16. D.	28. C.	40. MRI
17. C.	29. B.	41. CT scan
18. C.	30. A.	42. MRI
19. D.	31. C.	43. Neither
20. B.	32. B.	44. A.
21. A.	33. C.	45. D.

TABLE 2-1
Headache: Primary versus Secondary

Primary Headache	Secondary Headache
Not associated with other diseases, likely complex interplay of genetic, developmental, and environmental risk factors	Associated with or caused by other conditions, generally does not resolve until specific cause is diagnosed and addressed
Migraine, tension-type, cluster	Intracranial issue such as brain tumor, intracranial bleeding, or inflammation, viremia, or any condition that causes increased intracranial pressure

TABLE 2-2
Primary Headache: Clinical Presentation and Diagnosis

Headache Type	Headache Characteristics
Tension-type headache	Lasts 30 minutes to 7 days (usually 1–24 hours) with two or more of the following characteristics Pressing, nonpulsatile pain Mild to moderate in intensity Usually bilateral location Notation of 0–1 of the following (>1 suggests migraine): nausea, photophobia, or phonophobia Female:male ratio 5:4
Migraine without aura	Lasts 4–72 hours with two or more of the following characteristics Usually unilateral location, although occasionally bilateral Pulsating quality, moderate to severe in intensity Aggravation by normal activity such as walking, or causes avoidance of these activities During headache, one or more of the following Nausea/vomiting, photophobia, phonophobia Female:male ratio 3:1 Positive family history in 70%–90%
Migraine with aura	Migraine-type headache occurs with or after aura Focal dysfunction of cerebral cortex or brainstem causes one or more aura symptoms to develop over 4 minutes, or two or more symptoms occur in succession Symptoms include feeling of dread or anxiety, unusual fatigue, nervousness or excitement, GI upset, visual or olfactory alteration No aura symptom should last >1 hour. If this occurs, an alternative diagnosis should be considered Positive family history in 70%–90%

Continued

TABLE 2-2

Primary Headache: Clinical Presentation and Diagnosis—cont'd

Headache Type	Headache Characteristics
Cluster headache	Tendency of headache to occur daily in groups or clusters, hence the name cluster headache Clusters usually last several weeks to months, then disappear for months to years Usually occur at characteristic times of year, such as vernal and autumnal equinox with one to eight episodes per day, at the same time of day. Common time is ~1 hour into sleep; the pain awakens the person (hence the term "alarm clock" headache) Headache is often located behind one eye with a steady, intense ("hot poker in the eye" sensation), severe pain in a crescendo pattern lasting 15 minutes to 3 hours, with most in the range of 30–45 minutes. Pain intensity has helped earn the condition the name "suicide headache." Most often occurs with ipsilateral autonomic sign such as lacrimation, conjunctival injection, ptosis, and nasal stuffiness Female:male ratio ~1:3 to 1:8 (depending on source) Family history of cluster headache present in ~20%

Source: Standards of Care for Headache Diagnosis and Treatment. Chicago, National Headache Foundation, http://www.headaches.org/content/standards-care-headache-diagnosis-and-treatment

specific criteria, clinicians frequently misdiagnose migraine. One reason for error is the nature of these diagnostic criteria. The International Headache Society (IHS) criteria do not include all symptoms frequently observed in episodes of migraine. Consequently, migraine associated with muscle or neck pain, which is not an IHS migraine diagnostic criterion, is often diagnosed as tension-type headache, and migraine associated with nasal symptoms such as rhinorrhea and nasal congestion, also not included as IHS diagnostic criteria, is diagnosed as a "sinus" headache. In both cases, these headaches are usually migraine in nature.

Headache rarely can be the presenting symptom of a serious illness. The key points to consider in assessing a patient with headache are presented in Box 2–1 and Table 2–3. The question of whether to obtain neuroimaging with head CT or magnetic resonance imaging (MRI) to evaluate for underlying disease often arises in the care of a patient with nonacute primary headache. In the absence of a normal neurological examination, the results of neuroimaging yield little additional information but add significantly to health-care cost (Table 2–4 and Table 2–5).

BOX 2-1

Helpful Observations in Patients with Acute Headache

■ History of previous identical headaches
■ Intact cognition
■ Supple neck
■ Normal neurological examination results
■ Improvement in symptoms while under observation and treatment

TABLE 2-3

Headache "Red Flags"

Consider diagnosis other than primary headache if headache "red flags" are present
- **S**ystemic symptoms
  - Fever, weight loss, or secondary headache risk factors such as HIV, malignancy, pregnancy, anticoagulation
- **N**eurological signs, symptoms
  - Any newly acquired neurological finding including confusion, impaired alertness or consciousness, nuchal rigidity, hypertension, papilledema, CN dysfunction, abnormal motor function
- **O**nset
  - Sudden, abrupt, or split-second, the "thunderclap" headache
  - Onset of headache with exertion, sexual activity, coughing, sneezing
    - Suggests subarachnoid hemorrhage, sudden onset increased ICP
- **O**nset (age at onset of headache)
  - Older (>50 years) and younger (<5 years)
- **P**revious headache history
  - First headache in adult ≥30 years
    - Primary headache pattern usually established in youth/young adult years
  - New onset of different headache
    - Change in attack frequency, severity, or clinical features including progressive headache without headache-free period

Source: Dodick DW. Clinical clues and clinical rules: primary vs secondary headache. *Adv Stud Med* 3:S550–S555, 2003.

TABLE 2-4

Evidence-Based Guidelines in the Primary Care Setting: Neuroimaging in Patients with Nonacute Headache

Significantly increased odds of finding abnormality on neuroimaging
- Rapidly increasing headache frequency
- History
  - Dizziness or lack of coordination
  - Subjective numbness or tingling
  - Headache causing awakening from sleep
  - Headache worse with Valsalva maneuver
  - Accelerating, new-onset headache
- Abnormal neurological examination
- Increasing age
  - More likely nonacute finding such as old infarct, atrophy

Unlikely to correlate with abnormal neuroimaging; neuroimaging unlikely to yield helpful clinical information
- Neurological examination normal
- Long-standing history of similar headache
- "Worst headache of my life"

Consensus-based principles
- Testing should be avoided if it would not lead to a change in management
- Not recommended if individual no more likely than general population to have significant abnormality
- Testing not normally recommended as population policy, although may make sense at individual level (e.g., with patient or provider fear)

Source: http://www.aan.com/professionals/practice/pdfs/gl0088.pdf, American Academy of Neurology evidence-based guidelines in the primary care setting: Neuroimaging in nonacute headache

TABLE 2-5

Head CT Scan Versus MRI

CT Scan	MRI
Rapid imaging (~5–10 min; important if intracranial hemorrhage is suspected)	Longer procedure (~45 min)
Exposes patient to ionizing radiation (cancer risk)	No exposure to ionizing radiation
Greater risk of allergic reaction to contrast agent (iodine)	Contrast agent less likely to cause allergic reaction (gadolinium)
Can be used in patients with implantable devices	Cannot be used in patients with implantable devices
Better at detecting acute hemorrhage and bone abnormalities	Better at detecting small and subtle lesions
Less cost	More expensive

Migraine without aura affects about 80% of persons with migraine. On careful questioning, many patients report a migraine warning, however, such as agitation, jitteriness, disturbed sleep, or unusual dreams (see Table 2–2 for diagnostic criteria). Migraine with aura is found in about 20% of patients with migrainous disorders. The aura is a recurrent neurological symptom that arises from the cerebral cortex or brainstem. Typically, the aura develops over 5 to 20 minutes, lasts less than 1 hour, and is accompanied or followed by migraine. Patients who have migraines with aura do not have more severe headaches than patients without aura, but the former patients are more likely to be offered a fuller range of therapies. Patients without aura may be misdiagnosed as having tension-type headaches and are often not offered headache therapies specifically suited for migraines, such as the triptans.

Although much of headache care is focused on the relief and prevention of migraine, tension-type headaches are a significant source of suffering and lost function (see Table 2–2 for diagnosis). Abortive treatment options to relieve headache pain include the use of acetaminophen; NSAIDs; and combination products such as butalbital with acetaminophen and acetaminophen, aspirin, and caffeine. Prophylactic therapies are effective at limiting the number and frequency of tension-type headache. Consideration should also be given for coexisting migraine and tension-type headache; in this situation, triptan use is often helpful.

Cluster headaches, also known as migrainous neuralgia, are most common in middle-aged men, particularly men with heavy alcohol and tobacco use. Although cluster is the only primary headache type more common in men than women, more recent study reveals that the condition is likely underdiagnosed in women. Sometimes called the "suicide headache" because of the severity of the associated pain, cluster headache occurs periodically in clusters (hence its name) of several weeks, with associated lacrimation and rhinorrhea. Treatment includes reduction of triggers, such as tobacco and alcohol use, and initiation of prophylactic therapy and appropriate abortive therapy (triptans, high-dose NSAIDs, and high-flow oxygen).

Headache treatment is aimed at identifying and reducing headache triggers. Lifestyle modification is a highly effective and often underused headache therapy (Tables 2–6 and 2–7). In addition, abortive therapy should be offered. Prophylactic

TABLE 2-6

Potential Lifestyle, Health Status or Medication Triggers Influencing the Onset or Severity of Migraine Symptoms: A Comprehensive Headache Treatment Plan Includes Minimizing or Eliminating These Triggers Whenever Possible

Menses, ovulation, or pregnancy
Birth control/hormone replacement (progesterone) therapy
Illness of virtually any kind, whether acute or chronic
Intense or strenuous activity/exercise
Sleeping too much/too little/jet lag
Fasting/missing meals
Bright or flickering lights
Excessive or repetitive noises
Odors/fragrances/tobacco smoke
Weather/seasonal changes
High altitudes
Medications
Stress/stress letdown

Source: http://www.guideline.gov/summary/summary.aspx?ss=
15&doc_id=6578&nbr=4138

TABLE 2-7

Potential Dietary Triggers Influencing the Onset or Severity of Migraine Symptoms: A Comprehensive Headache Treatment Plan Includes Minimizing or Eliminating These Triggers Whenever Possible

Sour cream
Ripened cheeses (cheddar, Stilton, Brie, Camembert)
Sausage, bologna, salami, pepperoni, summer sausage, hot dogs
Pizza
Chicken liver, pâté
Herring (pickled or dried)
Any pickled, fermented, or marinated food
Monosodium glutamate (MSG) (soy sauce, meat tenderizers, seasoned salt)
Freshly baked yeast products, sourdough bread
Chocolate
Nuts or nut butters
Broad beans, lima beans, fava beans, snow peas
Onions
Figs, raisins, papayas, avocados, red plums
Citrus fruits
Bananas
Caffeinated beverages (tea, coffee, cola)
Alcoholic beverages (wine, beer, whiskey)
Aspartame/phenylalanine-containing foods or beverages

Source: http://www.guideline.gov/summary/summary.aspx?ss=
15&doc_id=6578&nbr=4138

therapy, aimed at limiting the number and severity of future headaches, is also often indicated. Rescue therapy is used when abortive therapy is ineffective in providing headache relief.

When a migraine abortive agent is chosen, a number of considerations should be kept in mind. These medications are available in many forms (i.e., oral, parenteral, nasal spray, rectal suppository). Migraine is also present in many forms. A thoughtful match between the presentation of typical migraine and the form of medication is helpful. Following are some examples:

• Oral products generally take ½ to 1 hour before there is significant relief of migraine pain. These products are best suited for patients with migraine who have a slowly developing headache with minimum GI distress. As with all migraine therapies, oral medications should be used as soon as possible after the onset of symptoms. The use of oral products to manage migraine is the least expensive option and facilitates patient self-care.

• Injectable products (e.g., sumatriptan (Imitrex) and dihydroergotamine (D.H.E. 45, Migranal) have a rapid onset of action, usually within 15 to 30 minutes. These products are best suited for patients with rapidly progressing migraines accompanied by significant GI upset. Sumatriptan is available as a self-injector for patient administration. Dihydroergotamine is usually given intravenously for severe migraine along with parenteral hydration. Injectables are usually the most expensive treatment option, and using these products sometimes means that a patient with migraine requires a provider visit to facilitate the use of the medication. Certain triptans (sumatriptan [Imitrex] and zolmitriptan [Zomig]) and the ergot derivative dihydroergotamine (Migranal) are available as nasal sprays, have a similarly rapid onset of action, and are tolerable in the presence of GI upset. Analgesics (aspirin, acetaminophen) or antiemetics (prochlorperazine [Compazine], promethazine [Phenergan] and ondansetron hydrochloride {Zofran}) can be used for pain control or treatment of GI upset, respectively.

- Triptans act as selective serotonin receptor agonists and work at the 5-HT1D serotonin receptor site, allowing an increased uptake of serotonin. Because of potential vasoconstrictor effect, their use is contraindicated in patients with Prinzmetal angina or established or high risk for coronary artery disease, in pregnant women, and in individuals who have recently used ergots. Because of the risk of serotonin syndrome, a condition of excessive availability of this neurotransmitter, triptans should be used with caution with monoamine oxidase inhibitors (MAOIs) or high-dose selective serotonin reuptake inhibitors. Although triptans are specifically labeled for use only in migraine, some patients with severe tension-type headache benefit from their use, which lends further support to the hypothesis that there is a shared mechanism in migraine and tension-type headache. Adding an analgesic such as an NSAID to the use of a triptan yields improved pain control in many migraineurs. An example of a combined triptan/NSAID product is Treximet (sumatriptan with naproxen sodium).

- Ergotamines are ergot derivatives that act as 5-HT1A and 5-HT1D receptor agonists and do not alter cerebral blood flow. Because of potential vasoconstrictor effect, their use should be avoided in the presence of coronary artery disease and pregnancy. Ergotamines are available in various forms, including oral and sublingual tablets, suppositories, injectables, and nasal sprays; examples include dihydroergotamine mesylate [Migranal, D.H.E. 45] and ergotamine tartrate with caffeine [Migergot]). These products are helpful in the treatment of migraine, but not tension-type headache.

- NSAIDs can be highly effective in tension-type and migraine headache. These products inhibit prostaglandin and leukotriene synthesis and are most helpful when used at the first sign of headache, when GI upset is not a significant issue. The National Health Foundation Guidelines advise the use of rapid-onset NSAIDs such as ibuprofen in high doses with booster doses. Plain naproxen (Naprosyn) has a relatively slow onset of analgesic activity, whereas naproxen sodium (Aleve, Anaprox) use is associated with a significantly more rapid onset of pain relief. Acetaminophen and aspirin can also provide relief in migraine and tension-type headache, but provide less analgesic effect.

- Fioricet is a combination medication consisting of caffeine, butalbital, and acetaminophen. Caffeine enhances the analgesic properties of acetaminophen, and butalbital's barbiturate action enhances select neurotransmitter action, helping to relieve migraine and tension-type headache pain. With infrequent use, this product offers an inexpensive and generally well-tolerated headache treatment. Frequent or excessive use of Fioricet should be discouraged because of the potential for barbiturate dependency from butalbital and analgesic rebound headache from the acetaminophen component of the product.

- Excedrin Migraine is an over-the-counter aspirin, acetaminophen, and caffeine combination product that is approved by the U.S. Food and Drug Administration (FDA) for migraine therapy and is effective in tension-type headache. Its advantages include ease of patient access to the product, excellent side-effect profile, and low cost; the product is available as a branded form as well as a less costly generic. Excessive acetaminophen use can lead to analgesic rebound headache.

- Neuroleptics are a class of medications historically used to treat major mental health problems; this class of drugs is also known as the first-generation antipsychotics. Examples of neuroleptics are prochlorperazine (Compazine) and promethazine (Phenergan). Because of their antiemetic effect, these products are occasionally used as adjuncts in migraine therapy. Because these drugs generally are highly sedating, using them in the clinician's office can make it difficult for patients to return home. Use should be limited to 3 days a week because of the risk of extrapyramidal movements (EPMs). Other antiemetics used in migraine include ondansetron (Zofran), a nonsedating, albeit more expensive, option that is helpful if the patient needs to return quickly to work or other responsibilities. Metoclopramide (Reglan), a prokinetic agent that is generally well tolerated with infrequent use, is helpful in relieving milder GI symptoms; this drug should not be used on a daily basis because of EPM risk.

- Use of systemic corticosteroids is helpful with intractable or severe migraine and in cluster headache. Owing to the well-known adverse effects of this drug class, corticosteroid use for this purpose is not recommended more often than once a month. Examples of corticosteroid types and doses include prednisone 20 mg qid for 2 days.

- Opioids such as hydrocodone and oxycodone can provide analgesia and are often prescribed for migraine rescue. These products are sedating and potentially habituating, in addition to being substances of abuse.

Use of prophylactic therapy for migraine, tension-type, or cluster headache should be considered if abortive headache therapy is used frequently or if inadequate symptom relief is obtained from appropriate use of these therapies. The goal of headache prophylactic therapy is a minimum of a 50% reduction in number of headaches in about two-thirds of all patients, along with easier-to-control headaches that respond more rapidly to standard therapies and likely require less medication. Most agents work through blockade of the 5HT2 receptor, and 1 to 2 months of use is needed before an effect is seen. Before headache prophylaxis is initiated, headache-provoking medications, such as estrogen, progesterone, and vasodilators, must be eliminated or limited. Lifestyle modification to minimize headache risk is also critical.

Beta blockers are commonly used in migraine prevention, though the exact mechanism of how they work is not clear. It was discovered by chance that patients taking beta blockers for angina and who also experienced migraines were found to have decreased frequency of migraine attacks while taking the beta blocker. Metoprolol and propranolol have the strongest evidence demonstrating preventive effects; however, atenolol and nadolol also demonstrate some effectiveness. However, the use of acebutolol has not demonstrated any effects in migraine prevention. Although select calcium channel blockers, in particular verapamil, have been recommended in the past for headache prevention, current evidence-based guidelines do not support the use of these products for this purpose. Antiepileptic drugs (AEDs), such as divalproex sodium, sodium valproate, and topiramate, have also demonstrated effectiveness in preventing migraines. These drugs have multiple modes of action on the central nervous system that likely impact the pathophysiology of migraines. However, the AED lamotrigine is not recommended for migraine prevention as evidence indicates that this agent is ineffective. Select antidepressants, including the tricyclic antidepressants such as nortriptyline and amitriptyline, as well as the selective serotonin norepinephrine inhibitors, including venlafaxine, can also be considered for migraine prophylaxis.

Evidence supports the use of certain herbal preparations, vitamins, and minerals for the prevention of migraine headaches. The strongest evidence supports the use of petasites (butterbur) for migraine prevention, although riboflavin, magnesium, and feverfew can also be helpful. Coenzyme Q10 (CoQ10) and estrogen supplementation, in particular during the premenstrual week, can also be considered for migraine prevention, though the evidence is weaker to support their use.

Secondary headaches are caused by an underlying disease process, often with increased ICP. The headache in increased ICP is usually reported as worst on awakening, which is when brain swelling is the most severe. The pain is less intense as the day progresses and as the pressure lessens, in contrast to a tension-type headache, which usually worsens as the day goes on. Because intervention is guided by the underlying cause, establishing the appropriate diagnosis in all forms of secondary headache is critical.

DISCUSSION SOURCES

Institute for Clinical Systems Improvement (ICSI). Diagnosis and treatment of headache. Bloomington (MN): Institute for Clinical Systems Improvement (ICSI); 2011.

Robbins L. http://www.headachedrugs.com/pdf/HA-2008.pdf, Headache 2008-2009.

Silberstein SD, Holland S, Freitag F, et al. Evidence-based guideline update: Pharmacologic treatment for episodic migraine prevention in adults. Report of the Quality Standards Subcommittee of the American Academy of Neurology and the American Headache Society. *Neurology* 78:1337–1345, 2012.

Meningitis and Encephalitis

46. An 18-year-old college freshman is brought to the student health center with a chief complaint of a 3-day history of progressive headache and intermittent fever. On physical examination, he has positive Kernig and Brudzinski signs. The most likely diagnosis is:
    A. viral encephalitis.
    B. bacterial meningitis.
    C. acute subarachnoid hemorrhage.
    D. epidural hematoma.

47. Of the following, which is the least likely bacterial source to cause meningitis?
    A. colonization of the skin
    B. colonization of the nose and throat
    C. extension of acute otitis media
    D. extension of bacterial rhinosinusitis

48. Risk factors for bacterial meningitis include all of the following except:
    A. over 25 years of age.
    B. living in a community setting.
    C. cigarette smoker.
    D. use of immunosuppressant drugs.

49. The average incubation period for the organism *N. meningitidis* is:
    A. 24 hours.
    B. 3 to 4 days.
    C. 12 to 14 days.
    D. 21 days.

50. A 19-year-old college sophomore has documented meningococcal meningitis. You speak to the school health officers about the risk to the other students on campus. You inform them that:
    A. the patient does not have a contagious disease.
    B. all students are at significant risk regardless of their degree of contact with the infected person.
    C. only intimate partners are at risk.
    D. individuals with household-type or more intimate contact are considered to be at risk.

51. When evaluating the person who has bacterial meningitis, the NP expects to find cerebrospinal fluid (CSF) results of:
A. low protein.
B. predominance of lymphocytes.
C. glucose at about 30% of serum levels.
D. low opening pressure.

52. When evaluating a patient who has aseptic or viral meningitis, the NP expects to find CSF results of:
A. low protein.
B. predominance of lymphocytes.
C. glucose at about 30% of serum levels.
D. low opening pressure.

53. Which of the following describes the Kernig sign?
A. Neck pain occurs with passive flexion of one hip and knee, which causes flexion of the contralateral leg.
B. Passive neck flexion in a supine patient results in flexion of the knees and hips.
C. Elicited with the patient lying supine and the hip flexed 90 degrees, it is present when extension of the knee from this position elicits resistance or pain in the lower back or posterior thigh.
D. Headache worsens when the patient is supine.

54. Physical examination findings in papilledema include:
A. arteriovenous nicking.
B. macular hyperpigmentation.
C. optic disk bulging.
D. pupillary constriction.

55. Which of the following organisms is a gram-negative diplococcus?
A. *Streptococcus pneumoniae*
B. *Neisseria meningitidis*
C. *Staphylococcus aureus*
D. *Haemophilus influenzae*

56. Which of the following signs and symptoms most likely suggests meningitis cause by *N. meningitidis*?
A. a purpura or a petechial rash
B. absence of fever
C. development of encephalitis
D. absence of nuchal rigidity

57. All of the following persons should receive a dose of the meningococcal vaccine except:
A. a 19-year-old who received a first dose at 12 years of age.
B. a 22-year-old who has not received the vaccine and will be moving to a college dormitory.
C. a 35-year-old who will be traveling to a country where meningococcal disease is hyperendemic.
D. a 14-year-old who received a first dose at 11 years of age.

58. During an outbreak of meningococcal meningitis, all of the following can be used as chemoprophylaxis except:
A. a single dose of ceftriaxone.
B. multiple doses of rifampin.
C. multiple doses of amoxicillin.
D. a single dose of meningococcal conjugate vaccine (MCV4 or Menactra).

Answers

46. B.	51. C.	56. A.
47. A.	52. B.	57. D.
48. A.	53. C.	58. C.
49. B.	54. C.	
50. D.	55. B.	

Meningitis is an infection of the meninges, CSF, and ventricles. The disease is typically defined further by its cause, such as bacterial (pyogenic), viral (aseptic), fungal, or other cause. Encephalitis is inflammation of the brain, most commonly caused by a virus. Encephalitis can cause flu-like symptoms, such as fever or severe headache, and can also result in confusion, seizures, and sensory or motor impairment.

In bacterial meningitis, the causative pathogens differ according to patient age and certain risk characteristics. Bacterial seeding usually occurs via hematogenous spread, when organisms can enter the meninges through the bloodstream from other parts of the body; the pathogen likely was asymptomatically carried in the nose and throat. Another mechanism of acquisition is local extension from another infection, such as acute otitis media or bacterial rhinosinusitis. Congenital problems and trauma can provide a pathway via facial fractures or malformation (e.g., cleft lip or palate). Common pathogens in bacterial meningitis in adults include *Streptococcus pneumoniae* (gram-positive diplococci), *Neisseria meningitidis* (gram-negative diplococci), *Staphylococcus* species (gram-positive cocci), and *Haemophilus influenzae* type b (Hib; gram-negative coccobacilli). Vaccines against certain bacterial strains that cause meningitis have been shown to be highly effective in preventing the infection. The pneumococcal conjugate vaccine (PCV13) results in 96% effectiveness in preventing invasive disease in healthy children, whereas the pneumococcal polysaccharide vaccine (PPV23) has been shown to be 50% to 85% effective in preventing invasive disease in healthy adults by the serotypes covered in the vaccine. Both meningococcal vaccines (MCV4 and MPSV4), when given at recommended schedules, are also about 90% effective in preventing meningococcal infection caused by strains covered in the vaccine.

The issue of meningitis contagion needs to be addressed. *N. meningitidis,* an organism normally carried in about 5% to 10% of healthy adults and 60% to 80% of individuals in closed populations, such as military recruits, is transmitted through direct contact or respiratory droplets from infected people. Meningococcal disease most likely occurs within a few days of acquisition of a new strain, before the development of specific serum antibodies. Individuals acquire the infection if they are exposed to virulent bacteria and have no protective bactericidal antibodies. Smoking and concurrent upper respiratory tract viral infection diminish the integrity of the respiratory mucosa and increase the likelihood of invasive disease. Other risk factors include less than 20 years of age, living in a community setting, pregnancy (for meningitis caused by listeriosis), and having a compromised immune system. The incubation period of the organism averages 3 to 4 days (range 1 to 10 days), which is the period of communicability. Bacteria can be found for 2 to 4 days in the nose and pharynx and for up to 24 hours after starting antibiotics. Public health authorities should be contacted when a person presents with suspected or documented bacterial meningitis.

The clinical presentation of bacterial meningitis in an adult usually includes the classic triad of fever, headache, and nuchal rigidity, or stiff neck. As with most forms of infectious disease, however, atypical presentation in older adults is common. In particular, nuchal rigidity and fever are often absent. Encephalitis is more likely viral in origin and usually manifests with fewer meningeal signs. Some common viruses that cause encephalitis include herpes simplex virus, other herpesviruses (e.g., Epstein-Barr virus, varicella-zoster virus), enteroviruses, mosquito- and tick-borne viruses, the rabies virus, and childhood viruses (e.g., measles and mumps). A virus can be acquired from mosquito or tick bites that transmit the virus or through contact with a person or object contaminated with the virus. In areas known to have mosquitoes that carry encephalitis-causing viruses, it is important to take measures to prevent being bitten.

To eliminate or support the diagnosis of meningitis, lumbar puncture with CSF evaluation should be part of the evaluation of a febrile adult or child who has altered findings on neurological examination. Pleocytosis, defined as a WBC count of more than 5 cells/mm³ of CSF, is an expected finding in meningitis caused by bacterial, viral, tubercular, fungal, or protozoan infection; an elevated CSF opening pressure is also a nearly universal finding. The typical CSF response in bacterial meningitis includes a WBC median count of 1200 cells/mm³ of CSF with 90% to 95% neutrophils; additional findings are a reduced CSF glucose amount below the normal level of about 40% of the plasma level, and an elevated CSF protein level. In viral or aseptic meningitis, CSF results include normal glucose level, normal to slightly elevated protein levels, and lymphocytosis. Further testing to ascertain the causative organism is warranted. Head CT or MRI should be considered before lumbar puncture is performed.

Brudzinski and Kernig signs, suggestive of nuchal rigidity and meningeal irritation, are often positive in children 2 years or older and adults with meningitis. The Brudzinski sign is elicited when passive neck flexion in a supine patient results in flexion of the knees and hips. The Kernig sign is elicited with the patient lying supine and the hip flexed at 90 degrees.

A positive sign is present when extension of the knee from this position elicits resistance or pain in the lower back or posterior thigh. Papilledema, or optic disk bulging, or absence of venous pulsations on funduscopic examination indicates increased ICP. Less common presenting symptoms include vomiting, seizures, and altered consciousness. In meningitis caused by *N. meningitidis*, a purpura or a petechial rash is noted in about 50% of patients. Patients with viral meningitis usually have less severe symptoms that have a gradual onset; skin rash is uncommon.

For patients with suspected encephalitis, brain imaging (MRI or CT) is often the first test used. This will reveal if the symptoms are caused by swelling of the brain or a tumor. Similar to meningitis, a lumbar puncture can be used to identify the causative virus or other infectious agent. An EEG may also be used to detect abnormal patterns of electrical activity in the brain that are consistent with a diagnosis of encephalitis. In rare cases, a brain biopsy may be used for patients with worsening symptoms and/or when treatment has no effect.

Vaccination against the organism can be used for close contacts of patients with meningococcal disease resulting from A, C, Y, or W135 serogroups to prevent secondary cases. No effective vaccine exists to protect individuals from meningococcal meningitis caused by serogroup B. Widespread or universal chemoprophylaxis is not recommended during a meningococcal meningitis outbreak. Chemoprophylaxis should be considered for individuals in close contact, including household-type contact when there is a potential for sharing glassware and dishes, with patients in an endemic situation but has limited efficacy interrupting transmission during an epidemic. Options include a single dose of oral ciprofloxacin or intramuscular ceftriaxone. An alternative is four oral doses of rifampin over 2 days. Given rifampin's ability to induce cytochrome 450 isoenzymes, this medication should only be used after a complete inventory of all medications the patient could be taking has been conducted and no potential interactions identified.

Immunization against *N. meningitidis* can also be used in an outbreak; this option is helpful against current and future outbreaks. In the United States, two vaccines against the organism are available: meningococcal polysaccharide vaccine (MPSV4 or Menomune-A/C/Y/W-135) and meningococcal conjugate vaccine (MCV4 or Menactra). Both vaccines can prevent four types of meningococcal disease, including two of the three types most common in the United States (serogroup C, Y, and W-135) and a type that causes epidemics in Africa (serogroup A); protection from all possible meningococcal strains is not provided by the vaccines.

MCV4 is recommended for all children as part of routine preadolescent visit (11 to 12 years old). For children who have never received MCV4 previously, a dose is recommended for all 13- to 18-year-olds. For those 19 to 21 years of age, the vaccine is not routinely recommended but can be administered as catch-up vaccination for those who have not received a booster dose after their 16th birthday. A booster dose is recommended at age 16 for children who received the MCV4 vaccine at ages 11 to 12 years. Other individuals at increased risk for whom routine vaccination is recommended are college freshmen living in dormitories, microbiologists who are routinely exposed to meningococcal bacteria, individuals who are functionally or surgically asplenic, individuals with immune system disorder, those with HIV (if another indication for vaccination exists), people who are likely to travel to countries that have an outbreak of meningococcal disease, and people who might have been exposed to meningitis during an outbreak. MCV4 is the preferred vaccine for individuals 11 to 55 years old in these risk groups, but MPSV4 can be used if MCV4 is unavailable. MPSV4 should be used for adults age 56 years and older who are at risk.

Meningitis caused by most other agents is a result of a patient rather than contagion factor; that is, the meningitis is a result of extension of an existing illness such as bacterial sinusitis and otitis media. Treatment of a patient with meningitis includes supportive care and the use of the appropriate anti-infective agents. Empiric therapy will depend on findings from the Gram stain, culture, or other CSF testing. If gram-positive diplococci are present, treatment should consist of ceftriaxone or cefotaxime plus vancomycin plus timed dexamethasone. For gram-negative diplococci, treatment should consist of cefotaxime or ceftriaxone. If gram-positive bacilli or coccobacilli are present, then treat with ampicillin with or without gentamicin. If gram-negative bacilli are present, treat with ceftazidime or cefepime with or without gentamicin. Susceptibility results can also be used to guide appropriate treatment selection. Acyclovir is an option in aseptic meningitis, pending identification of the offending virus. Prudent clinical practice requires keeping abreast of current trends in causative pathogens and microbial resistance.

DISCUSSION SOURCES

Centers for Disease Control and Prevention. Meningococcal disease. http://www.cdc.gov/meningococcal/about/index.html

Centers for Disease Control and Prevention. Viral meningitis. http://www.cdc.gov/meningitis/viral.html

Gondim F, Singh M, Croul S. http://emedicine.medscape.com/article/1165557, eMedicine: Meningococcal meningitis

Centers for Disease Control and Prevention. Prevention and control of meningococcal disease: Recommendations of the Advisory Committee on Immunization Practices (ACIP). *MMWR* 62(RR02):1–22, 2013.

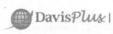
See full color images of this topic
on DavisPlus at
http://davisplus.fadavis.com |
Keyword: Fitzgerald

Multiple Sclerosis

59. The cause of multiple sclerosis is best described as:
   A. a destructive process of the nerve fiber protecting myelin.
   B. an intracranial viral infection.
   C. inflammation of the brain and/or spinal cord.
   D. an autoimmune disorder that destroys muscle fibers.

60. Common symptoms of MS include all of the following except:
   A. numbness or weakness in one or more limbs.
   B. double vision or blurring vision.
   C. facial weakness or numbness.
   D. cold sensitivity.

61. Risk factors for MS include all of the following except:
   A. older than 50 years of age.
   B. female gender.
   C. northern European ancestry.
   D. autoimmune disease.

62. The diagnosis of MS can typically involve all of the following approaches except:
   A. MRI.
   B. analysis of CSF.
   C. check for presence of Kernig sign.
   D. evoked potential test.

63. Treatment options in MS to attenuate disease progression include:
   A. interferon beta-1b.
   B. methylprednisolone.
   C. ribavirin.
   D. phenytoin.

Answers

59. A.	61. A.	63. A.
60. D.	62. C.	

Multiple sclerosis (MS), a recurrent, chronic demyelinating disorder of the central nervous system, is a disease characterized by episodes of focal neurological dysfunction, with symptoms occurring acutely, worsening over a few days, and lasting weeks, followed by a period of partial to full resolution. Symptoms of MS can vary and depend on the location of affected nerve fibers. Common symptoms include weakness or numbness of a limb, monocular visual loss, diplopia, vertigo, facial weakness or numbness, sphincter disturbances, ataxia, and nystagmus. Heat sensitivity is also common in persons with MS, with small increases in body temperature triggering or exacerbating MS symptoms. MS is usually classified into two forms: (1) relapsing, remitting MS (RRMS), in which episodes resolve with good neurological function between exacerbations and minimal to no cumulative defects, and which accounts for approximately 85% of patients with the condition; and (2) primary progressive MS, in which episodes do not fully resolve, and there are cumulative defects. Most patients with RRMS enter a stage referred to as secondary progressive MS.

MS can occur at any age but most commonly affects people between the ages of 20 and 40 years. Women are about twice as likely to develop MS compared with men. Other risk factors include family history of MS, ethnicity (highest incidence with northern European ancestry), certain viral infections (e.g., Epstein-Barr), and the presence of another autoimmune disease (e.g., thyroid disease, type 1 diabetes, or IBS).

The initial diagnosis of MS is often difficult to make because the signs of recurrent fatigue, muscle weakness, and other nonspecific signs and symptoms are often attributed to other diseases or simply to stress and fatigue. MRI can reveal demyelinating plaques, a typical finding in MS. However, these lesions can also be present with other conditions, such as lupus, migraines, or diabetes. A lumbar puncture is conducted to evaluate for abnormal findings in the CSF and can help rule out viral infections or other conditions that can cause neurological symptoms similar to MS. Characteristic CSF findings include pleocytosis with predominance of monocytes and abnormal protein levels, including a modest increase in total protein, a markedly increased gamma-globulin fraction, a high immunoglobulin G index, presence of oligoclonal bands, and an increase in myelin basic protein. Evoked potential testing can contribute to the development of the diagnosis by detecting lesions or nerve damage in the optic nerves, brainstem, or spinal cord. As with other conditions that have a complex origin and complicated course, expert consultation should be sought when diagnosing suspected MS and caring for the patient with the condition.

MS treatment generally falls into three categories: therapy for relapses, long-term disease-modifying medications, and symptomatic management. Triggers for exacerbations are varied, but often include onset of common infectious disease such as urinary tract infection; however, most exacerbations have no identifiable trigger. Treatment of exacerbations includes treatment of the underlying precipitating illness, if present, and systemic high-dose corticosteroids. Because most exacerbations improve without specific therapy, disagreement exists as to the utility of this treatment. This therapy seems to shorten the course of most exacerbations, but does not seem to have an impact on long-term disease progression. Some clinicians opt for lower-dose corticosteroid therapy with variable results.

Immunomodulatory therapy with interferon beta-1b (Betaseron, Extavia) or interferon beta-1a (Avonex, Rebif) has been shown to reduce significantly the frequency of exacerbations and long-term disability in RRMS. Immunosuppressive therapy with mitoxantrone (Novantrone) also has some utility in reducing the rate of progression. Natalizumab (Tysabri) is a monoclonal antibody with considerable clinical efficacy in treating MS, but this medication carries a warning about progressive multifocal leukoencephalopathy, a rare, destructive brain infection, associated with its use. Subcutaneous glatiramer acetate (Copaxone) may reduce the number of MS attacks by blocking the immune system's attack on myelin. Fingolimod (Gilenya) is an oral medication that traps immune cells in lymph nodes. Because of associated bradycardia with this drug, patients should have their heart rate monitored for 6 hours following the first dose. Teriflunomide (Aubagio), which inhibits the production of T- and B-cells, has been shown to reduce MS attacks and associated lesions. However, liver function must be closely monitored for patients taking this medication as it can cause serious liver damage. Symptom

management therapies are aimed at the specific needs of the individual patient and often include nondrug interventions, such as physical and occupational therapy, and management of urological problems such as altered bladder function. Expert consultation should be sought while providing care for the complex healthcare needs of patients with MS.

DISCUSSION SOURCE

Dangond, F. http://emedicine.medscape.com/article/1146199, eMedicine: Multiple sclerosis.

Parkinson Disease

64. Parkinson disease is primarily caused by:
    A. degradation of myelin surrounding nerve fibers.
    B. alteration in dopamine-containing neurons within the midbrain.
    C. deterioration of neurons in the brainstem.
    D. excessive production of acetylcholinesterase in the CSF.

65. Which of the following is most consistent with findings in patients with Parkinson disease?
    A. rigid posture with poor muscle tone
    B. masklike facies and continued cognitive function
    C. tremor at rest and bradykinesia
    D. excessive arm swinging with ambulation and flexed posture

66. The diagnosis of Parkinson disease relies on findings of:
    A. clinical evaluation of six cardinal features.
    B. head MRI or CT scan.
    C. pleocytosis in the CSF.
    D. a visual evoked potential test.

67. Dopamine or dopamine agonists used to treat Parkinson disease include all of the following except:
    A. levodopa.
    B. chlorpromazine.
    C. ropinirole.
    D. pramipexole.

68. In addition to dopamine agonists, other drug classes used to treat Parkinson disease include all of the following except:
    A. MAO B inhibitors.
    B. catechol O-methyltransferase (COMT) inhibitors.
    C. SSRIs.
    D. anticholinergics.

69. Surgical intervention such as deep brain stimulation can be helpful in the management of Parkinson disease-related symptoms:
    A. in early disease as a first-line therapy.
    B. in patients with advanced disease who have unstable medication responses.
    C. related to memory loss.
    D. only as a last resort when all other options have been exhausted.

70. Which of the following statements regarding "on" and "off" periods of Parkinson disease is false?

A. A person can move with relative ease during an "on" period.

B. An "off" period typically occurs at the C_{max} following levodopa dosing.

C. Medication adjustment can usually minimize "off" periods.

D. Surgical treatment may be needed to manage dyskinesia during "off" periods.

Answers

64. B.	67. B.	70. B.
65. C.	68. C.	
66. A.	69. B.	

Parkinson disease is a slowly progressive movement disorder that is largely caused by an alteration in dopamine-containing neurons of the pars compacta of the substantia nigra. Age at onset is usually in the sixth decade and older, but the onset can occur in much younger adults.

The diagnosis of Parkinson disease is made by clinical evaluation and consists of a combination of six cardinal features: tremor at rest, rigidity, bradykinesia (slowness in the execution of movement), flexed posture, loss of postural reflexes, and masklike facies. At least two of these, with one being tremor at rest or bradykinesia, must be present. Classically, an individual with Parkinson disease holds the arms rigidly at the sides with little movement during ambulation; forward falls are common. The parkinsonian gait usually consists of a series of rapid small steps; to turn, patients must take several small steps, moving forward and backward.

Because Parkinson disease is characterized by an alteration in the dopaminergic pathway, dopamine agonists such as ropinirole (Requip) and pramipexole (Mirapex) are usually the early disease treatment of choice, in part because of a proposed neuroprotective effect and a better adverse-effect profile than levodopa. Levodopa, a metabolic precursor of dopamine, continues to be used to minimize symptoms, but tends to be less effective with more adverse effects as the disease progresses; most patients who take levodopa for more than 5 to 10 years develop dyskinesia. Levodopa is often given with carbidopa in the fixed-dose combination known as Sinemet or Parcopa.

Amantadine (Symmetrel) is an antiviral drug with time-limited (usually less than 1 year) antiparkinsonian benefits, but it can be used in later stages of the disease to help reduce dyskinesias. Catechol O-methyltransferase (COMT) inhibitors including tolcapone (Tasmar) and entacapone (Comtan) are clinically helpful because these medications increase the half-life of levodopa by reducing its metabolism. Monoamine oxidase-B (MAO-B) inhibitors, such as selegiline (Eldepryl, Zelapar) or rasagiline (Azilect), also help increase levodopa's half-life by reducing its metabolism.

Apomorphine (Apokyn) is an injectable-only dopamine agonist that can be used in advanced Parkinson disease as a rescue therapy for the treatment of hypomobility or "off" periods. Other medications used in the treatment of Parkinson disease include anticholinergics, such as benztropine (Cogentin), to help with tremor; however, this class of drugs is well known to cause dry mouth, urinary retention, and altered mentation, particularly in older adults. In view of the complexity of prescribing Parkinson disease medications, the prescriber should be well versed in these products and seek expert consultation.

As Parkinson disease progresses, patients often develop variability in response to treatment, known as motor fluctuations, often referred to as "on" and "off" periods. During an "on" period, a person can move with relative ease. An "off" period describes times when a person has more difficulty with movement; this can be manifested either by significant difficulty in initiating movement or with uncontrolled body movements including dyskinesia. A common time for a person with Parkinson disease to experience an "off" period is toward the end of a levodopa dosing period, when the drug seems to be "wearing off." This problem can usually be managed with medication adjustment. If this approach is not helpful, surgical treatment offers another form of treatment for uncontrolled writhing movement (choreiform movement or dyskinesia) of the body or a limb.

For most people with Parkinson disease, "off" periods and dyskinesias can be managed with changes in medications. However, when medication adjustments do not improve mobility or when medications cause significant side effects, surgical treatment can be considered. Pallidotomy can be helpful in tremor, rigidity, bradykinesia, and levodopa-induced dyskinesias. Deep brain stimulation surgery for Parkinson disease is helpful in making the "off" state more like movement in the "on" state, and is helpful in the reduction of levodopa-induced dyskinesias. As with other therapies, expert consultation should be sought, and all options should be thoroughly discussed with the patient before pursuing surgical intervention.

DISCUSSION SOURCES

National Parkinson Foundation. http://www.parkinson.org/NET-COMMUNITY/Page.aspx?pid=226&srcid=216, Parkinson primer

Jankovic J, Poewe W. Therapies in Parkinson's disease. *Curr Opin Neurol* 25:433–447, 2012.

Seizure Disorders

71. Which of the following best describes patient presentation during an absence (petit mal) seizure?

A. blank staring lasting 3 to 50 seconds, accompanied by impaired level of consciousness

B. awake state with abnormal motor behavior lasting seconds

C. rigid extension of arms and legs, followed by sudden jerking movements with loss of consciousness

D. abrupt muscle contraction with autonomic signs

72. Which of the following best describes patient presentation during a simple partial seizure?
   A. blank staring lasting 3 to 50 seconds, accompanied by impaired level of consciousness
   B. awake state with abnormal motor behavior lasting seconds
   C. rigid extension of arms and legs, followed by sudden jerking movements with loss of consciousness
   D. abrupt muscle contraction with autonomic signs

73. Which of the following best describes patient presentation during a tonic-clonic (grand mal) seizure?
   A. blank staring lasting 3 to 50 seconds, accompanied by impaired level of consciousness
   B. awake state with abnormal motor behavior lasting seconds
   C. rigid extension of arms and legs, followed by sudden jerking movements with loss of consciousness
   D. abrupt muscle contraction with autonomic signs

74. Which of the following best describes patient presentation during a myoclonic seizure?
   A. blank staring lasting 3 to 50 seconds, accompanied by impaired level of consciousness
   B. awake state with abnormal motor behavior lasting seconds
   C. rigid extension of arms and legs, followed by sudden jerking movements with loss of consciousness
   D. brief, jerking contractions of arms, legs, trunk, or all of these

75. Treatment options for an adult with seizures include all of the following agents except:
   A. carbamazepine.
   B. phenytoin.
   C. gabapentin.
   D. tamsulosin.

76. Medications with narrow therapeutic indexes (NTIs) include all of the following except:
   A. topiramate.
   B. phenytoin.
   C. carbamazepine.
   D. valproate.

77. Which of the following statements about potential drug interactions with phenytoin is false?
   A. Phenytoin increases theophylline clearance by increasing cytochrome P-450 (CYP 450) enzyme activity.
   B. When taken with other highly protein-bound drugs, the free phenytoin concentration can increase to toxic levels.
   C. Phenytoin can increase the metabolic capacity of hepatic enzymes, thus leading to reduced drug levels.
   D. When phenytoin and theophylline are given together, the result is a higher concentration of both drugs than when given separately.

78. A patient taking phenytoin can exhibit a drug interaction when concurrently taking:
   A. cyclosporine.
   B. famotidine.
   C. acetaminophen.
   D. aspirin.

Answers

71. A.	**74.** D.	**77.** D.
72. B.	**75.** D.	**78.** A.
73. C.	**76.** A.	

The type of seizure directs the treatment of a seizure disorder. Knowledge of the presentation of common forms of seizures is critical (Table 2–8).

Numerous seizure therapies, including standard or older products such as phenytoin, carbamazepine, clonazepam, ethosuximide, and valproic acid, and more recently developed antiepileptic drugs (AEDs), such as gabapentin, lamotrigine, and topiramate, are now available. Expert knowledge of the indications and adverse reactions of these medications is needed before AED therapy is initiated or continued.

Certain AEDs, including phenytoin and carbamazepine, are narrow therapeutic index (NTI) drugs. A certain amount of such drugs is therapeutic, and just slightly more than this amount is potentially toxic. Conversely, a slightly lower dose might not be therapeutic. Other NTI drugs include warfarin, theophylline, and digoxin. Many of these drugs have high levels of protein binding and significant use of hepatic enzymatic pathways for drug metabolism, such as CYP 450. Phenytoin is highly protein bound (greater than 90%); when taken with other highly protein-bound drugs, it can potentially be displaced from its protein-binding site, leading to increased free phenytoin and a risk of toxicity. Carbamazepine and phenytoin can increase the metabolic capacity of hepatic enzymes, which leads to more rapid metabolism of the drug and reduced levels of this and other drugs. Phenytoin use increases theophylline clearance by increasing CYP 450 enzyme activity. Concomitant use of theophylline and phenytoin can lead to altered phenytoin pharmacokinetics. The net result is that when phenytoin and theophylline are given together, levels of both drugs can decrease by 40%. When taken with birth control pills, carbamazepine induces estrogen metabolism, potentially leading to contraceptive failure. The prescriber should be familiar with the drug interactions of all AEDs and monitor therapeutic levels and for adverse reactions.

DISCUSSION SOURCES

Indiana University School of Medicine Division of Clinical Pharmacology. http://medicine.iupui.edu/clinpharm/ddis/clinical-table/, P450 drug interaction table: Abbreviated clinically relevant table.

Jankovic SM, Dostic M. Choice of antiepileptic drugs for the elderly: Possible drug interactions and adverse effects. *Expert Opin Drug Metab Toxicol* 8:81–91, 2012.

TABLE 2-8

Description of Common Seizure Disorders

Seizure Type	Description of Seizure	Comments
Absence (petit mal)	Blank staring lasting 3–50 seconds accompanied by impaired level of consciousness	Usual age of onset 3–15 years
Myoclonic	Awake state or momentary loss of consciousness with abnormal motor behavior lasting seconds to minutes; one or more muscle groups causing brief jerking contractions of the limbs and trunk, occasionally flinging patient	Difficult to control; at least half also have tonic-clonic seizures. Usual age of onset 2–7 years
Tonic-clonic (grand mal)	Rigid extension of arms and legs followed by sudden jerking movements with loss of consciousness; bowel and bladder incontinence common with postictal confusion	Onset at any age; in adults, new onset may be found in brain tumor, post-head injury, alcohol withdrawal
Simple partial or focal seizure (jacksonian)	Awake state with abnormal motor, sensory, autonomic, or psychic behavior; movement can affect any part of body, localized or generalized	Typical age of onset 3–15 years
Complex partial	Aura characterized by unusual sense of smell or taste, visual or auditory hallucinations, stomach upset; followed by vague stare and facial movements, muscle contraction and relaxation, and autonomic signs; can progress to loss of consciousness	Onset at any age

Source: Epilepsy Foundation: http://www.epilepsyfoundation.org/about/types/types/index.cfm, Seizures and syndromes

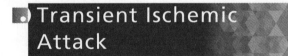

Transient Ischemic Attack

79. Risk factors for transient ischemic attack (TIA) include all of the following except:
A. atrial fibrillation.
B. carotid artery disease.
C. combined oral contraceptive use.
D. pernicious anemia.

80. A TIA is characterized as an episode of reversible neurological symptoms that can last:
A. 1 hour.
B. 6 hours.
C. 12 hours.
D. 24 hours.

81. When caring for a patient with a recent TIA, you consider that:
A. long-term antiplatelet therapy is likely indicated.
B. this person has a relatively low risk of future stroke.
C. women present with this disorder more often than men.
D. rehabilitation will be needed to minimize the effects of the resulting neurological insult.

82 to 84. Rank the following causes of stroke from the most common (1) to least common (3):
82. Cerebral hemorrhage
83. Cerebral ischemia
84. Subarachnoid hemorrhage

85. Antiplatelet agents commonly used in secondary prevention of stroke include all of the following except:
A. aspirin.
B. clopidogrel.
C. aspirin plus extended-release dipyridamole.
D. rivaroxaban.

86. Which of the following conditions is least likely to contribute to an increased risk of stroke?
A. hyperlipidemia
B. diabetes mellitus
C. Crohn's disease
D. hypertension

87 to 93. When considering the diagnosis of acute stroke, which of the following can be part of the presentation? (Answer yes or no.)

_____ **87.** partial loss of visual field

_____ **88.** unilateral hearing loss

_____ **89.** facial muscle paralysis

_____ **90.** vertigo

_____ **91.** diplopia

_____ **92.** headache

_____ **93.** ataxia

94. Acute cerebral hemorrhage is best identified with which of the following imaging techniques?
A. transesophageal echocardiogram
B. CT scan
C. cerebral angiogram
D. MR angiography

Answers

79.	D.	**85.**	D.	**91.**	Yes
80.	D.	**86.**	C.	**92.**	Yes
81.	A.	**87.**	Yes	**93.**	Yes
82.	2	**88.**	Yes	**94.**	B.
83.	1	**89.**	Yes		
84.	3	**90.**	Yes		

A TIA is an acute neurological event in which all signs and symptoms, including numbness, weakness, and flaccidity, and visual changes, ataxia, or dysarthria, resolve usually within minutes, but certainly by 24 hours after onset. If changes persist beyond 24 hours, the diagnosis of stroke should be considered. TIA should be considered a "stroke warning." Risk factors include carotid artery and other forms of atherosclerosis; structural cardiac problems, such as valvular problems that lead to increased risk of embolization; and hypercoagulable conditions, such as antiphospholipid antibody and combined oral contraceptive use. Intervention includes minimizing risk factors through lifestyle modification (e.g., smoking cessation; diet; exercise; cardiovascular and cerebrovascular disease risk reduction such as aggressive treatment of dyslipidemia, hypertension, and diabetes mellitus) and long-term antiplatelet therapy. Aspirin is the least expensive option for antiplatelet therapy and is associated with the fewest adverse effects. Clopidogrel (Plavix) or aspirin plus extended-release dipyridamole (Aggrenox) can be used as alternatives to aspirin.

Acute stroke is often thought of as manifesting with sudden-onset unilateral limb weakness and motor dysfunction. Although these findings are often part of the clinical presentation, other findings, such as changes in hearing and vision, seizure, and head and neck pain, are often noted (Table 2–9).

TABLE 2-9
Acute Stroke Presentation

Sign/Symptom	Clinical Presentation
Alteration in consciousness	Stupor Confusion Agitation Memory loss Delirium Seizures Coma
Headache	Intense or unusually severe, often with sudden onset, usually described as having different characteristics compared with patient's typical primary headache Altered level of consciousness or neurological deficit Unusual or severe neck or facial pain
Aphasia Facial weakness or asymmetry	Paralysis of facial muscles (e.g., when patient speaks or smiles) May be on same side (ipsilateral) or opposite side (contralateral) to limb paralysis
Altered coordination	Incoordination, weakness, paralysis, or sensory loss of one or more limbs (usually one half of the body and in particular the hand) Ataxia (poor balance, clumsiness, or difficulty walking)
Visual loss	Monocular or binocular Report of partial loss of the field
Miscellaneous	Vertigo Diplopia Unilateral hearing loss Nausea, vomiting Photophobia Phonophobia

Source: Internet Stroke Center: http://www.strokecenter.org/education/ais_evaluation/lt_rt_hemisphere.htm, Emergency stroke evaluation and diagnosis

About 80% of strokes are due to cerebral ischemia, about 15% are due to cerebral hemorrhage, and 5% are due to subarachnoid hemorrhage; in younger adults, carotid artery dissection can cause stroke, accounting for about 5% of all strokes. Acute stroke should be thought of as a "brain attack," in which a portion of the brain is acutely ischemic, a potentially reversible condition if blood flow is reestablished. If blood flow is not restored, the ischemic tissue will be compromised, and the ischemia evolves into a cerebral infarction, often with devastating long-term consequences. If acute stroke is suspected, the patient must undergo emergency neuroimaging and be evaluated for thrombolytic or revascularization therapy in the appropriate healthcare setting.

When utilizing neuroimaging for stroke, a head CT scan is helpful in identifying acute cerebral hemorrhage, whereas MRI is a more sensitive test in the acute phase of ischemic stroke. CT or MR angiography is helpful in showing stenosis or occlusion in the brain-supplying vessels. Carotid ultrasound, echocardiogram, and cerebral angiogram can help to identify or rule out concomitant and contributing conditions as well as identify the possible source of the blood clot. An echocardiogram can be used to find the source of clots in the heart that may have traveled to the brain to cause a stroke. A transesophageal echocardiogram can be used to obtain clear, detailed ultrasound images of the heart and any blood clots that are present.

Because atherosclerosis is a major contributor to stroke risk, prevention of the condition should be aimed at reducing atherosclerotic risk through control of hypertension, dyslipidemia, and diabetes mellitus. Patients with a history of TIA or ischemia are also at high risk for another cerebrovascular event, myocardial infarction, and sudden cardiac death, and benefit from aggressive measures to reduce atherosclerotic risk. Secondary prevention against ischemic stroke and TIA should include antiplatelet therapy with aspirin or aspirin with extended-release dipyridamole (Aggrenox); if these options are not tolerated or in the presence of peripheral arterial or multivessel atherosclerotic disease, clopidogrel (Plavix) should be prescribed. These agents inhibit platelet activation through different mechanisms of action. When TIA or stroke originates from cardiac embolus, oral anticoagulation (warfarin) therapy, with a goal international normalized ratio of 2.0 to 3.0, should be provided.

For those with hypertension, appropriate antihypertensive medications should be initiated to try to get the patient to goal. For adults older than age 60 year, the general recommended blood pressure goal is less than 150/90 mmHg. Agents commonly used to decrease blood pressure include thiazide diuretics (e.g. hydrochlorothiazide [HCTZ]), beta blockers, calcium antagonists, ACE inhibitors, and angiotensin receptor blockers (ARBs). Combination therapy that uses lower doses of medications can provide enhanced efficacy with decreased frequency of adverse effects.

DISCUSSION SOURCES

Cruz-Flores, S. http://emedicine.medscape.com/article/1160021-overview#aw2aab6b3, eMedicine: Stroke anticoagulation and prophylaxis

Internet Stroke Center. http://www.strokecenter.org/education/ais_evaluation/lt_rt_hemisphere.htm, Emergency stroke evaluation and diagnosis

Giant Cell Arteritis

95. Risk factors for giant cell arteritis include all of the following except:
    A. older age.
    B. female gender.
    C. osteoarthritis.
    D. Northern European descent.

96. Which of the following statements is false regarding giant cell arteritis?
    A. results in inflammation of temporal and other arteries
    B. normal sections of arteries can be found in between affected sections
    C. primarily impacts smaller-sized vessels
    D. results in a tender or nodular, pulseless vessel

97. Mrs. Lewis is a 74-year-old woman with well-controlled hypertension. She is taking hydrochlorothiazide and presents with a 3-day history of unilateral throbbing headache with difficulty chewing because of pain. On physical examination, you find a tender, noncompressible temporal artery. Blood pressure (BP) is 160/88 mm Hg, apical pulse is 98 bpm, and respiratory rate is 22/min; the patient is visibly uncomfortable. The optimal technique to confirm a diagnosis of giant cell arteritis is:
    A. check serum ALT/AST levels.
    B. biopsy of temporal artery.
    C. CT scan of the head.
    D. transesophageal echocardiogram.

98. Therapeutic interventions for Mrs. Lewis should include:
    A. systemic corticosteroid therapy.
    B. addition of an angiotensin-converting enzyme inhibitor (ACEI) to her antihypertensive regimen.
    C. warfarin therapy.
    D. initiation of topiramate (Topamax) therapy.

99. Headache associated with giant cell arteritis is least likely to occur in the:
    A. frontal area.
    B. temporal area.
    C. vertex.
    D. occipital area.

100. For a patient receiving standard therapy for giant cell arteritis, the use of all of the following concomitant therapies should be considered except:
    A. aspirin.
    B. nitrate.
    C. bisphosphonate and calcium/vitamin D.
    D. proton-pump inhibitor.

101. Concomitant disease seen with giant cell arteritis includes:
    A. polymyalgia rheumatica.
    B. acute pancreatitis.
    C. psoriatic arthritis.
    D. reactive arthritis.

102. One of the most serious complications of giant cell arteritis is:

A. hemiparesis.
B. arthritis.
C. blindness.
D. uveitis.

Answers

95. C.	**98.** A.	**101.** A.
96. C.	**99.** B.	**102.** C.
97. B.	**100.** B.	

See full color images of this topic on DavisPlus at
http://davisplus.fadavis.com |
Keyword: Fitzgerald

Giant cell or temporal arteritis is an autoimmune vasculitis that is most common in patients 50 to 85 years old; average age at onset is 70 years. A systemic disease affecting medium-sized and large-sized vessels, giant cell arteritis also causes inflammation of the temporal artery. Inflammation and swelling of the arteries causes decreased blood flow and its associated symptoms. The swelling normally affects just part of an artery with sections of normal artery in between. Extracranial branches of the carotid artery are often involved; this often results in a tender or nodular, pulseless vessel, usually the temporal artery, accompanied by a severe unilateral headache. On examination, the temporal artery is occasionally normal, however. Giant cell arteritis and polymyalgia rheumatica are thought to represent two parts of a spectrum of disease and are often found together. Other risk factors for giant cell arteritis include female gender and Northern European descent, particularly people of Scandinavian origin.

In an older adult, these clinical syndromes are often accompanied by respiratory tract symptoms (cough, sore throat, hoarseness) or mental status changes, rather than by the classically reported findings of headache, jaw claudication, and acute reduction or change in vision. The headache that is usually part of the presentation is occasionally reported as being located in the frontal, vertex, or occipital area, rather than in the temporal area.

Apart from relieving pain, treatment of giant cell arteritis helps minimize the risk of blindness, which is one of the most serious complications of the disease. Approximately 50% of patients with giant cell arteritis experience visual symptoms, including transient visual blurring, diplopia, eye pain, or sudden loss of vision; transient repeated episodes of blurred vision are usually reversible, but sudden loss of vision is an ominous sign and is almost always permanent. As soon as the diagnosis is made, high-dose systemic corticosteroid therapy should be initiated; this therapy typically involves prednisone, 1 to 2 mg/kg per day, until the disease appears to be under control, followed by a careful dose reduction until the lowest dose that can maintain clinical response can be determined. This dose is continued for 6 months to 2 years. When symptoms have been stable, and the corticosteroid therapy is going to be discontinued, a slow taper with close monitoring is warranted because of the risk of adrenal suppression and disease resurgence. Gastrointestinal cytoprotection with misoprostol or a proton pump inhibitor and bone protection with a bisphosphonate plus calcium/vitamin D supplement should also be provided to minimize these corticosteroid-related adverse effects. Aspirin can also be considered to reduce the risk of stroke. Corticosteroid-sparing agents, such as methotrexate, azathioprine, cyclophosphamide, and cyclosporine, can be helpful in reducing adverse effects associated with long-term steroid therapy. However, data are lacking on the effectiveness of these agents in treating giant cell arteritis.

Diagnosis of giant cell arteritis should include a confirmatory arterial biopsy. Color duplex ultrasonography of the temporal arteries has been used as an alternative or complement to superficial temporal artery biopsy. Because the disease frequently skips portions of the vessel, biopsy specimens of multiple vessel sites should be obtained. C-reactive protein (CRP) and erythrocyte sedimentation rate (ESR), although nonspecific tests of inflammation, are usually markedly elevated.

DISCUSSION SOURCES

Roque M. http://www.emedicine.com/OPH/topic254.htm, eMedicine: Giant cell arteritis

Barraclough K, Mallen CD, Helliwell T, et al. Diagnosis and management of giant cell arteritis. *Br J Gen Pract* 62:329–30, 2012.

Charlton R. Optimal management of giant cell arteritis and polymyalgia rheumatic. *Ther Clin Risk Manag* 8:173–179, 2012.

Skin Disorders

3

Skin Lesions

1 to 12. Match the following descriptions to the correct lesion or distribution name.

_____ **1.** multiple lesions blending together

_____ **2.** flat discoloration less than 1 cm in diameter

_____ **3.** circumscribed area of skin edema

_____ **4.** narrow linear crack into epidermis, exposing dermis

_____ **5.** vesicle-like lesion with purulent content

_____ **6.** flat discoloration greater than 1 cm in diameter

_____ **7.** raised lesion, larger than 1 cm, may be same or different color from the surrounding skin

_____ **8.** netlike cluster

_____ **9.** loss of epidermis and dermis

_____ **10.** loss of skin markings and full skin thickness

_____ **11.** skin thickening usually found over pruritic or friction areas

_____ **12.** in a ring formation

A. ulcer
B. atrophy
C. fissure
D. reticular
E. wheal
F. pustule
G. patch
H. plaque
I. macule
J. confluent or coalescent
K. annular
L. lichenification

Answers

1. J. confluent or coalescent
2. I. macule
3. E. wheal
4. C. fissure
5. F. pustule
6. G. patch
7. H. plaque
8. D. reticular
9. A. ulcer
10. B. atrophy
11. L. lichenification
12. K. annular

Identification of common dermatologic lesions is important to safe clinical practice (Table 3–1).

TABLE 3-1
Skin Lesions

Lesion	Description	Example
COMMON PRIMARY SKIN LESIONS		
Macule	Flat discoloration, usually <1 cm in diameter	Freckle
Patch	Flat area of skin discoloration, larger than a macule	Vitiligo
Papule	Raised lesion, <1 cm, may be same or different color than the surrounding skin	Raised nevus
Vesicle	Fluid-filled, <1 cm	Varicella
Plaque	Raised lesion, ≥ 1 cm, may be same or different color than surrounding skin	Psoriasis
Purpura	Lesions caused by red blood cells leaving circulation and becoming trapped in skin	Petechiae, ecchymosis
Pustule	Vesicle-like lesion with purulent content	Impetigo, acne
Wheal	Circumscribed area of skin edema	Hive
Nodule	Raised lesion, ≥1 cm, usually mobile	Epidermal cyst
Bullae	Fluid-filled, ≥1 cm	Blister with second-degree burn
COMMON SECONDARY SKIN LESIONS		
Excoriation	Marks produced by scratching	Seen in areas of pruritic skin diseases
Lichenification	Skin thickening resembling callus formation	Seen in areas of recurrent scratching
Fissure	Narrow linear crack into epidermis, exposing dermis	Split lip, athlete's foot
Erosion	Partial focal loss of epidermis; heals without scarring	Area exposed after bullous lesion opens
Ulcer	Loss of epidermis and dermis; heals with scarring	Pressure sore
Scale	Raised, flaking lesion	Dandruff, psoriasis
Atrophy	Loss of skin markings and full skin thickness	Area treated excessively with higher potency corticosteroids
TERMS DESCRIBING PATTERNS OF SKIN LESIONS		
Annular	In a ring	Erythema migrans in Lyme disease
Confluent or coalescent	Multiple lesions blending together	Multiple skin conditions
Reticular	Netlike cluster	Multiple skin conditions
Dermatomal	Along a neurocutaneous dermatome	Herpes zoster
Linear	In streaks	Poison ivy

Source: James, WD, Berger TG, Elston, DM. *Andrews' Diseases of the Skin: Clinical Dermatology*, ed. 11. Philadelphia: Saunders, 2011, pp. 8, 1–11.

DISCUSSION SOURCES

James WD, Berger TG, Elston DM. *Andrews' Diseases of the Skin: Clinical Dermatology*, ed. 11. Philadelphia: Saunders, 2011, pp. 12–17.

Czerkasij, V. A strategy for learning dermatology. *J Nurse Pract* 6: 555–556, 2010. http://www.dermatologylexicon.org

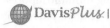 See full color images of this topic on DavisPlus at **http://davisplus.fadavis.com | Keyword: Fitzgerald**

Topical Medication Dispensing

13. How many grams of a topical cream or ointment are needed for a single application to the hands?
    A. 1
    B. 2
    C. 3
    D. 4

14. How many grams of a topical cream or ointment are needed for a single application to an arm?
    A. 1
    B. 2
    C. 3
    D. 4

15. How many grams of a topical cream or ointment are needed for a single application to the entire body?
    A. 10 to 30
    B. 30 to 60
    C. 60 to 90
    D. 90 to 120

Answers

13. B.   **14. C.**   **15. B.**

Knowledge of the amount of a cream or ointment needed to treat a dermatologic condition is an important part of the prescriptive practice (Table 3–2). Clinicians often write prescriptions for an inadequate amount of a topical medication with insufficient numbers of refills, possibly creating a situation in which treatment fails because of an inadequate length of therapy.

DISCUSSION SOURCE

Habif TP, Campbell JL, Chapman SM, et al. *Skin Disease: Diagnosis and Treatment*, ed. 3. Philadelphia: Elsevier Saunders; 2011.

Topical Medication Absorption

16. You write a prescription for a topical agent and anticipate the greatest rate of absorption when it is applied to the:
    A. palms of the hands.
    B. soles of the feet.
    C. face.
    D. abdomen.

17. You prescribe a topical medication and want it to have maximum absorption, so you choose the following vehicle:
    A. gel
    B. lotion
    C. cream
    D. ointment

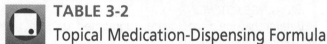

TABLE 3-2
Topical Medication-Dispensing Formula

	Amount Needed for One Application	Amount Needed in Twice-a-Day Application for 1 Week	Amount Needed in Twice-a-Day Application for 1 Month
Hands, head, face, anogenital region	2 g	28 g	120 g (4 oz)
One arm, anterior or posterior trunk	3 g	42 g	180 g (6 oz)
One leg	6 g	84 g	320 g (12 oz)
Entire body	30–60 g	420–840 g (14–28 oz)	1.8–3.6 kg (60–120 oz or 3.75–7.5 lb)

Source: Habif TP, Campbell JL, Chapman SM et al. *Skin Disease: Diagnosis and Treatment*, ed. 3. Philadelphia: Saunders, 2011, pp. 6, 644–645.

Answers

16. C.   **17.** D.

The safe prescription of a topical agent for patients with dermatologic disorders requires knowledge of the best vehicle for the medication. Certain parts of the body, notably the face, axillae, and genital area, are quite permeable, allowing greater absorption of medication than less permeable areas, such as the extremities and trunk. In particular, the thickness of the palms of the hands and soles of the feet creates a barrier so that relatively little topical medication is absorbed when applied to these sites. Cutaneous drug absorption is typically inversely proportional to the thickness of the stratum corneum. Hydrocortisone absorption from the forearm is less than one-third of the amount that is absorbed from the forehead.

In general, the less viscous the vehicle containing a topical medication, the less of the medication is absorbed. As a result, medication contained in a gel or lotion is absorbed in smaller amounts than medication contained in a cream or ointment. Besides enhancing absorption of the therapeutic agent, creams and ointments provide lubrication to the region, often a desirable effect in the presence of xerosis or lichenification.

DISCUSSION SOURCE

Robertson D. Mailbach H. Dermatologic pharmacology. In: Katzung, B (ed). *Katsung's Basic and Clinical Pharmacology*. ed. 12. New York: McGraw-Hill Medical; 2012, pp. 991–1008.

Topical Corticosteroids

18. One of the mechanisms of action of a topical corticosteroid preparation is as:
A. an antimitotic.
B. an exfoliant.
C. a vasoconstrictor.
D. a humectant.

19. To enhance the potency of a topical corticosteroid, the prescriber recommends that the patient apply the preparation:
A. to dry skin by gentle rubbing.
B. and cover with an occlusive dressing.
C. before bathing.
D. with an emollient.

20. Which of the following is the least potent topical corticosteroid?
A. betamethasone dipropionate 0.1% (Diprosone)
B. clobetasol propionate 0.05% (Cormax)
C. hydrocortisone 2.5%
D. fluocinonide 0.05% (Lidex)

Answers

18. C.   **19.** B.   **20.** C.

Corticosteroids are a class of drugs often used to treat inflammatory and allergic dermatologic disorders. Although corticosteroids reduce inflammatory and allergic reactions through numerous mechanisms (including immunosuppressive and inflammatory properties), their relative potency is based on vasoconstrictive activity; that is, the most potent topical steroids, such as betamethasone (class 1), have significantly greater vasoconstricting action than the least potent agents, such as hydrocortisone (class 7) (Table 3–3).

DISCUSSION SOURCES

James, WD, Berger TG, Elston DM. *Andrews' Diseases of the Skin: Clinical Dermatology*, ed. 11. Philadelphia: Saunders, 2011, pp. 136–137.

Robertson D, Mailbach H. Dermatologic pharmacology. In: Katzung B (ed). *Katzung's Basic and Clinical Pharmacology*, ed 12. New York: McGraw-Hill Medical, 2012, pp. 991–1008.

Stringer J. Adrenocortical hormones. In: Stringer J (ed). *Basic Concepts in Pharmacology*, ed 4. New York: McGraw-Hill Medical, 2011, pp. 185–188.

TABLE 3-3
Examples of Topical Corticosteroid Potency

LOW POTENCY
Hydrocortisone (0.5%, 1%, 2.5%)
Fluocinolone acetonide 0.01% (Synalar)
Triamcinolone acetonide 0.025% (Aristocort)
Fluocinolone acetonide 0.025% (Synalar)
Hydrocortisone butyrate 0.1%
Hydrocortisone valerate 0.2% (Westcort)
Triamcinolone acetonide 0.1%

MIDRANGE POTENCY
Betamethasone dipropionate, augmented, 0.05% (Diprolene AF cream)
Mometasone furoate 0.1% (Elocon ointment)

HIGH POTENCY
Fluocinolone acetonide 0.2% (Synalar-HP)
Desoximetasone 0.25% (Topicort)
Fluocinonide 0.05% (Lidex)

SUPER-HIGH POTENCY
Betamethasone dipropionate, augmented, 0.05% (Diprolene gel, ointment)
Clobetasol propionate 0.05% (Temovate)
Halobetasol propionate 0.05% (Ultravate 0.05%)

Source: Benson HA, Watkinson AC. *Topical and Transdermal Drug Delivery: Principles and Practice.* Hoboken, NJ: John Wiley & Sons, 2012, pp. 357–366.

Antihistamine

21. Antihistamines exhibit therapeutic effect by:
    A. inactivating circulating histamine.
    B. preventing the production of histamine.
    C. blocking activity at histamine receptor sites.
    D. acting as a procholinergic agent.

22. A possible adverse effect with the use of a first-generation antihistamine such as diphenhydramine in an 80-year-old man is:
    A. urinary retention.
    B. hypertension.
    C. tachycardia.
    D. urticaria.

23. Which of the following medications is likely to cause the most sedation?
    A. chlorpheniramine
    B. cetirizine
    C. fexofenadine
    D. loratadine

Answers

21. C.   **22. A.**   **23. A.**

Antihistamines prevent action of formed histamine, a potent inflammatory mediator, and can be used to control acute symptoms of itchiness and allergy. All antihistamines work by blocking histamine-1 (H_1) receptor sites, preventing the action of histamine.

Systemic antihistamines are usually divided into two groups: standard or first-generation products, such as diphenhydramine (Benadryl) or chlorpheniramine (Chlor-Trimeton), and newer or second-generation products, such as loratadine (Claritin), desloratadine (Clarinex), cetirizine (Zyrtec), fexofenadine (Allegra), and levocetirizine (Xyzal). The first-generation antihistamines readily cross the blood-brain barrier, causing sedation; as a result, these medications should be used with appropriate caution and should not be taken during activities when risk of accident or injury is significant. Their anticholinergic activity can result in drying of secretions, visual changes, and urinary retention; the last mentioned is most often a problem for older men with benign prostatic hyperplasia. The use of first-generation antihistamines by older adults, particularly in higher doses as a sleep aid, can result in negative cognitive effects. The second-generation antihistamines do not easily cross the blood-brain barrier, which results in lower rates of sedation. With little anticholinergic effect, the use of a product such as loratadine is likely to provide less drying of nasal secretions compared with diphenhydramine use, but also will have less negative effect on cognition, particularly in older adults.

DISCUSSION SOURCE

Robertson D, Mailbach H. Dermatologic pharmacology. In: Katzung B (ed), *Katzung's Basic and Clinical Pharmacology*, ed. 12. New York: McGraw-Hill Medical; 2012, pp. 991–1008.

Impetigo

24. Clinical features of bullous impetigo include:
    A. intense itch.
    B. vesicular lesions.
    C. dermatomal pattern.
    D. systemic symptoms such as fever and chills.

25. The likely causative organisms of nonbullous impetigo in a 6-year-old child include:
    A. *H. influenzae* and *S. pneumoniae*.
    B. group A streptococcus and *S. aureus*.
    C. *M. catarrhalis* and select viruses.
    D. *P. aeruginosa* and select fungi.

26. The spectrum of antimicrobial activity of mupirocin (Bactroban) includes:
    A. primarily gram-negative organisms.
    B. select gram-positive organisms.
    C. *Pseudomonas* species and anaerobic organisms.
    D. only organisms that do not produce beta-lactamase.

27. An impetigo lesion that becomes deeply ulcerated is known as:
    A. cellulitis.
    B. erythema.
    C. ecthyma.
    D. empyema.

28. First-line treatment of impetigo with less than 5 lesions of 1-2 centimeters in diameter on the legs in a 9-year-old girl is:
    A. topical mupirocin.
    B. topical neomycin.
    C. oral cefixime.
    D. oral doxycycline.

29. An oral antimicrobial option for the treatment of methicillin-sensitive *S. aureus* includes all of the following except:
    A. amoxicillin.
    B. dicloxacillin.
    C. cephalexin.
    D. cefadroxil.

30. Which of the following is an oral antimicrobial option for the treatment of a community-acquired methicillin-resistant *S. aureus* cutaneous infection?
    A. amoxicillin
    B. dicloxacillin
    C. cephalexin
    D. trimethoprim-sulfamethoxazole

31. You see a kindergartner with impetigo and advise that she can return _____ hours after initiating effective antimicrobial therapy.
A. 24
B. 48
C. 72
D. 96

Answers

24. B.	**27.** C.	**30.** D.
25. B.	**28.** A.	**31.** A.
26. B.	**29.** A.	

Impetigo is a contagious skin infection that usually consists of discrete purulent lesions. Although most common among children in tropical or subtropical regions, the prevalence increases in northern climates during the summer months. Its peak incidence is among children 2 to 5 years old, although older children and adults can also be affected. There is no sex or racial predilection for the condition. Impetigo skin lesions are nearly always caused by the gram-positive organisms group A streptococci, *Staphylococcus aureus,* or a mix of both.

Impetigo usually occurs on exposed areas of the body; the infection most frequently affects the face and extremities. The lesions remain well localized but are frequently multiple and can be either bullous or nonbullous. Bullous impetigo is usually caused by strains of *S. aureus* that produce a toxin causing cleavage in the superficial skin layer, with the causative pathogens usually present in the nose before the outbreak of the cutaneous disease. The bullous lesions usually appear initially as superficial vesicles that rapidly enlarge to form a bulla or blister that is often filled with a dark or purulent liquid and can take on a pustular appearance. The lesion ruptures, and a thin, lacquer-like crust typically forms quickly. The pattern of the lesion often reflects autoinoculation with the offending organism.

The lesions of nonbullous impetigo usually begin as papules that rapidly evolve into vesicles surrounded by an area of erythema. The pustules increase in size, breaking down in the next 4 to 6 days, forming characteristic thick crusts. About 70% of patients with impetigo have nonbullous lesions. In either form, the lesions heal slowly and leave depigmented areas.

Until more recently, nonbullous impetigo was usually caused by *Streptococcus* species. Now, most cases are caused by staphylococci alone or in combination with streptococci. Streptococci isolated from lesions are primarily group A organisms, but occasionally other serogroups (e.g., groups C and G) are responsible. Prospective studies of streptococcal impetigo have shown that the responsible microorganisms initially colonize the unbroken skin. As a result, personal hygiene has an influence on disease incidence in that colonization with a given streptococcal strain precedes the development of impetigo lesions by a mean duration of 10 days; inoculation of surface organisms into the skin by abrasions, minor trauma, or insect bites then ensues. Streptococcal strains can be transferred from the skin or impetigo lesions to the upper respiratory tract.

Rarely, an impetigo lesion can become deeply ulcerated, known as ecthyma. Although regional lymphadenitis occurs, systemic symptoms are usually absent.

When impetigo results in a few lesions, topical therapy is indicated with mupirocin (Bactroban or Centany) as the preferred agent. Mupirocin use is associated with higher cure rates compared with oral erythromycin, and both are noted to be superior to penicillin. Retapamulin (Altabax) ointment is also an effective, albeit more expensive, therapeutic option. Bacitracin and neomycin are less effective topical treatments; use of these products is not recommended for the treatment of impetigo.

Patients who have numerous lesions or who are not responding to topical agents should receive oral antimicrobials effective against *S. aureus* and *Streptococcus pyogenes.* In the past, penicillin was a common choice that was clinically effective because most cases were caused by *Streptococcus* species. Because *S. aureus* currently accounts for most cases of bullous impetigo and for a substantial portion of nonbullous infections, antimicrobials with a gram-positive spectrum of activity and stability in the presence of beta-lactamase, such as dicloxacillin or a first-generation or second-generation cephalosporin are now often used as a first-line choice, particularly if methicillin-sensitive *S. aureus* (MSSA) is considered to be the likely causative pathogen. Impetigo caused by methicillin-resistant *S. aureus* (MRSA) is increasing in frequency, however. In addition, nearly one-half of MRSA strains show resistance to mupirocin, These strains are generally macrolide-resistant as well; the macrolides are a class of antimicrobials including azithromycin, clarithromycin, and erythromycin. The advent of infection by these resistant pathogens requires that other options also be considered. These options include trimethoprim-sulfamethoxazole and clindamycin. Minocycline and doxycycline, both tetracycline forms, can also be helpful but should not be used in children younger than 11 years due to the risk of staining of the permanent teeth. Even in these times of resistant pathogens, most episodes of impetigo resolve without complication or need for a second-line agent. In many areas of the world, however, cutaneous infections with nephritogenic strains of group A streptococci are the major antecedent of poststreptococcal glomerulonephritis. No conclusive data indicate that treatment of streptococcal pyoderma prevents nephritis. At the same time, treatment of impetigo is important to minimize risk of infectious transmission. Children with impetigo should be kept out of school or daycare for 24 hours after initiation of antibiotic therapy, and family members should be checked for lesions.

DISCUSSION SOURCES

Gilbert D, Moellering R, Eliopoulos G, Chambers H, Saag M. *The Sanford Guide to Antimicrobial Therapy,* ed. 44. Sperryville, VA: Antimicrobial Therapy, Inc; 2014, pp. 55.

Lewis, LL. http://emedicine.medscape.com/article/965254-treatment, eMedicine: Impetigo

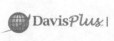

See full color images of this topic on DavisPlus at
**http://davisplus.fadavis.com |
Keyword: Fitzgerald**

Bolaji RS, Dabade TS, Gustafson CJ, Davis SA, Krowchuk DP, Feldman SR. Treatment of impetigo: Oral antibiotics most commonly prescribed. *J Drugs Dermatol* 11(4):489–494, 2012.

Acne Vulgaris

32. The use of which of the following medications contributes to the development of acne vulgaris?
  A. lithium
  B. propranolol
  C. sertraline
  D. clonidine

33. First-line therapy for acne vulgaris with closed comedones includes:
  A. oral antibiotics.
  B. isotretinoin.
  C. benzoyl peroxide.
  D. hydrocortisone cream.

34. When prescribing tretinoin (Retin-A), the NP advises the patient to:
  A. use it with benzoyl peroxide to minimize irritating effects.
  B. use a sunscreen because the drug is photosensitizing.
  C. add a sulfa-based cream to enhance antiacne effects.
  D. expect a significant improvement in acne lesions after approximately 1 week of use.

35. In the treatment of acne vulgaris, which lesions respond best to topical antibiotic therapy?
  A. open comedones
  B. cysts
  C. inflammatory lesions
  D. superficial lesions

36. You have initiated therapy for an 18-year-old man with acne vulgaris and have prescribed doxycycline. He returns in 3 weeks, complaining that his skin is "no better." Your next action is to:
  A. counsel him that 6 to 8 weeks of treatment is often needed before significant improvement is achieved.
  B. discontinue the doxycycline and initiate minocycline therapy.
  C. advise him that antibiotics are likely not an effective treatment for him and should not be continued.
  D. add a second antimicrobial agent such trimethoprim-sulfamethoxazole.

37. Who is the best candidate for isotretinoin (Accutane) therapy?
  A. a 17-year-old patient with pustular lesions and poor response to benzoyl peroxide
  B. a 20-year-old patient with cystic lesions who has tried various therapies with minimal effect
  C. a 14-year-old patient with open and closed comedones and a family history of "ice pick" scars
  D. an 18-year-old patient with inflammatory lesions and improvement with tretinoin (Retin-A)

38. In a 22-year-old woman using isotretinoin (Accutane) therapy, the NP ensures follow-up to monitor for all of the following tests except:
  A. hepatic enzymes
  B. triglyceride measurements
  C. pregnancy test
  D. platelet count

39. Leonard is an 18-year-old man who has been taking isotretinoin (Accutane) for the treatment of acne for the past 2 months. Which of the following is the most important question for the clinician to ask at his follow-up office visit?
  A. Are you having any problems remembering to take your medication?
  B. Have you noticed any dry skin around your mouth since you started using Accutane?
  C. Do you notice any improvement in your skin?
  D. Have you noticed any recent changes in your mood?

40. A 14-year-old male presents with acne consisting of 25 comedones and 20 inflammatory lesions with no nodules. This patient can be classified as having:
  A. mild acne.
  B. moderate acne.
  C. severe acne.
  D. very severe acne.

41. In a 13-year-old female patient with mild acne and who experiences an inadequate response to benzoyl peroxide treatment, an appropriate treatment option would be to:
  A. add a topical retinoid.
  B. add an oral antibiotic.
  C. consider isotretinoin.
  D. consider hormonal therapy.

Answers

32. A.	36. A.	40. B.
33. C.	37. B.	41. A.
34. B.	38. D.	
35. C.	39. D.	

Acne vulgaris is a common pustular disorder caused by a combination of factors. An increase in sebaceous activity causes plugging of follicles and retention of sebum, allowing an overgrowth of the organism *Propionibacterium acnes*. This overgrowth allows an inflammatory reaction with the resulting wide variety of lesions, including open and closed comedones, cysts, and pustules. Due to follicular plugging, the use of a keratolytic agent is advised as well as an antibacterial to minimize the inflammatory effects of *P. acnes*.

Benzoyl peroxide is an inexpensive, generally well tolerated antibacterial agent suitable for the treatment of mild to moderate acne; the product also has comedolytic activity. Topical and systemic antibiotics are also used to treat acne and are particularly helpful as therapy for pustular lesions.

The mechanism of action of antibiotics in acne therapy is probably not based solely on their antimicrobial action but is likely in part a result of antiinflammatory activity. Additional acne vulgaris agents include topical vitamin A derivatives such as tretinoin (Retin-A), synthetic retinoid (Accutane), and comedolytic (benzoyl peroxide). (Table 3–4). When selecting acne treatment, therapeutic options should be based on the severity of acne (mild, moderate, or severe) (Table 3–5).

Nearly all adolescents develop some acne vulgaris to some degree, with milder cases resolving by early adulthood. Only 15% seek treatment for this problematic condition, which affects teenagers at a time in their lives when body image and

TABLE 3-4
Acne Medications

Acne Medication	Mechanism of Action and Considerations for Use
Benzoyl peroxide gel, cream, lotion, various concentrations	• Antimicrobial against *P. acnes* and comedolytic effects • Safe and effective over-the-counter availability • Lower strength formulation often as effective as higher strength and likely to cause less skin irritation • Often given in combination with topical antibiotics, usually used with a keratolytic
Azelaic acid (Finacea, Azelex) 15% and 20% cream	• Likely antimicrobial against *P. acnes,* keratolytic, possibly alters androgen metabolism • Expect ~6 weeks of therapy before noting improvement • Mild skin irritation with redness and dryness common with initial use, improves over time • Less potent, but less irritating than tretinoin preparations
Tretinoin (retinoic acid) gel, cream, various concentrations Adapalene (Differin, Tazarotene) synthetic tretinoin	• Decreases cohesion between epidermal cells, kerotolytic, increases epidermal cell turnover, transforms closed to open comedones • Mild skin irritation with redness and dryness common with initial use, improves over time; expect ~6 weeks of therapy before noting improvement • Photosensitizing; advise patient to use sunscreen
Oral antibiotics (doxycycline, minocycline are primary, others include clindamycin, erythromycin, azithromycin, others)	• Antimicrobial against *P. acnes,* anti-inflammatory • Indicated for treatment of moderate papular inflammatory acne, usually when topical therapy has been inadequate • Once skin clears (usually about 3-6 months) , taper off slowly over a few months while adding topical antibiotic agents; rapid discontinuation results in return of acne • Long-term therapy is often needed
Topical antibiotics (clindamycin, erythromycin, tetracycline, others)	• Antimicrobial against *P. acnes,* antiinflammatory • Indicated in treatment of mild to moderate inflammatory acne vulgaris; less effective than oral antibiotics; often given in combination with benzoyl peroxide
Combined estrogen-progestin hormonal contraceptives such as birth control pills, ring, or patch	• Reduction in ovarian androgen production, decreased sebum production
Isotretinoin (Accutane, Ro-Accutane, Claravis, Sotret, Amnesteem, Absorica) capsules, various strengths	• Likely inhibits sebaceous gland function • Indicated for treatment of cystic acne that does not respond to other therapies • Usual course of treatment is 4–6 months; discontinue when nodule count is reduced by 70%; repeat course only if needed after 6 months off drug • Prescriber and patient must be properly educated in use of drug and fully aware of adverse reactions profile, including cheilitis, conjunctivitis, hypertriglyceridemia, xerosis, photosensitivity, and potent teratogenicity. Women must use two types of highly effective contraception while on isotretinoin. Careful monitoring for mood destabilization and suicidal thoughts is an important part of patient care during isotretinoin use.

Sources: Gilbert D, Moellering R, Eliopoulos G, Chambers H, Saag M. *The Sanford Guide to Antimicrobial Therapy.* ed. 44. Sperryville, VA: Antimicrobial Therapy, Inc., 2014, p. 51.
James, WD, Berger TG, Elston, DM. *Andrews' Diseases of the Skin: Clinical Dermatology*, ed. 11. Philadelphia: Saunders, 2011, pp. 8, 228–235.

TABLE 3-5
Combined Acne Severity Classification

Severity	Definition
Mild acne	Fewer than 20 comedones, or Fewer than 15 inflammatory lesions, or Total lesion count fewer than 30
Moderate acne	20–100 comedones, or 15–50 inflammatory lesions, or Total lesion count 30–125
Severe acne	More than 5 nodules, or Total inflammatory lesion count >50, or Total lesion count >125

Source: Liao DC. Management of acne. *J Fam Pract.* 52:43–51, 2003.

social acceptance are usually of greater influence than they are at any other time of life. Numerous effective and often inexpensive treatment options are available.

Acne-inducing drugs should be avoided, if possible. Certain medications, such as lithium and phenytoin (Dilantin), often cannot be discontinued because of underlying health problems. In any event, drug-induced acne can be treated with conventional therapy (see Table 3–4).

Isotretinoin (Accutane) is effective in cystic acne that does not respond to conventional therapy. Although most patients who take it have adverse effects related only to dry skin, the prescriber and patient need to be well aware of potentially serious problems associated with its use, including pseudotumor cerebri (idiopathic intracranial hypertension), hypertriglyceridemia, elevated hepatic enzymes, and cheilitis. The U.S. Food and Drug Administration (FDA) ruled that labeling for the use of isotretinoin be changed to reflect a possible connection between its use and altered mood. During isotretinoin treatment, the patient should be observed closely for symptoms of depression, such as sad mood, irritability, impulsivity, altered sleep, loss of interest or pleasure in previously enjoyable activities, change in weight or appetite, and new problems with school or work performance. In addition, the patient should be asked about suicidal ideation and altered mood at every office visit while taking the medication. Patients should stop isotretinoin use and they and/or their caregiver should contact the healthcare professional right away if the patient has any of the previously mentioned symptoms. Simply discontinuing the offending medication might be insufficient, and further evaluation is likely needed. Isotretinoin is also a potent teratogen; women taking the medication should have two negative pregnancy tests, including one on the second day of their normal menstrual period, before beginning the medication. In addition, women using isotretinoin should use two forms of highly effective contraception and have a pregnancy test done monthly during therapy.

Guidelines released from the American Academy of Pediatrics recommend various treatment options based on disease severity and response to initial treatment (Table 3–6).

DISCUSSION SOURCES

James, WD, Berger TG, Elston DM. *Andrews' Diseases of the Skin: Clinical Dermatology*, ed. 11. Philadelphia: Saunders, 2011, pp. 228–234.

Gilbert D, Moellering R, Eliopoulos G, Chambers H, Saag M. *The Sanford Guide to Antimicrobial Therapy*, ed. 44. Sperryville, VA: Antimicrobial Therapy, Inc., 2014, p. 51.

Robertson D, Mailbach H. Dermatologic pharmacology. In: Katzung B. *Katzung's Basic and Clinical Pharmacology.* ed. 12. New York: McGraw-Hill Medical, 2012, pp. 991–1008.

United States Food and Drug Administration. http://www.fda.gov/downloads/drugs/drugsafety/ucm085812.pdf

Eichenfield LF, Krakowski AC, Piggott C, et al. Evidence-based recommendations for the diagnosis and treatment of pediatric acne. *Pediatrics.* 131:S163, 2013, http://pediatrics.aappublications.org/content/131/Supplement_3/S163.full.html,

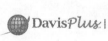 DavisPlus |

See full color images of this topic on DavisPlus at
**http://davisplus.fadavis.com |
Keyword: Fitzgerald**

TABLE 3-6
Treatment Recommendations for Acne

	Mild Acne (comedonal or inflammatory/ mixed lesions)	Moderate Acne (comedonal or inflammatory/ mixed lesions)	Severe Acne (inflammatory/mixed and/or nodular lesions)
Initial treatment	Benzoyl peroxide (BP) or topical retinoid	Topical combination therapy BP + retinoid or Retinoid + (BP + antibiotic) or (Retinoid + antibiotic) + BP	Combination therapy Oral antibiotic + topical retinoid + BP ± consider oral isotretinoin

Continued

TABLE 3-6

Treatment Recommendations for Acne—cont'd

	Mild Acne (comedonal or inflammatory/mixed lesions)	Moderate Acne (comedonal or inflammatory/mixed lesions)	Severe Acne (inflammatory/mixed and/or nodular lesions)
Initial treatment (alternative)	Topical combination therapy BP + antibiotic or BP + retinoid or BP + retinoid + antibiotic	Oral antibiotic + topical retinoid + BP or Topical retinoid + antibiotic + BP	
Inadequate response	Add BP or retinoid if not already prescribed or Change topical retinoid concentration, type, and/or formulation or Change topical combination therapy	Change topical retinoid concentration, type, and/or formulation and/or Change topical combination therapy and/or Add or change oral antibiotic* or Consider oral isotretinoin	Consider changing oral antibiotic and consider oral isotretinoin*

*For female patients, consider hormonal therapy.
Source: Eichenfield LF, Krakowski AC, Piggott C, et al. Evidence-based recommendations for the diagnosis and treatment of pediatric acne. *Pediatrics*. 131:S163–186, 2013.

◗ Bite Wounds

42. A common infective agent in domestic pet cat bites is:
    A. viridans streptococcus species.
    B. *Pasteurella multocida.*
    C. *Bacteroides* species.
    D. *Haemophilus influenzae.*

43. A 28-year-old woman presents to your practice with chief complaint of a cat bite sustained on her right ankle. Her pet cat had bitten her after she inadvertently stepped on its paw while she was in her home. Her cat is 3 years old, is up-to-date on immunizations, and does not go outside. Physical examination reveals pinpoint superficial puncture wounds on the right ankle consistent with the presenting history. She washed the wound with soap and water immediately and asks if she needs additional therapy. Treatment for this patient's cat bite wound should include standard wound care with the addition of:
    A. oral erythromycin.
    B. topical bacitracin.
    C. oral amoxicillin-clavulanate.
    D. parenteral rifampin.

44. A 24-year-old man arrives at the walk-in center. He reports that he was bitten in the thigh by a raccoon while walking in the woods. The examination reveals a wound that is 1 cm deep on his right thigh. The wound is oozing bright red blood. Your next best action is to:
    A. administer high-dose parenteral penicillin.
    B. initiate antibacterial prophylaxis with amoxicillin.
    C. give rabies immune globulin and rabies vaccine.
    D. suture the wound after proper cleansing.

45. A significant rabies risk is associated with a bite from all of the following except:
    A. humans.
    B. foxes.
    C. bats.
    D. skunks.

46. You see a 33-year-old male with a minor dog bite on his hand. The examination reveals a superficial wound on the left palm. The dog is up-to-date on immunizations. In deciding whether to initiate antimicrobial therapy, you consider that _____ of dog bites become bacterially infected.
    A. 5%
    B. 20%
    C. 50%
    D. 75%

47. You see a 52-year-old woman who was bitten by a rat while opening a Dumpster. The examination reveals a wound approximately 1 cm deep that is oozing bright red blood. Treatment of this patient should include standard wound care with the addition of:
A. rabies immune globulin.
B. rabies vaccine.
C. oral ciprofloxacin.
D. oral amoxicillin-clavulanate.

48. You see a 28-year-old man who was involved in a fight approximately 1 hour ago with another person. The patient states, "He bit me in the arm." Examination of the left forearm reveals an open wound consistent with this history. Your next best action is to:
A. obtain a culture and sensitivity of the wound site.
B. refer for rabies prophylaxis.
C. irrigate the wound and débride as needed.
D. close the wound with adhesive strips.

Answers

42. B.	**45.** A.	**48.** C.
43. C.	**46.** A.	
44. C.	**47.** D.	

Bite wounds should not be considered benign or inevitable. Intervention includes education to avoid further bites; a patient's history must include a complete documentation of events leading up to the bite.

All bites should be considered to carry infectious risk. This risk can vary from the relatively low rate of infection from dog bites (approximately 5%) to the very high rate from cat bites (approximately 80%). Initial therapy for all bite wounds should include vigorous wound cleansing with antimicrobial agents as appropriate and débridement if necessary. Starting short-term antimicrobial prophylactic therapy within 12 hours of the injury should be considered as directed by the location and origin of the bite wound, and tetanus immunization should be updated as needed (Table 3–7).

The clinician should check with local authorities for information on rabies when a bite involves domestic pets; because the rabies risk in this situation is usually negligible, rabies prophylaxis is not indicated. In recent years, there has been an increase in cases of rabies domestically, primarily from bites by usually docile, often nocturnal wild animals that attack without provocation. These include bats, foxes, woodchucks, squirrels, and skunks. Human bites carry no rabies risk.

DISCUSSION SOURCES

Gilbert D, Moellering R, Eliopoulos G, Chambers H, Saag M. *The Sanford Guide to Antimicrobial Therapy*, ed. 44. Sperryville, VA: Antimicrobial Therapy, Inc., 52:48–49, 2014.
Ballentine JR. http://www.emedicinehealth.com/human_bites/article_em.htmed.

TABLE 3-7
Infectious Agents and Treatment in Bites

Type of Bite	Infective Agent	Prophylaxis or Treatment of Infection
Bat, raccoon, skunk	Uncertain; significant rabies risk	For bacterial infection Primary: amoxicillin with clavulanate, 875 mg/125 mg bid or 500 mg/125 mg tid Alternative: doxycycline, 100 mg bid Animal should be considered rabid, and patients should be given rabies immune globulin and vaccine and consider tetanus prophylaxis
Cat	*Pasteurella multocida,* *Staphylococcus aureus*	Primary: amoxicillin with clavulanate, 875 mg/125 mg bid 500 mg/125 mg tid Alternative: cefuroxime, 0.5 g bid; doxycycline, 100 mg orally bid Switch to penicillin if *P. multocida* is cultured from wound Because 80% become infected, all wounds should be cultured and treated empirically
Dog	*P. multocida, S. aureus,* *Bacteroides* spp., others	Primary: amoxicillin with clavulanate, 875 mg/125 mg bid Alternative: clindamycin, 300 mg qid, plus a fluoroquinolone; or clindamycin with TMP-SMX (children) Only 5% become infected. Treat only if bite is severe, or if significant comorbidity such as diabetes mellitus or immunosuppression

Continued

TABLE 3-7

Infectious Agents and Treatment in Bites—cont'd

Type of Bite	Infective Agent	Prophylaxis or Treatment of Infection
Human	*Streptococcus viridans, Staphylococcus epidermidis, Corynebacterium, Eikenella corrodens, S. aureus, Bacteroides* spp., *Peptostreptococcus*	Early, not yet infected: amoxicillin with clavulanate, 875 mg/125 mg bid for 5 days Later (3–24 hours, signs of infection): parenteral therapy with ampicillin with sulbactam, cefoxitin, others Penicillin allergy: Clindamycin with ciprofloxacin or TMP-SMX
Rat	Streptobacillus moniliformis, Spirillum minus	Primary: amoxicillin with clavulanate, 875 mg/125 mg bid Alternative: doxycycline Rabies prophylaxis not indicated
Pig or swine	Polymicrobial gram-positive cocci, gram-negative bacilli, anaerobes, *Pasteurella* spp.	Primary: amoxicillin with clavulanate, 875 mg/125 mg bid Alternative: parenteral third-generation cephalosporin, others
Nonhuman primate	Herpesvirus simiae	Acyclovir

Source: Gilbert D, Moellering R, Eliopoulos G, Chambers H, Saag M. *The Sanford Guide to Antimicrobial Therapy*. ed. 44th. Sperryville, VA: Antimicrobial Therapy, Inc., 2014, p. 52.

Burn Wounds

49. A patient presents with a painful, blistering thermal burn involving the first, second, and third digits of his right hand. The most appropriate plan of care is to:
A. apply an anesthetic cream to the area and open the blisters.
B. apply silver sulfadiazine cream (Silvadene) to the area followed by a bulky dressing.
C. refer the patient to burn specialty care.
D. wrap the burn loosely with a nonadherent dressing and prescribe an analgesic agent.

50. Gram-negative bacteria that commonly cause burn wound infections include all of the following except:
A. *P. aeruginosa.*
B. *E. coli.*
C. *K. pneumoniae.*
D. *H. influenzae.*

51. Which of the following is recommended for preventing a burn wound infection?
A. topical corticosteroid
B. topical silver sulfadiazine
C. oral erythromycin
D. oral moxifloxacin

52. You examine a patient with a red, tender thermal burn that has excellent capillary refill involving the entire surface of the anterior right leg. The estimated involved body surface area (BSA) is approximately:
A. 5%.
B. 9%.
C. 13%.
D. 18%.

53. A burn that is about twice as large as an adult's palmar surface of the hand including the fingers encompasses a BSA of approximately _____%.
A. 1
B. 2
C. 3
D. 4

54. to 56. Match the following:

_____ **54.** First-degree burn

_____ **55.** Second-degree burn

_____ **56.** Third-degree burn

A. Affected skin blanches with ease.
B. Surface is raw and moist.
C. Affected area is white and leathery.

Answers

49. C.	**52.** B.	**55.** B.
50. D.	**53.** B.	**56.** C.
51. B.	**54.** A.	

As with bites, burn intervention includes asking for a complete history of the events leading up to the injury to develop a plan for avoiding future events. In addition, education for burn avoidance for high-risk individuals for burn injury, such as children, elderly adults, and smokers, should be a routine part of primary care.

Generally, smaller (less than 10% of body surface area), minor (second-degree or lower) burns not involving a high-function area such as the hand or foot and of minimal cosmetic consequence can be treated in the outpatient setting. Gram-positive bacteria, such as *Staphylococcus aureus* or coagulase-negative streptococci (CNS), can colonize the burn area within 48 hours of injury unless a topical antimicrobial is used. Eventually, colonization with other Gram-positive (e.g., enterococci) or Gram-negative bacteria (i.e., *Pseudomonas aeruginosa, Escherichia coli, Klebsiella pneumoniae*) can occur. Treatment options include prevention of infection by the use of a topical antibiotic such as mafenide acetate (Sulfamylon) or silver sulfadiazine (Silvadene). The use of systemic antibiotics for prophylaxis is generally not as effective as topical agents. An alternative is to use petroleum gauze dressing that provides protection to the affected area. Patients with any burn involving areas of high function such as the hands and feet, of significant cosmetic consequence such as the face, or any burns involving the genitalia should be referred promptly to specialty care.

First-degree and second-degree burns are characterized by erythema, hyperemia, and pain. With first-degree burns, the skin blanches with ease; skin with second-degree burns has blisters and a raw, moist surface. In third-degree burns, pain may be minimal, but the burns are usually surrounded by areas of painful first-degree and second-degree burns. The surface of third-degree burns is usually white and leathery. It is important to estimate the body surface area (BSA) affected by the burn (Fig. 3–1). The palmar surface of the hand including the fingers represents a BSA of 1% throughout the life span and can provide a helpful guide in estimating the extent of a burn.

DISCUSSION SOURCES

James, WD, Berger TG, Elston DM. *Andrews' Diseases of the Skin: Clinical Dermatology*, ed. 11. Philadelphia: Saunders, 2011, pp. 18–19.

Gilbert D, Moellering R, Eliopoulos G, Chambers H, Saag M. *The Sanford Guide to Antimicrobial Therapy*, ed. 44. Sperryville, VA: Antimicrobial Therapy, Inc., 2014, p. 53.

Plantz SH. http://www.emedicinehealth.com/wilderness_burns/article_em.htm, eMedicine: Burns

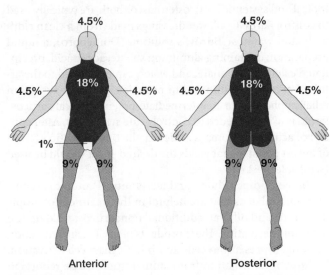

Figure 3-1 Rule of nines for calculating total burn surface area. *(Source: Adapted from Richard R, Staley M. Burn Care and Rehabilitation. Philadelphia: F.A. Davis, 1994, p. 109.* Wedro, BC. http://www.emedicinehealth.com/burn_percentage_in_adults_rule_of_nines/article_em.htm

Church D, Elsayed S, Reid O, Winston B, Lindsay R. Burn wound infections. *Clin Microbiol Rev.* 19:403–434, 2006.

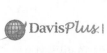

◗ Atopic Dermatitis

57. A mother brings to the clinic her 3-year-old daughter, who presents with dry red patches on her face around the eyes. The mother has observed her daughter constantly rubbing the area, which has caused swelling around the eyes. Physical examination is consistent with atopic dermatitis. The NP considers that this is a diagnosis that:
A. requires a skin culture to confirm contributing bacterial organisms.
B. should be supported by a biopsy of the affected area.
C. necessitates obtaining peripheral blood eosinophil level
D. Is usually made by clinical assessment alone.

58. Type I hypersensitivity reactions, such as atopic dermatitis, involve the action of which antibodies binding to receptor sites on mast cells?
A. IgG
B. IgM
C. IgE
D. IgA

59. During type I hypersensitivity reactions, histamine released from degraded mast cells causes all of the following except:
A. vasodilation.
B. mucous gland stimulation.
C. enhanced sebum production.
D. tissue swelling.

60. The most important aspect of skin care for individuals with atopic dermatitis is:
A. frequent bathing with antibacterial soap.
B. consistent use of medium-potency to high-potency topical steroids.
C. application of lubricants.
D. treatment of dermatophytes.

61. One of the most common trigger agents for contact dermatitis is:
A. exposure to nickel.
B. use of fabric softener.
C. bathing with liquid body wash.
D. eating spicy foods.

62. A common site for atopic dermatitis in an adult is on the:
A. dorsum of the hand.
B. face.
C. neck.
D. flexor surfaces.

63. A common site for atopic dermatitis in an infant is:
    A. the diaper area.
    B. the face.
    C. the neck.
    D. the posterior trunk.

64. In counseling a patient with atopic dermatitis, you suggest all of the following can be used to alleviate symptoms of a flare except:
    A. the use of oral antihistamines.
    B. applying a heating pad on the affected region for 30 minutes.
    C. the use of topical corticosteroids.
    D. applying cool, wet dressings made from a clean cloth and water to the affected area.

65. The mechanism of action of pimecrolimus (Elidel) in the treatment of atopic dermatitis is as a/an:
    A. immunomodulator.
    B. antimitotic.
    C. mast cell activator.
    D. exfoliant.

66. When counseling a patient about the use of tacrolimus (Protopic) or pimecrolimus (Elidel), you mention that:
    A. this is the preferred atopic dermatitis treatment in infants.
    B. there is a possibility of increased cancer risk with its use.
    C. the product is used interchangeably with topical corticosteroids.
    D. the product is a potent antihistamine.

67. You see a 34-year-old man with atopic dermatitis localized primarily on the arms who complains of severe itching. The condition becomes worse at night and interferes with his sleep. You recommend:
    A. taking a bedtime dose of antihistamine.
    B. taking a bedtime dose of acetaminophen.
    C. taking a hot shower prior to bedtime.
    D. applying a warm compress to the affected areas 30 minutes prior to bedtime.

Answers

57. D.	61. A.	65. A.
58. C.	62. D.	66. B.
59. C.	63. B.	67. A.
60. C.	64. B.	

Atopic dermatitis, or eczema, is one manifestation of a type I hypersensitivity reaction. This type of reaction results from immunoglobulin E (IgE) antibodies occupying receptor sites on mast cells. This causes a degradation of the mast cell and subsequent release of histamine, resulting in vasodilation, mucous gland stimulation, and tissue swelling. Type I hypersensitivity reactions are usually divided into two subgroups: atopy and anaphylaxis.

The atopy subgroup includes many common clinical conditions, such as allergic rhinitis, atopic dermatitis, allergic gastroenteropathy, and allergy-based asthma. Atopic diseases have a strong familial component and tend to cause localized rather than systemic reactions. Individuals with atopic disease are often able to identify allergy-inducing agents. Allergic contact dermatitis is a form of eczematous dermatitis. Common causes of contact dermatitis include exposure to metals including nickel, rubber additives to shoes and gloves, some toiletries, and topical medications.

A key symptom of atopic dermatitis is pruritus (itching). The disease typically has an intermittent course with flares and remissions occurring. The primary physical findings include xerosis (dry skin), lichenification, and eczematous lesions. The eczematous changes and morphology can occur at various body sites and will depend on the age of the patient (i.e., infant, child, or adult).

Criteria for the diagnosis of atopic dermatitis include the presence of itching and subsequent scratching plus three or more of the following: red or inflamed rash, presence of excessive dryness/scaling, and location in skin folds of arms or legs. With severe outbreaks, vesicles are often present. Additional findings include early age at initial onset (0 to 5 years) and elevated serum IgE and peripheral blood eosinophil levels. In infants, the face is often involved, whereas the diaper area, owing to the occlusive, damp environment, is usually spared. The diagnosis of atopic dermatitis is usually made by clinical assessment without the need for confirmatory testing.

Treatment for atopic dermatitis includes avoiding offending agents, minimizing skin dryness by limiting soap and water exposure, and using lubricants consistently. In general, the patient should be encouraged to treat the skin with care because it tends to be sensitive; the person with atopic dermatitis has an abnormal skin barrier that allows for loss of water and resulting dryness. When flares occur, the skin eruption is caused largely by histamine release. Antihistamines, topical and systemic corticosteroids, or both are typically used to control flares. Cool, wet dressings made from a clean cloth with cool water or Burow's solution (Domeboro), a liquid preparation containing aluminum sulfate, acetic acid, precipitated calcium carbonate, and water, can be applied to the affected area for 30 minutes to provide significant symptom relief; application of an intermediate-potency topical corticosteroid is usually needed to control acute symptoms. After control of acute symptoms is achieved, the topical corticosteroid of lowest potency that yields the desired effect should be used (see Table 3–3).

Pimecrolimus (Elidel) and tacrolimus (Protopic) are immunomodulators that are helpful in the treatment of atopic dermatitis and offer an additional, noncorticosteroid option for atopic dermatitis. These products block T-cell stimulation by antigen-presenting cells and inhibit mast cell activation. Because of information from animal studies, case reports in a small number of patients, and knowledge of how drugs in this class work, an advisory about the potential for increased cancer risk with the use of these products has been released. Tacrolimus and pimecrolimus should be used only as labeled and only if other prescription and supportive treatments have failed to work or cannot be tolerated. These products should not be used in children younger than age 2 years.

Itch (pruritus) is a distressing symptom; many patients say it is more bothersome than pain. Pruritus is a cardinal symptom of many forms of dermatitis. Histamine contributes to the development of itching; the use of an antihistamine can provide relief. Pruritus tends to be worst at night, often causing disturbance in sleep. In particular, providing the patient with a bedtime dose of antihistamine can yield tremendous relief from itching and improve sleep. Hydroxyzine (Atarax) seems to provide better relief of itching than other antihistamines. Cetirizine (Zyrtec) is a less sedating antihistamine that is a metabolite of hydroxyzine.

DISCUSSION SOURCES

James, WD, Berger TG, Elston, DM. *Andrews' Diseases of the Skin: Clinical Dermatology,* ed. 11. Philadelphia: Saunders, 2011, pp. 62–69.

Chamlin S. Atopic dermatitis. In: Rakel R, Bope E, eds. *Conn's Current Therapy 2013*. Philadelphia: Saunders, 2012, pp. 207–210.

Robertson D, Mailbach H. Dermatologic pharmacology. In: Katzung, B, *Katzung's Basic and Clinical Pharmacology*, ed. 12. New York: McGraw-Hill Medical, 2012, 991–1008.

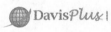 See full color images of this topic on DavisPlus at **http://davisplus.fadavis.com** | Keyword: Fitzgerald

Herpes Zoster

68. A 38-year-old woman with advanced human immunodeficiency virus (HIV) disease presents with a chief complaint of a painful, itchy rash over her trunk. Examination reveals linear vesicular lesions that do not cross the midline and are distributed over the posterior thorax. This presentation is most consistent with:
A. herpes zoster.
B. dermatitis herpetiformis.
C. molluscum contagiosum.
D. impetigo.

69. A Tzanck smear that is positive for giant multinucleated cells was taken from a lesion caused by:
A. herpesvirus.
B. *S. aureus.*
C. streptococci.
D. allergic reaction.

70. What is the most effective protection against shingles?
A. previous episode of chickenpox as a child
B. prior episode of shingles
C. receipt of varicella-zoster immunization
D. avoiding children and daycare centers

71. Shingles most commonly involve the dermatomes of the:
A. legs and pubic area.
B. face.
C. upper arms and shoulders.
D. thorax.

72. When caring for an adult with an outbreak of shingles, you advise that:
A. there is no known treatment for this condition.
B. during outbreaks, the chickenpox (varicella) virus is shed.
C. although they are acutely painful, the lesions heal well without scarring or lingering discomfort.
D. this condition commonly strikes young and old alike.

73. Analgesia options for a patient with shingles can include all of the following except:
A. topical lidocaine gel 5% with oral acetaminophen.
B. Burow's solution with a high-potency oral NSAID.
C. Burow's solution with an oral opioid.
D. fentanyl transdermal patch and a topical medium-potency corticosteroid on the affected area.

74. Risk factors for the development of postherpetic neuralgia include:
A. age younger than 50 years at the time of the outbreak.
B. severe prodromal symptoms.
C. lumbar location of lesions.
D. low volume of lesions.

75. Treatment options in postherpetic neuralgia include all of the following except:
A. injectable methylprednisolone.
B. oral pregabalin.
C. oral nortriptyline.
D. topical lidocaine.

76. The zoster vaccine (Zostavax) is a(n):
A. inactivated/killed virus vaccine.
B. conjugate vaccine containing a virus-like particle (VLP).
C. live, attenuated vaccine.
D. inactivated toxin vaccine.

Answers

68.	A.	**71.**	D.	**74.**	B.
69.	A.	**72.**	B.	**75.**	A.
70.	C.	**73.**	D.	**76.**	C.

Herpes zoster infection, commonly known as shingles, is an acutely painful condition caused by the varicella-zoster virus, the same agent that causes chickenpox. The virus lies dormant in the dorsal root ganglia of a dermatome. When activated, the characteristic blistering lesions occur along a dermatome, usually not crossing the midline. The resulting pain is burning, throbbing, or stabbing; intense itch is also occasionally described. The thoracic dermatomes are the most commonly involved sites, followed by the lumbar dermatomes.

Anyone who has had chickenpox is at risk for shingles, whereas recipients of varicella-zoster immunization have virtually no risk. Shingles is usually seen in elderly individuals, patients who are immunocompromised, and individuals with some other underlying health problem. When shingles is seen in younger adults, the possibility of HIV infection or other immunocompromised condition should be considered. During the acute attack, the chickenpox (varicella-zoster) virus is shed; patients can transmit this infection. Shingles is not communicable from person to person, however. Approximately 4% of patients with zoster develop a recurrent episode later in life.

Diagnosis of shingles is usually straightforward because of its characteristic lesions. If confirmation is needed, a Tzanck smear reveals giant multinucleated cells, a finding in all herpetic infections.

Scarring and postherpetic neuralgia are problematic sequelae of shingles. Initiating antiviral therapy with high-dose acyclovir (Zovirax), valacyclovir (Valtrex), or famciclovir (Famvir), preferably within the first 72 hours of herpes zoster outbreak, helps limit the severity of the lesions and minimize the risk of postherpetic neuralgia and scarring. Systemic corticosteroids are often prescribed during the acute stage of shingles along with antivirals. This combination therapy usually results in more rapid resolution of pain but not of zoster lesions.

Adequate analgesia should be offered to a person with shingles. Using topical agents such as topical lidocaine gel 5%, Burow's solution with a high-potency nonsteroidal antiinflammatory drug or opioid, or combination of these helps provide considerable relief. The patient should also be monitored for superinfection of lesions. Because of the risk of complication and possible compromise of vision, expert consultation should be sought if herpes zoster involves a facial or ocular dermatome. The rash usually resolves within 14 to 21 days.

Postherpetic neuralgia is defined as pain persisting at least 1 month after the rash has healed. Risk factors for the development of postherpetic neuralgia include the site of initial involvement, with greatest risk if outbreak involved the trigeminal or brachial plexus region; moderate risk with a thoracic outbreak; and lower risk with jaw, neck, sacral, and lumbar involvement. Additional risks include severe rash and intense prodromal pain. The incidence increases dramatically with age, with only 4% of adults 30 to 50 years old reporting postherpetic neuralgia and approximately 50% of adults older than 80 years reporting it. Tricyclic antidepressants (e.g., amitriptyline, nortriptyline), gabapentin (Neurontin), pregabalin (Lyrica), and topical lidocaine patches are effective and are often used in the treatment of postherpetic neuralgia.

Zoster vaccine (Zostavax) is an immunization for protection against herpes zoster (or shingles). The vaccine is prepared from a live, attenuated strain of varicella-zoster virus. Zostavax is designed to yield a more potent, higher titer than varicella virus live vaccine (Varivax), used in children for chickenpox. Because reactivation of the varicella virus appears to be related to a decline in varicella-zoster virus-specific immunity, the use of zoster vaccine significantly reduces shingles risk. This vaccine should be used even with a history of shingles. The clinician should check for the latest recommendations on candidates for the zoster vaccine.

DISCUSSION SOURCES

James, WD, Berger TG, Elston, DM. *Andrews' Diseases of the Skin: Clinical Dermatology*, ed. 11. Philadelphia: Saunders, 2011, pp. 372–376.

Krause R. http://www.emedicine.com/emerg/TOPIC823.HTM, eMedicine: Herpes zoster

McElveen WA, Gonzalez R, Sinclair D. http://www.emedicine.com/neuro/TOPIC317.HTM, eMedicine: Postherpetic neuralgia

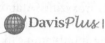 Davis*Plus* | See full color images of this topic on DavisPlus at **http://davisplus.fadavis.com** | Keyword: Fitzgerald

Onychomycosis

77. Characteristics of onychomycosis include all of the following except:
    A. it is readily diagnosed by clinical examination.
    B. nail hypertrophy.
    C. brittle nails.
    D. fingernails respond more readily to therapy than toenails.

78. Oral antifungal treatment options for onychomycosis include all of the following except:
    A. itraconazole.
    B. fluconazole.
    C. metronidazole.
    D. terbinafine.

79. When prescribing itraconazole (Sporanox), the NP considers that:
    A. the drug is a cytochrome P-450 3A4 inhibitor.
    B. one pulse cycle is recommended for fingernail treatment, and two cycles are needed for toenail therapy.
    C. continuous therapy is preferred in the presence of hepatic disease.
    D. taking the drug on an empty stomach enhances the efficacy of the product.

80. When prescribing pulse dosing with itraconazole for the treatment of fingernail fungus, the clinician realizes that:
    A. a transient increase in hepatic enzymes is commonly seen with its use.
    B. drug-induced leukopenia is a common problem.
    C. the patient needs to be warned about excessive bleeding because of the drug's antiplatelet effect.
    D. its use is contraindicated in the presence of iron-deficiency anemia.

81. When prescribing fluconazole, the NP considers that it is a cytochrome P-450:
    A. 3A4 inhibitor.
    B. 2CP inhibitor.
    C. 2D6 inducer.
    D. 1A2 inducer.

82. In diagnosing onychomycosis, the NP considers that:
   A. nails often have a single midline groove.
   B. pitting is often seen.
   C. microscopic examination reveals hyphae.
   D. Beau lines are present.

83. In counseling a patient on the use of topical products to treat nail fungal infections, the NP considers that:
   A. nail lacquers, such as ciclopirox olamine 8% solution (Penlac), offer similar effectiveness to oral antifungals.
   B. some herbal products, such as tea tree oil, can be an effective alternative to oral agents.
   C. topical products have limited penetration through the nail matrix to reach the site of infection.
   D. cream-based products are more effective than gel-based products in treating nail fungal infections.

Answers

77.	A.	80.	A.	83.	C.
78.	C.	81.	B.		
79.	A.	82.	C.		

Onychomycosis, or dermatophytosis of the nail, is a chronic disfiguring disorder. The nails are dull, thickened, and lusterless with a pithy consistency. Parts of the nail often break off. Because trauma and other conditions can cause a similar appearance, confirmation of the diagnosis with microscopic examination for hyphae of the nail scrapings mixed with potassium hydroxide (KOH) is important, although it has a high rate of false-negative results. Fungal cultures should be obtained from pulverized nail scrapings or clippings.

Antifungals such as itraconazole (Sporanox), terbinafine (Lamisil), and fluconazole (Diflucan) offer well-tolerated effective treatment for fingernail and toenail fungal infections. These medications can be used in pulse cycles, with times of drug use alternating with abstinent periods. An example of pulse dosing is itraconazole, 400 mg daily, for the first week of the month for 2 months to treat the fingernails and for 3 months to treat the toenails. The products are held within the nail matrix for months after therapy; this produces effective treatment at a considerably reduced cost compared with constant therapy. In addition, all oral antifungals have hepatotoxic potential and may cause an increase in hepatic enzyme levels. Pulse therapy reduces this risk considerably, however.

Caution is needed when itraconazole is prescribed because it inhibits cytochrome P-450 3A4, a pathway also used by drugs such as diazepam, digoxin, anticoagulants, and certain HIV protease inhibitors. In addition, fluconazole is a cytochrome P-450 2CP inhibitor, a pathway also used by drugs such as carbamazepine, some benzodiazepines, and calcium channel blockers. The concomitant use of these antifungals with the aforementioned medications can lead to significant drug interactions. Terbinafine has significantly less drug interaction potential.

Topical treatment has proved to be of little value because the antifungal agent is held within the nail matrix. Oral agents such as griseofulvin require months of therapy with a high rate of relapse. Topical over-the-counter creams and medications, such as Vicks VapoRub, thymol oil, and tree tea oil, are usually not effective as the nails are too thick and hard for external applications to penetrate to the site of infection.

Antifungal nail lacquers, consist of an antifungal agent (e.g., ciclopirox or amorolfine) in a clear, stable, film-forming lacquer vehicle. When applied to the nails, these products provide a hard, clear, water-resistant film containing the antifungal agent. However, the effectiveness of these products in treating nail fungal infections is limited and typically poorer than oral antifungal agents.

DISCUSSION SOURCES

James, WD, Berger TG, Elston, DM. *Andrews' Diseases of the Skin: Clinical Dermatology,* ed. 11. Philadelphia: Saunders, 2011, pp. 295–296.

Blumberg M. http://www.emedicine.com/derm/topic300.htm, eMedicine: Onychomycosis

Gilbert D, Moellering R, Eliopoulos G, Chambers H, Saag M. *The Sanford Guide to Antimicrobial Therapy,* ed. 44. Sperryville, VA: Antimicrobial Therapy, Inc., 2014, pp. 123–124.

Robertson D, Mailbach H. Dermatologic pharmacology. In: Katzung B. *Katzung's Basic and Clinical Pharmacology.* ed. 12. New York: McGraw-Hill Medical, 2012, pp. 991–1008.

Scabies

84. A 78-year-old resident of a long-term care facility complains of generalized itchiness at night that disturbs her sleep. Her examination is consistent with scabies. Which of the following do you expect to find on examination?
   A. excoriated papules on the interdigital area
   B. annular lesions over the buttocks
   C. vesicular lesions in a linear pattern
   D. honey-colored crusted lesions that began as vesicles

85. In counseling a patient with scabies, the NP recommends all of the following methods to eliminate the mite from bedclothes and other items except:
   A. wash items in hot water.
   B. run items through the clothes dryer for a normal cycle.
   C. soak items in cold water for at least 1 hour.
   D. place items in a plastic storage bag for at least 1 week.

86. Which of the following represents the most accurate patient information when using permethrin (Elimite) for treating scabies?
   A. To avoid systemic absorption, the medication should be applied over the body and rinsed off within 1 hour.
   B. The patient should notice a marked reduction in pruritus within 48 hours of using the product.
   C. Itch often persists for a few weeks after successful treatment.
   D. It is a second-line product in the treatment of scabies.

87. When advising the patient about scabies contagion, you inform her that:
A. mites can live for many weeks away from the host.
B. close personal contact with an infected person is usually needed to contract this disease.
C. casual contact with an infected person is likely to result in infestation.
D. bedding used by an infected person must be destroyed.

88. The use of lindane (Kwell) to treat scabies is discouraged because of its potential for:
A. hepatotoxicity.
B. neurotoxicity.
C. nephrotoxicity.
D. pancreatitis.

Answers

84. A.	**86.** C.	**88.** B.
85. C.	**87.** B.	

Scabies is a communicable skin disease caused by a host-specific mite, generally requiring close personal, skin-to-skin contact to achieve contagion. Contact with used, unwashed bedding and clothing from an affected person also can result in infection. Bedclothes and other items used by a person with scabies must be either washed in hot water or placed in the clothes dryer for a normal cycle. Alternatively, items can be placed in plastic storage bags for at least 1 week because mites do not survive for more than 3 to 4 days without contact with the host. The mites tend to burrow in areas of warmth, such as the finger webs, axillary folds, belt line, areolae, scrotum, penis, under the breasts, with lesions developing and clustering in these areas. The lesions often start with the characteristic burrows but in most cases progress to a vesicular or papular form, usually with excoriation caused by scratching.

Permethrin (Elimite) lotion is the preferred method of treatment for scabies. The lotion must be left on for 8 to 14 hours to be effective. Despite effective therapy, individuals with scabies often have a significant problem with pruritus after permethrin treatment because of the presence of dead mites and their waste trapped in the skin, which causes an inflammatory reaction. This debris is eliminated from the body over a few weeks; the distress of itchiness passes at that time. Oral antihistamines, particularly for nighttime use, and low-potency to medium-potency topical corticosteroids should be offered to help with this problem (Table 3–8). In the past, lindane (Kwell) was used, but the use of this product presents potential problems with neurotoxicity and a resulting seizure risk and lower efficacy. In particular, lindane should not be used by pregnant women, children, and elderly patients.

TABLE 3-8
Medications Used in the Treatment of Acute IgE-Mediated Hypersensitivity Reaction

Medications	Mechanism of Action	Comments
Antihistamines	Antagonize H$_1$-receptor sites. Prevent action of formed histamine, so helpful in treatment of acute allergic reaction	In acute reaction, give parenterally or in a quickly absorbed oral form such as chewable tablet or liquid First-generation products (diphenhydramine [Benadryl], chlorpheniramine [Chlor-Trimeton]) • Cross blood-brain barrier, causing sedation • Anticholinergic activity can cause blurred vision, dry mucous membranes Second-generation products (loratadine [Claritin], cetirizine [Zyrtec], fexofenadine [Allegra]) • Little transfer across blood-brain barrier. Low rates of sedation • Less anticholinergic effect
Epinephrine parenterally, usually given IM (preferred) or SC	Alpha-1, beta-1, beta-2 agonists. Potent vasoconstrictor, cardiac stimulant, bronchodilator	• Initial therapy for anaphylaxis because of its multiple modes of reversing airway and circulatory dysfunction • Anaphylaxis usually responds quickly to epinephrine given parenterally
Oral corticosteroids	Inhibit eosinophilic action and other inflammatory mediators	• In higher dose and with longer therapy (>2 weeks), adrenal suppression can occur • Taper usually not needed if use is short-term (<10 days) and at lower dose (prednisone, 40–60 mg/day) • Potential for causing gastropathy

Source: http://www.aaaai.org/conditions-and-treatments/library/at-a-glance/anaphylaxis.aspx

DISCUSSION SOURCES

James, WD, Berger TG, Elston, DM. *Andrews' Diseases of the Skin: Clinical Dermatology,* ed. 11. Philadelphia: Saunders, 2011, pp. 442–444.

Gunning K, Pippitt K, Kiraly B, et al. Pediculosis and scabies: treatment update. *Am Fam Physician,* 86(86):535–541, 2012.

Cordoro KM, Elston DM. http://emedicine.medscape.com/article/1109204-overview#showall, Dermatologic manifestations of scabies

Psoriasis Vulgaris

89. Psoriasis vulgaris is a chronic skin disease caused by:
A. bacterial colonization.
B. absence of melanin.
C. accelerated mitosis.
D. type I hypersensitivity reaction.

90. You examine a patient with psoriasis vulgaris and expect to find the following lesions:
A. lichenified areas in flexor areas
B. well-demarcated plaques on the knees
C. greasy lesions throughout the scalp
D. vesicular lesions over the upper thorax

91. Psoriatic lesions arise from:
A. decreased skin exfoliation.
B. rapid skin cell turnover, leading to decreased maturation and keratinization.
C. inflammatory changes in the dermis.
D. lichenification.

92. Anthralin (Drithocreme) is helpful in treating psoriasis because it has what kind of activity?
A. antimitotic
B. exfoliative
C. vasoconstrictor
D. humectant

93. Treatment options in generalized psoriasis vulgaris include all of the following except:
A. psoralen with ultraviolet A light (PUVA) therapy.
B. methotrexate.
C. cyclosporine.
D. systemic corticosteroids.

94. Which of the following is not a potential adverse effect with long-term high-potency topical corticosteroid use?
A. lichenification
B. telangiectasia
C. skin atrophy
D. adrenal suppression

95. Biological agents to treat psoriasis, such as infliximab and etanercept, work by blocking the action of:
A. IL-9.
B. CD4.
C. TNF-α.
D. IgG.

96. For severe, recalcitrant psoriasis that affects more than 30% of the body, all of the following treatments are recommended except:
A. methotrexate.
B. topical anthralin (Drithocreme).
C. tumor necrosis factor (TNF) modulators.
D. cyclosporine.

97. The use of TNF modulators for the treatment of psoriasis is associated with an increased risk for:
A. gastrointestinal disorders.
B. nephrotoxicity.
C. QTc prolongation.
D. reactivation of latent tuberculosis.

Answers

89. C	**92.** A	**95.** C
90. B	**93.** D	**96.** B
91. B	**94.** A	**97.** D

Psoriasis vulgaris is a chronic skin disorder caused by accelerated mitosis and rapid cell turnover, which lead to decreased maturation and keratinization. This process prevents the dermal cells from "sticking" together, allowing for a shedding of cells in the form of characteristic silvery scales and leaving an underlying red plaque. Psoriasis is typically found in extensor surfaces; the lesions are most often found in plaques over the elbows and knees. The scalp and other surfaces are occasionally involved.

Topical corticosteroids have antiinflammatory and mild antimitotic activity, which allows for regression of psoriatic plaques. A common treatment plan is to use a medium-potency to high-potency drug for short periods until the plaques resolve and then to use a lower potency product three to four times a week to maintain remission. As with all dermatoses, consistent use of high-potency topical steroids is discouraged because of potential risk of skin atrophy, telangiectasia formation, corticosteroid-induced acne, and striae. In addition, the extensive use of topical corticosteroids leads to significant systemic absorption and potential subclinical adrenal function suppression. Tar preparations can be helpful, but these products have a low level of patient acceptance because of the messiness and odor associated with these preparations.

Additional treatment options include use of anthralin (Drithocreme), a topical antimitotic, and calcipotriene, a topical vitamin D_3 derivative. Although offering effective psoriasis therapy, these products are significantly more expensive than topical corticosteroids and tars. Use should be reserved for corticosteroid-resistant conditions.

If psoriasis is generalized, covering more than 30% of body surface area, treatment with topical products is difficult and expensive. Ultraviolet A light exposure three times weekly is highly effective but is associated with an increase in skin cancer risk and photoaging. For severe, recalcitrant psoriasis, cyclosporine, methotrexate, systemic retinoids, and newer biological agents such as tumor necrosis factor (TNF) modulators etanercept (Enbrel), adalimumab (Humira), or ustekinumab (Stelara) are also used. TNF-α is a proinflammatory cytokine that amplifies inflammation through various pathways and has been implicated in psoriasis pathogenesis. TNF-α antagonists bind to the cytokine and block its proinflammatory action. Although these biologic agents can be effective in treating psoriasis, they are associated with significant adverse effects, including injection site and infusion reactions, infection, and reactivation of latent tuberculosis. The risk of infection is highest in patients with predisposing conditions, such as diabetes, heart failure, or concomitant use of immunosuppressive drugs. Referral to a clinician with expertise in prescribing these agents is indicated.

DISCUSSION SOURCES

James, WD, Berger TG, Elston, DM. *Andrews' Diseases of the Skin: Clinical Dermatology*, ed. 11. Philadelphia: Saunders, 2011, pp. 190–198.

Meffert J, O'Connor RE. http://emedicine.medscape.com/article/1943419-overview, accessed 7/20/13.

Robertson D, Mailbach H. Dermatologic pharmacology. In: Katzung, B, *Katzung's Basic and Clinical Pharmacology*, ed.12. New York: McGraw-Hill Medical, 2012, pp. 991–1008.

Taheri A, Feldman SR. Biologics in practice: How effective are biologics? *The Dermatologist*, November:34–37, 2012.

Weger W. Current status and new developments in the treatment of psoriasis and psoriatic arthritis with biological agents. *Br J Pharmacol*. 160:810–820, 2010.

Davis*Plus* | See full color images of this topic on DavisPlus at **http://davisplus.fadavis.com** | Keyword: Fitzgerald

Seborrheic Dermatitis

98. Seborrheic dermatitis is likely caused by:
A. accelerated mitosis of skin cells.
B. colonization of skin by *Staphylococcus aureus*.
C. an inflammatory reaction to *Malassezia* species on skin.
D. exposure to excessive UV radiation.

99. Which of the following best describes seborrheic dermatitis lesions?
A. flaking lesions in the antecubital and popliteal spaces
B. greasy, scaling lesions in the nasolabial folds
C. intensely itchy lesions in the groin folds
D. silvery lesions on the elbows and knees

100. Among the following, who is at greatest risk of developing seborrheic dermatitis?
A. a 15-year-old boy residing in a rural setting
B. a 34-year-old woman who smokes 2 packs per day (PPD)
C. a 48-year-old male truck driver
D. a 72-year-old man with Parkinson disease

101. In counseling a patient with seborrheic dermatitis on the scalp about efforts to clear lesions, you advise her to:
A. use ketoconazole shampoo.
B. apply petroleum jelly nightly to the affected area.
C. coat the area with high-potency corticosteroid cream three times a week.
D. expose the lesions periodically to heat by carefully using a hair dryer.

102. A 64-year-old man with seborrhea mentions that his skin condition is "better in the summer when I get outside more and much worse in the winter." You respond:
A. Sun exposure is a recommended therapy for the treatment of this condition.
B. Although sun exposure is noted to improve the skin lesions associated with seborrhea, its use as a therapy is potentially associated with an increased rate of skin cancer.
C. The lower humidity in the summer months noted in many areas of North America contributes to the improvement in seborrheic lesions.
D. Use high-potency topical corticosteroids during the winter months, tapering these off for the summer months.

103. You see a 67-year-old man with seborrheic dermatitis that has failed to respond to treatment with ketoconazole shampoo. An appropriate second-line treatment option can include all of the following except:
A. oral fluconazole.
B. a topical immune modulator.
C. topical propylene glycol.
D. high-potency topical corticosteroid.

Answers

98. C.	**100.** D.	**102.** B.
99. B.	**101.** A.	**103.** D.

Seborrheic dermatitis is a chronic, recurrent skin condition found in areas with a high concentration of sebaceous glands, such as the scalp, eyelid margins, nasolabial folds, ears, and upper trunk. Numerous theories are proposed for its cause. Because of the lesions' response to antifungal agents, the backbone of therapy for the condition, seborrheic dermatitis is most likely caused by an inflammatory reaction to *Malassezia* species (formerly *Pityrosporum* species), a yeast form present on the scalp of all humans. Further supporting this hypothesis is the fact that seborrhea is often found in patients who are immunocompromised or chronically ill (e.g., elderly adults and people with Parkinson disease). *Malassezia* organisms are likely a cofactor linked to T-cell depression, increased sebum levels, and an activation of the alternative complement pathway.

Skin lesions associated with seborrhea usually respond to topical antifungals such as ketoconazole. Class IV or lower corticosteroid creams, lotions, or solutions are also helpful during a flare (see Table 3–3); topical immune modulators such as pimecrolimus and tacrolimus, sulfur or sulfonamide combinations, and propylene glycol offer additional treatment options. The use of lubricants such as petroleum jelly can help remove stubborn lesions so that the lesions can be exposed to antifungal therapy (e.g., selenium sulfide or ketoconazole shampoo). Systemic ketoconazole or fluconazole is occasionally used if seborrheic dermatitis is severe or unresponsive.

As with any skin condition, high-potency topical corticosteroid use is discouraged because of the risk of subcutaneous atrophy, telangiectatic vessels, and other problems. Although seborrhea usually worsens in the winter and improves in the summer, exposing lesions to sunlight is not recommended because of the potential increase in skin cancer risk and photoaging.

DISCUSSION SOURCES

Selden S. http://emedicine.medscape.com/article/1108312-overview#showall, Seborrheic dermatitis

Schmidt, JA. Seborrheic dermatitis: A clinical practice snapshot. *Nurse Pract* (8):36, 32–37, 2011.

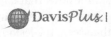 See full color images of this topic on DavisPlus at
http://davisplus.fadavis.com | Keyword: Fitzgerald

Skin Cancer

104. A 49-year-old man presents with a skin lesion suspicious for malignant melanoma. You describe the lesion as having:
A. deep black–brown coloring throughout.
B. sharp borders.
C. a diameter of 3 mm or less.
D. variable pigmentation.

105. The use of sunscreen has minimal impact on reducing the risk of which type of skin cancer?
A. squamous cell carcinoma
B. basal cell carcinoma
C. malignant melanoma
D. all forms of skin cancer

106. A 72-year-old woman presents with a newly formed, painless, pearly, ulcerated nodule with an overlying telangiectasis on the upper lip. This most likely represents:
A. an actinic keratosis.
B. a basal cell carcinoma.
C. a squamous cell carcinoma.
D. molluscum contagiosum.

107. Which of the following represents the most effective method of cancer screening?
A. skin examination
B. stool for occult blood
C. pelvic examination
D. chest radiography

108. When examining a mole for malignant melanoma, all of the following characteristics can indicate a melanoma except:
A. asymmetry with nonmatching sides.
B. color is not uniform.
C. a recently formed lesion.
D. a lesion that has been present for at least 2 years.

109. The most common sites for squamous and basal cell carcinoma include:
A. palms of hands and soles of feet.
B. pelvic and lumbar regions.
C. the abdomen.
D. the face and scalp.

110. A 56-year-old truck driver presents with a new nodular, opaque lesion with nondistinct borders on his left forearm. This most likely represents a(n):
A. actinic keratosis.
B. squamous cell carcinoma.
C. basal cell carcinoma.
D. malignant melanoma.

111. Risk factors for malignant melanoma include:
A. Asian ancestry.
B. history of blistering sunburn.
C. family history of psoriasis vulgaris.
D. presence of atopic dermatitis.

112. Definitive diagnosis of skin cancer requires:
A. skin examination.
B. CT scan.
C. biopsy.
D. serum antigen testing.

113. Nonsurgical options for the treatment of squamous and basal cell carcinoma include all of the following except:
A. cryotherapy.
B. electrodissection with curettage.
C. topical cancer chemotherapy.
D. oral hydroxyurea.

114. A skin biopsy results indicate the presence of malignant melanoma for a 53-year-old woman. You recommend:
A. excision of the entire lesion.
B. electrodissection with curettage.
C. initiating treatment with topical cancer chemotherapy.
D. consultation with a skin cancer expert to direct next best action.

115. Skin lesions associated with actinic keratoses can be described as:
A. a slightly rough, pink or flesh-colored lesion in a sun-exposed area.
B. a well-defined, slightly raised, red, scaly plaque in a skinfold.
C. a blistering lesion along a dermatome.
D. a crusting lesion along flexor aspects of the fingers.

116. Treatment options for actinic keratoses include topical:
A. vitamin D derivative cream.
B. 5-fluorouracil.
C. acyclovir.
D. doxepin.

117. Recommended nonpharmacological options to treat actinic keratosis include all of the following except:
A. chemical peel.
B. cryotherapy.
C. laser resurfacing.
D. Mohs micrographic surgery.

Answers

104. D.	109. D.	114. D.
105. C.	110. B.	115. A.
106. B.	111. B.	116. B.
107. A.	112. C.	117. D.
108. D.	113. D.	

As with any area of dermatology, accurate diagnosis of a condition depends on knowledge of the description of the lesion and its most likely site of occurrence. The most potent risk factor for any skin cancer is sun exposure; patients should be instructed on sun avoidance. The consistent use of high–sun protection factor (SPF) sunscreen is critical and helps reduce, but not eliminate, the risk of squamous or basal cell carcinoma. Sunscreen use likely does little to minimize malignant melanoma risk.

Skin examination has the benefit of enabling the examiner to detect premalignant lesions (e.g., actinic keratoses and other precursor lesions to squamous cell carcinoma including keratoacanthoma) and malignant lesions.

Malignant melanoma is a malignancy that arises from melanocytes, cells that make the pigment melanin, and is the most common fatal dermatologic malignancy. "ABCDE" is a mnemonic for assessing malignant melanoma:
A = asymmetric with nonmatching sides
B = borders are irregular
C = color is not uniform; brown, black, red, white, blue
D = diameter usually larger than 6 mm, or the size of a pencil eraser
E = evolving lesions, either new or changing (most melanomas manifest as new lesions)

The characteristics of basal cell carcinoma (BCC) include a long latency period and low metastatic risk. Depending on lesion location, untreated BCC can lead to significant deformity and possibly altered function. As a result, early recognition and intervention is recommended. To help with BCC, remember this mnemonic; "PUT ON" sunscreen":
P = pearly papule
U = ulcerating
T = telangiectasia
O = on the face, scalp, pinnae
N = nodules = slow growing

Compared with BCC, squamous cell carcinoma (SCC) tends to grow more rapidly and has a low but significant metastatic risk. Although difficult to distinguish from BCC

by skin examination alone, the mnemonic "NO SUN" can help with the identification of early SCC lesions:
N = nodular
O = opaque
S = sun-exposed areas
U = ulcerating
N = nondistinct borders

Later lesions may also include scale and firm margins.

Although the aforementioned mnemonics are helpful in identifying these lesions, diagnosis of cutaneous malignancy requires a biopsy. Intervention depends on biopsy results and final diagnosis. Therapy is usually surgical, involving removal of the lesion with a reasonable "clean" or disease-free margin. Mohs micrographic surgery is recommended in the presence of skin tumors with aggressive histologic patterns or invasive features. Nonsurgical options in BCC and SCC include destruction of the lesion with cryotherapy, electrodesiccation with curettage, focal radiation, and topical cancer chemotherapy. Intervention in malignant melanoma is based on additional factors including staging and sentinel node biopsy results; this requires expert opinion consultation.

Actinic keratoses are UV-induced skin lesions that can evolve into squamous cell carcinoma. Actinic keratoses begin as small rough spots that are easier felt than seen; the lesions are often best identified by rubbing the examining finger over the affected area and appreciating the sandpaper-like quality. Over time, the lesions enlarge, typically 3 to 10 mm in diameter, and usually become scaly and red, although color can vary. Treatment of actinic keratoses, also known as solar keratoses, includes cryotherapy with liquid nitrogen. This causes destruction of the lesions with resulting crust for about 2 weeks, revealing healed tissue and usually an excellent cosmetic outcome. Alternatives include the use of 1% to 5% fluorouracil creams once a day for 2 to 3 weeks until the lesions become crusted over. As another alternative, 5% fluorouracil cream can be used once a day for 1 to 2 days weekly for 7 to 10 weeks. This regimen yields a similar therapeutic outcome without crusting or discomfort. Additional options include 5% imiquimod cream, topical diclofenac gel, and photodynamic therapy (PDT) with topical delta-aminolevulinic acid. Resurfacing with chemical peels and laser are additional destructive treatment options for actinic keratoses.

DISCUSSION SOURCES

Latha MS, Martis J, Bellary S, et al. Sunscreening agents: A review. *J Clin Aesth Dermatol.* 6(1):16–26, 2013.

Ortel E, Bolotin D. Cancers of the skin. In: Rakel R, Bope E, eds. *Conn's Current Therapy 2013*. Philadelphia: Saunders, 2012, pp. 219–222.

James, WD, Berger TG, Elston, DM. *Andrews' Diseases of the Skin: Clinical Dermatology,* ed. 11. Philadelphia: Saunders, 2011, pp. 676, 685–690.

Spencer, JM. Elston, DM. http://emedicine.medscape.com/article/1099775-overview#showall

Rosen T, Lebwohl MG. Prevalence and awareness of actinic keratosis: barriers and opportunities. *J Am Acad Dermatol.* Jan;68(1 Suppl), 2013.

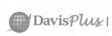
See full color images of this topic on DavisPlus at
http://davisplus.fadavis.com
Keyword: Fitzgerald

Urticaria

118. Type I hypersensitivity reaction is mediated through:
    A. TNF-α binding to T cells.
    B. IgG antibodies binding to T cells.
    C. IgE antibodies binding to mast cells.
    D. IL-10 binding to basophils.

119. Which of the following do you expect to find in the assessment of the person with urticaria?
    A. eosinophilia
    B. low erythrocyte sedimentation rate
    C. elevated thyroid-stimulating hormone level
    D. leukopenia

120. Common clinical conditions included in the atopy subgroup of type I hypersensitivity reactions include all of the following except:
    A. allergic rhinitis.
    B. rosacea.
    C. atopic dermatitis.
    D. allergic gastroenteropathy.

121. A 24-year-old woman presents with hive-form linear lesions that develop over areas where she has scratched. These resolve within a few minutes. This most likely represents:
    A. dermographism.
    B. contact dermatitis.
    C. angioedema.
    D. allergic reaction.

122. An urticarial lesion is usually described as a:
    A. wheal.
    B. plaque.
    C. patch.
    D. papule.

123. Common clinical manifestations of anaphylaxis can include all of the following except:
    A. upper airway edema.
    B. itch without rash.
    C. dizziness with syncope.
    D. hypertension.

124. Common triggers for anaphylaxis include exposure to certain types of all of the following except:
    A. medications.
    B. food.
    C. pet dander.
    D. insect bites.

125. You see a 28-year-old man who is having an anaphylactic reaction following a bee sting and is experiencing trouble breathing. Your initial response is to administer:
    A. oral antihistamine.
    B. injectable epinephrine.
    C. supplemental oxygen.
    D. vasopressor therapy.

Answers

118. C.	121. A.	124. C.
119. A.	122. A.	125. B.
120. B.	123. D.	

Urticaria is a condition in which eruptions of wheals or hives occur most often in response to allergen exposure. The most common cause is a type I hypersensitivity reaction. This type of reaction is caused when IgE antibodies occupy receptor sites on mast cells, causing degradation of the mast cell and subsequent release of histamine, vasodilation, mucous gland stimulation, and tissue swelling. As with most allergen-based conditions, eosinophilia, an increase in the number of circulating eosinophils, is usually present. Type I hypersensitivity reactions consist of two subgroups: atopy and anaphylaxis.

Urticarial lesions often develop as groups of intensely itchy wheals or hives. The lesions usually last less than 24 hours and often only 2 to 4 hours. New lesions can form, however, extending the outbreak to 1 to 2 weeks.

Many common clinical conditions are included in the atopy subgroup, such as allergic rhinitis, atopic dermatitis, allergic gastroenteropathy, and allergy-based asthma. Atopic diseases have a strong familial component and tend to cause localized rather than systemic reactions. The person with atopic disease is often able to identify allergy-inducing agents. In addition to avoidance of offending agents, treatment for systemic atopic disease includes antihistamines, topical corticosteroids, and leukotriene modifiers (zafirlukast [Accolate], montelukast [Singulair]); systemic corticosteroids are often needed for severe flares.

Anaphylaxis typically causes a systemic IgE-mediated reaction to exposure to an allergen, often a drug (e.g., penicillin), insect venom (e.g., bee sting), or food (e.g., peanuts). Anaphylaxis is characterized by a wide variation in presentation, ranging from an urticarial reaction being noted in its mildest form to the presence of widespread vasodilation, urticaria, angioedema, and bronchospasm creating a life-threatening condition of airway obstruction coupled with circulatory collapse. First-line treatment includes avoiding or discontinuing use of the offending agent. Parenteral epinephrine is the preferred initial drug therapy for anaphylaxis because of its multiple modes of reversing airway and circulatory dysfunction. In the presence of anaphylaxis, there are no contraindications to epinephrine use. Additional therapy is based on the clinical presentation. Simultaneously, maintaining airway patency and adequate circulation is critical. Angioedema and urticaria are subcutaneous anaphylactic reactions but are not life-threatening unless tissue swelling impinges on the airway (Tables 3–9 and 3–10).

DISCUSSION SOURCES

Linscott MS. http://www.emedicine.com/emerg/TOPIC628.HTM, eMedicine: Urticaria

American Academy of Allergy, Asthma & Immunology. Anaphylaxis: Tips to remember. http://www.aaaai.org/conditions-and-treatments/library/at-a-glance/anaphylaxis.aspx

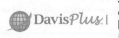 DavisPlus

See full color images of this topic on DavisPlus at
http://davisplus.fadavis.com |
Keyword: Fitzgerald

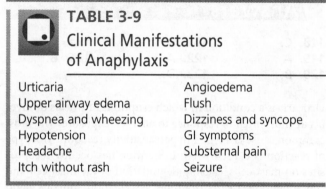

TABLE 3-9

Clinical Manifestations of Anaphylaxis

Urticaria	Angioedema
Upper airway edema	Flush
Dyspnea and wheezing	Dizziness and syncope
Hypotension	GI symptoms
Headache	Substernal pain
Itch without rash	Seizure

Note: Although urticaria and angioedema are most consistently reported, the clinical presentation of anaphylaxis can be quite variable.

Warts

126. When counseling a person who has a 2-mm verruca-form lesion on the hand, you advise that:
    A. bacteria are the most common cause of these lesions.
    B. lesions usually resolve without therapy in 12 to 24 months.
    C. there is a significant risk for future dermatologic malignancy.
    D. surgical excision is the treatment of choice.

127. The mechanism of action of imiquimod is as a/an:
    A. immunomodulator.
    B. antimitotic.
    C. keratolytic.
    D. irritant.

128. The most common human papillomavirus types associated with cutaneous, nongenital warts include:
    A. 1, 2, and 4.
    B. 6 and 11.
    C. 16 and 18.
    D. 32 and 36.

129. The human papillomavirus responsible for nongenital warts is mainly passed through:
    A. contact with infected surfaces.
    B. exposure to saliva from infected person.
    C. person-to-person contact.
    D. exposure to infected blood.

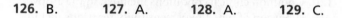

Answers

126. B.   **127.** A.   **128.** A.   **129.** C.

Verruca vulgaris lesions are also known as warts. Human papillomavirus types 1, 2, and 4 cause most nongenital warts; virus is passed through direct person-to-person contact. Over a 12- to 24-month period, nearly all lesions resolve without therapy. Surgical excision is rarely indicated. Intervention is warranted if warts interfere with function, such as with painful plantar warts on the soles of the feet, or if the lesions are cosmetically problematic (Table 3–11).

DISCUSSION SOURCES

Housman T, Williford P. Warts (verrucae). In: Rakel R, Bope E, eds. *Conn's Current Therapy 2008*. Philadelphia: Saunders, 2008, pp. 811–815.

Dall'oglio F, D'Amico V, Nasca MR, Micali G. Treatment of cutaneous warts: An evidence-based review. *Am J Clin Dermatol.* 13:73–96, 2012.

TABLE 3-10

Treatment of Anaphylaxis in Patient With Currently Patent Airway

Intervention	Comment
Immediate SC or IM administration of epinephrine	No contraindications to epinephrine use in anaphylaxis
	Failure to or delay in use associated with fatalities
Administer antihistamine such as diphenhydramine (Benadryl)	An important part of anaphylaxis treatment but should be used only with, not instead of, epinephrine
Additional measures as dictated by patient response	Airway maintenance including supplemental oxygen
	IV fluids, vasopressor therapy corticosteroids
	Repeat epinephrine every 5 minutes if symptoms persist or increase
	Repeat antihistamine with or without H_2 blocker if symptoms persist
	Observe as dictated by patient response, keeping in mind that anaphylaxis reactions often have a protracted or biphasic response
Arrange follow-up care	Provide instruction on avoidance of provoking agent
	Give epinephrine autoinjector (EpiPen) and safety of use prescription with appropriate education about indications

IM, intramuscular; IV, intravenous; SC, subcutaneous.
Source: http://www.aaaai.org/conditions-and-treatments/library/at-a-glance/anaphylaxis.aspx

TABLE 3-11
Treatment Options for Warts

Treatment	Instructions for Use	Comments
Liquid nitrogen	Apply to achieve a thaw time of 20–45 seconds Two freeze–thaw cycles may be administered every 2–4 weeks until lesion is gone	Usually good cosmetic results Can be painful, requires multiple treatments
Keratolytic agents (Cantharidin, Occlusal, Duofilm, DuoPlant, ViraSal, others)	Apply as directed until lesions resolve	Often needs long-term therapy before resolution Well tolerated With plantar warts, pare down lesion, then apply 40% salicylic acid plaster, changing every 5 days
Podophyllum resin (podofilox)	Patient applies three times a week for 4–6 weeks	Multiple cycles often needed Skin irritation common
Tretinoin	Apply bid to flat warts for 4–6 weeks	Needs consistent treatment for optimal results
Imiquimod (Aldara)	Frequency and duration of use depend on wart location	Immunomodulator Low rate of wart recurrence
Laser therapy	Used to dissect lesions	Needs 4–6 weeks to granulate tissue Best reserved for treatment-resistant warts

Source: Rosen AE. Warts (verrucae). In: Rakel R, Bope E, eds. *Conn's Current Therapy 2013*. Philadelphia: Saunders, 2012, p. 294.

Cellulitis

130. A 62-year-old woman presents 2 days after noticing a "bug bite" on her left forearm. Examination reveals a warm, red, edematous area with sharply demarcated borders. The patient is otherwise healthy with no fever. This most likely represents:
    A. contact dermatitis.
    B. an allergic reaction.
    C. cellulitis.
    D. erysipelas.

131. Which of the following statements is most accurate regarding cellulitis?
    A. Insect bites, abrasion, or other skin trauma can be the origin of cellulitis.
    B. Cellulitis most often occurs on the chest and abdomen.
    C. Necrosis is a common complication of cellulitis.
    D. Cellulitis often occurs spontaneously without any identifiable skin wound.

132. The most common causative organisms in cellulitis are:
    A. *Escherichia coli* and *Haemophilus influenzae*.
    B. *Bacteroides* species and other anaerobes.
    C. group A beta-hemolytic streptococci and *S. aureus*.
    D. pathogenic viruses.

133. Which of the following is the best treatment option for cellulitis when risk of infection with a methicillin-resistant pathogen is considered low?
    A. dicloxacillin
    B. amoxicillin
    C. metronidazole
    D. trimethoprim-sulfamethoxazole

Answers

130. C.   131. A.   132. C.   133. A.

Cellulitis is an acute infection of the subcutaneous tissue and skin, typically as part of a skin wound, such as an insect bite, surgical incision, abrasion, or other cutaneous trauma. The clinical presentation includes a warm, red, edematous area with sharply demarcated borders; lymphangitis, lymphadenitis, and, rarely, necrosis can also occur. Cellulitis is most commonly found in the extremities. The causative pathogen is usually a gram-positive organism such as group A beta-hemolytic streptococci and *S. aureus*. Rarely, particularly in immunocompromised individuals, certain gram-negative organisms are the causative agent.

Treatment for cellulitis involves the choice of an antimicrobial agent with strong gram-positive coverage (in streptococcal and staphylococcal infection); resistant pathogens, including methicillin-resistant *S. aureus* (MRSA), must be considered. Treatment options for cellulitis when MRSA risk is considered low include dicloxacillin. With significant

MRSA risk, or when cellulitis surrounds an area of furunculosis or abscess, treatment should be aimed at treating MRSA and streptococcal infection (see next section on MRSA). In addition to antimicrobial treatment, other actions that can help facilitate resolution of cellulitis include applying warm compresses to the affected area, keeping the affected limb rested, and elevating the affected area when possible.

DISCUSSION SOURCES

Gilbert D, Moellering R, Eliopoulos G, Chambers H, Saag M. *The Sanford Guide to Antimicrobial Therapy*, ed. 44. Sperryville, VA: Antimicrobial Therapy, Inc., 2014, pp. 254–256.

Stevens DL. Bacterial diseases of the skin. In: Rakel R, Bope E, eds. *Conn's Current Therapy 2013*. Philadelphia: Saunders, 2012, pp. 211–214.

DavisPlus | See full color images of this topic on DavisPlus at http://davisplus.fadavis.com | Keyword: Fitzgerald

Staphylococcus aureus Infection

134. You see a 36-year-old man with no chronic health problems who presents with two furuncles, each around 4 cm in diameter, on the right anterior thigh. These lesions have been present for 3 days, slightly increasing in size during this time. He has no fever or other systemic symptoms. You advise the following:
A. incision and drainage of the lesion
B. a systemic antibiotic empirically
C. a topical antibiotic
D. aspiration of the lesion contents and prescription of a systemic antibiotic based on culture results

135. A woman was treated as an inpatient for a serious soft tissue infection with parenteral linezolid and now is being seen on day 3 of her illness and is being discharged to home. She is feeling better and appears by examination to be clinically improved. Culture results reveal MRSA, sensitive to trimethoprim-sulfamethoxazole, linezolid, daptomycin, vancomycin, and clindamycin and resistant to cephalothin and erythromycin. Her antimicrobial therapy should be completed with:
A. oral cephalexin.
B. oral trimethoprim-sulfamethoxazole.
C. parenteral vancomycin.
D. oral linezolid.

Answer the following questions true or false

136. Skin lesions infected by community-acquired MRSA (CA-MRSA) often occur spontaneously on intact skin.

137. CA-MRSA is most commonly spread from one person to another via airborne pathogen transmission.

138. All CA-MRSA strains are capable of causing necrotizing infection.

139. The mechanism of resistance of MRSA is via the production of beta-lactamase.

140. If a skin and soft tissue infection does not improve in 48 to 72 hours with antimicrobial therapy, infection with a resistant pathogen is virtually the only cause.

141. Most acute-onset necrotic skin lesions reported in North America are caused by spider bites.

142. In an adult with BMI greater than 40 kg/m2 who is being treated with TMP-SMX for CA-MRSA, the recommended dose is two tablets bid.

Answers

134. A.	**137.** False	**140.** False
135. B.	**138.** False	**141.** False
136. False	**139.** False	**142.** True

Staphylococcus aureus is a ubiquitous gram-positive organism that normally grows on the skin and mucous membranes and is a common cause of skin and soft tissue infections. Strains of *S. aureus* that produce beta-lactamase, which is an enzyme capable of neutralizing penicillins, were first noted in the 1940s and became the dominant community and hospital pathogenic forms of the organism from the 1950s through the early 2000s. During that time, *S. aureus* skin and soft tissue infections were treated with antimicrobials possessing activity against gram-positive organisms and had stability in the presence of beta-lactamase, such as the macrolides (erythromycin, azithromycin, clarithromycin), certain cephalosporins (e.g., cephalexin, cefadroxil), and semisynthetic penicillin forms that possess beta-lactamase stability (dicloxacillin, methicillin [no longer used clinically], oxacillin, nafcillin). As a result, these strains are known as methicillin-sensitive *S. aureus* (MSSA). An additional treatment option was an antimicrobial with a beta-lactamase inhibitor, such as amoxicillin-clavulanate. In the past 3-4 decades, strains of *S. aureus* resistant to methicillin (MRSA) evolved into an important pathogen in infection associated with hospitals and long-term-care facilities. Until the early 2000s, however, MRSA was seldom noted in the community.

Across the United States, disease caused by MRSA acquired in the community (known as community-acquired or community-associated MRSA [CA-MRSA]) has been reported with increasing frequency. CA-MRSA is not simply an organism that has escaped the healthcare facility and taken up residence in the community; in contrast to healthcare-associated MRSA (HC-MRSA), in which numerous clones have been identified, two major clones are responsible for most CA-MRSA. One of these clones was implicated in a worldwide infectious disease outbreak more than 60 years ago. CA-MRSA infections usually involve the skin and soft tissues in the form of cellulitis, bullous impetigo, folliculitis, abscess, or an infected laceration. Less common is CA-MRSA–associated disease in the form of blood, bone, or joint infection or pneumonia. The Panton-Valentine leukocidin (PVL) toxin is present in approximately 77% of CA-MRSA strains and is less common in healthcare–associated MRSA strains. The PVL toxin promotes lysis of human leukocytes, and it is associated with severe necrotizing skin infections and hemorrhagic pneumonia.

CA-MRSA is usually acquired during person-to-person, skin-to-skin contact, but inanimate objects such as countertops or other surfaces also contribute to CA-MRSA transmission. Although MRSA acquired in healthcare facilities usually affects frail individuals, CA-MRSA is found predominately in otherwise healthy children and adults. Bearing this in mind, CA-MRSA infection does appear more common in low income populations and in certain ethnic groups, including African Americans and Native Americans. Additional risks include living in crowded conditions such as correctional facilities, participating in occupational or recreational activities with regular skin-to-skin contact such as wrestling, exposure to a person with CA-MRSA, and recent use of an antibiotic or recurrent skin infection (or both). Prevention of CA-MRSA includes appropriate hand hygiene, reduction of unnecessary skin-to-skin contact, and thorough cleaning of surfaces with a disinfectant solution.

The choice of therapy for skin and soft tissue infection must take into consideration issues of antimicrobial resistance and minimizing unnecessary antimicrobial use. In an afebrile patient with an abscess less than 5 cm in diameter, the first-line treatment of community-acquired skin and soft tissue infection is incision, drainage, and localized care such as warm soaks. A wound culture and sensitivity should be obtained to help guide treatment. If the abscess is equal to or greater than 5 cm in diameter, antimicrobial therapy should be added to the aforementioned localized treatment.

Given that the antimicrobials effective against MSSA (certain cephalosporins, penicillins, penicillin with beta-lactamase inhibitor combinations, and select macrolides) are ineffective in CA-MRSA, documentation of the organism's pattern of resistance can help direct therapy. Most strains of CA-MRSA remain sensitive to trimethoprim-sulfamethoxazole (TMP-SMX, Bactrim), doxycycline, or clindamycin. Given cost and efficacy, TMP-SMX is the primary antimicrobial therapy recommended, particularly in a person who is immunocompetent and without fever. Because successful therapy depends on achieving adequate concentration of the antimicrobial at the site of the infection, the recommended TMP-SMX dose is 1 double-strength tablets for 5 to 10 days, but duration should be individualized on the basis of the patient's clinical response; with BMI > 40 kg.m2, TMP-SMX 2 tablets bid is recommended.

In patients who are intolerant of sulfa drugs, alternatives to TMP-SMX therapy include doxycycline or minocycline.

Linezolid (Zyvox) is another effective, albeit expensive, oral treatment option, which is usually reserved for use when the aforementioned medications are not tolerated or ineffective. When parenteral treatment is needed, commonly used management options include linezolid, vancomycin, and daptomycin. Daptomycin is not indicated in the treatment of pneumonia.

Although TMP-SMX is usually active against CA-MRSA, its coverage against streptococcus is uncertain. If the causative pathogen of the skin and soft tissue infection is unclear and streptococcal infection is considered a possibility, such as is seen in cellulitis or erysipelas, the antimicrobial choice should be aimed at medications that provide coverage against staphylococci and streptococci. In this situation, using TMP-SMX with a beta-lactam such as a cephalosporin is recommended.

A person with CA-MRSA infection requires careful follow-up to ensure clinical resolution. Post-treatment cultures are unnecessary. Serious disease such as pneumonia or death resulting from CA-MRSA is, in many locations, a reportable disease.

As mentioned, the clinical presentation of CA-MRSA is usually as a cutaneous and soft tissue lesion in the form of boils and abscesses. Because a CA-MRSA lesion often has a dark or black center, the condition has often been attributed to a spider bite. In reality, spider bites are uncommon, usually occurring only when the arachnid is trapped in clothing or a shoe. In addition, few spider species have the capability of causing a significant bite. In particular, the brown recluse spider, or *Loxosceles reclusa,* can cause a necrotizing bite and is often blamed for lesions that are actually caused by CA-MRSA. Found primarily in the U.S. Midwest and Southeast, this arachnid hibernates during the winter, so bites, which are generally painless, occur between March and October. The term *recluse* depicts a shy creature that typically hides in shoes, boxes, and other small enclosed spaces. A single spider is occasionally spotted outside of its native region, having traveled in a suitcase or box. Only a small proportion of brown recluse spider bites become necrotic. When this occurs, a characteristic pattern known as the "red, white, and blue" sign follows, with a central purple-to-gray discoloration surrounded by a white ring of blanched skin and a large red halo. If necrosis occurs, a black eschar forms.

DISCUSSION SOURCES

Gilbert D, Moellering R, Eliopoulos G, Chambers H, Saag M. *The Sanford Guide to Antimicrobial Therapy,* ed. 44. Sperryville, VA: Antimicrobial Therapy, Inc., 2014, p. 52.

CA-MRSA Definition, symptoms, diagnosing, treatment, statistics-http://www.cdc.gov/mrsa/

James, WD, Berger TG, Elston, DM. *Andrews' Diseases of the Skin: Clinical Dermatology,* ed. 11. Philadelphia: Saunders, 2011, pp. 8, 414–447.

Herchline, TE. Cunha, BA. Staphylococcal infections. http://emedicine.medscape.com/article/228816-overview#showall, accessed 7/20/2013.

Centers for Disease Control. Venomous spider identification, prevention, symptoms and first aid for consumers. http://www.cdc.gov/niosh/topics/spiders/

Angular Cheilitis

143. An 88-year-old, community-dwelling man who lives alone has limited mobility because of osteoarthritis. Since his last office visit 2 months ago, he has lost 5% of his body weight and has developed angular cheilitis. You expect to find the following on examination:
    A. fissuring and cracking at the corners of the mouth
    B. marked erythema of the hard and soft palates
    C. white plaques on the lateral borders of the buccal mucosa
    D. raised, painless lesions on the gingival

144. A common cause of angular cheilitis is infection by:
    A. *Escherichia coli.*
    B. *Streptococcus pneumoniae.*
    C. *Candida* species.
    D. *Aspergillus* species.

145. Risk factors for angular cheilitis in adults include all of the following except:
    A. advanced age.
    B. HIV infection.
    C. alteration of facial vertical dimension due to loss of teeth.
    D. obesity.

146. First-line therapy for angular cheilitis therapy includes the use of:
    A. metronidazole gel.
    B. hydrocortisone cream.
    C. topical nystatin.
    D. oral ketoconazole.

Answers

143. A.   144. C.   145. D.   146. C.

Various oral and perioral infections are caused by *Candida* species, including angular cheilitis, also known as angular stomatitis, perlèche, or cheilosis. A major candidiasis risk factor is an immunocompromised state, whether resulting from advanced age, malnutrition, or HIV infection. In addition, physical characteristics can increase the risk for angular cheilitis, such as in an older adult who has a loss of vertical facial dimension because of loss of teeth, allowing for overclosure of the mouth; the resulting skin folds create a suitable environment for *Candida* growth.

Topical antifungals such as nystatin offer a reasonable first-line treatment for perioral and oral candidiasis. With particularly recalcitrant conditions and failure of topical therapy, systemic antifungals are occasionally needed. Treatment of the underlying condition is critical, as is maintenance of skin integrity through hygienic practices and skin lubrication.

DISCUSSION SOURCES

http://www.merckmanuals.com/home/mouth_and_dental_disorders/lip_and_toxngue_disorders/lip_disorders.html, Merck Manual online: Mouth, dental/lip and tongue disorders

Barankin B. http://www.ncbi.nlm.nih.gov/pmc/articles/PMC1949217/, National Institute of Health, angular cheilitis

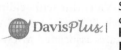

See full color images of this topic on DavisPlus at **http://davisplus.fadavis.com** | Keyword: Fitzgerald

Lyme Disease

147. A 29-year-old woman has a sudden onset of right-sided facial asymmetry. She is unable to close her right eyelid tightly or frown or smile on the affected side. Her examination is otherwise unremarkable. This likely represents paralysis of cranial nerve:
    A. III.
    B. IV.
    C. VII.
    D. VIII.

148. Which of the following represents the most important diagnostic test for the patient in the previous question?
    A. complete blood cell count with white blood cell differential
    B. serum testing for *Borrelia burgdorferi* infection
    C. computed tomography (CT) scan of the head with contrast enhancement
    D. serum protein electrophoresis

149. To transmit the bacterium that causes Lyme disease, an infected tick must feed on a human host for at least:
    A. 5 minutes.
    B. 30 minutes.
    C. 2 hours.
    D. 24 hours.

150. Lyme disease is caused by the bacterium:
    A. *Borrelia burgdorferi.*
    B. *Bacillus anthracis.*
    C. *Corynebacterium striatum.*
    D. *Treponema pallidum.*

151. Which of the following findings is often found in a person with stage 1 Lyme disease?
    A. peripheral neuropathic symptoms
    B. high-grade atrioventricular heart block
    C. Bell's palsy
    D. single painless annular lesion

152. Which of the following findings is often found in a person with stage 2 Lyme disease?
    A. peripheral neuropathic symptoms
    B. atrioventricular heart block
    C. conductive hearing loss
    D. macrocytic anemia

153. Stage 3 Lyme disease, characterized by joint pain and neuropsychiatric symptoms, typically occurs how long after initial infection?
A. 1 month
B. 4 months
C. 1 year
D. 5 years

154. Preferred antimicrobials for the treatment of adults with Lyme disease include all of the following except:
A. a tetracycline.
B. an aminoglycoside.
C. a cephalosporin.
D. a penicillin.

155. Which of the following would not be recommended to prevent Lyme disease when visiting a Lyme-endemic area?
A. Wear long pants and long-sleeved shirts.
B. Use insect repellent.
C. If a tick bite occurs, wait until after consulting a healthcare provider before removing the insect.
D. If a tick bite occurs and the tick is engorged, administer a single 200-mg dose of doxycycline.

● Answers

147. C.	**150.** A.	**153.** C.
148. B.	**151.** D.	**154.** B.
149. D.	**152.** B.	**155.** C.

Lyme disease is a multisystem infection caused by *B. burgdorferi,* a tick-transmitted spirochete. Although original reports of this disease, also known as Lyme borreliosis, were clustered through select areas of the United States, primarily in the Northeast and Mid-Atlantic states, it has now been diagnosed in every state. The disease's name comes from the town of Old Lyme, Connecticut, where it was first diagnosed after a community epidemic of rash and arthritis. Lyme disease is the most common vector-borne disease in the United States. Overdiagnosis of Lyme disease is a problem, as is the issue of significant but understandable anxiety about any tick exposure. Infected ticks must feed on the human host for more than 24 hours to transmit the spirochete. In addition, not all ticks are infected, with rates varying from 15% to 65% in areas where Lyme disease is endemic.

Lyme disease is typically divided into three stages:
Stage 1 (early localized disease): This is a mild flulike illness, often with a single annular lesion with central clearing (erythema migrans). The lesion is rarely pruritic or painful. Signs and symptoms can resolve in 3 to 4 weeks without treatment.
Stage 2 (early disseminated infection): Typically months later, the classic rash may reappear with multiple lesions, usually accompanied by arthralgias, myalgia, headache, and fatigue. Less commonly, cardiac manifestations such as heart block and neurological findings such as acute facial nerve paralysis (Bell's palsy) and aseptic meningitis may also be present. Individuals with Bell's palsy should undergo careful examination and serological testing for Lyme disease. Regression of symptoms can occur without treatment.
Stage 3 (late persistent infection): Starting approximately 1 year after the initial infection, musculoskeletal signs and symptoms usually persist, ranging from joint pain with no objective findings to frank arthritis with evidence of joint damage. Neuropsychiatric symptoms can appear, including memory problems, depression, and neuropathy.

Serum testing for *B. burgdorferi* by enzyme-linked immunosorbent assay and a confirmatory Western blot assay for IgM antibodies help to support the clinical diagnosis of Lyme disease; IgM antibodies decline to low levels after 4 to 6 months of illness, whereas IgG is noted about 6 to 8 weeks after onset of symptoms and often persists at low levels despite successful treatment. Careful correlation of patient history and physical examination and astute interpretation of laboratory diagnostics are critical to prevent overdiagnosing and underdiagnosing this condition.

Effective antimicrobials for treatment of Lyme disease include doxycycline, cefuroxime axetil (Ceftin), amoxicillin, and select macrolides. The clinician needs to be aware of the latest recommendation for dosage and duration of treatment with these products; recommendations include treatment for 14 to 21 days for earlier disease and up to 28 days with more advanced disease. Most adults with Lyme disease recover in weeks with appropriate treatment, although some have a late relapse.

Prevention of Lyme disease includes avoiding areas with known or potential tick infestation, wearing long-sleeved shirts and pants, and using insect repellents. Inspecting the skin and clothing for ticks with appropriate tick removal is also helpful. If a tick bite occurs, a single 200-mg dose of doxycycline taken orally appears to be effective in reducing Lyme disease risk if the tick is engorged and the patient lives or has visited a Lyme-endemic area; observation is also a reasonable option given the low rate of infection after tick bite, particularly with nonengorged tick bite in low risk areas.

DISCUSSION SOURCES

American Lyme Disease Foundation. http://www.aldf.com/lyme.shtml. Symptoms, diagnosis and treatment of Lyme disease
Centers for Disease Control and Prevention. http://www.cdc.gov/lyme/. Lyme disease, Symptoms, prevention, diagnosis, treatment and tick identification
Wormser GP, Dattwyler RJ, Shapiro ED, et al. The clinical assessment, treatment, and prevention of Lyme disease, human granulocytic anaplasmosis, and babesiosis: Clinical practice guidelines by the Infectious Diseases Society of America. *Clin Infect Dis.* 43:1089_1034, 2006. Available at: http://www.idsociety.org/uploadedFiles/IDSA/Guidelines-Patient_Care/PDF_Library/Lyme%20Disease.pdf, accessed 7/28/13.

Bed Bugs (*Cimex lectularius*)

156. All of the following characteristics about bed bugs are true except:
   A. they can be found in furniture, carpeting, and floorboards.
   B. their peak feeding time is at dawn.
   C. during feeding, they are attracted to body heat and carbon dioxide.
   D. they prefer to harbor unsanitary environments.

157. All of the following statements are true regarding skin reactions to bed bugs except:
   A. skin reactions are more common with repeated exposure to bed bug bites.
   B. skin reactions can typically involve papules, macules, or wheals.
   C. allergic reactions can be treated with topical corticosteroids.
   D. systemic skin reactions frequently occur following an initial exposure to bed bug bites.

158. You see a 42-year-old woman with a cluster of red, itchy spots on her left arm. She informs you that she recently stayed at a hotel that she later discovered was infested with bed bugs. You advise her that:
   A. she should immediately begin a regimen of oral antibiotics.
   B. the reaction is usually self-limiting and should resolve in 1 to 2 weeks.
   C. given that bed bug bites are usually not itchy, an alternative diagnosis should be considered.
   D. she should wash all of her clothes in cold water.

159. Signs that bed bugs are present in a home include all of the following except:
   A. small drops of fresh blood on floorboards.
   B. blood smears on bed sheets.
   C. presence of light brown exoskeletons.
   D. dark specks found along mattress seams.

160. Nonchemical means to eliminate bed bugs can include all of the following except:
   A. vacuuming crevices.
   B. washing bedding and other items in hot water.
   C. isolating the infested area from any hosts for at least 2 weeks.
   D. running bedding and other items in a dryer on high heat for 20 minutes.

Answers

156. D.	**158.** B.	**160.** C.
157. D.	**159.** A.	

Bed bugs (*Cimex lectularius*) are parasitic insects belonging to the family Cimicidae and are typically less than 1 cm in length and reddish brown in color. Bed bug infestations have been increasing worldwide, likely because of increased resistance to insecticides, such as pyrethroid insecticides, and a ban on the use of DDT. They can be found in furniture, floorboards, carpeting, peeling paint, areas of clutter, or other small spaces. Bed bugs do not have a preference for clean or unsanitary environments; they are found even in pristine homes and hotels. These parasites only need a warm host and hiding places. The insects come out at night to feed on the blood of a host, with peak feeding times just before dawn. They are typically attracted to body heat, carbon dioxide, vibration, sweat, and odor.

Confirming a diagnosis of a bed bug bite can be difficult, and a history of the home environment, work conditions, and presence of domestic animals should be obtained. Bed bug bites are usually red (often with a darker red spot in the middle); itchy; arranged in a rough line or in a cluster; and located on the face, neck, arms, and hands. Repeated exposure to bed bug bites can lead to skin reactions. Cutaneous reactions can include macules, papules, wheals, vesicles, bullae, and nodules. These reactions are typically self-limited and resolve within 1 to 2 weeks. Treatment of bites is not usually required. If a secondary infection occurs, treat with an antiseptic lotion or topical antibiotic. For allergic reactions, topical corticosteroids or oral antihistamines may be helpful. A disseminated bullous eruption with systemic reaction caused by bed bug bites may occur, but this is rare.

If bed bug bites are suspected, the home should be thoroughly inspected for insects. The inspection may need to be performed at night when the insects are active. Signs for the presence of bed bugs include dark specks typically found along the mattress seams, light brown empty exoskeletons, or bloody smears on bed sheets (due to crushing an engorged bed bug during sleep). Eliminating bed bugs can be difficult because they can live for weeks without feeding. If bed bugs are present in a home, professional extermination is recommended. A combination of pesticides and nonchemical treatments may be used. Nonchemical treatments can include vacuuming crevices where the insects may be present, washing clothes and other items in hot water (at least 120°F), placing items in a clothes dryer at medium to high heat for at least 20 minutes, or freezing items, preferably in a freezer that is set for 0 degrees F (-17°C), for at least 4 days.

DISCUSSION SOURCE

Studdiford JS, Conniff KM, Trayes KP, Tully AS. Bedbug infestation. *Am Fam Physician*. 86:653–658, 2012.

Rosacea

161. All of the following organisms have been implicated in the development of rosacea except:
   A. viruses.
   B. bacteria.
   C. yeast.
   D. mites.

162. Patients with rosacea are recommended to use daily:
    A. sunscreen.
    B. astringents.
    C. exfoliant.
    D. antimicrobial cream.

163. Topical therapies for the treatment of rosacea include all of the following except:
    A. metronidazole cream.
    B. azelaic acid gel.
    C. medium-potency corticosteroid cream.
    D. benzoyl peroxide.

164. Oral antimicrobial treatments recommended for rosacea include all of the following except:
    A. metronidazole.
    B. levofloxacin.
    C. erythromycin.
    D. doxycycline.

165. Which of the following is not a recommended option to make cosmetic improvements for phymatous rosacea?
    A. laser peel
    B. ablative laser surgery
    C. surgical shave technique
    D. mechanical dermabrasion

Answers

161. A.	163. C.	165. B.
162. A.	164. B.	

Rosacea is a common condition characterized by symptoms of facial flushing and a spectrum of clinical signs, including erythema, telangiectasia, and inflammatory papulopustular eruptions resembling acne. The symptoms are usually intermittent but can progressively lead to permanently flushed skin and, in some cases, permanent telangiectasia. The cause of rosacea is unknown, although inflammation plays a critical role in pathogenesis. Several organisms on the skin have been implicated in the development of rosacea. The *Demodex* species of mites that normally inhabit human hair follicles tend to prefer skin regions affected by rosacea. Bacterial species, such as *Helicobacter pylori* and *Staphylococcus aureus*, and yeast (*Malassezia* species) are also thought to contribute to the development of rosacea and would explain the effects of antimicrobials in the treatment of rosacea. Triggers for rosacea flares can be varied and specific for individual patients and can include UV/sunlight exposure, hot/cold exposure, exercise, stress, coffee, chocolate, caffeine, alcohol, spicy foods, and certain cosmetic products or medications.

The goal of treatment is to minimize the signs and symptoms of the disease. Rosacea can be classified into four subtypes with treatment selection guided by this classification. The erythematotelangiectatic type involves central facial flushing often accompanied by burning or stinging. Papulopustular rosacea typically affects middle-age women who present with a red central portion of their face that contains erythematous papules surmounted by pinpoint pustules. Phymatous rosacea is defined by marked skin thickenings and irregular surface nodularities of the nose, chin, forehead, one or both ears, and/or the eyelids. Ocular rosacea can include a variety of manifestations, including blepharitis, conjunctivitis, inflammation of the lids, and conjunctival telangiectasias.

Prior to initiating therapy for rosacea, the triggers for rosacea should be identified and lifestyle modifications should be made to minimize exposure to these triggers. The daily use of sunscreen is recommended for all patients with rosacea. Patients should also avoid the use of astringents, toners, menthols, camphor, exfoliants, waterproof cosmetics that require solvents for removal, or products containing sodium laurel sulfate. Nonablative lasers can be effective in remodeling the dermal connective tissue and improving the epidermal barrier. Typically, one to three treatment sessions are needed to achieve the best results. Mechanical dermabrasion, laser peel, and surgical shave techniques can be used to achieve cosmetic improvements of phymatous rosacea.

Effective treatment of rosacea may involve a combination of topical and oral medications. Topical treatments for rosacea include antimicrobials, immunosuppresants, and acne products. Metronidazole gel (0.75% or 1%) is commonly used as a first-line agent. Other topical antimicrobial options include erythromycin and clindamycin. Acne products can be effective for patients with papules, pustules, and the phymatous and glandular types of rosacea. Topical products can include azelaic acid, sulfacetamide products, benzoyl peroxide, or retinoid-like agents (i.e., isotretinoin and tretinoin). Dapsone can be considered in patients with severe, refractory rosacea or those who cannot take isotretinoin. Tacrolimus ointment (Protopic) inhibits immune reactions by blocking the release of cytokines from T-cells and can be helpful in reducing itching and inflammation. Tacrolimus should only be considered after other treatment options have failed. Use of topical medium and high-potency corticosteroids on the face should be avoided because it can produce rosacea-like symptoms or worsen pre-existing rosacea. Oral antibiotics may also be considered, more for their anti-inflammatory properties than for their antimicrobial activity. Oral antibiotic options include minocycline, doxycycline, tetracycline, metronidazole, or erythromycin. Oral isotretinoin may also be useful in patients whose rosacea does not respond to other therapies. However, the patient and provider need to be aware of potentially serious adverse effects associated with its use (see Table 3–4).

DISCUSSION SOURCES

Van Onselen J. Rosacea: Symptoms and support. *Br J Nurs.* 21: 1252–1255, 2012.
Baldwin HE. Diagnosis and treatment of rosacea: State of the art. *J Drugs Dermatol.* 11:725–730, 2012.

Eye, Ear, Nose, and Throat Problems

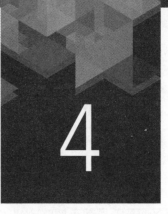

4

Conjunctivitis

1. A 19-year-old man presents with a chief complaint of a red, irritated right eye for the past 48 hours with eyelids that were "stuck together" this morning when he awoke. Examination reveals injected palpebral and bulbar conjunctiva and reactive pupils; vision screen with the Snellen chart evaluation reveals 20/30 in the right eye (OD), left eye (OS), and both eyes (OU); and purulent eye discharge on the right. This presentation is most consistent with:
   A. suppurative conjunctivitis.
   B. viral conjunctivitis.
   C. allergic conjunctivitis.
   D. mechanical injury.

2. A 19-year-old woman presents with a complaint of bilaterally itchy, red eyes with tearing that occurs intermittently throughout the year and is often accompanied by a rope-like eye discharge and clear nasal discharge. This is most consistent with conjunctival inflammation caused by a(n):
   A. bacterium.
   B. virus.
   C. allergen.
   D. injury.

3. Common causative organisms of acute suppurative conjunctivitis include all of the following except:
   A. *Staphylococcus aureus*.
   B. *Haemophilus influenzae*.
   C. *Streptococcus pneumoniae*.
   D. *Pseudomonas aeruginosa*.

4. Treatment options in suppurative conjunctivitis include all of the following ophthalmic preparations except:
   A. polymyxin B plus trimethoprim.
   B. levofloxacin.
   C. polymyxin.
   D. azithromycin.

5. Treatment options in acute and recurrent allergic conjunctivitis include all of the following except:
   A. cromolyn ophthalmic drops.
   B. oral antihistamines.
   C. ophthalmological antihistamines.
   D. corticosteroid ophthalmic drops.

6. The most common virological cause of conjunctivitis is:
   A. coronavirus.
   B. adenovirus.
   C. rhinovirus.
   D. human papillomavirus.

7. Treatment of viral conjunctivitis can include:
   A. moxifloxacin ophthalmic drops.
   B. polymyxin B ophthalmic drops.
   C. oral acyclovir.
   D. no antibiotic therapy needed.

Answers

1. A.	4. C.	7. D.
2. C.	5. D.	
3. D.	6. B.	

Because therapy in conjunctivitis is in part aimed at eradicating or eliminating the underlying causes, accurate diagnosis is critical. A patient with a presumptive diagnosis of suppurative conjunctivitis is usually treated with an ocular antimicrobial, though the presumptive bacterial infection will usually clear with local measures such as warm compresses and eye hygiene; the use of an ocular antimicrobial minimizes the risk of contagion and shortens the course of the illness. In viral conjunctivitis, the person usually also demonstrates signs and symptoms of viral upper respiratory tract infection; no antibacterial therapy is needed as the risk of superimposed bacterial infection is minimal. No treatment is needed for most cases of viral conjunctivitis as the virus will run its course over 2–3 weeks. For a person with allergic conjunctivitis, therapy should be focused on identifying and limiting exposure to specific allergens and the appropriate use of antiallergic agents (antihistamines or mast cell stabilizers) (Tables 4–1 and 4–2).

DISCUSSION SOURCES

Gilbert DN, Moellering RC, Eliopoulos GM, Chambers HF, Saag MS. *The Sanford Guide to Antimicrobial Therapy*. 44th ed. Sperryville, VA: Antimicrobial Therapy, Inc., 2014, p 12–13.

World Allergy Organization. http://www.worldallergy.org/educational_programs/gloria/us/materials.php, Allergic conjunctivitis 2009.

TABLE 4-1
Allergic Conjunctivitis: Defining Terms

Intermittent (seasonal) allergic conjunctivitis	IgE-mediated diseases related to seasonal allergens Common triggers—depend on time of year and geographic location (April/May, tree pollens; June/July, grass pollens; July/August, mold spores and weed pollens; others dependent on local environmental factors)
Persistent (perennial) allergic conjunctivitis	IgE-mediated diseases related to perennial allergens Common trigger—house dust mites (present in all geographic areas)

Source: US GLORIA. http://www.worldallergy.org/educational_programs/gloria/us/materials.php, Allergic conjunctivitis

TABLE 4-2
Treatment of Common Bacterial Eye, Ear, Nose, and Throat Infection

Site of Infection	Common Pathogens	Recommended Antimicrobial	Comments
Suppurative conjunctivitis (nongonococcal, non-chlamydial)	S. aureus, S. pneumoniae, H. influenzae Outbreaks due to atypical S. pneumoniae	Primary: Ophthalmic treatment with FQ ocular solution (gatifloxacin, levofloxacin, moxifloxacin) Alternative: Ophthalmic treatment with polymyxin B plus trimethoprim solution or azithromycin solution	Viral conjunctivitis ("pink eye," usually caused by adenovirus) often self-limiting. Relieve irritative symptoms with use of cold artificial tear solution Most S. pneumoniae is resistant to tobramycin, gentamicin
Otitis externa (swimmer's ear)	Pseudomonas spp., Proteus spp., Enterobacteriaceae Acute infection often S. aureus Fungi rare etiology	Otic drops with ofloxacin or ciprofloxacin with hydrocortisone or polymyxin B with neomycin and hydrocortisone For acute disease: dicloxacillin If MRSA is a concern: TMP-SMX, doxycycline, or clindamycin	Ear canal cleansing important. Decrease risk of reinfection by use of eardrops of 1:2 mixture or white vinegar and rubbing alcohol after swimming Do not use neomycin if tympanic membrane punctured
Malignant otitis externa in a person with diabetes mellitus, HIV/AIDS, on chemotherapy	Pseudomonas aeruginosa in >90%	Imipenem IV or meropenem IV ciprofloxacin (IV or PO) or ceftazidime IV or cefepime IV or (piperacillin IV pus tobramycin) or (ticarcillin plus tobramycin)	Surgical débridement usually needed. MRI or CT to evaluate for osteomyelitis often indicated Parenteral antimicrobial therapy possibly warranted for severe disease
Acute otitis media	S. pneumoniae, H. influenzae, M. catarrhalis, viral or no pathogen (approximately 55% bacterial, S. pneumoniae most common)	Patient has had no antibiotics in the prior month: • Amoxicillin high dose 1000 mg tid OR • Amoxicillin-clavulanate extended release 2000/125 mg po bid OR • Cefdinir 300 mg q12h or 600 mg q24h OR • Cefpodoxime proxetil 200 mg bid OR • Cefprozil 250-500 mg bid	Consider drug-resistant S. pneumoniae (DRSP) risk: antimicrobial therapy in past 1 month, age <2 years, day-care attendance. HD amoxicillin usually effective in DRSP Length of therapy: <2 years, 10 days; ≥2 years, 5–7 days. If allergy to beta-lactam drugs: TMP-SMX, clarithromycin, azithromycin; all less effective

TABLE 4-2
Treatment of Common Bacterial Eye, Ear, Nose, and Throat Infection—cont'd

Site of Infection	Common Pathogens	Recommended Antimicrobial	Comments
		Patient has had antibiotics in the prior month: • Amoxicillin-clavulanate extended release 2000/125 mg bid • Levofloxacin 750 mg q24h x 5 days • Moxifloxacin 400 mg q24h Duration of therapy if not mentioned, 5-7 days	against DRSP compared with other options. If penicillin allergy history is unclear or rash (no hive-form lesions), cephalosporins likely okay Clindamycin effective against DRSP, ineffective against *H. influenzae, M. catarrhalis* See Chapter 15, Pediatrics, for additional information
Exudative pharyngitis	Group A, C, G streptococcus, Fusobacterium (in research studies), infectious mononucleosis, primary HIV, *N. gonorrhea*, respiratory viruses	First-line for strep pharyngitis: penicillin V PO × 10 days or benzathine penicillin IM × 1 dose or (cefdinir or cefpodoxime) × 5 days. If penicillin allergy: clindamycin × 10 days. Azithromycin or clarithromycin are alternatives. Up to 35% *S. pyogenes* isolates resistant to macrolides.	Vesicular, ulcerative pharyngitis usually viral. Only 10% of adult pharyngitis due to group A streptococcus No treatment recommended for asymptomatic group A streptococcus carrier For recurrent, culture-proven *S. pyogenes*, primary treatment with cefdinir or cefpodoxime. Alternative with amoxicillin-clavulanate or clindamycin

Source: Gilbert DN, Moellering RC, Eliopoulos GM, Chambers HF, Saag MS. *The Sanford Guide to Antimicrobial Therapy.* 44th ed. Sperryville, VA: Antimicrobial Therapy, Inc, 2014.

Anterior Epistaxis

8. Anterior epistaxis is usually caused by:
A. hypertension.
B. bleeding disorders.
C. localized nasal mucosa trauma.
D. a foreign body.

9. First-line intervention for anterior epistaxis includes:
A. nasal packing.
B. application of topical thrombin.
C. firm pressure to the area superior to the nasal alar cartilage.
D. chemical cauterization.

10. The most common clinical finding in patients with severe or refractory epistaxis is:
A. type 2 diabetes mellitus.
B. hypertension.
C. acute bacterial sinusitis.
D. anemia.

11. A 22-year-old man with recurrent epistaxis episodes fails to respond to simple pressure. Alternative approaches include all of the following except:
A. initiating systemic prothrombotic therapy.
B. nasal packing.
C. chemical cautery.
D. topical antifibrinolytic agents.

Answers

8. C.   **9.** C.   **10.** B.   **11.** A.

Anterior epistaxis is usually the result of localized nasal mucosa dryness and trauma and is rarely a result of other causes such as hypertension or coagulation disorder. Hypertension is the most common associated finding in cases of severe or refractory epistaxis; there is not a particular blood pressure threshold when nose bleed risk is markedly increased. Most episodes can be easily managed with simple pressure—with firm pressure to the area superior to the nasal alar cartilage or an "entire nose pinched closed" position by the patient for a minimum of 10 minutes. If this action is ineffective, second-line therapies include nasal packing and cautery. Antifibri-nolytic agents are also available when other methods are not successful or for patients with a bleeding disorder. One such product contains a gel composed of collagen-derived particles and bovine-derived thrombin (Floseal). For refractory cases, arterial embolization or surgical therapy may be needed, including ligation of the internal maxillary artery, anterior ethmoid artery, and/or external carotid artery.

DISCUSSION SOURCES

Shukla PA, Chan N, Duffis EJ, et al. Current treatment strategies for epistaxis. *J Neuro Intervent Surg* 5:151–156, 2013. http://www.medscape.com/viewarticle/779484_1

Fatakia A, Winters R, Amedee RG. Epistaxis: A common problem. *Ochsner J* 10:176–178, 2010. http://www.ncbi.nlm.nih.gov/pmc/articles/PMC3096213

Ophthalmological Emergencies

12. All of the following are components of the classic ophthalmological emergency except:
    A. eye pain.
    B. purulent eye discharge.
    C. red eye.
    D. new onset change in visual acuity.

13. Mrs. Murphy is a 58-year-old woman presenting with a sudden left-sided headache that is most painful in her left eye. Her vision is blurred, and the left pupil is slightly dilated and poorly reactive. The left conjunctiva is markedly injected, and the eyeball is firm. Vision screen with the Snellen chart is 20/30 OD and 20/90 OS. The most likely diagnosis is:
    A. unilateral herpetic conjunctivitis.
    B. open-angle glaucoma.
    C. angle-closure glaucoma.
    D. anterior uveitis.

14. In caring for Mrs. Murphy, the most appropriate next action is:
    A. prompt referral to an ophthalmologist.
    B. to provide analgesia and repeat the evaluation when the patient is more comfortable.
    C. to instill a corticosteroid ophthalmic solution.
    D. to patch the eye and arrange for follow-up in 24 hours.

15. A 48-year-old man presents with a new-onset right eye vision change accompanied by dull pain, tearing, and photophobia. The right pupil is small, irregular, and poorly reactive. Vision testing obtained by using the Snellen chart is 20/30 OS and 20/80 OD. The most likely diagnosis is:
    A. unilateral herpetic conjunctivitis.
    B. open-angle glaucoma.
    C. angle-closure glaucoma.
    D. anterior uveitis.

16. Mrs. Allen is a 67-year-old woman with type 2 diabetes who complains of seeing flashing lights and floaters, decreased visual acuity, and metamorphopsia in her left eye. The most likely diagnosis is:
    A. open-angle glaucoma.
    B. central retinal artery occlusion.
    C. anterior uveitis.
    D. retinal detachment.

17. For Mrs. Allen, the most appropriate next course of action is:
    A. placement of an eye shield and follow-up in 48 hours.
    B. initiate treatment with an ophthalmic antimicrobial solution.
    C. initiate treatment with a corticosteroid ophthalmic solution.
    D. immediate referral to an ophthalmologist.

18. A 45-year-old man presents with eye pain. He reports that he was cutting a tree with a chain saw when some wood fragments hit his eye. You consider all of the following except:
    A. educating the patient on the use of appropriate eye protection for primary prevention of eye trauma.
    B. immediately removing any protruding foreign body from the eye.
    C. using fluorescein staining to detect small objects in the eye.
    D. prompt referral to an eye care specialist.

Answers

12. B.	15. D.	18. B.
13. C.	16. D.	
14. A.	17. D.	

The classic components of an ophthalmological emergency are a painful, red eye with a documented change in visual acuity. In the case of angle-closure glaucoma, the patient usually presents with all of these findings, and, without intervention, blindness ensues in 3 to 5 days. Prompt referral to expert ophthalmological care focused on relieving acute intraocular pressure is needed; laser peripheral iridectomy after reduction of intraocular pressure with appropriate medications is usually curative. In contrast, open-angle glaucoma, the disease's most common form, is a slowly progressive disease that seldom produces symptoms. In untreated open-angle glaucoma, the eventual visual loss is largely in the periphery, leading to the development of tunnel vision.

In anterior uveitis, another cause of an occasionally dully painful red eye with visual change, the pupil is usually constricted, nonreactive, and irregularly shaped. Treatment includes medications to assist in pupillary dilation and corticosteroids, administered topically, by periocular injection, or systemically. Evaluation for the underlying cause, including autoimmune and inflammatory diseases and ocular trauma, of this uncommon condition should also be done.

Mechanical trauma to the eye can cause globe rupture, which should be considered in all patients with eye injury. Primary prevention of trauma to the eye includes the use of appropriate protective eyewear or face shield. Eye injury from high-velocity trauma (e.g., flying object) should be treated as a penetrating injury. Injury from a small object is often detected only as a small corneal defect by fluorescein staining. Endophthalmitis and possible vision loss can result if not treated appropriately. If a protruding foreign body is present, it should not be removed if globe rupture is suspected. The use of an eye shield and immediate referral to an ophthalmologist is recommended.

Retinal detachment, the separation of the neurosensory layer of the retina from the choroid and retinal pigment epithelium, can lead to rapid degeneration of photoreceptors because of ischemia. Early diagnosis and treatment can prevent permanent vision loss. Risk factors include myopia (nearsightedness), cataract surgery, diabetic retinopathy, family history of retinal detachment, older age, and trauma. Patients with retinal detachment complain of unilateral photopsia, increasing number of floaters in the affected eye, decreased visual acuity, and metamorphopsia (wavy distortion of an object). If retinal detachment is suspected, immediate referral to an ophthalmologist is needed.

DISCUSSION SOURCES

Kilborne G. http://emedicine.medscape.com/article/798323, eMedicine: Iritis and uveitis

Romaniuk VM. Ocular trauma and other catastrophes. *Emerg Med Clin North Am* 31:399–411, 2013.

Primary Open-Angle Glaucoma

19. Which of the following is a common vision problem in the person with untreated primary open-angle glaucoma (POAG)?
    A. peripheral vision loss
    B. blurring of near vision
    C. difficulty with distant vision
    D. need for increased illumination

20. POAG is primarily caused by:
    A. hardening of the lens.
    B. elevated intraocular pressure.
    C. degeneration of the optic nerve.
    D. hypotension in the anterior maxillary artery.

21. Which of the following is most likely to be found on the funduscopic examination in a patient with untreated POAG?
    A. excessive cupping of the optic disk
    B. arteriovenous nicking
    C. papilledema
    D. flame-shaped hemorrhages

22. Risk factors for POAG include all of the following except:
    A. African ancestry.
    B. type 2 diabetes mellitus.
    C. advanced age.
    D. blue eye color.

23. Key diagnostic findings in POAG include which of the following?
    A. intraocular pressure greater than 25 mm Hg.
    B. papilledema.
    C. cup-to-disk ratio greater than 0.4
    D. sluggish pupillary response.

24. Adults at high risk for POAG should undergo a complete eye exam every:
    A. 1 to 2 years.
    B. 3 to 4 years.
    C. 5 to 6 years.
    D. 3 to 6 months.

25. Treatment options for POAG include all of the following topical ocular agents except:
    A. beta-adrenergic antagonists.
    B. alpha$_2$-agonists.
    C. prostaglandin analogues.
    D. mast cell stabilizers.

Answers

19. A.	22. D.	25. D.
20. B.	23. A.	
21. A.	24. A.	

Although the etiology of POAG is not completely understood, the result is elevated intraocular pressure caused by abnormal drainage of aqueous humor through the trabecular meshwork. POAG risk factors include African ancestry, diabetes mellitus, family history of POAG, history of certain eye trauma and uveitis, and advancing age. A gradual onset peripheral vision loss is most specific for open-angle glaucoma; this disease is the second most common cause of irreversible blindness in North America. Although all of these changes may be seen in patients with advanced open-angle glaucoma, changes in near vision are common as part of the aging process because of hardening of the lens (i.e., presbyopia) and the need for increased illumination. New onset of difficulty with distance vision can be found in patients with cataracts.

Glaucoma, either open-angle or angle-closure, is primarily a problem with excessive intraocular pressure. Tonometry reveals intraocular pressure greater than 25 mm Hg; in angle-closure glaucoma, the abnormal measurement is usually documented on more than one occasion. As a result, the optic disk and cup are "pushed in," creating the classic finding often called glaucomatous cupping. This creates a cup-to-disk ratio of greater than 0.3 or asymmetry of cup-to-disk ratio of 0.2 or more. Papilledema, in which the optic disk bulges and the margins are blurred, is seen when there is excessive pressure behind the eye, as in increased intracranial pressure (Fig. 4–1). Although the USP-STF has concluded that there is insufficient evidence to support routine screening for POAG in asymptomatic adults, some experts recommend a comprehensive eye exam including measurement of intraocular pressure for high-risk patients every 1 to 2 years.

Medication treatment options for primary open-angle or angle-closure glaucoma include topical beta-adrenergic antagonists such as timolol, alpha$_2$ agonists such as brimonidine, carbonic anhydrase inhibitors such as dorzolamide, and prostaglandin analogues such as latanoprost. Because of their ability to cause pupillary constriction, pilocarpine and similar medications are now seldom used. Laser trabeculoplasty and other surgical interventions are additional treatment options (Table 4–3).

DISCUSSION SOURCES

Mayo Clinic. Glaucoma. http://www.mayoclinic.com/health/glaucoma/DS00283

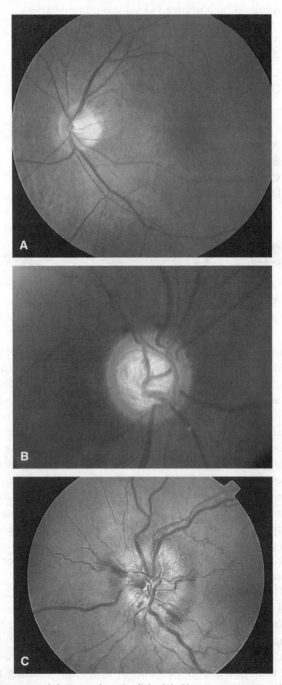

Figure 4-1 (A) Normal optic disk. (B) Glaucomatous cupping. (C) Bulging optic disk in papilledema.

Eyelid Disorders

26. A 22-year-old woman presents with a "pimple" on her right eyelid. Examination reveals a 2 mm pustule on the lateral border of the right eyelid margin. This is most consistent with:
    A. a chalazion.
    B. a hordeolum.
    C. blepharitis.
    D. cellulitis.

27. A 22-year-old woman presents with a "bump" on her right eyelid. Examination reveals a 2 mm, hard, non-tender swelling on the lateral border of the right eyelid margin. This is most consistent with:
    A. a chalazion.
    B. a hordeolum.
    C. blepharitis.
    D. cellulitis.

28. First-line treatment for uncomplicated hordeolum is:
    A. topical corticosteroid.
    B. warm compresses to the affected area.
    C. incision and drainage.
    D. oral antimicrobial therapy.

29. A potential complication of hordeolum is:
    A. conjunctivitis.
    B. cellulitis of the eyelid.
    C. corneal ulceration.
    D. sinusitis.

30. Initial treatment for a chalazion is:
    A. topical fluoroquinolone.
    B. topical corticosteroid.
    C. warm compresses of the affected area.
    D. surgical excision.

Answers

26. B.   28. B.   30. C.
27. A.   29. B.

A hordeolum is often called a stye and is usually caused by a staphylococcal infection of a hair follicle on the eyelid. An internal hordeolum points toward the conjunctival eye surface,

---

TABLE 4-3
Treatment Options in Glaucoma

Chronic, Primary Open-Angle Intervention (POAG)	Acute, Angle-Closure Intervention
• Reduce production of intraocular fluid • Topical beta-adrenergic antagonists • Topical alpha$_2$-agonist • Topical carbonic anhydrase inhibitors • Surgical intervention if needed to attain normal pressures • Photocoagulation • Increase fluid outflow – Prostaglandin analogues – Surgical intervention if needed to attain normal pressures • Trabeculoplasty • Trabeculectomy • Drainage implants	• Prompt ophthalmological referral • Relieve acute intraocular pressure – Reduce production of intraocular fluid • Topical beta-adrenergic antagonists • Topical alpha$_2$-agonist • Topical carbonic anhydrase inhibitors – Increase fluid outflow • Prostaglandin analogues • Surgical intervention when pressure normalized – Laser peripheral iridectomy

Source: Mayo Clinic. Glaucoma. http://www.mayoclinic.com/health/glaucoma/DS00283

---

whereas an external hordeolum is found on the lid margin. A chalazion is an inflammatory eyelid condition that may not involve infection but can follow hordeolum and is characterized by a hard, nontender swelling of the upper or lower lid. Because treatment regimens for each of these differ significantly, accurate diagnosis is critical. Cellulitis is a serious complication of a hordeolum and is evidenced by widespread redness and edema over the eyelid.

Treatment for a simple hordeolum, or stye, includes warm compresses to the affected eye for 10 minutes three to four times a day. Rarely, incision and drainage are needed. Oral antimicrobial therapy for an uncomplicated hordeolum is not warranted. An infrequently encountered complication of a hordeolum is cellulitis of the eyelid. If this occurs, ophthalmic consultation should be obtained, and appropriate systemic antimicrobial therapy should be promptly initiated. Because *S. aureus* is the most common pathogen, treatment options include the use of an antibiotic with gram-positive coverage and beta-lactamase stability with the possibility of methicillin-resistant strains. As a result, knowledge of local patterns of *S. aureus* is important.

Because this is an inflammatory, but not infectious disease, antimicrobial therapy for chalazion is not warranted. Treatment includes warm soaks of the area. If this is not helpful, referral to an ophthalmologist for intralesional corticosteroid injection or excision is recommended, particularly if the chalazion impairs lid closure or presses on the cornea.

DISCUSSION SOURCES

Gilbert DN, Moellering RC, Eliopoulos GM, Chambers HF, Saag MS. *The Sanford Guide to Antimicrobial Therapy.* 44th ed. Sperryville, VA: Antimicrobial Therapy, Inc., 2014, p 12.
http://www.merckmanuals.com/professional/eye_disorders/eyelid_and_lacrimal_disorders/chalazion_and_hordeolum_stye.html, Merck Manual online: Chalazion and hordeolum (stye)

Ménière's Disease/Syndrome

31 to 33. Indicate whether each case represents Ménière's disease (D) or Ménière's syndrome (S):

_____ **31.** A 24-year-old man who experienced trauma to the head during a car accident.

_____ **32.** A 45-year-old woman with no apparent underlying cause for the condition.

_____ **33.** A 17-year-old who received aminoglycoside therapy for an intraabdominal infection.

34. Which of the following is true concerning Ménière's disease?
A. Neuroimaging helps locate the offending cochlear lesion.
B. Associated high-frequency hearing loss is common.
C. This is largely a diagnosis of exclusion.
D. Tinnitus is rarely reported.

35. Alterations in the ear involved in Ménière's disease include all of the following except:
A. change in endolymphatic pressure.
B. breakage in the membrane separating the endolymph and perilymph fluids.
C. distension of the tympanic membrane causing low-tone roaring tinnitus.
D. sudden change in the vestibular nerve firing rate.

36 to 40. Indicate whether each of the following clinical findings would be present in a patient with Ménière's disease. (Answer yes or no.)

_____ **36.** The Weber tuning test lateralizes to the affected ear.

_____ **37.** The Rinne's test reveals that air exceeds bone conduction.

_____ **38.** Pneumatic otoscopy in the affected ear can elicit symptoms or cause nystagmus.

_____ **39.** The Romberg test is negative.

_____ **40.** A positive Fukuda marching step test.

41. When evaluating a patient with Ménière's disease, the procedure of observing for nystagmus while moving the patient from sitting to supine with the head angled 45 degrees to one side and then the other is called:
A. the Romberg test.
B. Dix-Hallpike test.
C. the Rinne's test.
D. the Fukuda test.

42. Prevention and prophylaxis in Ménière's disease include all of the following except:
A. avoiding ototoxic drugs.
B. protecting the ears from loud noise.
C. limiting sodium intake.
D. restricting fluid intake.

43. to 46. Match the following to the lettered descriptions:

_____ **43.** dizziness

_____ **44.** vertigo

_____ **45.** nystagmus

_____ **46.** tinnitus

A. perception that the person or the environment is moving
B. subjective perception of altered equilibrium
C. rhythmic oscillations of the eyes
D. perception of abnormal hearing or head noises

Answers

31. S.	37. yes	43. B.
32. D.	38. yes	44. A.
33. S.	39. no	45. C.
34. C.	40. yes	46. D.
35. C.	41. B.	
36. no	42. D.	

Ménière's disease, an idiopathic condition, and Ménière's syndrome, a condition with symptoms identical to those of Ménière's disease but in which an underlying cause has been identified, are believed to result from increased pressure within the endolymphatic system. In health, two fluids, one potassium-rich and the other potassium-poor, separated by a thin membrane, fill the chambers of the inner ear: endolymph and perilymph. Housed within the separating membrane is the nervous tissue of hearing and balance. Normally, the pressure exerted on these fluids is constant, allowing for normal balance and hearing. If the pressure of these fluids varies, the nerve-rich membranes are stressed, which causes disturbance in hearing, ringing in the ears,

imbalance, a pressure sensation in the ear, and vertigo. The reason for the pressure changes varies, but most often they are caused by an increase in endolymphatic pressure that causes a break in the membrane separating the two fluids. When these fluids mix, the vestibular nerve receptors are bathed in the new, abnormal chemical mix, which leads to depolarization blockade and sudden change in the vestibular nerve firing rate. This creates an acute vestibular imbalance and the resulting sense of vertigo. Symptoms improve after the membrane is repaired, and normal sodium and potassium concentrations are restored.

A distinction needs to be made between Ménière's disease, usually idiopathic in origin, and Ménière's syndrome, usually secondary to various processes that interfere with normal production or resorption of endolymph, such as endocrine abnormalities, trauma, electrolyte imbalance, autoimmune dysfunction, medications, parasitic infections, and hyperlipidemia. Ménière's disease is largely a diagnosis of exclusion; diagnosis is made after other possible causes for the recurrent and often debilitating symptoms of dizziness, tinnitus, and low-frequency hearing loss have been ruled out. A distinct causative lesion cannot be identified. This condition is common and is characterized by repeat attacks; risk factors include use of ototoxic drugs such as aminoglycosides, long-term, high-dose salicylate use, certain cancer chemotherapeutics, and exposure to loud noise.

Clinical presentation of Ménière's disease and Ménière's syndrome usually involves a history of episodes of vertigo with a sensation that the room is whirling about, often preceded by decreased hearing, low-tone roaring tinnitus, and a feeling of increased ear pressure. Particularly severe episodes are accompanied by nausea and vomiting. Attacks can last minutes to hours, with exhaustion often reported after the most severe symptoms have passed. Duration and frequency of attacks can vary, although common triggers include certain foods and drinks, mental and physical stress, and variations in the menstrual cycle.

Examination of a person with Ménière's disease typically reveals significant nystagmus or rhythmic oscillations of the eyes and slow movement toward one side, usually the side of the affected ear, with a rapid correction to the midline. The Weber tuning test result usually lateralizes to the unaffected ear, whereas the Rinne's test shows that air exceeds bone conduction, a normal finding. Performing pneumatic otoscopy in the affected ear can elicit symptoms or cause nystagmus, whereas the same maneuver to the unaffected ear yields little response. Objective measures of hearing often reveal diminished hearing. The Romberg test is positive, with the patient showing increased swaying and difficulty staying balanced when standing with the eyes closed. Additional findings include a positive Fukuda marching step test, in which a directional drift—usually toward the affected ear—is noted when the patient is asked to perform a march step with the eyes closed. This latter maneuver may be impossible for a patient with severe symptoms. The result of the Dix-Hallpike test (i.e., observation of nystagmus while moving a patient from sitting to supine with the head angled 45 degrees to one side and then to the other) is occasionally also positive, indicating coexisting benign positional vertigo. Neuroimaging is usually not warranted, unless the examination reveals additional findings, or the diagnosis is unclear.

Treatment of Ménière's disease is aimed at minimizing or preventing symptoms. Antihistamines such as meclizine (Antivert, Bonine), antiemetics, or benzodiazepines can minimize symptoms. Benzodiazepines can be used to help reinforce rest and minimize anxiety associated with severe symptoms; these options do not treat the underlying condition. Thiazide diuretics decrease fluid pressure load in the inner ear and can be used to prevent, but not treat, attacks; these medications do not help after the attack has been triggered. Corticosteroids also have been shown to be helpful, likely because of their antiinflammatory properties, causing a reduction in endolymph pressure and potentially ameliorating vertigo, tinnitus, and hearing loss.

When standard therapy is ineffective and severe symptoms persist, chemical labyrinthectomy with intratympanic gentamicin is a treatment option. Surgery is reserved for patients with frequent, severely debilitating episodes that are unresponsive to other, less radical therapies; options include endolymphatic sac decompression, vestibular neurectomy, and surgical labyrinthectomy. The possible risk of permanent hearing loss with these interventions must be reviewed with the patient. In Ménière's syndrome, symptomatic treatment and intervention for the underlying cause are warranted.

DISCUSSION SOURCES

http://www.merckmanuals.com/professional/ear_nose_and_throat_disorders/inner_ear_disorders/menieres_disease.html?qt=&sc=&alt=, Merck Manual online: Meniere's disease

Li J. http://www.emedicine.com/ent/TOPIC232.HTM, eMedicine: Inner ear, Meniere disease, medical treatment

Oral Cancer

47. You inspect the oral cavity of a 69-year-old man who has a 100-pack per year cigarette smoking history. You find a lesion suspicious for malignancy and describe it as:
  A. raised, red, and painful.
  B. a denuded patch with a removable white coating.
  C. an ulcerated lesion with indurated margins.
  D. a vesicular-form lesion with macerated margins.

48. A firm, painless, relatively fixed submandibular node would most likely be seen in the diagnosis of:
  A. herpes simplex.
  B. acute otitis media (AOM).
  C. bacterial pharyngitis.
  D. oral cancer.

49. Which of the following is the most common form of oral cancer?
  A. adenocarcinoma
  B. sarcoma-form
  C. squamous cell carcinoma
  D. basal cell carcinoma

50. An independent risk factor of oral cancer is infection with:
  A. human herpes virus type 1.
  B. human papillomavirus type 16.
  C. adenovirus type 16
  D. Epstein-Barr virus

51. Screening for oral cancer is recommended:
  A. for high-risk patients only.
  B. at regularly scheduled dental visits.
  C. every two years.
  D. to be conducted by qualified healthcare providers only.

Answers

47. C.	**49.** C.	**51.** B.
48. D.	**50.** B.	

Risk factors for oral cancer include male gender, advancing age, and tobacco and alcohol abuse. More recently, chronic infection with human papillomavirus type 16 has been appreciated as an oral cancer risk factor. Most commonly squamous cell carcinoma, an oral cancer is usually characterized by a relatively painless, firm ulceration or raised lesion. The lymphadenopathy associated with oral cancer consists of immobile nodes that are nontender when palpated. Self-limiting oral lesions, such as herpes simplex, oral candidiasis, and aphthous stomatitis, usually cause discomfort. With infection, the associated lymphadenopathy that follows drainage tracts is characterized by tenderness and mobility. Oral cancer screening can occur during regularly scheduled dental checkups that include an exam of the entire mouth. The American Cancer Society also recommends that healthcare providers examine the mouth and throat as part of a routine cancer-related checkup. If oral cancer is suspected, referral for a lesion biopsy is recommended.

DISCUSSION SOURCES

http://www.merckmanuals.com/professional/ear_nose_and_throat_disorders/tumors_of_the_head_and_neck/oral_squamous_cell_carcinoma.html, Merck Manual online: Oral squamous cell carcinoma

http://www.oralcancerfoundation.org/facts, The Oral Cancer Foundation: Oral cancer facts

Antibiotic Allergy

52. Which of the following medications is not a penicillin form?
  A. amoxicillin
  B. ampicillin
  C. dicloxacillin
  D. imipenem

53. A cutaneous reaction nearly always occurs with the use of amoxicillin in the presence of infection with:
A. human herpes virus type 1.
B. human papillomavirus type 11.
C. adenovirus type 20.
D. Epstein-Barr virus.

54. In a person with a well-documented history of systemic cutaneous reaction without airway impingement following penicillin use, the use of which of the following cephalosporins is most likely to result in an allergic response?
A. cephalexin
B. cefprozil
C. ceftriaxone
D. cefpodoxime

55. Which of the following antimicrobial classes is associated with the highest rate of allergic reaction?
A. the macrolides
B. the beta-lactams
C. the aminoglycosides
D. the sulfonamides

56. A 36-year-old man presents for his initial visit to become a patient in a primary care practice. He is generally in good health with a history of hyperlipidemia and is currently taking an HMG-CoA reductase inhibitor. He reports that he is "allergic to just about every antibiotic," and reports a variety of reactions including diffuse urticaria, gastrointestinal upset, and fatigue but without respiratory involvement. He is unclear as to which antibiotics have caused these reactions and states that much of what he knows is from his mother who "told me I always got sicker instead of better when I took an antibiotic." His last use of an antimicrobial was more than 10 years ago and was without reaction. He does not recall the name of this medication, but he remembers that he was being treated for a "sinus infection." The next most appropriate step in his care is to:
A. advise the patient to obtain a more detailed history of what antibiotics he was given during his childhood.
B. refer to allergy and immunology for evaluation.
C. inform the patient to start an antihistamine whenever he is given an antibiotic.
D. provide a prescription for a systemic corticosteroid to take if he develops a reaction to his next antimicrobial course.

57. Serious allergic reactions caused by the use of trimethoprim-sulfamethoxazole include all of the following except:
A. anaphylaxis.
B. Stevens-Johnson syndrome.
C. toxic epidermal necrolysis.
D. fixed drug eruptions.

58. A 27-year-old woman presents with acute bacterial rhinosinusitis that has failed to respond to 5 days of treatment with amoxicillin. She reports that she experienced an allergic reaction to levofloxacin a few years ago that caused a rash as well as swelling of the lips and tongue. In deciding on a new antimicrobial, you consider avoiding the use of:
A. amoxicillin-clavulanate.
B. azithromycin.
C. moxifloxacin.
D. cefpodoxime.

59. You prescribe a regimen of doxycycline to treat an acute exacerbation of chronic bronchitis for a 56-year-old man. This is his first exposure to this antimicrobial. You advise that:
A. he should not experience an allergic reaction since he has no reported penicillin allergy.
B. if he experiences any allergic reaction, he should stop taking the antibiotic and contact a healthcare provider immediately.
C. if he experiences an allergic reaction, he should continue taking the medication until he meets with a healthcare provider to avoid resistance development.
D. any allergic reaction will eventually resolve once the regimen is complete.

Answers

52. D.	55. B.	58. C.
53. D.	56. B.	59. B.
54. A.	57. D.	

The penicillins, including penicillin, amoxicillin, dicloxacillin, ampicillin, and many others, and the cephalosporins, including a number of antibiotics containing the ceph- or cef- prefix, share a common feature: a beta-lactam nucleus in their molecular structures. Additional antibiotics with this property include less commonly used products such as the carbapenems (e.g., imipenem, usually given with cilastatin [Primaxin]) and the monobactams (e.g., aztreonam [Azactam]). Collectively, these antibiotics are known as the beta-lactams, the antimicrobial class with the highest rate of allergic reaction.

The most common allergic reactions to antibiotics including the cephalosporins and penicillins are maculopapular skin eruptions, urticaria, and pruritus; more severe reactions include respiratory and cardiovascular compromise. The reaction's onset can occur rapidly post drug ingestion, particularly if the patient has been sensitized to the antibiotic by previous exposure; rapid-onset classic symptoms including urticaria, pruritus, anaphylaxis, and bronchospasm are usually considered to be IgE-mediated Type I reactions. Less common reaction includes a hypersensitivity syndrome characterized by fever, eosinophilia, and other extracutaneous manifestations. Approximately 10% of the general population report penicillin allergy. However, this is likely a significant overestimation of this condition's prevalence.

Conventional practice is to assume that a patient with allergy to penicillin will also exhibit this reaction to the cephalosporins. However, the assumption of a 100% cross-sensitivity rate is inaccurate, as historical data suggest that at best, approximately 8% of patients with penicillin allergy will exhibit cephalosporin sensitivity; when select cephalosporins are eliminated, the rate is likely less than 1%. Indeed, the majority of what has been reported about penicillin-cephalosporin allergy has been derived from older retrospective studies in which penicillin allergy was not routinely confirmed by skin testing. Also, many reported penicillin reactions are not allergic in nature. For example, a toddler who develops *Candida* diaper rash during amoxicillin therapy is brought in by the parents who now believe that since the rash occurred while taking an antibiotic, the baby must be penicillin allergic. Some post-penicillin–use reactions are not allergic in nature. For example, when certain penicillin forms, such as ampicillin and amoxicillin, are administered to a person with Epstein-Barr virus infection, the most common causative organism in mononucleosis, a cutaneous reaction nearly always occurs; this rash is thought to be the result of altered immune status during the infection and not indicative of penicillin allergy. In addition, these historic data were gathered during a time when cephalosporins were often contaminated with traces of penicillin, an obvious trigger for an allergic reaction.

More recent study supports that the rate of cross-reactivity between penicillins and cephalosporins is probably less than 1% and determined by similarity in side chains and not the beta-lactam ring structure. Simply put, the greatest rate of cross-reactivity to the penicillins appears to arise from the use of the first-generation cephalosporins, including cephalexin (Keflex) and cefadroxil (Duricef). As a result of Pichichero's meta-analysis, the use of certain second-, third-, and fourth-generation cephalosporins, including cefprozil (Ceftin), cefuroxime, cefpodoxime (Vantin), ceftazidime, and ceftriaxone (Rocephin), appears to result in lower allergic risk.

For patients with a history of penicillin allergy, whether to prescribe a cephalosporin or not requires careful data-gathering on the exact reaction that occurs post penicillin use. If the history is consistent with a severe, rapid-onset IgE-mediated-type response, referral for allergy testing is the most prudent course; this approach should also be considered if the penicillin allergy history is unclear. When testing is undertaken, confirmation of both the presence of penicillin allergy and the presence or absence of cephalosporin sensitivity is important. This advice extends to the use of carbapenems and the monobactams. With a history of less severe reactions, clinical judgment is warranted. Additional research is needed before the recommendation to use the second-, third-, and fourth-generation cephalosporins can be routinely recommended, although these medications are listed in a number of treatment guidelines for use in the person with a history of penicillin allergy.

Allergic reactions to other antibiotic classes can also occur, though typically less frequently than beta-lactams. Trimethoprim-sulfamethoxazole (TMP-SMX) can cause both immediate and delayed reactions. Delayed reactions can range from mild maculopapular exanthema and fixed drug eruptions to serious manifestations (i.e., anaphylaxis, Stevens Johnson syndrome, or toxic epidermal necrolysis). Immediate reactions to fluoroquinolones are uncommon (0.4% to 2.0%) and can involve IgE- or non-IgE-mediated reactions. In rare cases, serious hypersensitivity and/or anaphylactic reactions have been reported following the first dose of a fluoroquinolone. Cross reactivity has been demonstrated with the fluoroquinolones; thus, patients who are allergic to a fluoroquinolone should avoid use of this class. Allergic reaction to the macrolides is relatively uncommon (ranging from 0.4% to 3%). Symptoms can range from mild to life-threatening, including rash or hives, swelling of the face, lips, and tongue, as well as difficulty breathing or swallowing. At the first sign of an allergic reaction, patients should stop taking the medication and contact their healthcare provider.

When seeing a patient who reports being allergic to virtually all antibiotics, referral to allergy and immunology for antibiotic allergy testing is critical to confirm what medications are safe to use if the patient presents with an infectious disease where such therapy is warranted.

DISCUSSION SOURCES

Allergic cross-reactivity among beta-lactam antibiotics: An update. *Pharmacist's Letter/Prescriber's Letter* 25(4):250427, 2009.

Gruchalla R, Pirmohamed M. Antibiotic allergy. *N Engl J Med* 354:601–609, 2006.

James C, Gurk-Turner C. Cross-reactivity of beta-lactam antibiotics. http://www.ncbi.nlm.nih.gov/pmc/articles/PMC1291320/

Pichichero, ME. Use of selected cephalosporins in penicillin-allergic patients: A paradigm shift. http://www.ncbi.nlm.nih.gov/pubmed/17349459

Thong BYH. Update on the management of antibiotic allergy. *Allergy Asthma Immunol Res* 2:77–86, 2010.

● Otitis Externa

60. A 45-year-old man presents with otitis externa. Likely causative pathogens include all of the following except:
    A. Enterobacteriaceae.
    B. *P. aeruginosa.*
    C. *Proteus* spp.
    D. *M. catarrhalis.*

61. Risk factors for otitis externa include all of the following except:
    A. frequent air travel.
    B. vigorous use of a cotton swab.
    C. frequent swimming.
    D. cerumen impaction.

62. Appropriate oral antimicrobial therapy for otitis externa with an accompanying facial cellulitis suitable for outpatient therapy includes a course of an oral:
    A. macrolide.
    B. cephalosporin.
    C. fluoroquinolone.
    D. penicillin.

63. Physical examination findings in otitis externa include:
   A. tympanic membrane immobility.
   B. increased ear pain with tragus palpation.
   C. tympanic membrane erythema.
   D. tympanic membrane bullae.

64. A risk factor for malignant otitis externa includes:
   A. the presence of an immunocompromised condition.
   B. age younger than 21 years.
   C. a history of a recent upper respiratory tract infection (URI).
   D. a complicated course of otitis media with effusion.

65. Diagnostic approaches commonly used to identify malignant otitis externa include all of the following except:
   A. CT scan.
   B. x-ray imaging.
   C. radionucleotide bone scanning.
   D. gallium scanning.

Answers

60. D.	**62.** C.	**64.** A.
61. A.	**63.** B.	**65.** B.

Risk factors for otitis externa include a history of recent ear canal trauma, usually after vigorous use of a cotton swab or other item to clean the canal, and conditions in which moisture is frequently held in the ear canal, such as with cerumen impaction and frequent swimming. Otitis externa can be caused by numerous pathogens, including various gram-positive organisms and fungi such as *Candida* or *Aspergillus* species. *P. aeruginosa* is the most common causative agent and the most likely organism in refractory otitis externa or accompanying cellulitis; cellulitis is an occasional complication of otitis externa, particularly in the presence of protracted infection or comorbidity, such as diabetes mellitus or immunosuppression.

Clinical presentation includes redness and edema of the ear canal accompanied by purulent or serous discharge and the hallmark finding of pain on tragus palpation or with the application of traction to the pinna. Facial, neck, or auricular cellulitis and unilateral neck lymphadenopathy are noted with complicated infection. When otitis externa is fungal in origin, usually the clinical presentation includes a report of less pain but more itch; ear discharge is usually described as being thicker and white to gray in color.

Malignant or necrotizing otitis externa, in which infection invades the deeper soft tissue, is a complication that occurs in patients who are immunocompromised or in those who have received radiotherapy to the skull base; osteomyelitis of the temporal bone is often seen in this rare condition. Presentation includes the usual features of otitis externa and pain disproportionate to clinical findings. Radiography is often used to depict the extent of the infection. CT is preferred as this modality better depicts bony erosion; however, radionucleotide bone scanning and gallium scanning can also be used to make the diagnosis. MRI can be considered secondarily or if soft tissue extension is of concern. Surgical débridement is typically needed. Antipseudomonal antimicrobial therapy is usually reserved for severe cases. Parenteral antimicrobial therapy is often warranted for severe disease (Table 4–2).

Effective topical therapies for otitis externa include otic suspension of an antimicrobial, such as a fluoroquinolone (ofloxacin or ciprofloxacin), or polymyxin B plus neomycin, with or without hydrocortisone solution. When the ear canal is edematous to the point at which topical antimicrobial drops cannot be well distributed, an ear wick is usually inserted and left in place for 2 to 3 days. Aural hygiene using gentle suction to remove debris can be helpful; irrigation in the presence of acute infection is usually not advocated. Oral antibiotics should be prescribed in individuals with cellulitis of the face or neck skin, in persons in whom severe edema of the ear canal limits penetration of topical agents, and in immunocompromised persons. If this therapy proves ineffective or in the presence of severe disease, inpatient hospital admission and parenteral antimicrobial therapy are likely indicated.

DISCUSSION SOURCES

Gilbert DN, Moellering RC, Eliopoulos GM, Chambers HF, Saag MS. *The Sanford Guide to Antimicrobial Therapy.* 44th ed. Sperryville, VA: Antimicrobial Therapy, Inc., 2014, p 10.

Waitzman A. http://www.emedicine.com/ped/TOPIC1688.HTM, eMedicine: Otitis externa

Acute Otitis Media

66 to 69. Indicate which of the following viruses are implicated in causing acute otitis media (AOM). (Answer yes or no.)

_____ **66.** respiratory syncytial virus

_____ **67.** herpes simplex virus 2

_____ **68.** influenza virus

_____ **69.** rhinovirus

70 to 74. Indicate which of the following bacteria are commonly implicated in causing AOM. (Answer yes or no.)

_____ **70.** *S. pneumoniae*

_____ **71.** *H. influenzae*

_____ **72.** *E. coli*

_____ **73.** *M. catarrhalis*

74. Risk factors for AOM include all of the following except:
   A. upper respiratory tract infection.
   B. untreated allergic rhinitis.
   C. tobacco use.
   D. aggressive ear canal hygiene.

75. Expected findings in AOM include:
   A. prominent bony landmarks.
   B. tympanic membrane immobility.
   C. itchiness and crackling in the affected ear.
   D. submental lymphadenopathy.

76. A 25-year-old woman has a 3-day history of left ear pain that began after 1 week of URI symptoms. On physical examination, you find that she has AOM. She is allergic to penicillin (use results in a rapidly developing hive-form reaction accompanied by difficulty breathing). She took an oral antimicrobial for the treatment of a urinary tract infection 2 weeks ago. The most appropriate oral antimicrobial option for this patient is:
A. clarithromycin.
B. levofloxacin.
C. amoxicillin.
D. cefadroxil.

77. A reasonable treatment option for AOM in an adult who is develops GI upset while taking amoxicillin is:
A. cefpodoxime.
B. erythromycin.
C. cephalexin.
D. trimethoprim-sulfamethoxazole.

78. Drug-resistant *S. pneumoniae* is least likely to exhibit resistance to which of the following antimicrobial classes?
A. advanced macrolides
B. tetracycline forms
C. first-generation cephalosporins
D. respiratory fluoroquinolones

79. Characteristics of *M. catarrhalis* include:
A. high rate of beta-lactamase production.
B. antimicrobial resistance resulting from altered protein-binding sites.
C. often being found in middle ear exudate in recurrent otitis media.
D. gram-positive organisms.

80. Which of the following is a characteristic of *H. influenzae*?
A. Newer macrolides are ineffective against the organism.
B. Its antimicrobial resistance results from altered protein-binding sites within the wall of the bacteria.
C. Some isolates exhibit antimicrobial resistance via production of beta-lactamase.
D. This is a gram-positive organism.

81. Which of the following is a characteristic of *S. pneumoniae*?
A. mechanism of antimicrobial resistance primarily because of the production of beta-lactamase
B. mechanism of antimicrobial resistance usually via altered protein-binding sites held within the microbe's cell
C. organisms most commonly isolated from mucoid middle ear effusion
D. gram-negative organisms

82. Which of the following is absent in otitis media with effusion?
A. fluid in the middle ear
B. otalgia
C. fever
D. itch

83. Treatment of otitis media with effusion usually includes:
A. symptomatic treatment.
B. antimicrobial therapy.
C. an antihistamine.
D. a mucolytic.

Answers

66. yes	**72.** no	**78.** D.
67. no	**73.** yes	**79.** A.
68. yes	**74.** D.	**80.** C.
69. yes	**75.** B.	**81.** B.
70. yes	**76.** B.	**82.** C.
71. yes	**77.** A.	**83.** A.

Although often considered a disease limited to childhood, AOM still ranks among the most frequent diagnoses noted in adult office visits. *S. pneumoniae, H. influenzae, M. catarrhalis,* and various viruses contribute to the infectious and inflammatory process of the middle ear. Eustachian tube dysfunction usually precedes the development of AOM, allowing negative pressure to be generated in the middle ear; this negative pressure enables pharyngeal pathogens to be aspirated into the middle ear, and the infection takes hold. Avoiding conditions that can cause eustachian tube dysfunction, such as upper respiratory infection, untreated or undertreated allergic rhinitis, tobacco use, and exposure to air pollution, can lead to a reduction in the occurrence of AOM.

S. pneumoniae causes 40% to 50% of AOM. It is the least likely of the three major causative bacteria to resolve without antimicrobial intervention (~10% of cases), and infection with this organism usually causes the most significant otitis media symptoms. Numerous isolates of this organism exhibit resistance to many standard, well-tolerated, inexpensive antibiotic agents, including lower-dose amoxicillin, certain cephalosporins, and the macrolides (azithromycin, clarithromycin, erythromycin). The mechanism of resistance is an alteration of intracellular protein-binding sites, which can typically be overcome by using higher doses of amoxicillin and select cephalosporins. A major risk factor for infection with drug-resistant *S. pneumoniae* is recent systemic antimicrobial use.

H. influenzae and *M. catarrhalis* are gram-negative organisms capable of producing beta-lactamase, an enzyme that cleaves the beta-lactam ring found in the penicillin, amoxicillin, and ampicillin molecule, rendering these antibiotics ineffective against the pathogen. These two organisms have high rates of spontaneous resolution in AOM (50% and 90%, respectively); however, *H. influenzae* is the organism most commonly isolated from mucoid and serous middle ear effusion. Organisms producing beta-lactamase likely contribute less to AOM treatment failure than does prescribing inadequate dosages of amoxicillin needed to eradicate drug-resistant *S. pneumoniae*. Common viral agents that cause AOM include human rhinovirus, respiratory syncytial virus, adenovirus, and influenza virus. AOM caused by these viral agents usually resolves in 7 to 10 days with supportive care alone.

Appropriate assessment is critical for arriving at the diagnosis of AOM. The tympanic membrane may be retracted or bulging and is typically reddened with loss of translucency and mobility on insufflation. With recovery, tympanic membrane mobility returns in about 1 to 2 weeks, but middle ear effusion usually persists for 4 to 6 weeks. Itching and crackling in the ear is common in patients with AOM and in patients with serous otitis, also known as otitis media with effusion. The bony landmarks usually appear prominent when the tympanic membrane is retracted, a condition usually seen with eustachian tube dysfunction, which may not be present in patients with AOM. The submental node is not in the drainage tract of the middle ear and is not enlarged in patients with AOM. Rather, the nodes within the anterior cervical chain on the ipsilateral side of the infection are often enlarged and painful.

Initial antimicrobial selection will depend on whether the patients had recent prior antimicrobial use (within the past month). High-dose amoxicillin can be used if no prior antimicrobials have been used; otherwise, high-dose amoxicillin, high-dose amoxicillin-clavulanate, or certain cephalosporins are recommended for patients with recent prior antimicrobial use (Table 4–2).

DISCUSSION SOURCES

Cook K. http://www.emedicine.com/emerg/TOPIC351.HTM, eMedicine: Otitis media

Gilbert DN, Moellering RC, Eliopoulos GM, Chambers HF, Saag MS. *The Sanford Guide to Antimicrobial Therapy.* 44th ed. Sperryville, VA: Antimicrobial Therapy, Inc., 2014 , p 11.

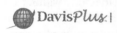

See full color images of this topic on DavisPlus at
**http://davisplus.fadavis.com |
Keyword: Fitzgerald**

Acute Pharyngitis

84. An 18-year-old woman has a chief complaint of a "sore throat and swollen glands" for the past 3 days. Her physical examination includes a temperature of 101° F (38.3° C), exudative pharyngitis, and tender anterior cervical lymphadenopathy. Right and left upper quadrant abdominal tenderness is absent. The most likely diagnosis is:
A. *Streptococcus pyogenes* pharyngitis.
B. infectious mononucleosis.
C. viral pharyngitis.
D. Vincent angina.

85. Treatment options for streptococcal pharyngitis for a patient with penicillin allergy include all of the following except:
A. azithromycin.
B. trimethoprim-sulfamethoxazole.
C. clarithromycin.
D. clindamycin.

86. *S. pyogenes* is transmitted primarily through:
A. sexual intercourse.
B. skin-to-skin contact.
C. saliva and droplet contact.
D. contaminated surfaces.

87. You are seeing a 25-year-old man with *S. pyogenes* pharyngitis. He asks if he can get a "shot of penicillin" for therapy. He has no history of drug allergy. You consider the following when counseling about the use of intramuscular penicillin:
A. There is nearly a 100% cure rate in streptococcal pharyngitis when it is used.
B. Treatment failure rates approach 20%.
C. This is the preferred agent in treating group G streptococcal infection.
D. Injectable penicillin has a superior spectrum of antimicrobial coverage compared with the oral version of the drug.

88. With regard to pharyngitis caused by group C streptococci, the NP considers that:
A. potential complications include glomerulonephritis.
B. appropriate antimicrobial therapy helps to facilitate more rapid resolution of symptoms.
C. infection with these organisms carries a significant risk of subsequent rheumatic fever.
D. acute infectious hepatitis can occur if not treated with an appropriate antimicrobial.

89. A 26-year-old man presents with a progressively worsening sore throat with dysphagia, trismus, and unilateral otalgia. His voice is muffled, and examination reveals an erythematous, swollen tonsil with contralateral uvular deviation. The most likely diagnosis is:
A. infectious mononucleosis.
B. viral pharyngitis.
C. peritonsillar abscess.
D. early-stage scarlet fever.

90. Patients with strep throat can be cleared to return to work or school after _____ hours of antimicrobial therapy.
A. 12
B. 24
C. 36
D. 48

91. Common causative organisms of peritonsillar abscess include all of the following except:
A. *Fusobacterium necrophorum.*
B. *Candida albicans.*
C. group C or G streptococcus.
D. group A beta-hemolytic streptococcus (GABHS).

92. When advising a patient with scarlet fever, the NP considers that:
A. there is increased risk for poststreptococcal glomerulonephritis.
B. the rash often peels during recovery.
C. an injectable cephalosporin is the preferred treatment option.
D. throat culture is usually negative for group A streptococci.

93. The incubation period for *S. pyogenes* is usually:
A. 1 to 3 days.
B. 3 to 5 days.
C. 6 to 9 days.
D. 10 to 13 days.

94. The incubation period for *M. pneumoniae* is usually:
A. less than 1 week.
B. 1 week.
C. 2 weeks.
D. 3 weeks.

95 to 97. Match the patient with the likely causative pathogen for pharyngitis.

_____ **95.** *S. pyogenes*

_____ **96.** *M. pneumoniae*

_____ **97.** respiratory virus

A. A 17-year-old man with a bothersome dry cough, lymphadenopathy, and tonsillar enlargement
B. A 34-year-old with cough, nasal discharge, hoarseness, conjunctival inflammation, and diarrhea
C. A 26-year-old woman with sore throat and fever, swollen tonsils covered with exudate, palatal petechiae, and anterior cervical lymphadenopathy

98. All of the following are common causes of penicillin treatment failure in streptococcal pharyngitis except:
A. infection with a strain of *Streptococcus* producing beta-lactamase.
B. failure to initiate or complete the antimicrobial course.
C. concomitant infection or carriage with an organism producing beta-lactamase.
D. inadequate penicillin dosage.

99. The symptoms of rheumatic fever include:
A. severe, intermittent headaches.
B. carditis and arthritis.
C. hepatic dysfunction.
D. generalized rash.

100. A 23-year-old man is diagnosed with pharyngitis caused by *S. pyogenes* serotype 4. Which of the following statements is false regarding this patient?
A. Antimicrobial therapy will reduce the risk of developing rheumatic fever.
B. Onset of glomerulonephritis symptoms can occur 1 to 3 weeks after pharyngeal infection.
C. Antimicrobial therapy minimizes the risk of glomerulonephritis.
D. Poststreptococcal glomerulonephritis is usually a self-limiting condition.

101. The rash associated with scarlet fever typically occurs how long after the start of the symptomatic infection?
A. 2 days
B. 4 days
C. 7 to 10 days
D. 2 to 3 weeks

102. Treatment of scarlet fever in a 19-year-old woman with no allergy to penicillin can include all of the following except:
A. penicillin.
B. cefdinir.
C. TMP-SMX.
D. cefpodoxime.

Answers

84. A.	91. B.	98. A.
85. B.	92. B.	99. B.
86. C.	93. B.	100. C.
87. B.	94. D.	101. A.
88. B.	95. C.	102. C.
89. C.	96. A.	
90. B.	97. B.	

S. pyogenes, also known as group A beta-hemolytic streptococcus, is the causative pathogen in 15% to 40% of sore throats in school-aged children but is less common in children younger than 3 years and in teenagers and adults. The organism is transmitted primarily via saliva and droplet contact. The incubation period lasts an average of 3 to 5 days, but can be up to 3 months. Clinical presentation of exudative pharyngitis caused by *S. pyogenes* includes complaints of sore throat and fever, and evidence of large, beefy tonsils, usually covered with exudate, palatial petechiae, and anterior cervical lymphadenopathy. Communicability gradually decreases over several weeks in untreated patients. Patients are no longer contagious within 24 hours of initiation of appropriate antimicrobial therapy and when without fever. Asymptomatic nasopharyngeal carriage is common.

S. pyogenes is not the sole cause of bacterial exudative pharyngitis. Another causative pathogen implicated is *Mycoplasma pneumoniae*. Infection with this organism is uncommon in children 5 years or younger and is most often seen in teenagers and younger adults. Clinical presentation includes inflammatory exudate, pharyngeal edema and erythema, cervical lymphadenopathy, and tonsillar enlargement. Because this organism is also a cause of acute bronchitis, the person with *M. pneumoniae* pharyngitis often has a bothersome dry cough; rapid streptococcal screen and standard throat culture fail to reveal the presence of this organism and yield negative results. The incubation period for *M. pneumoniae* is approximately 3 weeks, and it is usually contracted via cough and respiratory droplet.

Clinical findings most often associated with viral pharyngitis include cough, nasal discharge, hoarseness, pharyngeal ulcerations, conjunctival inflammation, and diarrhea. Groups C and G streptococci cause pharyngitis, but infection with these organisms carries minimal risk for rheumatic fever or glomerulonephritis. The infection and its resulting symptoms clear without antimicrobial therapy, but taking an appropriate antimicrobial helps minimize symptoms.

Complications of bacterial pharyngitis include peritonsillar abscess, rheumatic fever, and acute glomerulonephritis. Peritonsillar abscess is most commonly caused by *Fusobacterium necrophorum*, group A beta-hemolytic streptococcus (GABHS), or groups C and G streptococcus. Clinical presentation of peritonsillar abscess includes progressively worsening sore throat, often worse on one side; trismus (inability or difficulty in opening the mouth); drooling; a muffled, "hot potato" voice with an erythematous, swollen tonsil with contralateral uvular deviation; and cervical lymphadenopathy. Because airway compromise is a potentially life-threatening consequence of peritonsillar abscess, ultrasonography or CT of the affected region should be promptly obtained to confirm the diagnosis. Referral to emergency and specialty ENT care and treatment with appropriate antimicrobial therapy, needle aspiration, and airway maintenance must be initiated promptly. Antimicrobial therapy initiated early in the course of acute pharyngitis minimizes peritonsillar abscess risk.

Rheumatic fever is usually caused by *S. pyogenes* serotypes 1, 3, 5, 6, 14, 18, 19, and 24; on average, onset of symptoms of carditis and arthritis begins about 19 days (range 7 to 35 days) after the onset of sore throat symptoms. Antimicrobial treatment is helpful in minimizing rheumatic fever risk. Acute glomerulonephritis is also a complication of *S. pyogenes*, usually serotypes 1, 3, 4, 12, and 25 when associated with pharyngitis and serotypes 2, 4, 9, 55, 57, 59, and 60 when associated with skin infection. Onset of glomerulonephritis symptoms is usually 1 to 3 weeks after pharyngeal or skin infection. Although poststreptococcal glomerulonephritis is usually a self-limiting condition, patients can develop renal scarring with chronic proteinuria or hematuria. Antimicrobial therapy does not minimize glomerulonephritis risk. Infrequently seen but potentially purulent complications of streptococcal pharyngitis include otitis media, sinusitis, peritonsillar and retropharyngeal abscess, and suppurative cervical adenitis.

Scarlet fever is the clinical condition seen when a scarlatiniform rash with a fine sandpaper-like texture erupts during streptococcal pharyngitis, usually on the second day of illness. The rash starts on the trunk and spreads widely, usually sparing the palms and soles, and usually peels during recovery. Treatment of scarlet fever is identical to treatment of streptococcal pharyngitis and carries no increased risk of complications or sequelae.

A positive throat culture for *Streptococcus pyogenes* is considered the diagnostic standard in streptococcal pharyngitis. A potential drawback is that a positive result does not distinguish between acute viral pharyngitis with group A streptococcus carriage and acute streptococcal pharyngitis. Despite this, all patients with a positive throat culture should be treated with an appropriate antimicrobial. Rapid antigen detection tests detect the presence of the group A streptococcus carbohydrate antigen and can be completed in minutes, but with lower sensitivity and specificity than standard throat culture. As a result, many authorities advocate treating in the presence of a positive rapid streptococcal screen and following up negative studies with a throat culture in a patient in whom there is a high index of suspicion. If a rapid streptococcal test result is positive, antimicrobial treatment should be initiated immediately.

If a rapid strep screen is negative and a throat culture is performed, the question is raised as to whether treatment should be initiated while awaiting results. In delaying therapy until throat culture results are available, treatment for patients with positive cultures is delayed by 2 days. This delay poses little risk in an otherwise well person.

In the treatment of bacterial pharyngitis caused by *S. pyogenes*, penicillin remains highly effective. When the total daily dosage is given in equally divided twice-daily doses, treatment outcomes are equivalent to regimens of three or four times daily with significantly improved adherence. A single dose of injectable penicillin given intramuscularly offers a one-time treatment option. Limitations include increased risk of serious reaction with penicillin allergy and a treatment failure rate similar to that of a completed course of oral therapy. For patients with a penicillin allergy, azithromycin, clarithromycin, or clindamycin are alternatives (Table 4–2). Of group A beta-hemolytic streptococcus isolates, 35% are resistant to macrolides or clindamycin; these drugs should be used only when a patient has a penicillin allergy. Advice on the use of symptomatic treatment with salt-water gargles, throat lozenges, and analgesics should also be given.

When penicillin therapy fails, it is seldom because of a resistant *S. pyogenes* strain. Rather, oropharyngeal carriage with an organism producing beta-lactamase, such as *H. influenzae*, is often the problem; the presence of beta-lactamase renders the penicillin ineffective. Treatment with an antimicrobial stable in the presence of beta-lactamase, such as amoxicillin-clavulanate or a cephalosporin, is likely to be effective. If the streptococcal test result is negative, and the patient continues to have symptoms, infection with *M. pneumoniae* or *Chlamydophila* (*Chlamydia*) *pneumoniae* should be considered, particularly if cough is present. A macrolide or fluoroquinolone should be prescribed because beta-lactams (penicillins, cephalosporins) are less effective.

The treatment of *S. pyogenes* carriage, defined as a positive throat culture in an individual who has no symptoms, warrants mention. Antimicrobial therapy for *S. pyogenes* carriage is indicated only when an outbreak of rheumatic fever or glomerulonephritis is in progress, when there is a family history of acute rheumatic fever, when multiple documented pharyngitis episodes occur within a family over several weeks despite therapy, or when there is an outbreak of streptococcal pharyngitis in a closed or semi-closed environment, such as a correctional facility or college dormitory. First-line therapy includes treatment with clindamycin or amoxicillin with clavulanate; rifampin with penicillin can also be used.

DISCUSSION SOURCES

Gilbert DN, Moellering RC, Eliopoulos GM, Chambers HF, Saag MS. *The Sanford Guide to Antimicrobial Therapy*. 44th ed. Sperryville, VA: Antimicrobial Therapy, Inc., 2014 , pp 48–49.

University of Michigan Health System: Acute pharyngitis in children 2–18 years old. Ann Arbor, MI: University of Michigan Health System, 2011. http://www.guideline.gov/content.aspx?id=25757

Gerber MA, Baltimore RS, Eaton CB, et al. Prevention of rheumatic fever and diagnosis and treatment of acute streptococcal pharyngitis (American Heart Association guidelines). *Circulation* 119: 1541–1551, 2009.

◗ Allergic Rhinitis

103. A 25-year-old woman who has seasonal allergic rhinitis likes to spend time outdoors. She asks you when the pollen count is likely to be the lowest. You respond:
A. "Early in the morning."
B. "During breezy times of the day."
C. "After a rain shower."
D. "When the sky is overcast."

104. The physiological response causing allergic rhinitis is primarily mediated through:
A. IL-10.
B. IgE antibodies.
C. anti-IgM antibodies.
D. anti-TNF antibodies.

105 to 108. Match each allergen with the appropriate characteristic. *An answer can be used more than once.*

____ **105.** pollens
____ **106.** pet dander
____ **107.** dust mites
____ **108.** mold spores

A. most common perennial allergen
B. most common seasonal allergen
C. common indoor allergen

109. You prescribe nasal corticosteroid spray for a patient with perennial allergic rhinitis. What is the anticipated onset of symptom relief with its use?
A. immediately with the first spray
B. 1 to 2 days
C. a few days to a week
D. 2 or more weeks

110. Which of the following medications is most appropriate for allergic rhinitis therapy in an acutely symptomatic 24-year-old machine operator?
A. nasal cromolyn
B. diphenhydramine
C. flunisolide nasal spray
D. loratadine

111. Antihistamines work primarily through:
A. vasoconstriction.
B. action on the histamine-1 (H_1) receptor sites.
C. inflammatory mediation.
D. peripheral vasodilation.

112. Decongestants work primarily through:
A. vasoconstriction.
B. action on the H_1 receptor sites.
C. inflammatory mediation.
D. peripheral vasodilation.

113. Which of the following medications affords the best relief of acute nasal itch?
A. anticholinergic nasal spray
B. oral decongestant
C. corticosteroid nasal spray
D. oral antihistamine

114. According to the Allergic Rhinitis and Its Effects on Asthma (ARIA) treatment guidelines, which of the following medications affords the best relief of acute nasal congestion?
A. anticholinergic nasal spray
B. decongestant nasal spray
C. corticosteroid nasal spray
D. oral antihistamine

115. According to the ARIA treatment guidelines, which of the following medications affords the least control of rhinorrhea associated with allergic rhinitis?
A. anticholinergic nasal spray
B. antihistamine nasal spray
C. corticosteroid nasal spray
D. cromolyn nasal spray

116. Ipratropium bromide (Atrovent) helps control nasal secretions through:
A. antihistaminic action.
B. anticholinergic effect.
C. vasodilation.
D. vasoconstriction.

117. Oral decongestant use should be discouraged in patients with:
A. allergic rhinitis.
B. migraine headache.
C. cardiovascular disease.
D. chronic bronchitis.

118. Cromolyn's mechanism of action is as a/an:
A. anti–immunoglobulin E antibody.
B. vasoconstrictor.
C. mast cell stabilizer.
D. leukotriene modifier.

119. In the treatment of allergic rhinitis, leukotriene modifiers should be used as:
A. an agent to relieve nasal itch.
B. an inflammatory inhibitor.
C. a rescue drug.
D. an intervention in acute inflammation.

120. According to the Global Resources in Allergy (GLORIA) guidelines, which of the following is recommended for intervention in persistent allergic conjunctivitis?
A. topical mast cell stabilizer with a topical antihistamine
B. ocular decongestant
C. topical nonsteroidal antiinflammatory drug
D. topical corticosteroid

121. Allergen subcutaneous immunotherapy should be considered in all of the following except:
A. when allergy symptoms are controlled with environmental management.
B. when allergy symptoms persist despite optimal use of appropriate medications.
C. when there is a desire to reduce the use of allergy medications.
D. to prevent progression or development of asthma.

122. Which of the following is most appropriate for the treatment of moderate-to-severe allergic rhinitis and conjunctivitis when symptoms are not controlled with current therapy?
A. short course of an oral corticosteroids
B. single dose of a long-acting parenteral or IM corticosteroids
C. daily dose of oral first-generation antihistamine
D. immediate initiation of allergy immunotherapy

◗ Answers

103. C.	110. D.	117. C.
104. B.	111. B.	118. C.
105. B.	112. A.	119. B.
106. C.	113. D.	120. A.
107. A.	114. B.	121. A.
108. C.	115. D.	122. A.
109. C.	116. B.	

Allergic rhinitis is due to genetic-environmental interactions. A person with a genetic predisposition to allergens has environmental influences that cause the immune system to shift from a Th1 (non-allergic) state to a predominantly Th2 (allergic) state, which then promotes IgE production. Upon re-exposure to an allergen he/she has been sensitized to (development of allergen-specific IgE antibodies), an allergic response will occur with release of histamine and inflammatory mediators from the mast cells.

Allergic rhinitis is due to both indoor and outdoor aeroallergens. Dust mites are the most common trigger of perennial allergy symptoms. Pets, cockroaches, and mold spores are other indoor allergens found to cause nasal and ocular allergy symptoms. Pollens (trees, grasses, and ragweed) are major triggers in seasonal allergic rhinitis and allergic conjunctivitis. Pollen counts are generally the highest early in the morning, released shortly after dawn. Pollen travels best on warm, dry, breezy days and is lowest during chilly, wet periods. Some outdoor mold spores can also cause allergy symptoms. Certain spores are highest in dry, breezy weather. Others need high humidity to release spores, and their counts are highest during rainy periods.

The most important component of allergic rhinitis and allergic conjunctivitis therapy is avoidance of the allergen or reduction if avoidance cannot be achieved. Second-line therapy includes pharmacotherapy agents designed to relieve and/or to control symptoms. Medications that are used to acutely relieve symptoms ("relievers") include antihistamines, decongestants, and, in severe cases, oral corticosteroids. Medications used to control allergy symptoms ("controllers") include intranasal corticosteroids, leukotriene modifiers, and mast cell stabilizers.

According to ARIA guidelines, "reliever" medications recommended to treat allergy symptoms include antihistamines, decongestants, and a short course of oral corticosteroids for severe uncontrolled symptoms. Antihistamines work by blocking H_1 receptor sites. These medications prevent the action of formed histamine, a potent inflammatory mediator, and can be used to treat acute allergy symptoms. Second-generation antihistamines, such as loratadine (Claritin), are to be given first-line. They are effective in relieving symptoms and have little or no sedation. ARIA recommends avoiding first-generation antihistamines, such as diphenhydramine (Benadryl), due to their sedative and anticholinergic adverse effects. Nasal antihistamines have first-line benefits with seasonal allergic rhinitis associated with nasal congestion. Decongestants act as vasoconstrictors, opening edematous nasal passages and relieving congestion. ARIA guidelines suggest limiting topical decongestant use to less than 5 days and avoiding use in preschoolers. Regular use of oral decongestants is to be avoided due to potential adverse effects. Intranasal anticholinergic sprays work to inhibit parasympathetic transmission to submucosal glands. Their use is limited to relieving refractory rhinorrhea. A short course of oral corticosteroids is recommended in moderate-to-severe allergic rhinitis and conjunctivitis when symptoms are not controlled with current therapy. ARIA strongly recommends avoiding intramuscular administration of glucocorticoids. The oral route is equally effective and parenteral administration could cause unwanted adverse events (Tables 4–4 and 4–5; Figs. 4–2 and 4–3).

DISCUSSION SOURCES

Allergic Rhinitis and its Impact on Asthma Report, www.whiar. org/docs/ARIAReport_2010.pdf

Wallace, D. & Dykewicz, M., et al. Diagnosis and Management of Rhinitis: An update practice parameter. Joint Task Force on Practice Parameters (AAAAI, ACAAI & The Joint Council of Allergy, Asthma & Immunology). *J Allergy Clin Immunol* 122: S1–S84, 2008.

■) Acute Bacterial Rhinosinusitis

123. Which of the following findings is most consistent with the diagnosis of acute bacterial rhinosinusitis (ABRS)?
   A. upper respiratory tract infection symptoms persisting beyond 7 to 10 days
   B. mild midfacial fullness and tenderness
   C. preauricular lymphadenopathy
   D. marked eyelid edema

TABLE 4-4
Allergic Conjunctivitis Treatment

Nondrug therapies for all classifications	• Nondrug therapies • Avoidance of allergen • Cool compresses • Preservative-free artificial tears • Sunglasses to ameliorate photosensitivity, and possibly provide a degree of barrier protection against air-borne allergens

For intermittent, seasonal allergic conjunctivitis	• Controller therapy with
	  • Topical antihistamine or topical cromolyn *or*
	  • Topical antihistamine with mast cell stabilizer *or*
	  • Topical antihistamine with vasoconstrictor *or*
	  • Topical NSAID
	• If inadequate control for intermittent, seasonal
	  • Oral antihistamine

Specific allergen immunotherapy (allergen vaccination)	• Helpful in managing persistent allergic rhinitis and conjunctivitis • Of value in patients with multiorgan symptoms of IgE-mediated allergic sensitization • Risk-to-benefit ratio must be considered in all cases • Highly effective in selected patients • Evaluation and treatment must be made by a clinician with background in allergen immunotherapy with facilities to treat anaphylaxis

OTC and older pharmacotherapies	• Can be helpful, but should not be overused or abused. These products generally treat the presenting problem (eye redness or itch), but do not fully address the underlying problem (allergy)
	  • Ocular vasoconstrictors, helpful at reducing eye redness, but not recommended for regular use. OTC products are often combined with an antihistamine
	  • Topical NSAID such as ketorolac, helpful in reducing ocular itch and redness

Topical ocular corticosteroids	• Topical ocular corticosteroids should be prescribed and monitored only by a suitably qualified clinician, such as a specialist in allergy or ophthalmology, and only in the presence of severe allergic ocular disease for short-term use • Prolonged use can lead to secondary bacterial infection, glaucoma, and cataracts. With short-term use, increased risk for ocular viral or fungal infection

Source: US GLORIA. http://www.worldallergy.org/educational_programs/gloria/us/materials.php, Allergic conjunctivitis

TABLE 4-5
Medications Used in the Treatment of Allergic Rhinitis

Therapeutic Goal	Intervention	Comment
Controller therapy to prevent formation of inflammatory mediators	• Corticosteroid nasal spray (beclomethasone [Beconase], fluticasone [Flonase], others) • Leukotriene modifiers (montelukast [Singulair], zafirlukast [Accolate]) • Mast cell stabilizer (intranasal and optic cromolyn [NasalCrom])	• Controller therapy usually needs to be used for a few days to 2 weeks before maximum effect noted. Little effect on acute symptoms
Rescue therapy by inactivating formed inflammatory mediators	• Oral antihistamines (first-generation [chlorpheniramine, diphenhydramine, others], second-generation [loratadine, cetirizine, fexofenadine, levocetirizine, others]) • Antihistamine nasal spray (azelastine [Astelin] nasal spray) • Antihistamine optic drops (ketotifen [Zaditor] optic drops) • Short-term oral corticosteroids if needed for severe allergic symptoms	• Using only antihistamine rescue therapy usually not as effective on overall disease control as consistent use of controller therapy with rescue therapy as an adjunct
Rescue therapy and symptom relief by minimizing nasal discharge	• Anticholinergic nasal spray (Ipratropium bromide [Atrovent]) • Antihistamine nasal spray (Astelin, others)	• Helpful adjuncts as part of rescue therapy for patient with bothersome profuse nasal discharge
Rescue therapy and symptom relief by minimizing nasal congestion	Oral and nasal decongestants (alpha-adrenergic agonists such as pseudoephedrine [Sudafed])	• Potential for vasoconstriction and increased blood pressure and heart rate. Avoid or use with caution in hypertension, cardiovascular disease

ARIA Classification

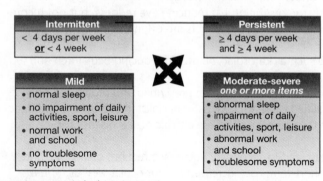

Intermittent
< 4 days per week
or < 4 week

Persistent
• ≥ 4 days per week and ≥ 4 week

Mild
• normal sleep
• no impairment of daily activities, sport, leisure
• normal work and school
• no troublesome symptoms

Moderate-severe
one or more items
• abnormal sleep
• impairment of daily activities, sport, leisure
• abnormal work and school
• troublesome symptoms

symptoms reported prior to treament

Figure 4-2 ARIA classification. (*Source: Bousquet J, Van Cauwenberge P, Khaltaev N. Allergic rhinitis and its impact on asthma. J Allergy Clin Immunol 108 [Suppl]:S147–S334, 2001.*)

Treatment of allergic rhinitis: ARIA Guidelines

moderate severe persistent

mild persistent

moderate severe intermittent

mild intermittent

intranasal corticosteroid

local chromone/mast cell stabilizer

oral or local non-sedative H1-blocker

intra-nasal decongestant (<10 days) or oral decongestant

allergen and irritant avoidance

immunotherapy

Figure 4-3 Treatment of allergic rhinitis according to ARIA guidelines. (*Source: http://www.whiar.org/docs/ARIA_PG_08_View_WM.pdf, ARIA Workshop Report: management of allergic rhinitis and its impact on asthma: global primary care education*)

124. The most common causative bacterial pathogen in ABRS in a 40 year-old adult is:
A. *M. pneumoniae*.
B. *S. pneumoniae*.
C. *M. catarrhalis*.
D. *E. coli*.

125. Risk factors for ABRS include all of the following except:
A. viral infection.
B. allergies.
C. tobacco use.
D. recent history of epistaxis.

126. Which of the following is a first-line therapy for the treatment of ABRS in an adult with no recent antimicrobial use?
A. amoxicillin-clavulanate
B. trimethoprim-sulfamethoxazole
C. clarithromycin
D. moxifloxacin

127. Which of the following represents a therapeutic option for ABRS in an adult patient with no recent antimicrobial care with treatment failure after 72 hours of appropriate doxycycline therapy?
A. clindamycin
B. clarithromycin
C. trimethoprim-sulfamethoxazole
D. high-dose amoxicillin with clavulanate

128. A 34-year-old man with penicillin allergy presents with ABRS. Three weeks ago, he was treated with doxycycline for "bronchitis." You now prescribe:
A. clarithromycin.
B. moxifloxacin.
C. cephalexin.
D. amoxicillin.

129. A 45-year-old person with severe ABRS has shown no clinical improvement after a total of 10 days of antimicrobial therapy. Initially treated with doxycycline for 5 days, he was then switched to levofloxacin for the past 5 days. This is his third episode of ABRS in the past 12 months. You consider:
A. initiating a course of oral corticosteroid.
B. switching treatment to moxifloxacin.
C. prompt referral for sinus imaging with a CT scan.
D. discontinuing antimicrobial therapy, performing a nasal swab for culture and sensitivity, and treatment dependent on these results.

130. According to the latest evidence, all of the following have demonstrated efficacy in relieving symptoms of ABRS except:
A. saline nasal spray.
B. nasal corticosteroid.
C. oral decongestant.
D. acetaminophen.

Answers

123. A.	**126.** A.	**129.** C.
124. B.	**127.** D.	**130.** C.
125. D.	**128.** B.	

ABRS is a clinical condition resulting from inflammation of the lining of the membranes of the paranasal sinuses caused by bacterial infection. Risk factors include any condition that alters the normal cleansing mechanism of the sinuses, including viral infection, allergies, tobacco use, and abnormalities in sinus structure. Inhaled tobacco use disturbs normal sinus mucociliary action and drainage, causing secretions to pool, and increases the risk of superimposed bacterial infection. In addition, viral URI and poorly controlled allergic rhinitis cause similar dysfunction, increasing ABRS risk. The observation of purulent discharge from one of the nasal turbinates is a highly sensitive finding in ABRS. Midfacial fullness is common in patients with uncomplicated URI, and anterior cervical lymphadenopathy is often found in many infectious and inflammatory conditions involving the head and pharynx. Marked eyelid edema is found only when the infection has extended beyond the sinuses and an orbital cellulitis has developed; a potentially life-threatening complication of ABRS.

Because ABRS is a clinical diagnosis based on patient presentation, with findings also reported in patients with a viral URI, the problem arises as to how to differentiate these two common conditions. The physical examination during ABRS, including sinuses tender to palpation and purulent nasal discharge, is often quite similar to what is seen during viral URI and therefore contributes little to the diagnosis. Since viral infections typically improve after 5 to 7 days, guidelines recommend that the diagnosis of ABRS be considered only in patients with URI-like symptoms with persistent or worsening symptoms for 7-10 days who continue to have: 1) maxillary/facial pain; and 2) purulent nasal discharge. For patients with severe illness (pain and fever), treatment should begin earlier but not before 3-4 days post onset of symptoms. In addition, the patient with a report of "double sickening," that is, approximately 3-4 days or more of URI-like symptoms that gradually improve then suddenly worsen, is suggestive of superimposed bacterial sinus infection. (See Table 4–6 and the algorithm on the management of acute bacterial rhinosinusitis.)

Most cases of ABRS do not require radiographic imaging since it is nonspecific and cannot distinguish between viral or bacterial infection. Advanced imaging via CT or MRI scan can be helpful for recurrent or complicated cases or when suppurative complications are suspected.

S. pneumoniae is the causative organism in most ABRS; this pathogen is also the least likely of the three major causative bacteria to resolve without antimicrobial intervention, and it causes the most significant symptoms. This organism exhibits resistance to numerous antibiotic agents, including lower dose amoxicillin, certain cephalosporins,

TABLE 4-6
Causative Pathogens in ABRS (ABS)

Organism	Description	Resistance
S. pneumoniae	Gram-positive diplococci, ABRS causative organism in adults=38%, children=21–33%	≥25% drug-resistant (DRSP) via altered protein-binding sites that limit antibiotic's ability to bind to the pathogen
H. influenzae	Gram-negative bacillus, ABRS causative organism in adults=36%, children=31–32%	≥30% penicillin-resistant via production of beta-lactamase that cleaves to beta-lactam ring
M. catarrhalis	Gram-negative coccus, ABRS causative organism in adults=16%, children=8–11%	≥90% penicillin-resistant via beta-lactamase production

Algorithm for the Management of Acute Bacterial Rhinosinusitis

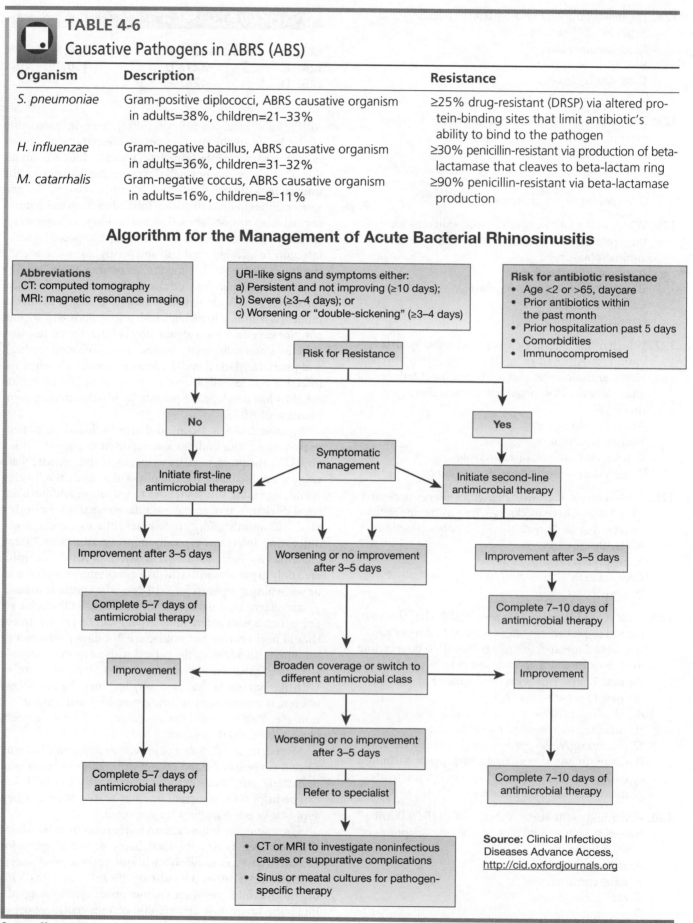

Abbreviations
CT: computed tomography
MRI: magnetic resonance imaging

URI-like signs and symptoms either:
a) Persistent and not improving (≥10 days);
b) Severe (≥3–4 days); or
c) Worsening or "double-sickening" (≥3–4 days)

Risk for antibiotic resistance
• Age <2 or >65, daycare
• Prior antibiotics within the past month
• Prior hospitalization past 5 days
• Comorbidities
• Immunocompromised

Risk for Resistance

No → Initiate first-line antimicrobial therapy

Yes → Initiate second-line antimicrobial therapy

Symptomatic management

Improvement after 3–5 days → Complete 5–7 days of antimicrobial therapy

Worsening or no improvement after 3–5 days

Improvement after 3–5 days → Complete 7–10 days of antimicrobial therapy

Broaden coverage or switch to different antimicrobial class

Improvement → Complete 5–7 days of antimicrobial therapy

Improvement → Complete 7–10 days of antimicrobial therapy

Worsening or no improvement after 3–5 days

Refer to specialist

• CT or MRI to investigate noninfectious causes or suppurative complications
• Sinus or meatal cultures for pathogen-specific therapy

Source: Clinical Infectious Diseases Advance Access, http://cid.oxfordjournals.org

Source: Chow AW, Benninger MS, Brook I, et al. IDSA clinical practice guideline for acute bacterial rhinosinusitis in children and adults. *Clin Infect Dis* 54:e72–112, 2012.

and macrolides. The mechanism of resistance is alterations of intracellular protein-binding sites, which can typically be overcome by using higher doses of amoxicillin, certain cephalosporins, and respiratory fluoroquinolones (levofloxacin [Levaquin] or moxifloxacin [Avelox]). Recent antimicrobial use is the major risk for infection with drug-resistant *S. pneumoniae*.

H. influenzae and *M. catarrhalis* are gram-negative organisms capable of producing beta-lactamase; the presence of this enzyme renders the penicillins ineffective. Although these two organisms have relatively high rates of spontaneous resolution without antimicrobial intervention in AOM, infections caused by these pathogens seldom resolve without antimicrobial therapy in ABRS (see Table 4–6). Empiric antimicrobial therapy in ABRS should be aimed at choosing an agent with significant activity against gram-positive (*S. pneumoniae*) and gram-negative organisms (*H. influenzae*, *M. catarrhalis*), with consideration for drug-resistant *S. pneumoniae* risk and possible need for stability in the presence of beta-lactamase. If there is treatment failure, the choice of a new antimicrobial depends on the initial medication that failed to eradicate the infection

and patterns of recent antimicrobial use (Table 4–7). Intervention in underlying contributory causes, such as treating allergic rhinitis and encouraging the cessation of tobacco use, is crucial to treatment success.

Treatments should also be considered to reduce the symptoms associated with ABRS. Saline via nasal spray or neti pot can be used to rinse nasal passages while a nasal corticosteroid (fluticasone [Flonase], mometasone [Nasonex], budesonide [Rhinocort Aqua], or triamcinolone [Nasacort], others) can be used to reduce inflammation. According to EBP recommendations, the use of decongestants, either oral or nasal sprays, is not recommended as adjunctive treatment for patients with ABRS as their use has little to no influence on patient outcomes. However, an individual patient can find a degree of symptom relief with these adjunctive therapies. OTC pain relievers (acetaminophen or ibuprofen) can help alleviate pain.

DISCUSSION SOURCES

Chow AW, Benninger MS, Brook I, et al. IDSA clinical practice guideline for acute bacterial rhinosinusitis in children and adults. *Clin Infect Dis* 54:e72–e112, 2012.

TABLE 4-7
Antimicrobial Regimens for Acute Bacterial Rhinosinusitis in Adults

Indication	Daily dose	Comments
Initial empiric therapy	First-line • Amoxicillin-clavulanate 500 mg/125 mg PO TID, or 875 mg/125 mg PO BID Second-line • Amoxicillin-clavulanate 2000 mg/125 mg PO BID • Doxycycline 100 mg PO BID or 200 mg PO daily	High dose (HD, 3-4 g/d) amoxicillin needed against DRSP Clavulanate as a beta-lactamase inhibitor, allows amoxicillin to have activity against beta-lactamase producing organisms such as *H. influenzae, M. catarrhalis* Doxycycline: DRSP treatment failure risk, activity against gram-negative organisms, stable in presence of beta-lactamase Pregnancy risk category D
β-lactam allergy (Allergy to antimicrobials with beta-lactam ring such as penicillins, cephalosporins)	Doxycycline 100 mg PO BID or 200 mg PO daily Levofloxacin 500 mg PO daily Moxifloxacin 400 mg PO daily	Respiratory fluoroquinolones (FQ)-Activity against DRSP, gram-negative organisms, stable in presence of beta-lactamase
Risk for antibiotic resistance or failed initial therapy	Amoxicillin-clavulanate 2000 mg/125 mg PO BID Levofloxacin 500 mg PO daily Moxifloxacin 400 mg PO daily	All options with activity against DRSP, gram-negative organisms, stable in presence of and/or active against beta-lactamase

Source: Chow AW, Benninger MS, Brook I, et al. IDSA clinical practice guideline for acute bacterial rhinosinusitis in children and adults. *Clin Infect Dis* 54:e72–112, 2012.

Infectious Mononucleosis

131. An 18-year-old woman presents with a chief complaint of a 3-day history of "sore throat and swollen glands." Her physical examination includes exudative pharyngitis, minimally tender anterior and posterior cervical lymphadenopathy, and maculopapular rash. She is diagnosed with infectious mononucleosis and was likely infected with the causative organism how many days ago?
    A. 5 to 10
    B. 20 to 30
    C. 30 to 50
    D. more than 100

132. The Epstein-Barr virus is primarily transmitted via:
    A. skin-to-skin contact.
    B. contact with blood.
    C. oropharyngeal secretions.
    D. genital contact.

133. Which of the following is most likely to be found in the laboratory data of a person with infectious mononucleosis?
    A. neutrophilia with reactive forms
    B. lymphocytosis with atypical lymphocytes
    C. thrombocytosis
    D. macrocytosis

134. You examine a 25-year-old man who has infectious mononucleosis with tonsillar hypertrophy, exudative pharyngitis, poor fluid intake due to difficulty swallowing, and a patent airway. You prescribe:
    A. amoxicillin.
    B. prednisone.
    C. ibuprofen.
    D. acyclovir.

135. In patients with infectious mononucleosis, which medication should be avoided due to a risk of rash development?
    A. acetaminophen
    B. sulfamethoxazole
    C. erythromycin
    D. amoxicillin

136. What percentage of patients with infectious mononucleosis has splenomegaly during the acute phase of the illness?
    A. at least 10%
    B. about 25%
    C. at least 50%
    D. nearly 100%

137. The size of a normal spleen is approximately:
    A. 1" × 1" × 3".
    B. 1" × 3" × 5".
    C. 2" × 4" × 6".
    D. 3" × 5" × 7".

138. Because of a risk for splenic rupture, persons who have recovered from infectious mononucleosis should wait how long before participating in collision or contact sports?
    A. at least 2 weeks
    B. at least 1 month
    C. at least 3 months
    D. at least 6 months

Answers

131. C.	134. B.	137. B.
132. C.	135. D.	138. B.
133. B.	136. C.	

Infectious mononucleosis is an acute systemic viral illness usually caused by Epstein-Barr virus, a DNA herpes virus that typically enters the body via oropharyngeal secretions and infects B lymphocytes. After an incubation period of 30 to 50 days, an intense T cell-mediated response develops and coincides with the onset of clinical illness. A 3- to 5-day prodrome of headache, malaise, myalgias, and anorexia is followed by acute symptoms that last about 5 to 15 days. The clinical presentation of acute infectious mononucleosis includes fatigue, exudative pharyngitis and tonsillar enlargement, fever, headache, with anterior and posterior cervical lymphadenopathy. Splenomegaly develops in more than 50% of patients, and hepatomegaly develops in about 10%; these organs are also tender to palpation. Additional findings include jaundice, periorbital edema, soft palatal petechiae, generalized adenopathy, rubella-like rash, and a 30% incidence of concurrent streptococcal pharyngitis. Full recovery time varies, but is usually about 4 to 6 weeks.

Diagnostic testing for patients with infectious mononucleosis usually includes obtaining a heterophile antibody test (Monospot), which has a sensitivity of 85% and specificity of 100%. The test does have limitations. Positivity increases during the first 6 weeks of illness, with only 60% of patients positive by the second week of illness. Furthermore, false negatives occur in 10% of adults and 50% of children. To complicate this issue further, acute infection with cytomegalovirus, adenovirus, *Toxoplasma gondii*, HIV, and other agents can cause an infectious mononucleosis-like illness with a risk of heterophile antibody cross reactivity and a resulting infectious mononucleosis false positive rate of 5% to 15%. Leukopenia with lymphocytosis is present. The presence of atypical lymphocytes is not unique to infectious mononucleosis and is commonly found in systemic viral infection. Mild thrombocytopenia is seen in 50% of patients; 85% of infected individuals develop a two-fold to three-fold elevation in hepatic enzymes (aspartate and alanine aminotransferases) by the second and third weeks of the illness.

Treatment of infectious mononucleosis is usually supportive, with recovery slow but complete. There is a potential, however, for upper pharyngeal obstruction and respiratory distress when enlarged tonsils and lymphoid tissue impinge on the upper airway. A use of a systemic corticosteroid such as prednisone, 40 to 60 mg/day for 3 days, is the treatment of choice, although little evidence exists to support this practice. However, the use of prednisone in a person with infectious mononucleosis who is having difficulty swallowing due to pharyngeal edema often provides symptomatic relief. In uncomplicated infectious mononucleosis, neither the use of antiviral agents such as acyclovir nor routine prescribing of systemic corticosteroid agents is indicated. Use of amoxicillin or ampicillin should be avoided as this can cause a cutaneous reaction (rash) in patients with Epstein-Barr virus infection. This rash is thought to be the result of altered immune status during the infection and not indicative of penicillin allergy.

In a person who participates in contact or collision sports or other activities, the risk of splenic rupture, the most common cause of mortality and morbidity in patients with infectious mononucleosis, needs to be considered during acute and convalescent stages. The risk for splenic rupture is greatest in the second and third weeks of illness—hence the mandate of abstaining from collision or contact sports for at least one month. The risk of rupture is greatest in the enlarged spleen; the size of the normal spleen can be recalled by the "rules of odds": $1 \times 3 \times 5$ inches in size, weighing 7 oz. (about 200 g), and lying between ribs 9 and 11. When the spleen is easily palpated, its size is usually increased by two or more times normal. The physical examination is a relatively insensitive measure of splenic size, however. Obtaining an ultrasound examination may be a prudent measure to ensure splenic regression before approving return to sports play. All persons with infectious mononucleosis are at risk of splenic rupture, however, regardless of spleen size.

DISCUSSION SOURCE

Singer-Leshinsky S. Pathogenesis, diagnostic testing, and management of mononucleosis. *JAAPA* 25:58–62, 2012.

Cardiac Disorders

5

Hypertension

1. You examine a 38-year-old woman who has presented for an initial examination and Papanicolaou test. She has no complaint. Her blood pressure (BP) is 154/98 mm Hg bilaterally and her body mass index (BMI) is 31 kg/m². The rest of her physical examination is unremarkable. Your next best action is to:
   A. initiate antihypertensive therapy.
   B. arrange for at least two additional BP measurements during the next 2 weeks.
   C. order blood urea nitrogen, creatinine, and potassium ion measurements and urinalysis.
   D. advise her to reduce her sodium intake.

2. You see a 68-year-old woman as a patient who is transferring care into your practice. She has a 10-year history of hypertension, diabetes mellitus, and hyperlipidemia. Current medications include hydrochlorothiazide, glipizide, metformin, simvastatin, and daily low-dose aspirin. Today's BP reading is 158/92 mm Hg, and the rest of her history and examination is unremarkable. Documentation from her former healthcare provider indicates that her BP has been in the range for the past 12 months. Your next best action is to:
   A. prescribe an angiotensin-converting enzyme inhibitor (ACEI).
   B. have her return for a BP check in 1 week.
   C. advise that her current therapy is adequate.
   D. add therapy with an aldosterone antagonist.

3. You examine a 78-year-old woman with long-standing, poorly controlled hypertension. When evaluating her for hypertensive target organ damage, you look for evidence of:
   A. lipid abnormalities.
   B. insulin resistance.
   C. left ventricular hypertrophy.
   D. clotting disorders.

4. Diagnostic testing for a patient with newly diagnosed primary hypertension diagnosis should include all of the following except:
   A. hematocrit.
   B. uric acid.
   C. creatinine.
   D. potassium.

5. In the person with hypertension, which of the following would likely yield the greatest potential reduction in BP in a patient with a BMI of 30 kg/m²?
   A. 10-kg (22-lb) weight loss
   B. dietary sodium restriction to 2.4 g (6 g NaCl) per day
   C. regular aerobic physical activity, such as 30 minutes of brisk walking most days of the week
   D. moderation of alcohol consumption

6 to 10. Match the antihypertension medication with its appropriate class.

6. amlodipine	A. beta-adrenergic receptor antagonist
7. diltiazem	B. nondihydropyridine calcium channel blocker
8. trandolapril	C. dihydropyridine calcium channel blocker
9. telmisartan	D. angiotensin receptor antagonist
10. pindolol	E. ACE inhibitor

11. You see a 38-year-old African-American male with hypertension who is currently being treated with thiazide-type diuretic. His current blood pressure reading is 156/94 mm Hg and he has no history of diabetes mellitus or chronic kidney disease. Following current best evidence, you consider adding which of the following medications?
   A. ACE inhibitor
   B. angiotensin receptor blocker
   C. beta-adrenergic receptor antagonist
   D. calcium channel blocker

12. Nondihydropyridine calcium channel blockers are contraindicated in patients with:
    A. type 1 diabetes mellitus.
    B. history of venous thromboembolism.
    C. severe left ventricular dysfunction.
    D. concomitant treatment with an ACEI.

13. In obtaining an office BP measurement, which of the following is most reflective of the best practice?
    A. Patient should sit in chair with feet flat on floor for at least 5 minutes before obtaining the reading.
    B. The BP cuff should not cover more than 50% of the upper arm.
    C. The patient should sit on the edge of the examination table without arm support to enhance reading accuracy.
    D. Obtaining the BP reading immediately after the patient walks into the examination room is recommended.

14. A BP elevation noted only at an office visit is commonly known as _____ hypertension.
    A. provider-induced
    B. clinical
    C. white coat
    D. pseudo

15. The most important long-term goal of treating hypertension is to:
    A. strive to reach recommended numeric BP measurement.
    B. avoid disease-related target organ damage.
    C. develop a plan of care with minimal adverse effects.
    D. treat concomitant health problems often noted in the person with this condition.

16. You start a patient with hypertension who is already receiving an ACEI on spironolactone. You advise the patient to return in 4 weeks to check which of the following laboratory parameters?
    A. sodium
    B. calcium
    C. potassium
    D. chloride

17. A 68-year-old woman presents with hypertension and BP of 152–158/92–96 mm Hg documented over 2 months on three different occasions. Electrocardiogram (ECG) and creatinine are normal, and she has no proteinuria. Clinical findings include the following: BMI 26.4 kg/m²; no S_3, S_4, or murmur; and point of maximal impulse at fifth intercostal space, mid-clavicular line. Which of the following represents the best intervention?
    A. Initiate therapy with metoprolol.
    B. Initiate therapy with hydrochlorothiazide.
    C. Initiate therapy with methyldopa.
    D. Continue to monitor BP, and start drug therapy if evidence of target organ damage.

18. Which of the following can have a favorable effect on a comorbid condition in a person with hypertension?
    A. chlorthalidone in gout
    B. propranolol with airway disease
    C. aldosterone antagonist in heart failure
    D. methyldopa in an older adult

19. According to JNC-8 guidelines, all of the following medications are first-line agents for use in a middle-aged white man without diabetes mellitus except:
    A. lisinopril.
    B. hydrochlorothiazide.
    C. metoprolol.
    D. amlodipine.

20. You see a 59-year-old man with poorly controlled hypertension. On physical examination, you note grade 1 hypertensive retinopathy. You anticipate all of the following will be present except:
    A. patient report of acute visual change.
    B. narrowing of the terminal arterioles.
    C. sharp optic disc borders.
    D. absence of retinal hemorrhage.

21. According to JNC-8, a 52-year-old well woman with a healthy BMI whose blood pressure is consistently 130–135/82–86 mm Hg is considered to have:
    A. normal blood pressure.
    B. hypertension requiring therapy with a CCB.
    C. hypertension requiring therapy with an alpha blocker.
    D. hypertension requiring therapy with a thiazide-type diuretic.

22. Which of the following is associated with the highest risk of ischemic heart disease?
    A. presence of microalbuminuria plus heavy alcohol intake
    B. absence of microalbuminuria plus use of a thiazolidinedione
    C. absence of microalbuminuria plus chronic physical inactivity
    D. presence of microalbuminuria plus cigarette smoking

23. When compared with Caucasians, African Americans tend to have a reduced effect with monotherapy with all of the following blood pressure medications except:
    A. ACEIs.
    B. ARBs.
    C. calcium channel blockers.
    D. beta blockers.

24 to 29. Match the recommended blood pressure goal for each patient according to JNC-8 guidelines. *An answer can be used more than once.*

24. a 57-year-old white male with no history of diabetes mellitus (DM) or chronic kidney disease (CKD)

25. a 62-year-old African-American male with diabetes mellitus

26. a 67-year-old female with CKD

27. a 62-year-old female with no history of DM or CKD

28. an 82-year-old male with no history of DM or CKD

29. a 72-year-old female with DM and CKD

A. <130/80 mm Hg
B. <140/80 mm Hg
C. <140/90 mm Hg
D. <150/90 mm Hg

30. You see a 62-year-old man without chronic kidney disease or diabetes mellitus who is currently being treated with low dose HCTZ and losartan. His blood pressure is currently 162/88 mm Hg. All of the following are appropriate next courses of action except:
A. increasing the dose of losartan.
B. adding a beta-adrenergic receptor antagonist.
C. adding a calcium channel blocker.
D. increasing the dose of HCTZ.

31. Which of the following statements concerning postural hypotension in the elderly is false?
A. It increases the risk of falls and syncope.
B. It is characterized by a drop in blood pressure when going from a standing to a sitting position.
C. It increases the risk of cardiovascular events.
D. It is associated with the use of vasodilating medications.

32 to 37. According to American College of Cardiology Foundation/American Heart Association (ACCF/AHA) guidelines, when treating elderly patients with hypertension, which of the following medications have a compelling indication for use in the following patient conditions? *(The medications listed can be used more than once. A given condition can have more than one medication indicated.)*

_____ **32.** Heart failure

_____ **33.** Diabetes mellitus

_____ **34.** Angina pectoris B

_____ **35.** Coronary artery disease

_____ **36.** Aortic aneurysm

_____ **37.** Recurrent stroke prevention

A. thiazide diuretic
B. beta blocker
C. ACEI
D. angiotensin receptor blocker (ARB)
E. aldosterone antagonist
F. calcium channel blocker

Answers

1. B.	**14.** C.	**27.** D.
2. A.	**15.** B.	**28.** D.
3. C.	**16.** C.	**29.** C.
4. B.	**17.** B.	**30.** B.
5. A.	**18.** C.	**31.** B.
6. C.	**19.** C.	**32.** A, B, C, D, E, F.
7. B.	**20.** A.	**33.** A, B, C, D, F.
8. E.	**21.** A.	**34.** B, F.
9. D.	**22.** D.	**35.** A, B, C, F.
10. A.	**23.** C.	**36.** A, B, C, F.
11. D.	**24.** C.	**37.** A, C, D, F.
12. C.	**25.** C.	
13. A.	**26.** C.	

Hypertension (HTN) is a complex disease with a core defect of vascular dysfunction that leads to select target organ damage (TOD); the target organs include the brain, eye, heart, and kidneys (Table 5–1). Appropriate HTN treatment significantly reduces TOD risk. When a BP reading of 115/75 mm Hg is used as a starting point, cardiovascular disease risk doubles with each increment of 20/10 mm Hg. HTN control leads to a reduction of stroke incidence by 35% to 40%, reduction of

myocardial infarction (MI) by 20% to 25%, and reduction of heart failure by 50%. Long-standing poorly controlled HTN is the leading cause of new-onset heart failure.

Evidence-based guidance for the diagnosis, prevention, and treatment of HTN include the following recommendations.

• Accurate clinical assessment depends on proper measurement of BP. The patient should be seated in a chair with feet flat on floor, without crossed legs, with arm supported

TABLE 5-1

Hypertension: A Complex Disease With a Core Defect of Vascular Dysfunction That Leads to Select Target Organ Damage

Target Organ	Potential Damage Outcome With Known Moderation as a Result of Effective Antihypertension Therapy
Brain	Stroke, vascular (multi-infarct) dementia
Cardiovascular system	Atherosclerosis, myocardial infarction, left-ventricular hypertrophy, heart failure
Kidney	Hypertensive nephropathy, renal failure
Eye	Hypertensive retinopathy with risk for blindness

at heart level, for at least 5 minutes before taking the BP measurement, not on an examination table with feet dangling. Failure to perform these measures can lead to an artificially elevated reading and lack of standardization from visit to visit. The BP cuff should be wide enough to cover more than 80% of the upper arm, and the cuff's bladder should be approximately 40% of the arm circumference. The use of a cuff that does not meet these qualifications can lead to a falsely elevated BP reading (Table 5–2).

- Lifestyle modification can yield significant improvement in BP measurements (Table 5–3).
- JNC-8 limits the preferred first-line and later-line medications to four classes: thiazide-type diuretics, calcium channel blockers (CCBs), angiotensin-converting enzyme inhibitors (ACEIs), and angiotensin receptor blockers (ARBs). Second- and third-line alternatives can include higher doses or combinations of agents in these four classes.
- Prior to using beta blockers, aldosterone antagonist or other classes of agents, JNC-8 recommends patients first receive a dose adjustment and combination of the four first-line agents. Triple therapy with an ACEI/ARB, CCB, and thiazide-type diuretic would precede use of a beta blocker, aldosterone antagonist or other alternative agent.
- The most important goal of HTN treatment is the avoidance of target organ damage (TOD). JNC-8 recommends

initiating pharmacologic therapy in the general population ≥60 years when SBP is ≥150 mm Hg or DBP ≥90 mm Hg, with a treatment goal of <150/90 mm Hg. For those <60 years, pharmacologic therapy should be initiated when SBP is ≥140 mm Hg or DBP ≥90 mm Hg, with a treatment goal of <140/90 mm Hg.

- JNC-8 recommendations for BP goals include less than 140/90 mm Hg in the presence of chronic kidney disease (CKD) or diabetes mellitus. In those with CKD and ≥18 years (regardless of race or diabetes status), initial or add-on therapy should include an ACEI or ARB to improve kidney outcomes.
- In more than two-thirds of individuals with hypertension, their HTN cannot be controlled on one drug, and they require two or more antihypertensive agents selected from different drug classes.
- Along with the traditional risks, microalbuminuria (MA) or glomerular filtration rate of less than 60 mL/min is identified as a cardiovascular risk factor. When adjusted for other risk factors, the relative risk of ischemic heart disease associated with MA is increased twofold. An interaction between MA and cigarette smoking has been noted, and the presence of MA more than doubled the predictive effect of the conventional atherosclerotic risk factors for development of ischemic heart disease. MA not only is an independent predictor of ischemic heart disease, but it also substantially increases the risk associated

TABLE 5-2

Keys to an Accurate Blood Pressure Measurement

- Take ≥2 measurements per visit (auscultatory method preferred)
- Have patient be seated comfortably for ≥5 minutes with back supported, feet on floor, and arm supported in horizontal position
- Blood pressure cuff placed at heart level

To detect postural hypotension or hypertension

- Take blood pressure measurement with patient standing for 1–3 minutes

TABLE 5-3
Lifestyle Modification in Hypertension

Modification	Recommendation	Average Systolic Blood Pressure Reduction Rate
Weight reduction	Maintain normal body weight (body mass index 18.5–24.9 kg/m²)	5–20 mm Hg/10 kg
DASH eating plan	Adopt a diet rich in fruits, vegetables, and low-fat dairy products with reduced content of saturated and total fat	8–14 mm Hg
Dietary sodium reduction	Reduce dietary sodium intake to <100 mmol/d (2.4 g sodium or 6 g sodium chloride)	2–8 mm Hg
Aerobic physical activity	Regular aerobic physical activity (e.g., brisk walking) at least 30 min per day, most days of the week	4–9 mm Hg
Moderation of alcohol consumption	Men: limit to ≤2 drinks* per day Women and lighter weight persons: limit to ≤1 drink* per day	2–4 mm Hg

*1 drink = ½ oz or 15 mL ethanol (e.g., 12 oz beer, 5 oz wine, 1.5 oz 80-proof whiskey).
Source: National Heart, Blood and Lung Institute: The Seventh Report of the Joint National Committee on Prevention, Detection, Evaluation, and Treatment of High Blood Pressure (JNC7). Available at www.nhlbi.nih. gov/guidelines/hypertension

with other established risk factors. Because the person with MA has significant cardiovascular disease risk, recommendations for HTN treatment include thiazide diuretics, beta blockers, ACEIs, and calcium channel blockers, particularly nondihydropyridine; in the presence of chronic renal disease, as manifested by MA, recommendations also include the use of an ACEI and an ARB.

- People of African ancestry show reduced BP responses to monotherapy with ACEIs, ARBs, and beta blockers compared with diuretics or calcium channel blockers. Although complete explanations for these racial differences are unknown, what is known is that HTN is the most common cause of renal failure in African Americans.
- In the presence of CKD, JNC-8 recommends an ACEI or an ARB should be prescribed to minimize renal disease risk regardless of race. Using an ACEI or an ARB as part of multidrug therapy, including a calcium channel blocker and thiazide diuretic, is likely to be needed. ACEIs and ARBs should not be used in combination.
- Nondihydropyridine calcium channel blockers (verapamil, diltiazem) are particularly helpful for BP control and renal protection. However, these drugs are potent inhibitors of cytochrome P450 3A4 isoenzyme and should be used with caution with other medications that are substrates of this isoenzyme, such as calcineurin inhibitors. Nondihydropyridines also reduce the heart rate as they induce bradycardic and negatively inotropic effects

and thus should be limited to patients with normal left ventricular function. These agents are contraindicated in patients with severe left ventricular dysfunction and in those with second- or third-degree AV block in the absence of a pacemaker.

The prevalence of hypertension increases in older populations. In the elderly, hypertension is characterized by an elevated systolic blood pressure with normal or low diastolic blood pressure, which is a consequence of age-associated stiffening of the large arteries. The therapeutic target blood pressure goal in the elderly is <140/90 mm Hg in persons aged 65–79 years and a systolic blood pressure of 140–145 mm Hg in persons aged 80 years, if reasonable. When considering blood pressure medications, healthcare providers must be vigilant about treatment-related adverse effects due to a high prevalence of cardiovascular and noncardiovascular comorbidities among the elderly. Some major concerns with the use of blood pressure medications include electrolyte disturbances, renal dysfunction, and excessive orthostatic blood pressure decline. Postural hypotension, defined as a fall in blood pressure of ≥20 mm Hg systolic, ≥10 mm Hg diastolic, or both within 3 minutes of standing upright, increases the risk of falls, syncope, and cardiovascular events in the elderly. Similar to younger adults, a combination of medications is often needed to control hypertension in the elderly, and initiation with combination therapy should be considered if blood pressure is >20/10 mm Hg above goal. Many conditions provide compelling indications to use certain drugs in the elderly (Table 5–4).

TABLE 5-4
Compelling Indications for Individual Drug Classes in Elder Patients

	Thiazide Diuretic	Beta-adrenergic Receptor Antagonist (Beta Blocker)	Angiotensin Converting Enzyme Inhibitor (ACEI)	Angiotensin Receptor Blocker (ARB)	Calcium Antagonist (Calcium Channel Blocker)	Aldosterone Antagonist
Heart failure	√	√	√	√	√	√
Post myocardial infarction		√	√	√		√
CAD or high CVD risk	√	√	√		√	
Diabetes	√	√	√	√	√	
Angina pectoris		√			√	
Aortopathy/aortic aneurysm	√	√	√		√	
Recurrent stroke prevention	√		√	√	√	

Source: Aronow WS, Fleg JL, Pepine CJ, et al. ACCF/AHA 2011 Expert consensus document on hypertension in the elderly. *J Am Coll Cardiol.* 57:2037–2114, 2011. Available at: http://www.medpagetoday.com/upload/2011/4/25/j.jacc.2011.01.008v1.pdf

DISCUSSION SOURCES

National Heart, Blood and Lung Institute. http://www.nhlbi.nih.gov/guidelines/hypertension/, The Seventh Report of the Joint National Committee on Prevention, Detection, Evaluation, and Treatment of High Blood Pressure (JNC7).

Prisant M. Hypertension. In: Bope ET, Kellerman RD, eds. *Conn's Current Therapy 2014.* Philadelphia: Saunders Elsevier, 2014, pp. 349–360.

Recarti C, Unger T. Prevention of coronary artery disease: Recent advances in the management of hypertension. *Curr Atheroscler Rep.* 15:311, 2013.

Aronow WS, Fleg JL, Pepine CJ, et al. ACCF/AHA 2011 Expert consensus document on hypertension in the elderly. *J Am Coll Cardiol.* 57:2037–2114, 2011. Available at: http://www.medpagetoday.com/upload/2011/4/25/j.jacc.2011.01.008v1.pdf, accessed 11/26/13.

James PA, Oparil S, Carter BL, et al. 2014 Evidence-based guideline for the management of high blood pressure in adults. Report from the panel members appointed to the Eighth Joint National Committee (JNC 8). *JAMA.* 2014. Available at: http://jama.jamanetwork.com/article.aspx?articleid=1791497

■) Heart Murmurs

38. You examine a 24-year-old woman with mitral valve prolapse (MVP). Her physical examination findings may also include:
    A. pectus excavatum.
    B. obesity.
    C. petite stature.
    D. hyperextensible joints.

39. In performing a cardiac examination in a person with MVP, you expect to find:
    A. an early- to mid-systolic, crescendo–decrescendo murmur.
    B. a pansystolic murmur.
    C. a low-pitched, diastolic rumble.
    D. a mid- to late-systolic murmur.

40. A risk factor for MVP includes a history of:
    A. rheumatic fever.
    B. rheumatoid arthritis.
    C. Kawasaki disease.
    D. Marfan syndrome.

41. Additional findings in MVP include:
    A. an opening snap.
    B. a mid-systolic click.
    C. a paradoxical splitting of the second heart sound (S_2).
    D. a fourth heart sound (S_4).

42. Intervention for patients with MVP often includes advice about which of the following?
    A. restricted activity because of low cardiac output
    B. control of fluid intake to minimize risk of volume overload
    C. routine use of beta-adrenergic antagonists to control palpitations
    D. encouragement of a regular program of aerobic activity

43. When a heart valve fails to open to its normal orifice size, it is said to be:
A. stenotic.
B. incompetent.
C. sclerotic.
D. regurgitant.

44. When a heart valve fails to close properly, it is said to be:
A. stenotic.
B. incompetent.
C. sclerotic.
D. regurgitant.

45. Upon detection of a suspected pathologic cardiac murmur, the next step in obtaining a diagnostic procedures usually includes a:
A. ventilation perfusion scan.
B. echocardiogram.
C. pulmonary artery angiography.
D. cardiac CT scan.

46. You are evaluating a patient who has rheumatic heart disease. When assessing her for mitral stenosis, you auscultate the heart, anticipating finding the following murmur:
A. systolic with wide radiation over the precordium
B. localized diastolic with little radiation
C. diastolic with radiation to the neck
D. systolic with radiation to the axilla

47. In evaluating mitral valve incompetency, you expect to find the following murmur:
A. systolic with radiation to the axilla
B. diastolic with little radiation
C. diastolic with radiation to the axilla
D. localized systolic

48. In evaluating the person with aortic stenosis, the NP anticipates finding 12-lead ECG changes consistent with:
A. right bundle branch block.
B. extreme axis deviation.
C. right atrial enlargement.
D. left ventricular hypertrophy.

49. Signs and symptoms consistent with endocarditis include all of the following except:
A. bradycardia.
B. Osler's nodes.
C. hematuria.
D. petechiae.

50. From the list below, the most helpful test in suspected bacterial endocarditis includes:
A. urine culture.
B. blood culture.
C. chest X-ray.
D. myocardial biopsy.

51. Of the following patients, who is in greatest need of endocarditis prophylaxis when planning dental work?
A. a 22-year-old woman with MVP with trace mitral regurgitation noted on echocardiogram
B. a 54-year-old woman with a prosthetic aortic valve
C. a 66-year-old man with cardiomyopathy
D. a 58-year-old woman who had a three-vessel coronary artery bypass graft with drug-eluting stents 1 year ago

52. Of the following people, who has no significant increased risk for developing bacterial endocarditis?
A. a 43-year-old woman with a bicuspid aortic valve
B. a 55-year-old man who was diagnosed with a Still's murmur during childhood
C. a 45-year-old woman with a history of endocarditis
D. a 75-year-old man with dilated cardiomyopathy

53. You are examining an 85-year-old woman and find a grade 3/6 crescendo–decrescendo systolic murmur with radiation to the neck. This is most likely caused by:
A. aortic stenosis.
B. aortic regurgitation.
C. anemia.
D. mitral stenosis.

54. Aortic stenosis in a 15-year-old male is most likely:
A. a sequela of rheumatic fever.
B. a result of a congenital defect.
C. calcific in nature.
D. found with atrial septal defect.

55. A risk factor for acquired aortic stenosis is:
A. history of pulmonary embolism.
B. COPD.
C. type 2 diabetes.
D. prior rheumatic fever.

56. Management of mild aortic stenosis in a 12-year-old boy usually includes:
A. ongoing monitoring with ECG and echocardiogram.
B. use of a balloon catheter to separate fused valve leaflets.
C. valve replacement.
D. use of warfarin or other anticoagulant.

57. A physiological murmur has which of the following characteristics?
A. occurs late in systole
B. is noted in a localized area of auscultation
C. becomes softer when the patient moves from supine to standing
D. frequently obliterates S_2

58. You are examining an 18-year-old man who is seeking a sports clearance physical examination. You note a mid-systolic murmur that gets louder when he stands. This may represent:
A. aortic stenosis.
B. hypertrophic cardiomyopathy.
C. a physiologic murmur.
D. a Still's murmur.

59. According to recommendations of the American Heart Association (AHA), which of the following antibiotics should be used for endocarditis prophylaxis in patients who are allergic to penicillin?
    A. erythromycin
    B. dicloxacillin
    C. azithromycin
    D. ofloxacin

60. A grade III systolic heart murmur is usually:
    A. softer than the S_2 heart sound.
    B. about as loud as the S_1 heart sound.
    C. accompanied by a thrill.
    D. heard across the precordium but without radiation.

61. The S_3 heart sound has all of the following characteristics except:
    A. heard in early diastole
    B. a presystolic sound
    C. noted in the presence of ventricular overload
    D. heard best with the bell of the stethoscope

62. The S_4 heart sound has which of the following characteristics?
    A. After it is initially noted, it is a permanent finding.
    B. It is noted in the presence of poorly controlled hypertension.
    C. It is heard best in early diastole.
    D. It is a high-pitched sound best heard with the diaphragm of the stethoscope.

63. Of the following individuals, who is most likely to have a physiological split S_2 heart sound?
    A. a 19-year-old healthy athlete
    B. a 49-year-old with well-controlled hypertension
    C. a 68-year-old with stable heart failure
    D. a 78-year-old with cardiomyopathy

64. Idiopathic hypertrophic subaortic stenosis (IHSS) is inherited in a:
    A. sex-linked recessive manner.
    B. sex-linked dominant manner.
    C. autosomal-recessive manner.
    D. autosomal-dominant manner.

Answers

38. A.	47. A.	56. A.
39. D.	48. D.	57. C.
40. D.	49. A.	58. B.
41. B.	50. B.	59. C.
42. D.	51. B.	60. B.
43. A.	52. B.	61. B.
44. B.	53. A.	62. B.
45. B.	54. B.	63. A.
46. B.	55. D.	64. D.

Heart murmurs are caused by the sounds produced from turbulent blood flow. Blood traveling through the chambers and great vessels is usually silent. When the flow is sufficient to generate turbulence in the wall of the heart or great vessel, a murmur occurs.

Murmurs are often benign; the examiner simply hears the blood flowing through the heart, but no cardiac structural abnormality exists. Certain cardiac structural problems, such as valvular and myocardial disorders, however, can contribute to the development of a murmur (Table 5–5).

Normal heart valves allow one-way, unimpeded, forward blood flow through the heart. The entire stroke output is able to pass freely during one phase of the cardiac cycle (diastole with the atrioventricular valves, systole with the others), and there is no backflow of blood. When a heart valve fails to open to its normal orifice, it is stenotic. When it fails to close appropriately, the valve is incompetent, causing regurgitation of blood to the previous chamber or vessel. Both of these events place a patient at significant risk for embolic disease.

Physiologic murmurs are heard in the absence of cardiac pathology. The term *physiologic* implies that the reason for murmur is something other than obstruction to flow and that the murmur is present with a normal gradient across the valve. This murmur is heard in 80% of thin adults or children if the cardiac examination is performed in a soundproof booth, and it is best heard at the left sternal border. The physiological murmur occurs in early to mid systole, leaving the S_1 and S_2 heart sounds intact. In addition, an individual with a benign systolic ejection murmur denies having cardiac symptoms and has an otherwise normal cardiac examination, including an appropriately located point of maximum impulse and full pulses. Because no cardiac pathology is present with a physiologic murmur, no endocarditis prophylaxis is needed. Once a heart murmur is detected, an ECG is used to detect heart rhythm and structure problems including chamber hypertrophy. A transthoracic or transesophageal echocardiogram is used to create moving images of the heart to identify abnormal heart valves, such as those that are calcified or leaking, as well as other heart defects. A cardiac CT or MRI can also be used to visualize heart defects that may cause the murmur; its use is typically limited to clinical situations where the echocardiogram results require clarification.

Aortic stenosis (AS) is the inability of the aortic valves to open to an optimal orifice. The aortic valve normally opens to 3 cm²; AS usually does not cause significant symptoms until the valvular orifice is limited to 0.8 cm². The disease is characterized by a long symptom-free period with rapid clinical deterioration at the onset of symptoms, including dyspnea, syncope, chest pain, and heart failure (HF). Low pulse pressure, the difference between the systolic and diastolic blood pressure, is a characteristic of severe AS.

When AS is present in adults who are middle-aged and older, it is most often the acquired form. Risk factors for acquired AS include older age and previous rheumatic fever. In an older adult, the problem is usually calcification, leading to the inability of the valve to open to its normal orifice.

TABLE 5-5
Assessment of Common Cardiac Murmurs in Adults

WHEN EVALUATING AN ADULT WITH CARDIAC MURMUR

Ask about major symptoms of heart disease: chest pain, heart failure symptoms, palpitations, syncope, activity intolerance

The bell of the stethoscope is most helpful for auscultating lower pitched sounds, whereas the diaphragm is most helpful for higher pitched sounds

Systolic murmurs are graded on a 1–6 scale, from barely audible to audible with stethoscope off the chest. Grade 3 murmur is about as loud as S_1 or S_2, whereas grade 2 murmur is slightly softer; grade 1 murmur is difficult to hear. Grade ≥4 murmurs are usually accompanied by a thrill, or the feel of turbulent blood flow. Diastolic murmurs are usually graded on the same scale but abbreviated to grades 1–4 because these murmurs are not loud enough to reach grades 5 and 6.

A critical part of the evaluation of a person with a heart murmur is to decide to offer antimicrobial prophylaxis. No prophylaxis is needed with benign murmurs. Please refer to the American Heart Association's Guideline for the latest advice.

Murmur	Important Cardiac Examination Findings	Additional Findings	Comments
Physiological (also known as innocent, functional)	Grade 1–3/6 early- to mid-systolic murmur heard best at left sternal border, but usually audible over precordium	No radiation beyond precordium. Softens or disappears with standing, increases in intensity with activity, fever, anemia. S_1, S_2 intact, normal PMI	Etiology probably flows over aortic valve. May be heard in ~80% of thin adults if examined in sound-proof room. Asymptomatic with no report of chest pain, heart failure symptoms, palpitations, syncope, activity intolerance
Aortic stenosis	Grade 1–4/6 harsh systolic murmur, usually crescendo–decrescendo pattern, heard best at second right intercostal space, apex, softens with standing	Radiates to carotids, may have diminished S_2, slow filling carotid pulse, narrow pulse pressure, loud S_4, heaving PMI. The greater the degree of stenosis, the later the peak of murmur	In younger adults, usually congenital bicuspid valve. In older adults, usually calcific, rheumatic in nature. Dizziness and syncope ominous signs, pointing to severely decreased cardiac output
Aortic sclerosis	Grade 2–3/6 systolic ejection murmur heard best at second right intercostal space	Carotid upstroke full, not delayed, no S_4, absence of symptoms	Benign thickening or calcification, or both, of aortic valve leaflets. No change in valve pressure gradient. Also known as "50 over 50" murmur as found in >50% adults >50 y.o.
Aortic regurgitation	Grade 1–3/4 high-pitched blowing diastolic murmur heard best at third left intercostal space	May be enhanced by forced expiration, leaning forward. Usually with S_3, wide pulse pressure, sustained thrusting apical impulse	More common in men, usually from rheumatic heart disease, but occasionally due to latent syphilis
Mitral stenosis	Grade 1–3/4 low-pitched late diastolic murmur heard best at the apex, localized. Short crescendo–decrescendo rumble, similar to a bowling ball rolling down an alley or distant thunder	Often with opening snap, accentuated S_1 in the mitral area. Enhanced by left lateral decubitus position, squat, cough, immediately after Valsalva	Nearly all rheumatic in origin. Protracted latency period, then gradual decrease in exercise tolerance leading to rapid downhill course owing to low cardiac output. Atrial fibrillation common

Continued

TABLE 5-5
Assessment of Common Cardiac Murmurs in Adults—cont'd

Murmur	Important Cardiac Examination Findings	Additional Findings	Comments
Atrial septal defect (uncorrected)	Grade 1–3/6 systolic ejection murmur at the pulmonic area	Widely split S_2, right ventricular heave	Typically without symptoms until middle age, then present with congestive heart failure. Persistent ostium secundum in mid septum
Pulmonary hypertension	Narrow splitting S_2, murmur of tricuspid regurgitation	Report of shortness of breath nearly universal	Seen with right ventricular hypertrophy, right atrial hypertrophy as identified by ECG, echocardiogram. Secondary pulmonary hypertension may be a consequence of dexfenfluramine (Redux), "phen/fen" (phentermine with fenfluramine) use (Dexfenfluramine and fenfluramine no longer available on the North American market due to safety issues.)
Mitral regurgitation	Grade 1–4/6 high-pitched blowing systolic murmur, often extending beyond S_2. Sounds like long "haaa," "hooo." Heard best at right lower scapular border	Radiates to axilla, often with laterally displaced PMI. Decreased with standing, Valsalva maneuver. Increased by squat, hand grip	Found in ischemic heart disease, endocarditis, RHD. With RHD, often with other valve abnormalities (aortic stenosis, mitral stenosis, aortic regurgitation)
Mitral valve prolapse	Grade 1–3/6 late-systolic crescendo murmur with honking quality heard best at apex. Murmur follows mid-systolic click	With Valsalva or standing, click moves forward into earlier systole, resulting in a longer sounding murmur. With hand grasp, squat, click moves back further into systole, resulting in a shorter murmur	Often seen with minor thoracic deformities such as pectus excavatum, straight back, and shallow anterior–posterior diameter. Chest pain is sometimes present, but there is a question as to whether mitral valve prolapse itself is cause

PMI, point of maximal impulse; RHD, rheumatic heart disease.
Source: Mangione S. *Physical Diagnosis Secrets*. ed. 2. St. Louis, MO: Elsevier Health Sciences, 2007.

Valvular changes in middle-aged adults without congenital AS are usually the sequelae of rheumatic fever and represent about 30% of valvular dysfunction seen in rheumatic heart disease.

AS may be present in children and younger adults and is usually caused by a congenital bicuspid (rather than tricuspid) valve or by a three-cusp valve with leaflet fusion. This defect is most often found in boys and young men and is commonly accompanied by a long-standing history of becoming excessively short of breath with increased activity such as running. The physical examination is usually normal except for the associated cardiac findings. For mild AS, treatment is not necessary, but ongoing monitoring is important to detect any change toward moderate to severe level. This may involve ECG, echocardiogram, exercise stress test, CT scan, or MRI. Surgical correction or replacement of the valve is often needed for moderate to severe AS.

The heart murmur of mitral regurgitation (MR) arises from mitral valve incompetency or the inability of the mitral valve to close properly. This incompetency allows a retrograde flow from a high-pressure area (left ventricle) to an area of lower pressure (left atrium). MR is most often caused by the degeneration of the mitral valve, commonly by rheumatic fever, endocarditis, calcific annulus, rheumatic heart disease, ruptured chordae, or papillary muscle dysfunction. In MR resulting from rheumatic heart disease, there is usually some degree of mitral stenosis. After the person becomes symptomatic, the disease progresses in a downhill course leading to HF over the next 10 years.

Mitral valve prolapse (MVP) is likely the most common valvular heart problem; it is present in perhaps 10% of the population. The degree of distress (chest pain, dyspnea) may depend in part on the degree of MR, although some studies have failed to reveal any difference in the rates of chest pain in patients with or without MVP. Potentially the greatest threat is the rupture of chordae, usually seen only in those with connective tissue disease, especially Marfan syndrome.

Most patients with MVP have a benign condition in which one of the valve leaflets is unusually long and buckles or prolapses into the left atrium, usually in mid systole. At that time, a click occurs that is followed by a short murmur caused by regurgitation of blood into the atrium. Cardiac output is usually uncompromised, and the event goes unnoticed by the patient; however, the clinician may detect this on examination. Echocardiography fails to reveal any abnormality, simply noting the valve buckling followed by a small-volume MR. If there are no cardiac complaints and the rest of the cardiac examination, including the ECG, is normal, no further evaluation is needed.

One way of describing this variation from the norm is to inform the patient that one leaflet of the mitral valve is a bit longer than usual. The "holder" (valve orifice) is of average size, however. This discrepancy causes the valve to buckle a bit, just as a person's foot would if forced into a shoe that is one or two sizes too small. As a result, the heart makes an extra set of sounds (click and murmur) but is not diseased or damaged. MVP is often found in patients with minor thoracic deformities such as pectus excavatum, a dish-shaped concave area at T1, and scoliosis. The exact nature of this correlation of findings is not understood.

The second and much smaller group of patients with MVP has systolic displacement of one or both of the mitral leaflets into the left atrium alone with valve thickening and redundancy, usually accompanied by mild to moderate MR. This group typically has additional health problems, such as Marfan syndrome or other connective tissue disease. There is a risk of bacterial endocarditis in this group because structural cardiac abnormality is present.

Barring other health problems, patients with MVP usually have normal cardiac output and tolerate a program of aerobic activity. This activity should be encouraged to promote health and well-being. The degree of MVP is increased, however, which increases intensity of the murmur, when circulating volume is low. Maintaining a high level of fluid intake should be encouraged for patients with MVP. Treatment with a beta-adrenergic antagonist (beta blocker) is indicated only when symptomatic recurrent tachycardia or palpitations is an issue.

Hypertrophic cardiomyopathy is a disease of the cardiac muscle. The ventricular septum is thick and asymmetrical, leading to potential blockage of the outflow tract. Patients often exhibit symptoms of cardiac outflow tract blockage with activity because the hypertrophic ventricular walls better approximate with the increased force of myocardial contraction associated with exercise. The presentation of hypertrophic cardiomyopathy can be sudden cardiac death. Idiopathic hypertrophic subaortic stenosis is a type of cardiomyopathy. A mutation in one of several genes can cause the condition. The mutation is inherited in an autosomal-dominant pattern, thus requiring only one copy of the mutant gene to cause the disorder. In most cases, an affected person has one parent with the condition. Patients with this disorder are usually young adults with a history of dyspnea with activity, but they are often asymptomatic.

Infective endocarditis is an infection of the inner lining of the heart, most commonly occurring in persons with damaged heart valves, prosthetic heart valves, or other heart defects. Risk factors also include a history of endocarditis or injected drug use. The infection can develop slowly or rapidly, depending on the causative pathogen, and signs and symptoms can vary accordingly. The most common include fever, chills, a new or altered heart murmur, fatigue, aching joints and muscles, shortness of breath, edema, persistent cough, unexplained weight loss, hematuria, tenderness of the spleen, Osler's nodes, and petechiae. Diagnosis involves a blood culture to detect the infection as well as a transesophageal echocardiogram to identify vegetation formation or infected tissue in the heart. An ECG can be used to detect alteration to heart function, whereas a chest X-ray, CT scan, or MRI may be used to detect spread of the infection to other sites. Endocarditis is treated with high doses of intravenous antibiotics that should be tailored to the causative pathogen and susceptibility profile. Treatment lasts at least 4–6 weeks to eradicate the infection. Surgery is occasionally required to repair or replace a damaged valve caused by infective endocarditis.

The American Heart Association (AHA) has developed guidelines for the evaluation of infectious endocarditis risk. Although in the past, infectious endocarditis prophylaxis was used liberally for most individuals with a past or current history of heart murmur or structural cardiac abnormality, the AHA has long advocated for restraint in this practice, recognizing that infectious endocarditis is much more likely to result from frequent exposure to random bacteremias associated with daily activities than from bacteremia caused by a dental, gastrointestinal tract, or genitourinary tract procedure; maintenance of optimal oral health and hygiene is likely more important than prophylactic antibiotics for a dental procedure in reducing infectious endocarditis risk. Infectious endocarditis prophylaxis is considered a reasonable option, however, for people at highest risk, including individuals with an infectious endocarditis history or a prosthetic heart valve (Table 5–6).

Heart sound abnormalities are commonly noted in poorly controlled hypertension (S_4) and heart failure (S_3). Knowledge of the timing and qualities of these sounds is an important component of safe and effective practice (Table 5–7).

DISCUSSION SOURCES

Goolsby MJ, Grubbs L. *Advanced Assessment: Interpreting Findings and Formulating Differential Diagnoses*, ed. 2. Philadelphia: F.A. Davis; 2011

Wilson W, Taubert KA, Gewitz M, et al. Prevention of infective endocarditis: Guidelines from the American Heart Association. *Circulation.* 116:1736–1754, 2007. Available at http://circ.ahajournals.org/content/116/15/1736.full.pdf

TABLE 5-6
Prevention of Endocarditis: Guidelines from the American Heart Association

PRIMARY REASONS FOR REVISIONS OF INFECTIOUS ENDOCARDITIS (IE) PROPHYLAXIS GUIDELINES

IE is much more likely to result from frequent exposure to random bacteremias associated with daily activities than from bacteremia caused by a dental, gastrointestinal (GI) tract, or genitourinary (GU) tract procedure.
Prophylaxis may prevent very few, if any, cases of IE in individuals who undergo a dental, GI tract, or GU tract procedure.
The risk of antibiotic-associated adverse events exceeds the benefit, if any, from prophylactic antibiotic therapy.
Maintenance of optimal oral health and hygiene may reduce incidence of bacteremia from daily activities and is more important than prophylactic antibiotics for a dental procedure to reduce the risk of IE.

CARDIAC CONDITIONS ASSOCIATED WITH HIGHEST RISK OF ADVERSE OUTCOME FROM ENDOCARDITIS FOR WHICH PROPHYLAXIS WITH DENTAL PROCEDURES IS REASONABLE

Prosthetic cardiac valve or prosthetic material used for cardiac valve repair
Previous IE
Congenital heart disease (CHD)*
- Unrepaired cyanotic CHD, including palliative shunts and conduits
- Completely repaired congenital heart defect with prosthetic material or device, whether placed by surgery or by catheter intervention, during the first 6 mo after the procedure[†]
- Repaired congenital heart disease with residual defects at the site or adjacent to the site of a prosthetic patch or prosthetic device (which inhibits endothelialization)
- Cardiac transplantation recipients who develop cardiac valvulopathy

DENTAL, ORAL, OR RESPIRATORY TRACT OR ESOPHAGEAL PROCEDURES: GIVE 30–60 MINUTES BEFORE PROCEDURE

Adults	Children
Amoxicillin 2 g PO	Amoxicillin 50 mg/kg PO
IF UNABLE TO TAKE ORAL MEDICATION	
Ampicillin 2 g IM or IV Cefazolin or ceftriaxone 1 g IM or IV	Ampicillin 50 mg/kg IM or IV
	Cefazolin or ceftriaxone 50 mg/kg IM or IV
ORAL, IF PENICILLIN OR AMPICILLIN ALLERGIC	
Clindamycin 600 mg	Clindamycin 20 mg/kg
Cephalexin[‡,§] 2 g	Cephalexin[§] 50 mg/kg
Azithromycin or clarithromycin 500 mg	Azithromycin or clarithromycin 15 mg/kg
IF PENICILLIN OR AMPICILLIN ALLERGIC AND UNABLE TO TAKE ORAL MEDICATION	
Cefazolin[§] or ceftriaxone[§] 1 g IM or IV	Cefazolin[§] or ceftriaxone[§] 50 mg/kg IM or IV
Clindamycin 600 mg IM or IV	Clindamycin 20 mg/kg IM or IV

*Except for the conditions listed, antibiotic prophylaxis is no longer recommended for any other form of CHD.
[†]Prophylaxis is reasonable because endothelialization of prosthetic material occurs within 6 mo after the procedure.
[‡]Or other first-generation or second-generation oral cephalosporin in equivalent adult or pediatric dosage.
[§]Cephalosporins should not be used in an individual with a history of anaphylaxis, angioedema, or urticaria with penicillins or ampicillin.
Source: Wilson W, Taubert KA, Gewitz M, et al. Prevention of infective endocarditis: Guidelines from the American Heart Association. *Circulation.* 116:1736–1754, 2007. Available at http://circ.ahajournals.org/content/116/15/1736.full.pdf

TABLE 5-7
Heart Sounds

Heart Sound	Significance	Comment	Heard Best
S_1	Marks beginning of systole. Produced by events surrounding closure of mitral and tricuspid valve.	Best heard at apex with the diaphragm	"**Lub** dub" heard nearly simultaneous with carotid upstroke
S_2	Marks end of systole. Produced by events surrounding closure of aortic and pulmonic valves	Best heard at base with diaphragm	"Lub **dub**" heard
Physiological split S_2	Widening of normal interval between aortic and pulmonic components of S_2. Caused by delay in pulmonic component	Heard best in pulmonic region	The split *in*creases on patient *in*spiration. Found in most adults <30 y.o., fewer beyond this age. Benign finding
Pathological split S_2	Fixed split—no change with inspiration Paradoxical split—narrows or closes with inspiration	Heard best in pulmonic region	Fixed split often found in uncorrected septal defect Paradoxical split often found in conditions that delay aortic closure, such as left bundle branch block Finding can resolve with treatment of underlying condition
Pathological S_3	Marker of ventricular overload, systolic dysfunction, or both	Heard in early diastole, can sound like it is "hooked on" to the back of S_2 Low pitch, best heard with bell, might miss with diaphragm	For diagnosis of heart failure, correlate with additional findings such as dyspnea, tachycardia, crackles Finding can resolve with treatment of underlying condition
S_4	Marker of poor diastolic function, most often found in poorly controlled hypertension or recurrent myocardial ischemia	Heard late in diastole, can sound like it is "hooked on" to the front of S_1 Sometimes called a presystolic sound Soft, low pitch (higher pitch than S_3), best heard with bell	Finding can resolve with treatment of underlying condition

Acute Coronary Syndrome

65. Causes of unstable angina include all of the following except:
    A. ventricular hypertrophy.
    B. vasoconstriction.
    C. nonocclusive thrombus.
    D. inflammation or infection.

66. Which of the following is most consistent with a person presenting with unstable angina?
    A. a 5-minute episode of chest tightness brought on by stair climbing and relieved by rest
    B. a severe, searing pain that penetrates the chest and lasts about 30 seconds
    C. chest pressure lasting 20 minutes that occurs at rest
    D. "heartburn" relieved by position change

67. The initial manifestation of coronary heart disease in men is most commonly:
   A. unstable angina.
   B. myocardial infarction.
   C. intracranial hemorrhage.
   D. stable angina.

68. In assessing a woman with or at risk for acute coronary syndrome (ACS), the NP considers that the patient will likely present:
   A. in a manner similar to that of a man with equivalent disease.
   B. at the same age as a man with similar health problems.
   C. more commonly with angina and less commonly with acute MI.
   D. less commonly with HF.

69. Rank the following signs and symptoms in the order of most common to least common in a 60-year-old woman in the time preceding an ACS event.
   A. dyspnea
   B. anxiety
   C. sleep disturbance
   D. unusual fatigue

70. The cardiac finding most commonly associated with unstable angina is:
   A. physiological split S_2.
   B. S_4.
   C. opening snap.
   D. summation gallop.

71. Which of the following changes on the 12-lead ECG do you expect to find in a patient with acute coronary syndrome?
   A. flattened T wave
   B. R wave larger than 25 mm
   C. ST segment deviation (>0.05 mV)
   D. fixed Q wave

72. Beta-adrenergic antagonists are used in ACS therapy because of their ability to:
   A. reverse obstruction-fixed vessel lesions.
   B. reduce myocardial oxygen demand.
   C. enhance myocardial vessel tone.
   D. stabilize arterial volume.

73. Nitrates are used in ACS therapy because of their ability to:
   A. reverse fixed vessel obstruction.
   B. reduce myocardial oxygen demand.
   C. cause vasodilation.
   D. stabilize cardiac rhythm.

74. Which of the following is most consistent with a patient presenting with acute MI?
   A. a 5-minute episode of chest tightness brought on by stair climbing
   B. a severe, localized pain that penetrates the chest and lasts about 3 hours
   C. chest pressure lasting 20 minutes that occurs at rest
   D. retrosternal diffuse pain for 30 minutes accompanied by diaphoresis

75 to 78. Match the clinical syndrome with its pathophysiologic characteristic.

75. unstable angina
76. stable angina
77. non–ST-elevated myocardial infarction (NSTEMI)
78. ST-elevated myocardial infarction (STEMI)

A. new onset of chest pain and discomfort at rest or worsening of symptoms with activities that previously did not provoke symptoms
B. predictable onset of chest pain or discomfort, usually with physical exertion
C. results from full thickness (transmural) necrosis of the myocardium and total occlusion of coronary artery
D. results from severe coronary artery narrowing, transient occlusion, or microembolization of thrombus and/or atheromatous material

79. Which of the following changes on the 12-lead ECG would you expect to find in a patient with history of acute transmural MI 6 months ago?
   A. 2-mm ST segment elevation
   B. R wave larger than 25 mm
   C. T wave inversion
   D. deep Q waves

80. Which of the following changes on the 12-lead ECG would you expect to find in a patient with myocardial ischemia?
   A. 2-mm ST segment elevation
   B. S wave larger than 10 mm
   C. T wave inversion
   D. deep Q waves

81. Thrombolytic therapy is indicated in patients with chest pain and ECG changes such as:
   A. 1-mm ST segment depression in leads V1 and V3.
   B. physiologic Q waves in leads aVF, V5, and V6.
   C. 3-mm ST segment elevation in leads V1 to V4.
   D. T wave inversion in leads aVL and aVR.

82. An abnormality of which of the following is the most sensitive marker for myocardial damage?
   A. aspartate aminotransferase
   B. creatine phosphokinase (CPK)
   C. troponin I (cTnI)
   D. lactate dehydrogenase

83. All of the following should be prescribed as part of therapy in ACS except:
   A. aspirin.
   B. metoprolol.
   C. lisinopril.
   D. nisoldipine.

84. You see a 54-year-old man who reports acute angina episodes with significant exertion. He is currently taking a beta blocker and clopidogrel. You consider the use of which of the following at the start of anginal symptoms?
   A. an oral dose of a calcium channel blocker
   B. a dose of nitroglycerin via oral spray
   C. an extra dose of the beta blocker
   D. a sustained-effect nitroglycerin patch

85. Which of the following is an absolute contraindication to the use of thrombolytic therapy?
   A. history of hemorrhagic stroke
   B. BP of 160/100 mm Hg or greater at presentation
   C. current use of warfarin
   D. active peptic ulcer disease

86. For a patient with a history of MI and who demonstrates intolerance to aspirin, an acceptable alternative antiplatelet medication is:
   A. ibuprofen.
   B. clopidogrel.
   C. warfarin.
   D. rivaroxaban.

87. Routine use of the treadmill exercise tolerance test is most appropriate for:
   A. a healthy 34-year-old woman.
   B. a 56-year-old man following coronary artery angioplasty who remains to establish activity tolerance.
   C. an 84-year-old man with stable angina who uses a walker.
   D. a 52-year-old woman with dyslipidemia and no history of ACS.

88. According to the recommendations of the American Association of Clinical Endocrinologists, the recommended low-density lipoprotein goal for a 64-year-old man with diabetes mellitus who presented with a history of ACS 2 years ago should be less than:
   A. 70 mg/dL (<1.8 mmol/L).
   B. 100 mg/dL (< 2.6 mmol/L).
   C. 130 mg/dL (< 3.4 mmol/L).
   D. 160 mg/dL (< 4.1 mmol/L).

89. Which of the following is least likely to be reported in ACS?
   A. newly noted pulmonary crackles
   B. transient MR murmur
   C. hypotension
   D. pain reproduced with palpation

Answers

65. A.	**74.** D.	**83.** D.
66. C.	**75.** A.	**84.** B.
67. B.	**76.** B.	**85.** A.
68. C.	**77.** D.	**86.** B.
69. D, C, A, B.	**78.** C.	**87.** B.
70. B.	**79.** D.	**88.** A.
71. C.	**80.** C.	**89.** D.
72. B.	**81.** C.	
73. C.	**82.** C.	

Acute coronary syndrome (ACS) and angina pectoris, most often caused by atherosclerosis, result from an imbalance in the ability to supply the myocardium with sufficient oxygen to meet its metabolic demands. ACS includes an umbrella of cardiovascular conditions that include ST-elevated myocardial infarction (STEMI), non–ST-elevated myocardial infarction (NSTEMI), and unstable angina. Typically, STEMI is associated with transmural myocardial infarction (full-thickness necrosis of the myocardium in the region of the MI), subsequent development of Q waves on the ECG, and total occlusion of a coronary artery. NSTEMI involves non-transmural MI, no Q-wave evolution of the ECG, and subtotal occlusion of the vessel.

The discomfort associated with an anginal episode is described with many terms—*pressure, pain, tightness, heaviness,* and *suffocation*. In stable angina, patterns of symptom provocation are usually predictable, with exertion often causing discomfort that is promptly relieved with rest, use of sublingual (tablet or spray) nitroglycerin, or both. Unstable angina is defined as a new onset of symptoms at rest or worsening symptoms with activities that did not previously provoke symptoms. The clinical presentation of unstable angina represents an emergency and should be handled accordingly. Testing to support the angina diagnosis includes a resting 12-lead ECG (although this is normal in about 50% of individuals with the disease) and exercise tolerance or other form of stress testing, often with myocardial nuclear imaging. Computed tomography to document coronary artery calcification is another non-invasive test.

Certain characteristics increase or decrease the likelihood of ACS (Tables 5–8 and 5–9). Women usually have onset of coronary heart disease at significantly older ages and are likely to present differently than men. Dyspnea is often an anginal equivalent in older women. In a study of 515 women with ACS, 95% reported new or different symptoms in weeks before the event, including unusual fatigue (70%), sleep disturbance (48%), shortness of breath (42%), indigestion (39%), and anxiety (35%). Symptoms experienced by the women during ACS included shortness of breath (58%), weakness (55%), unusual fatigue (43%), diaphoresis (39%), dizziness (39%), and chest pain or pressure (30%); 43% of the woman had no chest discomfort during the event.

TABLE 5-8

Chest Pain, Typical of Myocardial Ischemia or Myocardial Infarction

- Substernal compression or crush
- Pressure, tightness, heaviness, cramping, aching sensation
- Unexplained indigestion, belching, epigastric pain
- Radiating pain to neck, jaw, shoulders, back, or one or both arms
- Dyspnea, nausea/vomiting, diaphoresis

Source: American College of Cardiology/American Heart Association 2007 Guidelines for the Management of Patients with Unstable Angina/Non–ST-Elevation Myocardial Infarction. http://circ.ahajournals.org/cgi/content/short/CIRCULATIONAHA.107.185752v1, Executive summary: A report of the American College of Cardiology/American Heart Association Task Force on Practice Guidelines (Writing Committee to Revise the 2002 Guidelines for the Management of Patients with Unstable Angina/Non–ST-Elevation Myocardial Infarction)

Men often have their first manifestation of coronary heart disease in the form of MI, whereas women initially present first with angina pectoris, which often leads to MI. Women younger than 60 years often have a presentation similar to that of men, however. Atypical MI presentation is often noted in both sexes when patients are older than 80 years, which can include confusion and cognitive impairment.

Drug therapy in ACS includes beta blockers because these agents reduce myocardial workload through lowering heart rate, lowering stroke volume, and blunting catecholamine response and aspirin therapy; most patients with angina also have an indication for ACEI use. A calcium channel blocker (CCB) is often added if anginal symptoms occur two or more times per week and no contraindications to calcium channel blocker use exist. A CCB may be useful to relieve ischemia, lower blood pressure, or control the ventricular response rate to atrial fibrillation in patients who are intolerant of beta blockers. Caution, however, is advised for use in patients with left ventricular systolic dysfunction. Dihydropyridine CCBs (e.g., nifedipine, amlodipine) tend

TABLE 5-9

Likelihood That Signs and Symptoms Represent Acute Coronary Syndrome Secondary to Coronary Artery Disease

Features	High Likelihood: Any of the Following Present	Intermediate Likelihood: Absence of High-Likelihood Features and Presence of Any of the Following	Low Likelihood: Absence of High- or Intermediate-Likelihood Features but Many Have the Following
History	Chest or left arm pain or discomfort as chief symptom producing documented angina	Chest or left arm pain or discomfort as chief symptom Age >70 yr at onset Male sex Diabetes mellitus	Probable ischemic symptoms in absence of any intermediate-likelihood characteristics Recent cocaine use
Examination	Pulmonary edema New rales or crackles Transient mitral regurgitation murmur Hypotension	Extracardiac vascular disease	Chest discomfort reproduced by palpation
ECG findings	New or presumably new transient ST segment deviation (≥0.05 mV) or T wave inversion (≥0.2 mV) with symptoms	Fixed Q waves Abnormal ST segments or E waves not documented as new	T wave flattening or inversion in leads with dominant R waves ECG
Cardiac markers	Elevated cTnT, cTnI, or CPK-MB	Normal	Normal

Source: American College of Cardiology/American Heart Association 2007 Guidelines for the Management of Patients with Unstable Angina/Non–ST-Elevation Myocardial Infarction. http://circ.ahajournals.org/cgi/content/short/CIRCULATIONAHA.107.185752v1, Executive summary: A report of the American College of Cardiology/American Heart Association Task Force on Practice Guidelines (Writing Committee to Revise the 2002 Guidelines for the Management of Patients with Unstable Angina/Non–ST-Elevation Myocardial Infarction)

to be more potent vasodilators than nondihydropyridines (e.g., verapamil, diltiazem), whereas the latter tend to have more marked inotropic effects. Sustained-effect nitroglycerin via the oral or topical route (patch or ointment) can be added, particularly if nocturnal symptoms are present. Nitroglycerin via sublingual tablet or spray should be prescribed with advice on its use for acute symptoms and education to monitor frequency of use to detect patterns of anginal triggers and disease instability. Use of nitrates enhances myocardial perfusion through peripheral and central vasodilation. Overall cardiovascular risk reduction is also important with the use of appropriate dyslipidemia agents, with HMG-CoA reductase inhibitor therapy (statin) therapy nearly always indicated. Coronary angiography should be considered if exercise tolerance is poor, significant abnormality is noted on resting or exercise ECG or myocardial imaging, or symptoms become less stable. An exercise tolerance test can be performed on a routine basis for patients at high risk to check the effectiveness of procedures done to improve coronary circulation and can predict the risk of future cardiovascular events, such as a myocardial infarction.

S_4 is often heard with myocardial ischemia and poorly controlled angina pectoris. This sound of poor myocardial relaxation (compliance) and diastolic dysfunction may potentially cause decreased cardiac output. The third heart sound (S_3) is that of poor myocardial contractility and systolic dysfunction and usually leads to decreased cardiac output; this abnormal heart sound is often heard in the presence of heart failure.

MI/ACS most commonly occurs when an atherosclerotic plaque ruptures, leading to the formation of an occlusive thrombus. Coronary artery spasm can also occur, adding to the vessel obstruction. A patient with suspected ACS needs to be assessed promptly and accurately because therapy to reinstitute vessel patency (e.g., thrombolysis, percutaneous angioplasty, stent placement, coronary artery bypass grafting) should be initiated early in the process to limit myocardial damage. The 12-lead ECG should be assessed for changes consistent with myocardial ischemia, myocardial injury, and MI.

In approximately 75% of patients admitted to the hospital for MI, this condition is ruled out. At least 25% of all MIs are clinically silent, however. To reduce unneeded hospitalization and to detect asymptomatic MI/ACS, diagnostic tests that are highly sensitive and specific for myocardial damage are needed. An electrocardiogram (ECG) is typically the first test done to diagnose MI and is often performed while the patient is en route to the hospital by EMT to activate the cardiac team. This can be critical in reducing the arrival-to-catheterization time. Other tests may be used to determine the extent of heart damage caused by a myocardial infarction or to determine if symptoms are from another cause. These tests include a chest X-ray, echocardiogram, nuclear scan, CT angiogram, or coronary angiogram. Blood tests are also used to detect specific enzymes produced in the presence of heart damage induced by MI.

Troponin is a regulatory protein of the myofibril with three major subtypes: C, I, and T. Subtypes I (cTnI) and T (cTnT) are released in the presence of myocardial damage. Both increase rapidly within the first 12 hours after MI; cTnT typically remains elevated for about 168 hours, and cTnI remains elevated for about 192 hours. cTnI is the more cardiac-specific measure and is sensitive for small-volume myocardial damage. CTnT levels can be elevated in chronic renal failure, muscle trauma, and rhabdomyolysis. cTnI is more sensitive and specific than ECG and creatine phosphokinase isoenzyme MB (CK-MB) in diagnosing unstable angina and non–Q-wave MI. In addition, cTnI results are available quickly through a rapid assay. Protracted elevation of cTnI after MI or unstable angina is a predictor of increased mortality. People with angina without documented MI have a significantly higher risk of death within 42 days if cTnI is persistently elevated.

CK-MB has long been used as a serum marker of myocardial damage. CK-MB level increases within 6 to 12 hours of MI, begins to decrease within 24 to 48 hours, and usually returns to normal in about 60 hours. Because CK-MB clears quickly, its use in late detection of MI is limited. In addition, false-positive and false-negative results are noted.

The AHA periodically publishes guidelines for the management of patients with ST segment elevation MI, unstable angina, and non–ST segment elevation MI developed from consensus of nursing and medical experts and evidence-based health care. The AHA recommends the following therapy:

- Nitroglycerin via sublingual spray or tablet should be given, followed by parenteral nitroglycerin.
- Supplemental oxygen should be administered to patients with cyanosis or respiratory distress, and pulse oximetry or arterial blood gas determination should be done to confirm adequate arterial SaO_2 (>90%).
- Adequate analgesia should be provided with intravenous morphine sulfate when symptoms are not immediately relieved by nitroglycerin or when pulmonary congestion or severe agitation or both are present.
- A beta blocker should be given if there are no contraindications. The first dose should be administered intravenously. An ACEI should be given if no contraindications exist.
- Aspirin (160 to 325 mg orally in a chewable, nonenteric form) should be given as soon as possible after hospital presentation and continued indefinitely in patients who can tolerate it. Other antiplatelet agents, such as clopidogrel (Plavix), may be used if aspirin allergy or intolerance is present or as adjunctive therapy.
- A history, physical examination, 12-lead ECG, and cardiac marker tests should be performed promptly.

With a diagnosis of ACS and ST segment elevation, the patient should be evaluated for reperfusion; the examiner should look for ST segment elevation greater than 1 mm in contiguous leads. The presence of these changes usually indicates acute coronary artery occlusion, usually from thrombosis. In addition, clinically significant ST segment elevation largely dictates reperfusion therapy with the use of thrombolytic therapy, primary percutaneous transluminal coronary angioplasty, or other revascularization options. These therapies have the best effect on clinical outcomes if used within 6 hours after onset of chest pain but may be helpful 7 to 12 hours or more after MI symptoms begin. Percutaneous coronary intervention (PCI) is recommended in the presence of STEMI and ischemic symptoms of less than 12 hours duration. If fibrinolytic therapy is contraindicated, PCI should be performed in patients with STEMI and ischemic symptoms of less than 12 hours duration, irrespective of any time delay in first medical contact. Following PCI, dual antiplatelet therapy (aspirin plus clopidogrel, prasugrel, or ticagrelor) should be given for at least 12 months. When thrombolysis is used, heparin is usually given for at least 48 hours to ensure continued vessel patency. Before giving a thrombolytic agent such as tissue plasminogen activator or streptokinase, the prescriber must be aware of absolute and relative contraindications to thrombolytic therapy (Table 5–10).

If left bundle branch block is evident on ECG and the clinical scenario is consistent with acute MI, standard acute MI care should be offered. Patients with a presentation suggestive of MI but without ST segment changes should not receive thrombolysis. These patients should be hospitalized and placed on continuous ECG monitoring for rhythm disturbances; disturbances that are noted should be appropriately treated. Serial 12-lead ECGs should be obtained, and results should be correlated with clinical measures of myocardial necrosis, such as CK isoenzymes and troponin. Aspirin therapy should be continued, and heparin use should be considered, particularly in the presence of a large anterior MI or left ventricular mural thrombus because of increased risk of embolic stroke.

If no contraindications are present, beta blocker and ACEI therapy should be initiated promptly because the use of these products is associated with reduced mortality and morbidity after MI. Beta blocker and ACEI therapy should be continued indefinitely. Before hospital discharge, patients should undergo standard exercise testing to assess functional capacity, efficacy of current medical regimen, and risk stratification for subsequent cardiac events.

Ongoing care includes a goal of reducing low-density lipoprotein cholesterol to less than 100 mg/dL (<2.6 mmol/L) and in some patients at very high risk, including individuals with diabetes mellitus and established coronary artery disease, reducing it to less than 70 mg/dL (<1.8 mmol/L) using diet; exercise; and, as is typically needed, drug therapy. This

TABLE 5-10
Contraindications and Cautions for Fibrinolysis in ST Segment Elevation Myocardial Infarction*

Absolute Contraindications	Any prior intracranial hemorrhage
	Known structural cerebral vascular lesion (e.g., arteriovenous malformation)
	Known malignant intracranial neoplasm (primary or metastatic)
	Ischemic stroke within 3 mo *except* acute ischemic stroke within 4.5 hr
	Suspected aortic dissection
	Active bleeding or bleeding diathesis (excluding menses)
	Significant closed-head or facial trauma within 3 mo
	Intracranial or intraspinal surgery within 2 mo
	Severe uncontrolled hypertension (unresponsive to emergency therapy)
	For streptokinase, prior treatment within the previous 6 mo
Relative Contraindications	History of chronic, severe, poorly controlled hypertension
	Significant hypertension on presentation (systolic blood pressure >180 mm Hg or diastolic blood pressure >110 mm Hg)
	History of prior ischemic stroke <3 mo, dementia, or known intracranial pathology not covered in absolute contraindications
	Traumatic or prolonged (>10 min) CPR
	Major surgery (within past 3 weeks)
	Recent (within 2–4 weeks) internal bleeding
	Noncompressible vascular punctures
	Pregnancy
	Active peptic ulcer
	Oral anticoagulant therapy

*Viewed as advisory for clinical decision making and may not be all-inclusive or definitive.
INR, international normalized ratio.
Source: American College of Cardiology/American Heart Association (ACC/AHA) Task Force on Practice Guidelines. 2013 ACCF/AHA Guideline for the Management of ST-Elevation Myocardial Infarction. *J Am Coll Cardiol.* 61:e78-e140, 2013. Available at: http://content.onlinejacc.org/article.aspx?articleid=1486115.

ongoing care is in keeping with an overall plan to reduce or eliminate all cardiac risk factors, including inactivity, smoking, and obesity. At the same time, other sources advocate that a ≥ 50% reduction in LDL cholesterol from baseline via intensive statin therapy is preferred over a strict number goal. See the Endocrine Chapter for further information on this important topic.

DISCUSSION SOURCES

American Association of Clinical Endocrinologists' Comprehensive Diabetes Management Algorithm 2013 Consensus Statement, *Endocr Pract* 2013;19 (Suppl 1):1-48. https://www.aace.com/files/consensus-statement.pdf

American College of Cardiology/American Heart Association 2007 Guidelines for the Management of Patients with Unstable Angina/Non–ST-Elevation Myocardial Infarction: Executive Summary. http://circ.ahajournals.org/cgi/content/short/CIRCULATIONAHA.107.185752v1, A Report of the American College of Cardiology/American Heart Association Task Force on Practice Guidelines (Writing Committee to Revise the Guidelines for the Management of Patients with Unstable Angina/Non–ST-Elevation Myocardial Infarction)

American College of Cardiology/American Heart Association (ACC/AHA) Task Force on Practice Guidelines. http://circ.ahajournals.org/cgi/content/full/116/23/2762, 2007 Chronic Angina Focused Update of the ACC/AHA Guidelines for the Management of Patients with Chronic Stable Angina

American College of Cardiology/American Heart Association (ACC/AHA) Task Force on Practice Guidelines. 2012 ACCF/AHA Focused Update of the Guideline for the Management of Patients with Unstable Angina/Non-ST-Elevation Myocardial Infarction (Updating the 2007 Guideline and Replacing the 2011 Focused Update). *Circulation.* 126:875–910, 2012. http://content.onlinejacc.org/article.aspx?articleid=1217906, accessed 12/2/13.

American College of Cardiology/American Heart Association (ACC/AHA) Task Force on Practice Guidelines. 2013 ACCF/AHA Guideline for the Management of ST-Elevation Myocardial Infarction. *J Am Coll Cardiol.* 61:e78–e140, 2013. http://content.onlinejacc.org/article.aspx?articleid=1486115, accessed 12/2/13.

McSweeney J, Cody M, O'Sullivan P, Elberson K, Moser D, Garvin B. Women's early warning symptoms of acute myocardial infarction. *Circulation.* 108:2619–2623, 2003.

Heart Failure

90. Heart failure pathophysiology is characterized by:
   A. impaired atrial filling and ejection of blood.
   B. incomplete closure of tricuspid valve.
   C. near normal ventricular function.
   D. inadequate cardiac output to meet oxygen and metabolic demands of the body.

91. A leading cause of heart failure is:
   A. hypertensive heart disease.
   B. atrial fibrillation.
   C. pulmonary embolism.
   D. type 2 diabetes.

92 to 94. Match each of the following conditions with its mechanism for contributing to heart failure:

   92. pneumonia   A. increase in circulating volume of blood
   93. anemia
   94. high sodium intake   B. increased right-sided heart workload

   C. decreased oxygen-carrying capacity of blood

95. The condition of a sudden shortness of breath that usually occurs after 2-3 of hours of sleep that leads to sudden awakening followed by a feeling of severe anxiety and breathlessness is known as:
   A. dyspnea.
   B. orthopnea.
   C. resting dyspnea.
   D. paroxysmal nocturnal dyspnea.

96. You examine an 82-year-old woman who has a history of heart failure (HF). She is in the office because of increasing shortness of breath. When auscultating her heart, you note a tachycardia with a rate of 104 beats per minute and a single extra heart sound early in diastole. This sound most likely represents:
   A. summation gallop.
   B. S_3.
   C. opening snap.
   D. S_4.

97. You examine a 65-year-old man with dilated cardiomyopathy and HF. On examination, you expect to find all of the following except:
   A. jugular venous distention.
   B. tenderness on right upper-abdominal quadrant palpation.
   C. point of maximal impulse at the fifth intercostal space, mid-clavicular line.
   D. peripheral edema.

98. In patients with heart failure, the point of maximum impulse:
   A. remains unchanged near the fourth intercostal space.
   B. remains unchanged near the fifth intercostal space.
   C. shifts lower on the mid-clavicular line.
   D. shifts laterally by one or more intercostal spaces

99 to 101. Match the term with the correct impact on the heart.

   99. inotropic   A. cardiac rate
   100. chronotropic   B. cardiac conduction
   101. dromotropic

   C. force of the cardiac contraction

102. The rationale for using beta blocker therapy in treating a patient with HF is to:
A. increase myocardial contractility.
B. reduce the effects of circulating catecholamines.
C. relieve concomitant angina.
D. stabilize cardiac rhythm.

103. An ECG finding in a patient who is taking digoxin in a therapeutic dose typically includes:
A. shortened P-R interval.
B. slightly depressed, cupped ST segments.
C. widened QRS complex.
D. tall T waves.

104. A potential adverse effect of ACEI when used with spironolactone therapy is:
A. hypertension.
B. hyperkalemia.
C. renal insufficiency.
D. proteinuria.

105. ECG findings in a patient with digoxin toxicity would most likely include:
A. atrioventricular heart block.
B. T wave inversion.
C. sinus tachycardia.
D. pointed P waves.

106. Patients reporting symptoms of digoxin toxicity are most likely to include:
A. anorexia.
B. disturbance in color perception.
C. blurred vision.
D. diarrhea.

107. Which of the following is among the most common causes of HF?
A. dietary indiscretion
B. COPD
C. hypertensive heart disease
D. anemia

108. Which of the following medications is an aldosterone antagonist?
A. clonidine
B. spironolactone
C. hydrochlorothiazide
D. furosemide

109. Which of the following best describes orthopnea?
A. shortness of breath with exercise
B. dyspnea that develops when the individual is recumbent and is relieved with elevation of the head
C. shortness of breath that occurs at night, characterized by a sudden awakening after a couple of hours of sleep, with a feeling of severe anxiety, breathlessness, and suffocation
D. dyspnea at rest

110. Which of the following is unlikely to be noted in the person experiencing HF?
A. elevated serum B-type natriuretic peptide (BNP)
B. Kerley B lines noted on chest X-ray
C. left-ventricular hypertrophy on ECG
D. evidence of hemoconcentration on hemogram

111. Which of the following medications is an alpha/beta-adrenergic antagonist?
A. atenolol
B. metoprolol
C. propranolol
D. carvedilol

112. Which of the following best describes the patient presentation of New York Heart Association stage III heart disease?
A. Ordinary physical activity does not cause undue fatigue, dyspnea, or palpitations.
B. Ordinary physical activity results in fatigue, palpitations, dyspnea, or angina.
C. Less-than-ordinary activity leads to fatigue, dyspnea, palpitations, or angina.
D. Discomfort increases with any physical activity.

113. The risk for digoxin toxicity increases with concomitant use of all of the following medications except:
A. amiodarone.
B. clarithromycin.
C. cyclosporine.
D. levofloxacin.

) Answers

90. D.	98. D.	106. A.
91. A.	99. C.	107. C.
92. B.	100. A.	108. B.
93. C.	101. B.	109. B.
94. A.	102. B.	110. D.
95. D.	103. B.	111. D.
96. B.	104. B.	112. C.
97. C.	105. A.	113. D.

Heart failure (HF) occurs as a result of altered cardiac function that leads to inadequate cardiac output and a resulting inability to meet the oxygen and metabolic demands of the body. HF results from any structural or functional impairment of ventricular filling or ejection of blood. Hypertensive heart disease and atherosclerosis are the leading causes of HF. Less common causes in the at-risk adult include pneumonia (as a result of increased right-sided heart workload), anemia (because of the resulting decreased oxygen-carrying capability of the blood), and increased sodium intake (because of the resultant increase in circulating volume).

Clinical presentation of an acute exacerbation of HF includes dyspnea, or shortness of breath (SOB), that increases in severity, seen in a spectrum from exertional dyspnea (SOB with exercise), orthopnea (SOB that typically develops quickly when the individual is recumbent and is relieved with elevation of the head), paroxysmal nocturnal dyspnea (SOB that occurs at night, characterized by a sudden awakening after a couple hours of sleep, with a feeling of severe anxiety, breathlessness, and suffocation), and dyspnea at rest to acute pulmonary edema. Additional reported history often includes nocturia, fatigue, and weakness. Except for the mildest cases, crackles heard over the lung bases are characteristic; in severe cases, there is wheezing and expectoration of frothy, blood-tinged sputum. S_3 is usually noted, typically disappearing on resolution of the acute event. Additional findings usually include tachycardia, diaphoresis, pallor, and peripheral cyanosis with pallor. Although edema is considered a classic finding in HF, a substantial gain of extracellular fluid volume (i.e., a minimum of 5 L in adults) must occur before peripheral edema is manifested. As a result of liver engorgement from elevated right-sided heart pressures, hepatojugular reflux, hepatic engorgement, and tenderness are typically noted. The point of maximal impulse is normally at the fifth intercostal space, mid-clavicular line. This shifts laterally and perhaps over more than one intercostal space in the presence of dilated cardiomyopathy and its resultant increase in cardiac size.

Patients with HF are often assigned a classification of heart disease from either the ACCF/AHA (Stages A–D) or the New York Heart Association (NYHA I–IV). The ACCF/AHA stages of HF emphasize development and progression of disease, whereas the NYHA classes focus on exercise capacity and symptomatic status of the disease (Table 5–11). In treating an acute HF exacerbation, a patient often is initially consistent with a higher classification category (NYHA III or IV).

After treatment, the assignment of lower category (NYHA I or II) is likely noted and should be a clinical goal.

ECG helps to identify the presence of left atrial enlargement, left ventricular hypertrophy, and dysrhythmias often noted in HF but not specific to the diagnosis. ECG changes consistent with acute myocardial ischemia or MI as the cause of HF may also be revealed.

Laboratory testing in HF usually includes evaluation to rule in or rule out potential underlying causes (e.g., anemia, infection, renal insufficiency). B-type natriuretic peptide (BNP) is an amino acid structure common to all natriuretic peptides. The cardiac ventricles are the major source of plasma BNP; the amount in circulation is in proportion to ventricular volume expansion and pressure overload. As part of the evaluation of a patient with dyspnea and suspected HF, an elevated BNP level helps to support the diagnosis. The increased circulating volume found in HF can occasionally lead to evidence of hemodilution on hemogram; this corrects as circulating volume is normalized.

Findings on chest radiograph in HF include cardiomegaly and alveolar edema with pleural effusions and bilateral infiltrates in a butterfly pattern. Additional findings are loss of sharp definition of pulmonary vasculature; haziness of hilar shadows; and thickening of interlobular septa, also known as Kerley B lines. As part of the evaluation of heart valve function and competency, an echocardiogram is usually obtained. Radionuclide evaluation of left ventricular function provides helpful information on global heart function. Angiography and further studies should be directed by clinical presentation and other health risks.

The goal of HF therapy is threefold: reduction of preload, reduction of systemic vascular resistance (afterload reduction),

TABLE 5-11
Comparison of HF Classification Criteria for ACCF/AHA and NYHA

ACCF/AHA Stages of HF		NYHA Functional Classification	
A	At high risk for HF but without structural heart disease or symptoms of HF	I	No limitation of physical activity. Ordinary physical activity does not cause symptoms of HF.
B	Structural heart disease but without signs or symptoms of HF	II	Slight limitation of physical activity. Comfortable at rest, but ordinary physical activity results in symptoms of HF.
C	Structural heart disease with prior or current symptoms of HF	III	Marked limitation of physical activity. Comfortable at rest, but less than ordinary activity causes symptoms of HF.
D	Refractory HF requiring specialized interventions	IV	Unable to carry on any physical activity without symptoms of HF, or symptoms of HF at rest.

Source: Yancy CW, Jessup M, Bozkurt B, et al. 2013 ACCF/AHA guideline for the management of heart failure: A report of the American College of Cardiology Foundation/American Heart Association Task Force on Practice Guidelines. *Circulation*. 128:e240–e327, 2013. Available at: http://circ.ahajournals.org/content/128/16/e240. extract.

and inhibition of the renin and sympathetic nervous system. Because ACEIs and angiotensin receptor blockers (ARBs) cause central and peripheral vasodilation, these medications result in a reduction in cardiac workload and improvement in cardiac output. Although ACEIs and ARBs are the cornerstone of HF therapy, their use can be associated with adverse effects. Most common is hypotension, particularly when one of these agents is prescribed for a person who is currently taking a diuretic or vasodilator. To avoid hypotension, ACEI or ARB therapy should be started at low dosages and increased slowly to achieve a therapeutic response. Renal insufficiency can be precipitated by ACEI or ARB therapy; this usually occurs only in the presence of renal artery stenosis or underlying renal disease. Hyperkalemia with ACEI or ARB use is usually seen only with concurrent use of a potassium-sparing diuretic/aldosterone antagonist, such as spironolactone (Aldactone); in advancing renal disease; or in a poor hydration state, including overly aggressive diuretic use.

Diuretics assist with circulating volume and preload reduction. Unless contraindicated, a potassium-sparing diuretic such as spironolactone should be used because of its neurohumoral effects, allowing sodium excretion and enhanced vasodilation. These effects are achieved by the drug's ability to bind competitively at receptors found in aldosterone-dependent sodium-potassium exchange sites in the renal tubule.

Beta-adrenergic blockers are used to inhibit chronotropic and inotropic responses to beta-adrenergic stimulation; the use of an alpha/beta blocker such as carvedilol (Coreg) can provide the additional benefit of a vasodilating effect through its action blockade at the alpha receptors. Long-term beta-adrenergic antagonist (beta blocker) use has been shown to improve cardiac function, to reduce myocardial ischemia, to decrease myocardial oxygen consumption, and possibly to reduce the incidence of sudden cardiac death. This drug class is underused in HF therapy.

Digoxin has a positive inotropic effect and slows conduction through the atrioventricular node. A prolongation of the P-R interval and cupping of the ST segment are typically seen in ECGs of patients taking a therapeutic dose of digoxin. Because it is a medication with narrow therapeutic index and with significant drug–drug interactions and a potential proarrhythmic effect, clinical vigilance is needed with digoxin use. Drugs that interact with digoxin include amiodarone, diltiazem, select macrolides (clarithromycin and erythromycin), azole antifungals, cyclosporine, and verapamil. Drugs that can cause potassium loss, such as many diuretics, can also increase the risk of digoxin toxicity. In digoxin toxicity, numerous cardiac effects can be seen; atrioventricular block is the most common, whereas anorexia is the most commonly reported by patients. Visual changes are rarely reported. Digoxin use for 1 to 3 months is associated with reduced hospital admissions along with improved symptoms of HF, quality of life, and exercise tolerance in patients with mild to moderate HF. Long-term use of digoxin in patients with more severe HF (NYHA II or III) has been shown to have no effect on mortality but can reduce hospitalizations.

DISCUSSION SOURCES

Yancy CW, Jessup M, Bozkurt B, et al. 2013 ACCF/AHA guideline for the management of heart failure: a report of the American College of Cardiology Foundation/American Heart Association Task Force on Practice Guidelines. *Circulation.* 128:e240–e327, 2013. Available at: http://circ.ahajournals.org/content/128/16/e240.extract

Dumitru I. eMedicine. http://emedicine.medscape.com/article/163062-overview, Heart failure

Respiratory Disorders

6

Asthma

1. Which of the following best describes asthma?
   A. intermittent airway inflammation with occasional bronchospasm
   B. a disease of bronchospasm that leads to airway inflammation
   C. chronic airway inflammation with superimposed bronchospasm
   D. relatively fixed airway constriction

2. The patient you are evaluating is having a severe asthma flare. You have assessed that his condition is appropriate for office treatment. You expect to find the following on physical examination:
   A. tripod posture
   B. inspiratory crackles
   C. increased vocal fremitus
   D. hyperresonance on thoracic percussion

3. A 44-year-old man has a long-standing history of moderate persistent asthma that is normally well controlled by fluticasone with salmeterol (Advair) via metered-dose inhaler, one puff twice a day, and the use of albuterol 1 to 2 times a week as needed for wheezing. Three days ago, he developed a sore throat, clear nasal discharge, body aches, and a dry cough. In the past 24 hours, he has had intermittent wheezing that necessitated the use of albuterol, two puffs every 3 hours, which produced partial relief. Your next most appropriate action is to obtain a:
   A. chest radiograph.
   B. measurement of oxygen saturation (SaO_2).
   C. spirometry measurement.
   D. sputum smear for white blood cells (WBCs).

4. You examine Jane, a 24-year-old woman who has an acute asthma flare following a 3-day history of upper respiratory tract symptoms (clear nasal discharge, dry cough, no fever). She has a history of moderate persistent asthma that is in good control and an acceptable peak expiratory flow (PEF). She is using budesonide (Pulmicort) and albuterol as directed and continues to have difficulty with coughing and wheezing. At home, her PEF is 55% of personal best. In the office, her forced expiratory volume at 1 second (FEV1) is 65% of predicted. Her medication regimen should be adjusted to include:
   A. theophylline.
   B. salmeterol (Serevent).
   C. prednisone.
   D. montelukast (Singulair).

5. For Jane in the above question, you also prescribe:
   A. amoxicillin.
   B. azithromycin.
   C. levofloxacin.
   D. no antimicrobial therapy.

6. Peak expiratory flow meters:
   A. should only be used in the presence of a medical professional.
   B. provide a convenient method to check lung function at home.
   C. are as accurate as spirometry.
   D. should not be used more than once daily.

7. Which of the following is most likely to appear on a chest radiograph of a person during an acute severe asthma attack?
   A. hyperinflation
   B. atelectasis
   C. consolidation
   D. Kerley B signs

8. A 36-year-old man with asthma also needs antihypertensive therapy. Which of the following products should you avoid prescribing?
   A. hydrochlorothiazide
   B. propranolol
   C. amlodipine
   D. enalapril

9. Which of the following is inconsistent with the presentation of asthma that is not well controlled?
   A. a troublesome nocturnal cough at least 2 nights per week
   B. need for albuterol to relieve shortness of breath at least twice a week
   C. morning sputum production
   D. two or more exacerbations/year requiring oral corticosteroids

10. The cornerstone of moderate persistent asthma drug therapy is the use of:
    A. oral theophylline.
    B. mast cell stabilizers.
    C. short-acting beta2-agonists (SABA).
    D. inhaled corticosteroids.

11. Sharon is a 29-year-old woman with moderate persistent asthma. She is not using prescribed inhaled corticosteroids, but is using albuterol PRN to relieve her cough and wheeze with reported satisfactory clinical effect. Currently she uses about two albuterol metered-dose inhalers per month and is requesting a prescription refill. You consider that:
    A. her asthma is well controlled and albuterol use can continue.
    B. excessive albuterol use is a risk factor for asthma death.
    C. her asthma is not well controlled and salmeterol (Serevent) should be added to relieve bronchospasm and reduce her albuterol use.
    D. her asthma has better control with albuterol than inhaled corticosteroids.

12. In the treatment of asthma, leukotriene receptor antagonists should be used as:
    A. controllers to prevent bronchospasm.
    B. controllers to inhibit inflammatory responses.
    C. relievers to treat acute bronchospasm.
    D. relievers to treat bronchospasm and inflammation.

13. According to the National Asthma Education and Prevention Program Expert Panel Report-3 (NAEPP EPR-3) guidelines, which of the following is not a risk for asthma death?
    A. hospitalization or an emergency department visit for asthma in the past month
    B. current use of systemic corticosteroids or recent withdrawal from systemic corticosteroids
    C. difficulty perceiving airflow obstruction or its severity
    D. rural residence

14. An 18-year-old high school senior presents, asking for a letter stating that he should not participate in gym class because he has asthma. The most appropriate action is to:
    A. write the note because gym class participation could trigger asthma symptoms.
    B. excuse him from outdoor activities only to avoid pollen exposure.
    C. assess his level of asthma control and make changes in his treatment plan if needed so he can participate.
    D. write a note excusing him from gym until his follow-up exam in 2 months.

15. You see a 34-year-old man with moderate persistent asthma who has a severe asthma flare and a regimen of oral prednisone is being considered. Which of the following is true?
    A. A taper is needed for prednisone therapy lasting longer than 4 days.
    B. A taper is not needed if the prednisone regimen is for 7 days or less.
    C. A taper is not needed regardless of duration of prednisone therapy.
    D. A taper is needed if the patient is taking concomitant inhaled corticosteroids.

16. After inhaled corticosteroid is initiated, improvement in control is usually seen:
    A. on the first day of use.
    B. within 2 to 8 days.
    C. in about 3 to 4 weeks.
    D. in about 1 to 2 months.

17. Compared with albuterol, levalbuterol (Xopenex) has:
    A. a different mechanism of action.
    B. the ability potentially to provide greater bronchodilation with a lower dose.
    C. an anti-inflammatory effect similar to that of an inhaled corticosteroid.
    D. a contraindication to use in elderly patients.

18. Which of the following is consistent with the NAEPP comment on the use of inhaled corticosteroids (ICS) for a child with asthma?
    A. The potential but small risk of delayed growth with ICS is well balanced by their effectiveness.
    B. ICS should be used only if leukotriene modifiers fail to control asthma.
    C. Permanent growth stunting is consistently noted in children using ICS.
    D. Leukotriene modifiers are equal in therapeutic effect to the use of a long-acting beta2-agonist.

19. A potential adverse effect from ICS use is:
    A. oral candidiasis.
    B. tachycardia.
    C. gastrointestinal upset.
    D. insomnia.

20. Clinical findings characteristic of asthma include all of the following except:
  A. a recurrent spasmodic cough that is worse at night.
  B. recurrent shortness of breath and chest tightness with exercise.
  C. a congested cough that is worse during the day.
  D. wheezing with and without associated respiratory infections.

21. Which of the following best describes the mechanism of action of short-acting beta2-agonists?
  A. reducer of inflammation
  B. inhibition of secretions
  C. modification of leukotrienes
  D. smooth muscle relaxation

22. Regarding the use of long-acting beta2-agonists (LABAs), which of the following is true?
  A. LABAs enhance the antiinflammatory action of corticosteroids.
  B. Use of LABAs is associated with a small increase in risk of asthma death.
  C. LABA use reduces the risk of asthma exacerbations.
  D. LABAs can be used as monotherapy to relieve bronchospasms in asthma.

23. Which of the following is the therapeutic objective of using inhaled ipratropium bromide?
  A. as an antiinflammatory.
  B. an increase in vagal tone in the airway
  C. inhibition of muscarinic cholinergic receptors
  D. an increase in salivary and mucous secretions

24. Which of the following is true regarding the use of systemic corticosteroids in the treatment of asthma?
  A. Frequent short bursts are preferred over daily inhaled corticosteroids.
  B. The oral corticosteroid should be started at day 3-4 of the asthma flare for optimal effect.
  C. The oral route is preferred over parenteral therapy.
  D. The adult dose to treat an asthma flare should not exceed the equivalent of prednisone 40 mg daily.

25. Compared with short-acting beta2-agonists, long-acting beta2-agonists:
  A. are recommended as a first-line therapy in mild intermittent asthma.
  B. have a significantly different pharmacodynamic profile.
  C. have a rapid onset of action across the drug class.
  D. should be added to therapy only when ICS use does not provide adequate asthma control.

26. Which of the following statements is false regarding the use of omalizumab (Xolair)?
  A. Its use is recommended for patients with mild persistent asthma to prevent asthma flares.
  B. The medication selectively binds to IgE to reduce exacerbations.
  C. Labeled indication is for patients with poorly controlled asthma with frequent exacerbations.
  D. Special evaluation is required prior to its use and ongoing monitoring is needed during use.

27. Subcutaneous immunotherapy is recommended for use in patients:
  A. with well-controlled asthma and infrequent exacerbations.
  B. with allergic-based asthma.
  C. with moderate persistent asthma who are intolerant of ICS.
  D. with poorly-controlled asthma who fail therapy with omalizumab.

Answer the following questions true or false.

_____ **28.** Most prescribers are well versed in the relative potency of ICS and prescribe an appropriate dose for the patient's clinical presentation.

_____ **29.** Approximately 80% of the dose of an ICS is systemically absorbed.

_____ **30.** Leukotriene modifiers and ICS are interchangeable clinically because both groups of medications have equivalent anti-inflammatory effect.

_____ **31.** Little systemic absorption of mast cell stabilizers occurs with inhaled or intranasal use.

_____ **32.** Due to safety concerns, mast cell stabilizers are no longer available.

■) Answers

1. C.	**12.** B.	**23.** C.
2. D.	**13.** D.	**24.** C.
3. C.	**14.** C.	**25.** D.
4. C.	**15.** B.	**26.** A.
5. D.	**16.** B.	**27.** B.
6. B.	**17.** B.	**28.** False
7. A.	**18.** A.	**29.** False
8. B.	**19.** A.	**30.** False
9. C.	**20.** C.	**31.** True
10. D.	**21.** D.	**32.** False
11. B.	**22.** D.	

Asthma is a common chronic disorder of the airways that is complex and characterized by variable and recurring symptoms, airflow obstruction, bronchial hyperresponsiveness, and underlying inflammation. Risk factors contributing to the development of asthma include atopy, genetic-environmental interactions, and viral respiratory tract infections. Historical data consistent with asthma include a family history of asthma or allergies, personal history of allergies, recurrent symptoms and triggers, and improvement of symptoms and lung function with asthma therapies, especially a short-acting beta2-agonist (Table 6–1).

Asthma is a lower airway obstructive disease that can have clinical findings that are consistent with air trapping (Table 6–2). In asthma exacerbations, breath sounds may be reduced and hyperinflation is present on a chest radiograph due to significant air trapping. At the same time, chest x-ray is not required when treating a person with an asthma flare unless there is a suspicion of pneumonia. However, particularly in primary care, the physical exam is often normal and does not correlate well with asthma severity. Though wheezing can occur with asthma, it is not required for the diagnosis. Variable degrees of cough and/or difficulty breathing may be present without wheezing. The patient may be asymptomatic, have a normal exam and yet have a lung function 50% of personal best. A poor perception of symptoms, use of two or more short-acting beta2-agonist canisters/month, and prior severe exacerbations are

important risk factors for death from asthma and should influence decisions regarding asthma management (Table 6–3). The history and measurement of lung function is essential and more reliable than the physical exam. A decrease in forced expiratory volume at 1 second (FEV_1) predicted best or peak expiratory flow rate (PEFR) is usually noted before the onset of clinical obstructive findings. Various devices can be used to test for lung function. Spirometry is the most common lung function test used to diagnose and monitor asthma and provides a rapid method to evaluate lungs and

TABLE 6-1
Making the Diagnosis: Is it Asthma?

- Symptoms consistent with asthma
  - Recurrent cough, wheeze, shortness of breath and/or chest tightness
  - Symptoms occur or worsen at night, exercise, viral respiratory infections, aeroallergens and/or pulmonary irritants (such as second-hand smoke)
- Airflow obstruction is at least partially reversible
  - Increase in $FEV_1 \geq 12\%$ from baseline
  - Increase in $FEV_1 \geq 12\%$ post-short-acting beta2-agonist

Per EPR-3:

- Consider the diagnosis of asthma and perform spirometry if any of these indicators are present. These indicators are not diagnostic by themselves but the presence of multiple key indicators increases the probability of the diagnosis of asthma.
- Spirometry is needed to make the diagnosis of asthma.
  - Peak flow meter is used for monitoring, not for diagnosing, asthma.

Source: Expert Panel Report Guideline for the Diagnosis and Management of Asthma, EPR-3, p. 42. Available at www.nhlbi.nih.gov/guidelines/asthma/asthgdln.htm

TABLE 6-2
Clinical Findings in Asthma or Chronic Obstructive Pulmonary Disease Flare

Condition	Physical Examination Findings
Lower airway disease with resulting air trapping as found in asthma or chronic obstructive pulmonary disease flare or poor disease control	Hyperresonance on thoracic percussion Decreased tactile fremitus wheeze (expiratory first, inspiratory later) Prolonged expiratory phase of forced exhalation Low diaphragms Increased anterior-posterior diameter Reduction in forced expiratory volume at 1 second (FEV_1) or peak expiratory flow rate (early finding) Reduction in arterial oxygen saturation (SaO_2) (later finding)

Source: Mangione S. *Physical Diagnosis Secrets*, 2nd ed. St. Louis, MO: Elsevier Health Sciences, 2007.

TABLE 6-3
Risk Factors for Death from Asthma

- Infants <1 year old
- Previous severe exacerbations
- ≥2 hospitalizations in past year
- ≥3 ED visits in past year
- Hospitalization/ED visit in past month
- >2 canisters SABA use per month
- Poor patient perception of symptoms
- Lack of written asthma care plan
- Sensitivity to *Alternaria*
- Low socioeconomic status
- Illicit drug use
- Major psychosocial problems
- Comorbidities (CV disease, Other chronic lung disease)
- Major psychological disease

airways. Peak expiratory flow meters are less accurate than spirometry, but allow patients a convenient method to regularly test lung function at home.

According to the NAEPP EPR-3, the goals of therapy for achieving asthma control are to reduce impairment and to reduce risk. Reduction of impairment is achieved by the prevention of symptoms, use of a short-acting beta2-agonist limited to 2 or fewer days/week (unless for prevention of exercise-induced bronchospasm), maintenance of normal pulmonary function and normal activity levels, and meeting patients' and families' expectations of and satisfaction with asthma care. Reduction of risk is achieved by the prevention of exacerbations, prevention of lung function loss, and minimal or no adverse effects from medications.

Upon initial diagnosis of asthma, the level of asthma severity is assessed to guide decisions regarding therapeutic interventions. Asthma severity is classified as intermittent or persistent and is determined by the level of impairment and level of risk. Persistent asthma is subdivided as mild, moderate, and severe. The emphasis on follow-up visits is assessment of asthma control. The level of control (well controlled, not well controlled, or very poorly controlled) determines whether to maintain therapy, step-up therapy, or step-down therapy (Figures 6-1 to 6-3).

Because of the wide range of asthma medications currently available, the NP, patient, and family can work together to find a lifestyle and treatment regimen that provide optimal care with minimal to no adverse medication effects. Therapies are divided into two groups: relievers and controllers. Relievers consist of short-acting beta2-agonists (SABA), short-acting muscarinic agents (SAMA), and oral corticosteroids (OCS) (Table 6-4).

SABAs include albuterol (Proventil, Ventolin, ProAir), levalbuterol (Xopenex), and pirbuterol (Maxair). SABAs are the drug of choice for all age groups to relieve acute asthma symptoms including bronchoconstriction and to prevent exercise-induced bronchoconstriction. SABA use more than 2 days/week (unless for prevention of exercise-induced bronchospasm) indicates a need for better asthma control. SABAs work by binding to the beta2 adrenergic receptor, causing smooth muscle relaxation and bronchodilation. This effect occurs within 3 to 5 minutes. Compared with albuterol and pirbuterol, levalbuterol, a single isomer of the racemic albuterol, may be better tolerated than the other short-acting beta2-agonists, because of greater bronchodilation at a reduced dose.

Ipratropium bromide (Atrovent) is a short-acting muscarinic agent indicated for the treatment of moderate or severe asthma exacerbations to provide additional bronchodilation to albuterol. This anticholinergic inhaled agent inhibits muscarinic cholinergic receptors, reducing vagal tone in the airway, decreasing mucus secretion and blocking reflex bronchoconstriction because of reflex esophagitis. Its additive benefit to albuterol is primarily in the outpatient setting. Studies have not shown additional benefit to albuterol once hospitalized. The role of inhaled anticholinergics in the treatment of asthma is evolving.

Systemic corticosteroids are indicated in moderate to severe asthma exacerbations and when there is partial response to initial SABA use in exacerbations. Oral prednisone is preferred over parenteral corticosteroids. These medication forms are equally effective, and there is less risk of serious adverse reaction with oral corticosteroids. Duration of oral corticosteroids for asthma is usually 5 to 10 days. There is no need to taper the dose for a 7-day course and usually no need to taper for a 10-day course, particularly if a patient is on an inhaled corticosteroid (Table 6-5).

The backbone of persistent asthma therapy is medications that prevent and/or reduce airway inflammation to gain and maintain asthma control. Asthma controllers consist of inhaled corticosteroids (ICS), leukotriene modifiers (LTM) and inhaled corticosteroids combined with long-acting beta2-agonist (ICS/LABA). ICS (i.e. fluticasone [Flovent], mometasone [Asmanex], budesonide [Pulmicort], others) have proved to be most effective in preventing airway inflammation and are the preferred controller treatment for all levels of persistent asthma. Improvement in asthma control is seen within 2 to 8 days. Risk of asthma exacerbations are reduced with routine use of ICS. Local adverse effects include sore throat, oral candidiasis, and hoarseness. Rinsing the mouth after ICS use and use of a spacer can help reduce these effects. Primary care providers are often poorly informed as to the relative potency of a given ICS and prescribe too low a dose for the asthma severity; this is a major issue and impacts the attainment of asthma control (Table 6-6). Systemic absorption varies among the ICS agents but is usually much less than thought; at the recommended dose it can be less than 1% for certain ICS molecules, such as mometasone (Asmanex). It is advised, however, to monitor for systemic adverse effects, particularly if a patient is chronically on a high-dose ICS or has frequent oral corticosteroid use. Use the lowest ICS dose possible and implement corticosteroid-sparing strategies.

There is a potential but small risk of delayed growth and a potential in select children, such as those at high risk, for a small reduction (0.2 cm) in final adult height with ICS use. However, this potential risk is well balanced by the effectiveness of these medications. Interpretations of study results evaluating linear growth in childhood asthma are difficult because of the unknown influence from the uncontrolled disease itself versus the treatment.

Leukotriene modifiers (LTM), such as montelukast (Singulair) and zafirlukast (Accolate) are used to control asthma by inhibiting the inflammatory actions of leukotrienes. These medications are indicated as an alternative to ICS in mild persistent asthma and as add-on therapy to ICS in moderate and severe persistent asthma. Zileuton (Zyflo) is a seldom-used LTM used in uncontrolled asthma; periodic hepatic enzyme monitoring is required during use.

Long-acting beta2-agonists, including salmeterol (Serevent) and formoterol (Foradil), have a pharmacodynamic profile identical to SABAs, but with a significantly different pharmacokinetic profile. LABAs improve symptoms, improve

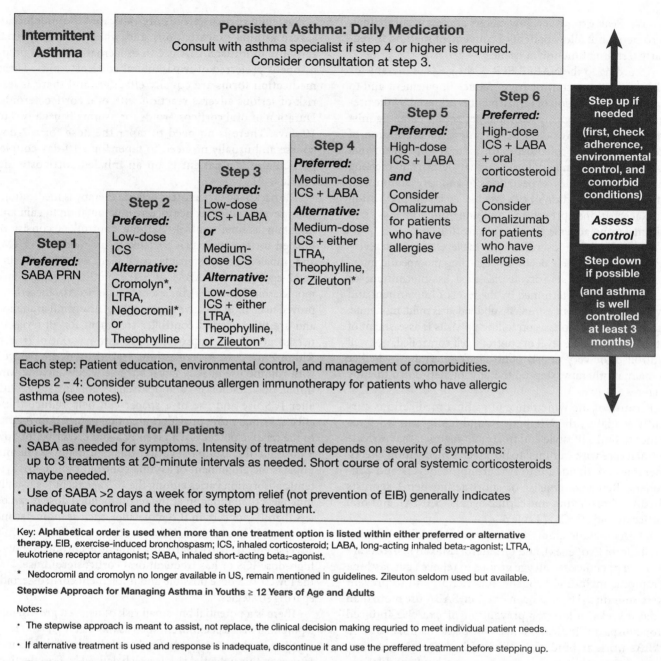

Each step: Patient education, environmental control, and management of comorbidities.

Steps 2 – 4: Consider subcutaneous allergen immunotherapy for patients who have allergic asthma (see notes).

Quick-Relief Medication for All Patients

• SABA as needed for symptoms. Intensity of treatment depends on severity of symptoms: up to 3 treatments at 20-minute intervals as needed. Short course of oral systemic corticosteroids maybe needed.

• Use of SABA >2 days a week for symptom relief (not prevention of EIB) generally indicates inadequate control and the need to step up treatment.

Key: **Alphabetical order is used when more than one treatment option is listed within either preferred or alternative therapy.** EIB, exercise-induced bronchospasm; ICS, inhaled corticosteroid; LABA, long-acting inhaled beta₂-agonist; LTRA, leukotriene receptor antagonist; SABA, inhaled short-acting beta₂-agonist.

* Nedocromil and cromolyn no longer available in US, remain mentioned in guidelines. Zileuton seldom used but available.

Stepwise Approach for Managing Asthma in Youths ≥ 12 Years of Age and Adults

Notes:

• The stepwise approach is meant to assist, not replace, the clinical decision making requried to meet individual patient needs.

• If alternative treatment is used and response is inadequate, discontinue it and use the preffered treatment before stepping up.

• Zileuton is a less desirable alternative due to limited studies as adjunctive therapy and the neeed to monitor liver function. Theophylline requires monitoring of serum concentration levels.

• In step 6, before oral systemic corticosteroids are introduced, a trial of high-dose ICS + LABA + either LTRA, theophylline, or zileuton may be considered, although this approach has not been studied in clinical trials.

• Step 1, 2, and 3 preferred therapies are based on Evidence A; step 3 alternative therapy is based on Evidence A for LTRA, Evidence B for theophylline, and Evidence D for zileuton. Step 4 preferred therapy is based on Evidence B, and alternative therapy is based on Evidence B for LTRA and theophylline and Evidence D for zileuton. Step 5 preferred therapy is based on Evidence B. Step 6 preferred therapy is based on the Expert Panel Report Guideline for the Diagnosis and Management of Asthma (EPR-2, 1997), and Evidence B for omalizumab.

• Immunotherapy for steps 2–4 is based on Evidence B for house-dust mites, animal danders, and pollens; evidence is weak or lacking for molds and cockroaches. Evidence is strongest for immunotherapy with single allergens. The role of allergy in asthma is greater in children than in adults.

• Clinicians who administer immunotherapy or omalizumab should be prepared and equipped to identify and treat anaphylaxis that may occur.

Figure 6-1 Stepwise approach for managing asthma in patients 12 years of age and older. (*Source: https://www.nhlbi.nih.gov/guidelines/asthma/asthgdln.pdf*)

Components of Severity		Classification of Asthma Severity (Youths ≥12 years of age or adults)			
			Persistent		
		Intermittent	**Mild**	**Moderate**	**Severe**
Impairment **Normal** **FEV1/FVC:** **8–19 yr 85%** **20–39 yr 80%** **40–59 yr 75%** **60–80 yr 70%**	Symptoms	≤2 days/week	>2 days/week but not daily	Daily	Throughout the day
	Nighttime awakenings	≤2x/month	3–4x/month	>1x/week but not nightly	Often 7x/week
	Short-acting beta₂-agonist use for symptom control (not prevention of EIB)	≤2 days/week	>2 days/week but not daily	Daily	Several times per day
	Interference with normal activity	None	Minor limitation	Some limitation	Extremely limited
	Lung function	• Normal FEV_1 between exacerbations • FEV_1 >80% predicted • FEV_1/FVC normal	• $FEV_1 \geq 80\%$ predicted • FEV_1/FVC normal	• FEV_1 = 60–80% predicted • FEV_1/FVC reduced 5%	• FEV_1 <60% predicted • FEV_1/FVC reduced 5%
Risk	Exacerbations requiring oral systemic corticosteroids	0–1/year (see note)	≥2/year (see note) →→→→		
		←← Consider severity and interval since last exacerbation. →→ Frequency and severity may fluctuate over time for patients in any severity category.			
		Relative annual risk of exacerbations may be related to FEV_1.			
Recommended Step for Initiating Therapy		Step 1	Step 2	Step 3	Step 4
				and consider short course of oral systemic corticosteroids	
		In 2–6 weeks, evaluate level of asthma control that is achieved, and adjust therapy accordingly.			

• Level of severity is determined by assessment of both impairment and risk. Assess impairment domain by patient's/caregiver's recall of previous 2–4 weeks and spirometry. Assign severity to the most severe category in which any feature occurs.

• At present, there are inadequate data to correspond frequencies of exacerbations with different levels of asthma severity. In general, more frequent and intense exacerbations (e.g., requiring urgent, unscheduled care, hospitalization or ICU admission) indicate greater underlying disease severity. For treatment purposes, patients who had 2 exacerbations requiring oral systemic corticosteroids in the past year may be considered the same patients who have persistent asthma, even in the absence of impairment levels consistent with persistent asthma.

Figure 6-2 Classifying asthma severity in youths ≥12 years of age and adults.

lung function, reduce exacerbations, and enhance the anti-inflammatory action of corticosteroids. Adding a LABA to an ICS is the preferred treatment for moderate and severe asthma. The LABA class received a boxed warning from the U.S. Food and Drug Administration (FDA) because LABA use is associated with increased risk of death in certain patient groups and should not be used without an ICS in asthma. Prescribe combination ICS/LABA only for patients with asthma not adequately controlled on a long-term asthma control medication, such as an inhaled corticosteroid, or whose disease severity clearly warrants initiation of treatment with both inhaled corticosteroid and LABA. Once asthma control is achieved and maintained, assess the patient at regular intervals and step down therapy (discontinue LABA) if possible without loss of asthma control, while maintaining the patient on a long-term asthma control medication, such as an inhaled corticosteroid. The NAEPP EPR-3 guidelines recommend achieving and maintaining control for at least 3 months before trying to step down. Many factors contribute to the decision-making process with individualization of care and consideration of the risk for future exacerbation being crucial.

Mast cell stabilizers (cromolyn and nedocromil) are mentioned in EPR-3; however, these agents are no longer available in the United States because of superior agents on the market. These are older inhalation agents that are safe, but inferior in potency to the newer agents such as ICS, and require multiple dosing daily. Theophylline is also mentioned, however rarely used due to superior agents now available, and its significant drug-drug interaction potential, a narrow therapeutic index, and requirement for periodic serologic drug level monitoring (Table 6–7).

Components of Control		Classification of Asthma Severity (Youths ≥12 years of age or adults)		
		Well-controlled	**Mild**	**Severe**
Impairment	**Symptoms**	≤2 days/week	>2 days/week	Throughout the day
	Nighttime awakenings	≤2x/month	1–3x/month	≥4x/week
	Interference with normal activity	None	Some limitation	Extremely limited
	Short-acting beta$_2$-agonist use for symptom control (not prevention of EIB)	≤2 days/week	>2 days/week	Several times per day
	Normal FEV$_1$ or peak flow	>80% predicted/ personal best	60–80% predicted/ personal best	<60% predicted/ personal best
	Validated Questionnaires ATAQ ACQ ACT	0 ≤0.75* ≥20	1–2 ≥1.5 16–19	3–4 N/A ≤15
Risk	Exacerbations	0–1/year	≥2/year (see note)	
		Consider severity and interval since last exacerbation.		
	Progressive loss of lung function	Evaluation requires long-term follow-up care.		
	Treatment-related adverse effects	Medication side effects can vary in intensity from none to very troublesome and worrisome. The level of intensity does not correlate to specific levels of control but should be considered in the overall assessment of risk.		
Recommended Action for Treatment		• Maintain current step • Regular follow-ups every 1–6 months to maintain control • Consider step down if well-controlled for at least three months	• Step up 1 step and reevaluate 2–6 wks • For side effects, consider alternative treatment options	• Consider short course of oral systemic corticosteroids • Step up 1-2 steps and reevaluate in 2 weeks • For side effects, consider alternative treatment options

*ACQ values 0.76-1.4 are indeterminant regarding well-controlled asthma.
Key: EIB, exercise-induced bronchospasm; FEV$_1$, forced expiratory volume in 1 second.

Figure 6-3 Assessing asthma control in youths ≥12 years of age and adults.

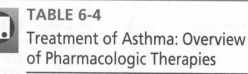

TABLE 6-4

Treatment of Asthma: Overview of Pharmacologic Therapies

- Relievers
  - Short-acting beta2- agonists (SABA)
  - Short-acting muscarinic agents (SAMA)
  - Oral corticosteroids (OCS)
- Controllers
  - Inhaled corticosteroids (ICS)
  - Leukotriene modifiers (LTM)
  - Inhaled corticosteroid/long-acting beta2-agonists (ICS/LABA)

Omalizumab (Xolair) is a humanized monoclonal antibody, indicated for those 12 years of age and older with moderate-severe persistent allergic asthma uncontrolled on ICS. The patient usually has poorly controlled asthma with recurrent exacerbations and quality of life limitations, despite optimal asthma treatment. Omalizumab is delivered by subcutaneous injection and acts by selectively binding to IgE, reducing exacerbations, symptoms, and corticosteroid use. This medication requires specialized evaluation prior to initiation and ongoing monitoring during its use.

Subcutaneous immunotherapy is another recommendation for asthma treatment in the NAEPP EPR-3 guidelines. Numerous well-documented studies have shown it to be an effective treatment for allergic asthma. It relieves allergic reactions that trigger asthma episodes and improves lung function.

Common causes for asthma flares are aeroallergen exposure, viral respiratory infections, and non-adherence to controller medications. It is important to identify triggers and develop a plan for avoiding or minimizing them. The patient should have an individualized asthma action plan to guide care during an exacerbation. Severe exacerbations can occur at all asthma severity levels.

TABLE 6-5

Relative Potency of Systemic Corticosteroids

Higher potency corticosteroids (equipotent doses)	Betamethasone, 0.6–0.75 mg Dexamethasone, 0.75 mg	Half-life 36–54 hr
Medium potency corticosteroids (equipotent doses)	Methylprednisolone, 4 mg Triamcinolone, 4 mg Prednisolone, 5 mg Prednisone, 5 mg	Half-life 18–36 hr
Lower potency (equipotent doses)	Hydrocortisone, 20 mg Cortisone, 25 mg	Half-life 8–12 hr

Source: Drug Facts and Comparisons. Philadelphia, PA: Wolters Kluwer Health, 2013.
www.factsandcomparisons.com.

TABLE 6-6

Estimated Comparative Daily Doses for Inhaled Corticosteroid (ICS) Therapy in Patients 12 Years and Older

	Low Daily Dose	Medium Daily Dose	High Daily Dose
Beclomethasone HFA (Qvar) 40 or 80 mcg/puff	80–240 mcg	>240–480 mcg	>480 mcg
Budesonide DPI (Pulmicort Flexhaler) 180 mcg/inhalation	180–540 mcg	>540–1080 mcg	>1080 mcg
Fluticasone HFA MDI (Flovent HFA) 44, 110, or 220 mcg/puff	88–264 mcg	264–440 mcg	>440 mcg
Fluticasone DPI (Flovent Diskus) 50, 100, or 250 mcg/puff	100–300 mcg	300–500 mcg	>500 mcg
Mometasone DPI (Asmanex) 200 mcg/puff	200 mcg	400 mcg	>400 mcg

Source: NAEPP. www.nhlbi.nih.gov/guidelines/asthma/epr3/resource.pdf

TABLE 6-7

Medications Used for Treating Patients With Asthma and Chronic Obstructive Pulmonary Disease (COPD)

Medication	Mechanism of Action	Indication	Comment
Short-acting bronchodilators ***Short-acting beta2-agonists (SABA) albuterol (Proventil,** Ventolin, ProAir) & pirbuterol (Maxair) levalbuterol (Xopenex) ***Short-acting muscarinic agents (SAMA)** iptratropium (Atrovent)	SABA: bronchodilation via stimulation of beta2 receptor site SAMA: anticholinergic and muscarinic antagonist; yielding bronchodilation	SABA: reliever drug; treatment of acute asthma and COPD symptoms SAMA: Reliever drug for COPD; add-on for asthma exacerbation	Onset of action within 15 minutes SABA, 30 minutes SAMA Duration 4–6 hrs

Continued

TABLE 6-7

Medications Used for Treating Patients With Asthma and Chronic Obstructive
Pulmonary Disease (COPD)—cont'd

Medication	Mechanism of Action	Indication	Comment
Long-acting bronchodilators *Long-acting beta2-agonists (LABA)** (salmeterol (Serevent), formoterol (Foradil), indacaterol (Onbrez) ***Long-acting muscarinic agents (LAMA):** tiotropium (Spiriva), aclidium (Pressair)	LABA: bronchodilation through stimulation of receptor site beta2 LAMA:	LABA: controller drug; treatment and prevention of bronchospasm in asthma and COPD LAMA: treatment of bronchospasm in COPD	LABA: Onset of action 1 hr (15–30 min for formoterol) Duration of action 12 hr Not to be used as monotherapy in asthma
Inhaled corticosteroids mometasone (Asmanex) fluticasone (Flovent) budesonide (Pulmicort) beclomethasone (Qvar), ciclesonide (Alvesco)	Block late-phase activation to allergen, inhibit inflammatory cell migration and activation	Controller drug, preferred treatment for persistent asthma to prevent and control inflammation In COPD, routine use recommended with FEV_1 <60% predicted and/or with recurrent exacerbations.	Need consistent use to be helpful. Cornerstone medication of most asthma levels
Leukotriene receptor antagonist, also known as leukotriene modifier (montelukast [Singulair], zafirlukast [Accolate], (zileuton [Zyflo])	Inhibit action of inflammatory mediator (leukotriene) by blocking select receptor sites	Controller drug, prevention of inflammation in asthma	Likely less effective than inhaled corticosteroids Particularly effective add-on medication with inhaled corticosteroid and with allergic rhinitis. In mild persistent asthma, an alternative, although not preferred
Systemic corticosteroids	Inhibit eosinophilic action and other inflammatory mediators	Treatment of acute inflammation such as in asthma flare or COPD exacerbation	Oral route preferred whenever possible. Indicated in treatment of acute asthma flare to reduce inflammation In higher dose and with longer therapy (>2 weeks), adrenal suppression may occur No taper needed if use is short-term (<10 days) and at lower dose (prednisone, 40–60 mg/d or less)
Mast cell stabilizers Cromolyn sodium (Intal) nedocromil (Tilade)	Halts degradation of mast cells and release of histamine and other inflammatory mediators	Controller drug, prevention of inflammation in asthma	No longer available in United States Need consistent use to be helpful Less effective than other controller therapies

TABLE 6-7
Medications Used for Treating Patients With Asthma and Chronic Obstructive Pulmonary Disease (COPD)—cont'd

Medication	Mechanism of Action	Indication	Comment
Theophylline	Mild bronchodilator via non-phosphodiesterase inhibitor. Possible mild anti-inflammatory effect	Prevention of bronchospasm in asthma and COPD	Narrow therapeutic index drug with numerous potential drug interactions. Monitor carefully for toxicity by checking drug levels and clinical presentation
Phosphodiesterase-4 inhibitors Roflumilast (Daliresp)	Not well defined; thought to be because of the effects of increased intracellular cAMP in lung cells	Indicated as a treatment to reduce the risk of COPD exacerbations in patients with severe COPD associated with chronic bronchitis and a history of exacerbations.	Is not a bronchodilator and is not indicated for the relief of acute bronchospasm.

Source: Report of the Expert Panel. www.nhlbi.nih.gov/guidelines/asthma/, Guidelines for the diagnosis and management of asthma (EPR-3), accessed 12/3/13.

DISCUSSION SOURCES

Cox, et al. Allergen immunotherapy: A practice parameter third update. 2010. Available at www.aaaai.org (American Academy of Allergy, Asthma and Immunology), accessed 1/28/13.

Guilbert TW, et al. Growth of preschool children at high risk for asthma 2 years after discontinuation of fluticasone. *J Allergy Clin Immunol* 128:956–963, 2011.

National Asthma Education and Prevention Program. Guidelines for the Diagnosis and Management of Asthma-update on Selected Topics. NIH-NHLBI. Available at www.nhlbi.nih.gov/guidelines/asthma

Skoner DP. Balancing safety and efficacy in pediatric asthma management. *Pediatrics* 109:381–392, 2002.

Strunk R, et al. Long-term budesonide or nedocromil treatment, once discontinued, does not alter the course of mild-moderate asthma in children and adolescents. *J Pediatr* 154:682–687, 2009.

Thomas A, et al. Approaches to stepping up and stepping down care in asthmatic patients. *J Allergy Clin Immunol* 128:915–924, 2011.

▶ COPD

33. When discussing immunizations with a 67-year-old woman with chronic obstructive pulmonary disease (COPD), you advise that she:
A. receive live attenuated influenza virus vaccine.
B. avoid immunization against influenza because of the risk associated with the vaccine.
C. receive inactivated influenza virus vaccine.
D. take an antiviral for the duration of the influenza season.

34 to 37. Indicate whether each statement is true or false.

____ **34.** Seasonal influenza vaccination is generally recommended for all persons over the age of 6 months.

____ **35.** A 66-year-old woman is an acceptable candidate for the high-dose inactivated influenza vaccine shot.

____ **36.** Cigarette smokers should not receive the pneumococcal vaccine until 65 years of age.

____ **37.** A 52-year-old immunocompetent patient with COPD who receives the pneumococcal vaccine should get revaccinated in 5 years.

38. When used in treating COPD, ipratropium bromide (Atrovent) is prescribed to achieve which of the following therapeutic effects?
A. increase mucociliary clearance
B. reduce alveolar volume
C. bronchodilation
D. mucolytic action

39. What is the desired therapeutic action of inhaled corticosteroids when used to treat COPD?
A. reversal of fixed airway obstruction
B. improvement of central respiratory drive
C. reduction of airway inflammation
D. mucolytic activity

40. Which is most consistent with the diagnosis of COPD?
    A. FEV_1/FVC ratio equal to or less than 0.70 after properly timed SABA use
    B. dyspnea on exhalation
    C. elevated diaphragms noted on x-ray
    D. polycythemia noted on complete blood cell count

41. The most effective nonpharmacologic method to prevent exacerbations in patients with COPD is:
    A. weight loss for those with a BMI greater than 25 kg/m^2.
    B. avoid exposure to children or day-care centers.
    C. brisk walking for at least 5 minutes 3-5 times a day as tolerated.
    D. avoid exposure to pulmonary irritants, such as cigarette smoke.

42. When managing patients with COPD who continue to smoke cigarettes, a discussion on the importance of smoking cessation should occur:
    A. at the initial diagnosis visit.
    B. with each COPD flare.
    C. once inhaled corticosteroid therapy is initiated.
    D. at every office visit.

43. According to the Global Initiative for Chronic Obstructive Lung Disease (GOLD) COPD guidelines, which of the following medications is indicated for use in all COPD stages?
    A. short-acting inhaled beta2-agonist
    B. inhaled corticosteroid
    C. long-acting anticholinergic
    D. long-acting beta2-agonist

44. According to the GOLD COPD guidelines, the goal of inhaled corticosteroid use in stage III or severe COPD is to:
    A. minimize the risk of repeated exacerbations.
    B. improve cough function.
    C. reverse alveolar hypertrophy.
    D. help mobilize secretions.

45. Which of the following systemic corticosteroid doses is most potent?
    A. methylprednisolone 8 mg
    B. triamcinolone 10 mg
    C. prednisone 15 mg
    D. hydrocortisone 18 mg

46. Which of the following pathogens is often implicated in a COPD exacerbation caused by respiratory tract infection?
    A. *Legionella* species
    B. *Streptococcus pyogenes*
    C. Respiratory tract viruses
    D. *Staphylococcus aureus*

47. Which is the most appropriate choice of therapy in the treatment of a mild acute COPD exacerbation in a 42-year-old man?
    A. A 5-day course of levofloxacin
    B. A 7-day course of amoxicillin
    C. A 10-day course of doxycycline
    D. Antimicrobial therapy is usually not indicated.

48. Which is the most appropriate statement about therapy for a severe COPD exacerbation in a 52-year-old man?
    A. A 5-day course azithromycin should be prescribed.
    B. A 10-day course of amoxicillin/clavulanate is advisable,
    C. A 7-day course of trimethoprim-sulfamethoxazole is recommended.
    D. The role of antimicrobial therapy is debated, even for severe disease.

49. You see a 67-year-old man with stage IV (very severe) COPD who asks, "When should I use my home oxygen?" You respond:
    A. as needed when short of breath.
    B. primarily during sleep hours.
    C. preferably during waking hours.
    D. for at least 15 hours a day.

50. With a COPD exacerbation, a chest x-ray should be obtained:
    A. routinely in all patients
    B. when attempting to rule out a concomitant pneumonia.
    C. if sputum volume is increased.
    D. when work of breathing is increased.

51. Which of the following best describes the role of theophylline in COPD treatment?
    A. indicated in moderate to very severe COPD
    B. use limited by narrow therapeutic profile and drug-drug interaction potential
    C. a potent bronchodilator
    D. available only in parenteral form

52. All of the following are consistent with the GOLD COPD recommendation for pulmonary rehabilitation except:
    A. reserved for very severe COPD.
    B. goals include improvement in overall well-being.
    C. an underused therapeutic option.
    D. components aimed at reducing the deconditioning common in COPD.

Answers

33. C.	40. A.	47. D.
34. True	41. D.	48. D.
35. True	42. D.	49. D.
36. False	43. A.	50. B.
37. False	44. A.	51. B.
38. C.	45. C.	52. A.
39. C.	46. C.	

Chronic obstructive pulmonary disease (COPD) is a preventable and treatable disease with significant extrapulmonary effects that can contribute to the severity in individual patients. The pulmonary component is characterized by airflow limitation that is not fully reversible. The airflow limitation is usually progressive and associated with an abnormal inflammatory response of the lung to noxious particles or gases. This response results in a decrease in the ratio of forced expiratory volume at 1 second (FEV_1) to forced vital capacity (FVC).

Historically, the hallmark symptom of chronic bronchitis is a chronic productive cough, whereas for emphysema it is shortness of breath. However, these terms are not used as part of the Global Obstructive Lung Disease (GOLD) guidelines for the diagnosis and management of COPD. Instead, emphasis is on the symptoms of dyspnea, chronic cough, and sputum production with the understanding that airway inflammation, smooth muscle constriction, and altered lung mechanics occurs. Patients with COPD typically present for care in the fifth and sixth decades of life, usually after having symptoms for more than a decade.

Diagnosis should be considered in any patient with progressive dyspnea, chronic cough or sputum production, and/or with a history of risk factors, such as tobacco use. Dyspnea is typically persistent and progressive and is worse with exercise and exacerbations. Cough can be intermittent and is often unproductive. However, often the cough is productive and chronic. Spirometry should then be performed and is required to make the clinical diagnosis of COPD. The forced expiratory volume in the first second of expiration (FEV_1):forced vital capacity (FVC) ratio is considered the most sensitive indicator of early airflow limitation. The presence of a post-bronchodilator FEV_1:FVC less than 70% confirms persistent airflow obstruction. The degree of spirometric abnormality generally reflects the severity of COPD. However, symptoms often do not correlate well with objective measurements and/or patients may deny symptoms and meet diagnostic criteria for COPD. The COPD Assessment Test (CAT) is a useful adjunct to symptoms, spirometry abnormality, and identification of risk for exacerbations for the assessment of the level of COPD severity and choosing pharmacologic therapy (Tables 6–8 to 6–10).

TABLE 6-8

Classification of Severity of Airflow Limitation in COPD Based on Post-bronchodilator FEV_1

IN PATIENTS WITH FEV_1/FVC<0.70:

GOLD 1	Mild	$FEV_1 \geq 80\%$ predicted
GOLD 2	Moderate	$50\% \leq FEV_1 < 80\%$ predicted
GOLD 3	Severe	$30\% \leq FEV_1 < 50\%$ predicted
GOLD 4	Very severe	$FEV_1 < 30\%$ predicted

Source: Global Initiative for Chronic Obstructive Lung Disease, Pocket Guide to COPD Diagnosis, Management and Prevention, www.goldcopd.org/guidelines-pocket-guide-to-copd-diagnosis.html, accessed 12/3/13.

TABLE 6-9

Global Initiative for Chronic Obstructive Pulmonary Disease (GOLD) Pharmacologic Therapy for Stable COPD

Patient group	First choice	Second choice	Alternative choice**
A Low Risk Less Symptoms	SA anticholinergic (ipratropium [Atrovent]) PRN *or* SA beta2-agonist (albuterol [Ventolin HFA, Proventil HFA]) PRN	LA anticholinergic (tiotropium [Spiriva]) *or* LA beta2-agonist (salmeterol [Serevent]) *or* SA beta2-agonist *and* SA anticholinergic (ipratropium bromide with albuterol [Combivent Respimat])	Theophylline
B Low Risk More Symptoms	LA anticholinergic (tiotropium [Spiriva]) *or* LA beta2-agonist (salmeterol [Serevent])	LA anticholinergic (tiotropium [Spiriva]) *and* LA beta2-agonist (salmeterol [Serevent])	SA beta2-agonist (albuterol [Ventolin HFA, Proventil HFA]) *and/or* SA anticholinergic (ipratropium [Atrovent]) (ipratropium bromide with albuterol [Combivent Respimat])

Continued

TABLE 6-9

Global Initiative for Chronic Obstructive Pulmonary Disease (GOLD) Pharmacologic Therapy for Stable COPD—cont'd

Patient group	First choice	Second choice	Alternative choice**
C High Risk Less Symptoms	ICS (fluticasone, budesonide) + LA beta2-agonist (salmeterol, formoterol [Advair, Symbicort]) *or* LA anticholinergic (tiotropium [Spiriva])	LA anticholinergic (tiotropium [Spiriva]) *and* LA beta2-agonist (salmeterol [Serevent])	PDE-4 inhibitor (roflumilast [Daliresp***]) SA beta2-agonist (albuterol [Ventolin HFA, Proventil HFA]) *and/or* SA anticholinergic (ipratropium [Atrovent]) Theophylline (do not use w/roflumilast)
D High Risk More Symptoms	ICS (fluticasone, budesonide) + LA beta2-agonist (salmeterol, formoterol [Advair, Symbicort]) *or* LA anticholinergic (tiotropium [Spiriva])	ICS (fluticasone [Flovent HFA], budesonide [Pulmicort Flexhaler]) and LA anticholinergic (tiotropium [Spiriva]) *or* ICS (fluticasone, budesonide) + LA beta2-agonist (salmeterol, formoterol [Advair, Symbicort]) *and* LA anticholinergic (tiotropium [Spiriva]) *or* ICS + LA beta2-agonist (Advair, Symbicort) *and* PDE-4 inhibitor (roflumilast [Daliresp***]) *or* LA anticholinergic (tiotropium [Spiriva]) *and* LA beta2-agonist (salmeterol [Serevent]) *or* LA anticholinergic (tiotropium [Spiriva]) *and* PDE-4 inhibitor (roflumilast [Daliresp***])	Carbocysteine (mucolytic) SA beta2-agonist (albuterol [Ventolin HFA, Proventil HFA]) *and/or* SA anticholinergic (ipratropium [Atrovent]) Theophylline

*Medications in each box are mentioned in alphabetical order and therefore not necessarily in order of preference.

**Medications in this column can be used alone or in combination with other options in the First and Second choice columns

Source: Global Initiative for Chronic Obstructive Lung Disease, Pocket Guide to COPD Diagnosis, Management, and Prevention 2011.

***Roflumilast (Daliresp) {phosphodiesterase 4 (PDE4) inhibitor}, therapeutic option to reduce the risk of COPD exacerbations in patients with severe and very severe COPD associated with chronic bronchitis who have a history of exacerbations. Not a bronchodilator and not indicated for relief of acute bronchospasm. Adverse effects include unintended weight loss, changes in mood, thinking, and behavior. Not to be used with theophylline.

Medications mentioned represent examples of the given drug class not a comprehensive list of all options.

Source: Global Initiative for Chronic Obstructive Lung Disease, Pocket Guide to COPD Diagnosis, Management and Prevention, www.goldcopd.org/guidelines-pocket-guide-to-copd-diagnosis.html, accessed 11/20/13.

TABLE 6-10
Combined Assessment of COPD

Patient	Characteristic	Spirometric classification	Exacerbations per year	CAT
A	Low Risk Less Symptoms	GOLD 1–2	≤1	<10
B	Low Risk More Symptoms	GOLD 1–2	≤1	≥10
C	High Risk Less Symptoms	GOLD 3–4	≥2	<10
D	High Risk More Symptoms	GOLD 3–4	≥2	≥10

The goals of COPD treatment are to relieve symptoms, reduce the impact of the symptoms, and reduce future adverse health events including exacerbations. Nonpharmacologic achievement of these goals includes smoking cessation and avoidance of other pulmonary irritants. Because 80% of all cases of COPD can be attributed directly to tobacco use, encouraging the patient to stop smoking is an important clinical goal. Despite symptoms, many patients continue to smoke. Raising the issue of smoking cessation at every visit and offering assistance with this is an important part of the ongoing care of the person with COPD. Counseling about general hygiene should also be provided, including information on minimizing exposure to passive smoking, allergens, and air pollution, and advice on hydration, nutrition, and avoiding respiratory tract infection.

Patients with COPD are at higher risk of a number of vaccine-preventable diseases and immunization should be encouraged. Routine seasonal influenza vaccination is recommended for all persons older than 6 months of age and should be encouraged and given annually for COPD patients. There are currently a variety of influenza vaccines that can be used. The trivalent or quadrivalent inactivated vaccine administered intramuscularly can be used for all patients 6 months and older with no contraindications. The live, attenuated influenza vaccine (LAIV) administered via a nasal spray is approved for most individuals aged 2 through 49 years but should not be used in individuals with airway disease. Meanwhile, a high-dose inactivated vaccine is available for those 65 years and older that is likely to improve the immune response in this older patient population. Pneumococcal vaccination is currently recommended for all adults 65 years and older as well as younger adults considered at higher risk of disease, including cigarette smokers, people with asthma, and anyone with COPD. Two pneumococcal vaccines are approved for use in adults. Pneumovax is a 23-valent polysaccharide vaccine that protects against 23 pneumococcal serotypes and is recommended for adults 65 years and older, as well as younger adults at high risk for disease. PCV13 or Prevnar 13 is a pneumococcal conjugate vaccine that is approved for adults 50 years and older and protects against 13 serotypes. Check label recommendations for the use of pneumococcal vaccine.

The backbone of pharmacologic therapy for COPD is the inhaled bronchodilators. Patients at all levels of COPD severity should be prescribed a short-acting beta2-agonist for acute relief of symptoms. Routine, daily bronchodilators are begun at the moderate severity stage COPD (Stage 2) and continued throughout very severe COPD (Stage 4). Options include a long-acting anticholinergic agent (tiotropium [Spiriva], aclidium bromide [Turdoza Pressair]), a long-acting beta2-agonist (salmeterol [Serevent], formoterol [Foradil], arformoterol [Brovana], indacaterol [Onbrez]), or a short-acting anticholinergic agent dosed several times daily (ipratropium [Atrovent]). The long-acting bronchodilators are preferred over the multi-dosed, short-acting agents due to superior effectiveness and convenience. The choice between the long-acting bronchodilators depends on availability of the drug, the patient's individual response in terms of symptom relief, and adverse effects. Combining bronchodilators of different pharmacologic classes may improve efficacy. Routine use of inhaled corticosteroids in COPD patients with FEV_1 less than 60% predicted improves symptoms and lung function, and reduces the frequency of exacerbations. Combination inhaled corticosteroid/long-acting bronchodilator is more effective in improving symptoms and lung function, and reducing exacerbations in patients with moderate to very severe COPD than either individual component. Long-term treatment with oral corticosteroids is not recommended. Theophylline is less effective and less well tolerated than other bronchodilators. There is a risk for drug-drug interactions, and it has a narrow therapeutic index. Roflumilast (Daliresp) is a phosphodiesterase-4 inhibitor indicated for the reduction of exacerbations in severe and very severe chronic bronchitis.

Patients at all severity levels of COPD benefit from exercise training and pulmonary rehabilitation. The goal of this intervention is to improve quality of life, decrease symptoms, and increase physical participation in activities of daily living. Components of a pulmonary rehabilitation program include reversing the effects of physical deconditioning, social isolation, weight loss, muscle wasting, and altered mood often noted with COPD. Improvements in exercise tolerance and symptoms of dyspnea and fatigue can be sustained even after a single pulmonary rehabilitation program. Because of issues of funding, access, and lack of provider and patient knowledge of this helpful intervention, pulmonary rehabilitation is an underused, yet helpful intervention.

Long-term oxygen therapy for patients with COPD should be considered, particularly as the disease progresses, or when a patient presents with advanced disease (Table 6–11). The goal of therapy is to ensure adequate oxygen delivery to the vital organs by increasing the baseline PaO_2 at rest to 60 mm Hg or greater at sea level, or producing SaO_2 equal to or greater than 90%, or both. In patients with chronic respiratory failure, oxygen therapy administered more than 15 hours per day has been shown to increase survival. Many patients wait until they are breathless, then attempt to correct this with as-needed oxygen use and fail to achieve maximum benefit; these benefits include not only improved overall well-being, but also increased survival.

Exacerbations of respiratory symptoms that necessitate treatment are important clinical events in COPD. The most common causes of an exacerbation are infection of the tracheobronchial tree and air pollution, but the cause of at least one-third of severe exacerbations cannot be identified. Inhaled bronchodilators (beta2-agonists or anticholinergics or both) are effective for the treatment of COPD exacerbation. Consider adding a long-acting bronchodilator if the patient is not currently using one and adding an inhaled corticosteroid to reduce the risk of future exacerbations. If baseline FEV_1 is less than 60% of predicted, a systemic corticosteroid, with oral route preferred, such as prednisone 40 mg daily for 5 to 10 days, should be added; knowledge of the relative potency of these drugs is important to safe and effective clinical practice. (See Table 6–5). Although a 10-day course of systemic corticosteroid therapy has been advised, recent study supports the efficacy and safety of a shorter 5-day course.

Antimicrobial therapy is not always needed as part of treatment of a COPD exacerbation because the cause can be nonbacterial in origin, such as an environmental problem or viral infection. Use of an antibiotic is likely indicated, however, when symptoms of breathlessness and cough are accompanied by altered sputum characteristics that suggest bacterial infection, such as increased purulence or change in volume. The therapeutic choice should be dictated by antimicrobial coverage for the major bacterial pathogens involved in COPD exacerbation, while taking into account local patterns of bacterial resistance (Table 6–12). Because of the possibility of a concomitant pneumonia, a chest x-ray should be obtained when the patient presents with fever or unusually low SaO_2 or both; in the absence of these findings, a chest x-ray is not usually needed.

DISCUSSION SOURCES

Gilbert D, Moellering R, Eliopoulos G, Chambers H, Saag M. *The Sanford Guide to Antimicrobial Therapy*, 44th ed. Sperryville, VA: Antimicrobial Therapy, Inc., 2014.

Global Initiative for Chronic Obstructive Lung Disease. Pocket Guide to COPD Diagnosis, Management and Prevention, http://www.goldcopd.org/Guidelines/guidelines-resources.html

Tuberculosis

53. You examine a 28-year-old woman who has emigrated from a country where tuberculosis (TB) is endemic. She has documentation of receiving Bacille Calmette-Guérin (BCG) vaccine as a child. With this information, you consider that:
    A. she will always have a positive tuberculin skin test (TST) result.
    B. biannual chest radiographs are needed to assess her health status accurately.
    C. a TST finding of 10 mm or more induration should be considered a positive result.
    D. isoniazid therapy should be given for 6 months before TST is undertaken.

TABLE 6-11
Long-term Oxygen Therapy in Chronic Obstructive Pulmonary Disease

Goal	To ensure adequate oxygen delivery to vital organs by increasing baseline PaO_2 at rest to ≥60 mm Hg at sea level or producing SaO_2 ≥90%, or both
Indications to Initiate Long-Term (>15 Hours/Day) Oxygen Therapy	PaO_2 <55 mm Hg *or* SaO_2 <88% with or without hypercapnia PaO_2 55–69 mm Hg *or* SaO_2 89% in the presence of cor pulmonale, right heart failure, or polycythemia (hematocrit >56%)

Source: Global Initiative for Chronic Obstructive Lung Disease, Pocket Guide to COPD Diagnosis, Management and Prevention, www.goldcopd.org/guidelines-pocket-guide-to-copd-diagnosis.html

TABLE 6-12
Etiology and Recommendations for Antimicrobial Therapy in Chronic Obstructive Pulmonary Disease (COPD) Exacerbations

ETIOLOGY	Viruses (20%–50%) Bacteria: • Aside from bacterial infection, tobacco use, air pollution, and viruses common contributing factors • Causative pathogens (30-50%) include *Haemophilus influenzae, Haemophilus parainfluenzae, Streptococcus pneumoniae, Moraxella catarrhalis.* • Less common pathogens include atypical pathogens, other gram-positive and -negative organisms.
MILD-TO-MODERATE DISEASE	Antimicrobial therapy usually not indicated. If prescribed, consider using the following agents: • Amoxicillin • Doxycycline
SEVERE DISEASE (INCREASED DYSPNEA, INCREASED SPUTUM VISCOSITY/ PURULENCE, AND INCREASED SPUTUM VOLUME) *Role of antimicrobial therapy debated even for severe disease.*	Use one of the following agents: • Amoxicillin-clavulanate • Cephalosporin • Azithromycin • Clarithromycin • Fluoroquinolone with activity against drug-resistant *S. pneumoniae*

Source: Gilbert DN, Moellering RC, Eliopoulos GM, Chambers HF, Saag MS. *The Sanford Guide to Antimicrobial Therapy,* 44th ed. Sperryville, VA: Antimicrobial Therapy, Inc., 2014.

54. A 33-year-old woman works in a small office with a man recently diagnosed with active pulmonary TB. Which of the following would be the best plan of care for this woman?
   A. She should receive TB chemoprophylaxis if her TST result is 5 mm or more in induration.
   B. Because of her age, TB chemoprophylaxis is contraindicated even in the presence of a positive TST result.
   C. If the TST result is positive but the chest radiograph is normal, no further evaluation or treatment is needed.
   D. Further evaluation is needed only if the TST result is 15 mm or more in induration.

55. Compared with TST, potential advantages of the QuantiFERON-TB Gold test (QTF-G) include all of the following except:
   A. ability to have entire testing process complete with one clinical visit.
   B. results are available within 24 hours.
   C. interpretation of test is not subject to reader bias.
   D. provides a prediction as to who is at greatest risk for active disease development.

For the following questions, answer "yes" or "no" in response to the question, "Does this patient have a reactive TST?"

____ 56. A 45-year-old woman with type 2 diabetes mellitus and chest radiograph finding consistent with previous TB and a 7-mm induration

____ 57. A 21-year-old man with no identifiable TB risk factors and a 10-mm induration

____ 58. A 31-year-old man with HIV and a 6-mm induration

____ 59. A 45-year-old woman from a country in which TB is endemic who has an 11-mm induration

____ 60. A 42-year-old woman with rheumatoid arthritis who is taking etanercept (Enbrel) who has a 7-mm induration

61. Risk factors for development of infection reactivation in patients with latent TB infection include all of the following except:
   A. diabetes mellitus.
   B. immunocompromise.
   C. long-term oral corticosteroid therapy.
   D. male gender.

62. Clinical presentation of progressive primary TB most commonly includes all of the following except:
   A. malaise.
   B. fever.
   C. dry cough.
   D. frank hemoptysis.

Answers

53. C.	57. No	61. D.
54. A.	58. Yes	62. D.
55. D.	59. Yes	
56. Yes	60. Yes	

Pulmonary tuberculosis (TB) is a chronic bacterial infection, caused by *Mycobacterium tuberculosis* and transmitted through aerosolized droplets. With an estimated 20% to 43% of the world's population infected, the disease occurs disproportionately in disadvantaged populations, such as the homeless, the malnourished, and people living in overcrowded and substandard housing. About 30% of individuals exposed to the causative organism become infected. In an immunocompetent host, when the organism is acquired, an immune reaction ensues to help contain the infection within granulomas. This stage, known as primary TB, is usually symptom-free. Viable organisms can lie dormant within the granulomas for years, however; this stage is known as latent TB infection (LTBI). A person with LTBI does not have active disease and is not contagious.

Without treatment, individuals with LTBI have a 10% lifetime risk of reactivation of the disease, known as postprimary TB, with 50% of the reactivations occurring within the first 2 years of primary infection. This increases to a risk of 10% per year in the presence of HIV infection; increased rates of reactivation are also noted with other forms of immunocompromise (systemic corticosteroid or other immunosuppressive drug use, many chronic illnesses) or diabetes mellitus. After primary infection, about 5% of patients do not mount a containing immune response and develop progressive primary TB.

Public health measures to ensure adequate shelter, hygiene, and nutrition for the vulnerable public are an important primary prevention measure against the spread of TB infection. TST is an effective method of identifying individuals infected with *M. tuberculosis*. This test, when performed on an asymptomatic patient, is an example of secondary prevention or health screening. The test is performed by injecting 0.1 mL of purified protein derivative transdermally. The results should be checked within 48 to 72 hours, with the transverse measurement of any change in the test site measured in millimeters of induration, not simply redness. A positive TST result is usually noted within 2 to 10 weeks of acquiring the organism. Thresholds for a positive TST result vary in different clinical conditions (Table 6–13). The interpretation of the test is the same in the presence or absence of Bacille Calmette-Guérin (BCG) vaccination history. In certain circumstances, two-step testing and anergy testing should be considered.

The TST has limitations, including the need for multiple visits, one to inject the PPD then a return visit to read or interpret the test, and a low sensitivity in the people with immunosuppression, a group at high risk for reactivation. In addition, test results can be compromised by poor injection technique or the use of an inferior purified protein derivative product. As a result, alternative testing has been developed and is gaining increased acceptance. A blood test, known by its trade name QuantiFERON-TB, detects interferon-γ, which is released by T lymphocytes in response to *M. tuberculosis*-specific antigens. This test can be performed from a blood sample obtained on a single provider visit, with results available within 24 hours. In addition, its sensitivity is greater in patients with immunocompromise or with a history of receiving BCG vaccine.

Any patient with a positive TST or QuantiFERON-TB test result should have a chest x-ray to help exclude the diagnosis of active pulmonary tuberculosis. In addition, a careful evaluation for clinical evidence of active disease, including malaise, weight loss, fever, night sweats, and chronic cough, should be carried out; these findings often evolve over 4 to 6 weeks in a person with active TB, and atypical presentation is common in immunocompromised individuals. Although blood-tinged sputum is occasionally reported, the cough associated with TB is often dry; frank hemoptysis is rarely

TABLE 6-13

Classification of Tuberculin Skin Test Reaction

An induration of ≥5 mm is considered positive in:	**An induration of ≥10 mm** is considered positive in:	**An induration of ≥15 mm** is considered positive in any
• HIV-infected persons • A recent contact of a person with tuberculosis (TB) disease • Persons with fibrotic changes on chest radiograph consistent with prior TB • Patients with organ transplants • Persons who are immunosuppressed for other reasons (e.g., taking the equivalent of >15 mg/d of prednisone for ≥1 mo, taking TNF-α antagonists)	• Recent immigrants (<5 yr) from high-prevalence countries • Injection drug users • Residents and employees of high-risk congregate settings • Mycobacteriology laboratory personnel • Persons with clinical conditions that place them at high risk • Children <4 y.o. • Infants, children, and adolescents exposed to adults in high-risk categories	person, including persons with no known risk factors for TB. Targeted skin testing programs should be conducted only in high-risk groups, however

reported. The chest examination is usually normal, with dyspnea seldom reported unless disease is extensive.

Chemoprophylaxis therapy with isoniazid and other agents to prevent the development of active pulmonary TB should be considered for patients with latent tuberculosis—that is, positive tuberculin test results, but negative chest radiograph results and no suspicion of disease revealed by health history or physical examination. The duration of isoniazid therapy is 6 to 9 months, depending on the dosing regimen. Rifampin is an alternative choice if isoniazid cannot be taken or is poorly tolerated. Although the risk of liver toxicity with anti-TB drug use increases with age, age alone is not a contraindication to its use, particularly in individuals at higher risk.

In the presence of active pulmonary TB, multiple antimicrobial therapies are administered that are aimed not only at eradicating the infection, but also at minimizing the risk of developing a resistant pathogen. In this era of multidrug-resistant TB, it is prudent to consult with local TB experts to ascertain the local patterns of susceptibility. With latent and active disease, public health involvement is critical to maximize the patient outcome and minimize risk to the general population.

DISCUSSION SOURCES

National Center for HIV/AIDS, Viral Hepatitis, STD and TB Prevention, Division of Tuberculosis Elimination. www.cdc.gov/tb/

Sharma S, Mohan A. Tuberculosis and other mycobacterial diseases. In: Rakel R, Bope E (eds): *Conn's Current Therapy 2014.* Philadelphia, PA: Saunders Elsevier.

Community-Acquired Pneumonia

63 to 68. According to the American Thoracic Society/Infectious Disease Society of American (ATS/IDSA) Consensus Guidelines on the Management of Community-Acquired Pneumonia in Adults, which of the following is the most appropriate antimicrobial for treatment of community-acquired pneumonia (CAP) in:

63. A 42-year-old man with no comorbidity, no reported drug allergy, and no recent antimicrobial use?
A. azithromycin
B. cefpodoxime
C. trimethoprim-sulfamethoxazole
D. ciprofloxacin

64. A 46-year-old well woman with a history of a bilateral tubal ligation who is macrolide intolerant?
A. clarithromycin
B. amoxicillin
C. doxycycline
D. fosfomycin

65. A 78-year-old woman with a history of COPD, hypertension, and dyslipidemia who is taking lovastatin and a dihydropyridine calcium channel blocker?
A. clindamycin
B. high-dose amoxicillin with doxycycline
C. clarithromycin
D. ceftriaxone

66. A 69-year-old man with heart failure, prior myocardial infarction, and type 2 diabetes?
A. respiratory fluoroquinolone
B. amoxicillin with a beta-lactamase inhibitor
C. cephalosporin
D. beta-lactam plus macrolide

67. A 28-year-old woman with a severe beta-lactam allergy who has a dry cough, headache, malaise, no recent antimicrobial use, and no comorbidity who takes no medication?
A. clarithromycin
B. amoxicillin
C. levofloxacin
D. ceftriaxone

68. A 47-year-old woman who was recently treated within the past two months with a beta-lactam for acute bacterial sinusitis?
A. amoxicillin-clavulanate
B. high-dose amoxicillin
C. clarithromycin
D. moxifloxacin

69. Criteria to distinguish if pneumonia is community-acquired include all of the following except:
A. lives in the community.
B. not a resident of a long-term care facility.
C. no prior antimicrobial use in the previous 3 months.
D. no recent hospitalization.

70. Common symptoms of community-acquired pneumonia in otherwise well adults include all of the following except:
A. cough.
B. altered mental status.
C. dyspnea.
D. pleuritic chest pain.

71. A diagnosis of pneumonia is confirmed by:
A. sputum culture.
B. sputum gram stain.
C. bronchoalveolar lavage.
D. chest radiograph.

72. Which of the following is a quality of respiratory fluoroquinolones?
A. activity against drug-resistant *S. pneumoniae* (DRSP)
B. poor activity against atypical pathogens
C. predominantly hepatic route of elimination
D. poor activity against beta-lactamase producing organisms.

73. The mechanism of resistance of DRSP is through the cell's:
    A. beta-lactamase production.
    B. hypertrophy of cell membrane.
    C. alteration in protein-binding sites.
    D. failure of DNA gyrase reversal.

74. The primary mechanism of antimicrobial resistance of *H. influenzae* is through the organism's:
    A. beta-lactamase production.
    B. hypertrophy of cell membrane.
    C. alteration in protein-binding sites.
    D. failure of DNA gyrase reversal.

75. Which of the following characteristics applies to macrolides?
    A. consistent activity against DRSP
    B. contraindicated in pregnancy
    C. effective against atypical pathogens
    D. unstable in the presence of beta-lactamase

76. According to the ATS/IDSA guidelines, what is the usual length of antimicrobial therapy for the treatment of CAP for outpatients?
    A. less than 5 days
    B. 5 to 7 days
    C. 7 to 10 days
    D. 10 to 14 days

77 to 79. Based on the CURB-65 criteria, indicate which patients should be treated as an inpatient (I) or outpatient (O).

77. A 47-year-old man with no confusion, BUN = 17 mg/dL, respiratory rate = 32/min, and blood pressure = 110/72 mm Hg

78. A 56-year-old woman with no confusion, BUN = 22 mg/dL, respiratory rate = 27/min, blood pressure = 88/56 mm Hg

79. A 72-year-old man with confusion, BUN = 18 mg/dL, respiratory rate = 35/min, blood pressure = 102/66 mm Hg

80. Risk factors for pneumonia caused by *P. aeruginosa* include all of the following except:
    A. mechanical ventilation.
    B. cystic fibrosis.
    C. community residence.
    D. chronic tracheostomy.

81. Which of the following most accurately describes sputum analysis in the evaluation of the person with community-acquired pneumonia?
    A. Gram stain is routinely advised.
    B. Antimicrobial therapy should not be initiated until sputum specimen for culture has been obtained.
    C. Sputum analysis is not recommended in the majority of patients with community-acquired pneumonia.
    D. If required, chest physical therapy can be used to facilitate sputum production.

82. Which of the following best describes the mechanism of transmission in an atypical pneumonia pathogen?
    A. microaspiration
    B. respiratory droplet
    C. surface contamination
    D. aerosolized contaminated water

83. Risk factors for death resulting from pneumonia include:
    A. viral origin.
    B. history of allergic reaction to multiple antimicrobials.
    C. renal insufficiency.
    D. polycythemia.

84. All of the following antimicrobial strategies help facilitate the development of resistant pathogens except:
    A. longer course of therapy.
    B. lower antimicrobial dosage.
    C. higher antimicrobial dosage.
    D. prescribing a broader spectrum agent.

85. Findings of increased tactile fremitus and dullness to percussion at the right lung base in the person with CAP likely indicate an area of:
    A. atelectasis.
    B. pneumothorax.
    C. consolidation.
    D. cavitation.

86. You are caring for a 52-year-old man who is currently smoking 1.5 PPD, has a 40-pack-year cigarette smoking history, and has CAP. It is the third day of his antimicrobial therapy, and he is without fever, is well hydrated, and is feeling less short of breath. His initial chest x-ray revealed a right lower lobe infiltrate. Physical examination today reveals peak inspiratory crackles with increased tactile fremitus in the right posterior thorax. Which of the following represents the most appropriate next step in this patient's care?
    A. His current plan of care should continue because he is improving by clinical assessment.
    B. A chest radiograph should be taken today to confirm resolution of pneumonia.
    C. Given the persistence of abnormal thoracic findings, his antimicrobial therapy should be changed.
    D. A computed tomography scan of the thorax is needed today to image better any potential thoracic abnormalities.

87. While seeing a 62-year-old who is hospitalized with CAP, the NP considers that:
    A. pneumococcal vaccine should be given when antimicrobial therapy has been completed.
    B. pneumococcal vaccine can be given today, and influenza vaccine can be given in 2 weeks.
    C. influenza vaccine can be given today, and antipneumococcal vaccine can be given in 2 weeks.
    D. influenza and antipneumococcal vaccines should be given today.

88. Risk factors for infection with DRSP include all of the following except:
   A. systemic antimicrobial therapy in the previous 3 months.
   B. exposure to children in day care.
   C. age older than 65 years.
   D. use of inhaled corticosteroids.

89. The mechanism of transmission of *Legionella* species is primarily via:
   A. respiratory droplet.
   B. inhalation of aerosolized contaminated water.
   C. contact with a contaminated surface.
   D. hematogenous spread.

90. Which pneumococcal vaccine offers protection against the greatest number of serotypes?
   A. Pneumovax
   B. Prevnar
   C. PCV7
   D. LAIV

Identify the following organisms as a gram-positive, gram-negative, or atypical pathogen.

_____ **91.** *Streptococcus pneumoniae*

_____ **92.** *Haemophilus influenzae*

_____ **93.** *Legionella* species

_____ **94.** *Chlamydophila pneumoniae*

_____ **95.** *Mycoplasma pneumoniae*

Answers

63. A.	75. C.	87. D.
64. C.	76. B.	88. D.
65. B.	77. O	89. B.
66. A.	78. I	90. A.
67. A.	79. I	91. gram-positive
68. D.	80. C.	
69. C.	81. C.	92. gram-negative
70. B.	82. B.	
71. D.	83. C.	93. atypical
72. A.	84. C.	94. atypical
73. C.	85. C.	95. atypical
74. A.	86. A.	

Pneumonia is the most common cause of death from infectious disease and is the eighth leading cause of overall mortality in the United States. Although pneumonia is often considered a disease primarily of older adults and persons with chronic illness, most episodes occur in immunocompetent community-dwelling individuals; about 20% of children develop pneumonia by age 5 years. Most often caused by bacteria or virus, pneumonia is an acute lower respiratory tract infection involving lung parenchyma, interstitial tissues, and alveolar spaces. The term *community-acquired pneumonia* (CAP) is used to describe the onset of disease in a person who resides within the community, not in a nursing home or other care facility, with no recent (less than 2 weeks) hospitalization.

Patients with pneumonia usually present with cough (more than 90%), dyspnea (66%), sputum production (66%), and pleuritic chest pain (50%), although nonrespiratory symptoms, including fatigue and gastrointestinal upset, are also commonly reported. As with other infectious diseases, elderly patients often report fewer symptoms and often present with an elevated resting respiratory rate and generally feeling ill; altered mental status is often noted in the older adult with pneumonia.

Chest x-ray is helpful in the assessment of the person with CAP. Characteristic infiltrate patterns are typically seen with certain pathogens, such as interstitial infiltrates with atypical pathogens or viruses and areas of consolidation with *Streptococcus pneumoniae*. Therapy should be based on patient characteristics and risk factors, however, rather than the pattern of the radiographic abnormality. According to the recommendations of the IDSA/ATS Consensus Guidelines, an abnormal chest radiograph and clinical findings are required to confirm the diagnosis of pneumonia.

Although numerous organisms are capable of causing pneumonia, relatively few are seen with frequency. *S. pneumoniae*, also known as the pneumococcal organism, is a gram-positive diplococcus, is the most common CAP pathogen in adults, and is found in most deaths caused by CAP. *H. influenzae* is a predominant pathogen in CAP patients with COPD. *Mycoplasma pneumoniae* and *Chlamydophila* (formerly *Chlamydia*) *pneumoniae* are common causative pathogens of CAP. These organisms are transmitted by coughing and are often found among people living in closed communities, such as households, college dormitories, military barracks, and residential centers, including long-term care facilities. *M. pneumoniae, C. pneumoniae, Legionella* species and respiratory viruses are often referred to as atypical pathogens (causing atypical pneumonia) because these organisms are not detectable via gram stain, cannot be cultured on standard bacterial media, and clinically do not present with a classic pneumonia presentation. Usually contracted by inhaling mist or aspirating liquid that comes from a water source contaminated with the organisms, pulmonary infection with *Legionella* species can result in pneumonia ranging from mild to severe disease; there is no evidence for person-to-person spread of the disease. Risk factors for severe disease with *Legionella* species, capable of causing the most serious illness of the atypical pathogens, include tobacco use, airway disease, and diabetes mellitus. With airway impairment, pneumonia is often caused by anaerobic gram-negative bacilli or mixed gram-negative organisms.

Successful community-based care of a person with pneumonia depends on many factors. The patient must have intact gastrointestinal function and be able to take and tolerate oral medications and adequate amounts of fluids. A competent caregiver must be available. Also, the patient should be able to return for follow-up examination and evaluation.

Certain patient characteristics increase the likelihood of death from pneumonia and should alert the NP to consider hospitalization and aggressive therapy. These include age older than 65 years and severe electrolyte or hematological disorder, such as serum sodium concentration of less than 130 mEq/L, hematocrit less than 30%, or absolute neutrophil count of less than 1000/mm^3. The CURB-65 criteria can assist the clinician in determining whether a patient should be hospitalized. CURB-65 allocates one point for each of the following five criteria: confusion; BUN greater than19 mg/dL; respiratory rate greater than 30/minutes; blood pressure less than 90/60 mm Hg; and 65 years of age and older. A score of one or less indicates that the patient can be treated as an outpatient, whereas a score greater than 1 indicates hospitalization is needed. The presence of a comorbid disease—such as impaired renal function, diabetes mellitus, heart failure, immunosuppression, and airway dysfunction—poses increased risk, as do abnormalities in vital signs, such as fever, tachycardia, tachypnea, and hypotension.

The pathogen responsible for pneumonia also needs to be considered because pneumonia death risk is increased when *S. aureus*, often seen in postinfluenza pneumonia, or gram-negative rods such as *Klebsiella pneumoniae* or Pseudomonas aeruginosa, cause infection. Risk factors for pneumonia caused by gram-negative bacilli include alcoholism, underlying chronic bronchiectasis (e.g., cystic fibrosis), chronic tracheostomy and/or mechanical ventilation, and febrile neutropenia. Sputum analysis for Gram stain or culture is not recommended for the majority of patients with community-acquired pneumonia though is commonly obtained during the evaluation of a person with pneumonia who is treated in hospital.

Because definitive identification of the organism is unlikely, the choice of antimicrobial agent to treat pneumonia is largely empirical, directed at the most likely causative organism in view of patient characteristics, such as age and comorbidity. Since pneumococcal pneumonia, caused by *S. pneumoniae*, carries a significant risk for mortality, the chosen antimicrobial should always be effective against this pathogen, regardless of patient presentation. Choosing an antimicrobial with activity against atypical organisms (*M. pneumoniae, C. pneumoniae, Legionella* species) and gram-positive and gram-negative organisms (*S. pneumoniae, H. influenzae* if patient risk is present) helps ensure optimal outcome.

An additional consideration is antimicrobial resistance. Factors that facilitate the development of resistant microbes include repeated exposure to a given agent, underdosing (eradicating more sensitive organisms, leaving more resistant pathogens untouched), and an unnecessarily prolonged period of treatment. Shorter course high-dose therapy maximizes and exploits concentration-dependent killing by achieving higher maximum concentration and area under the curve/minimal inhibitory concentration values; allowing treatment of difficult pathogens, increased tissue penetration, and improved patient adherence to the regimen; and minimizing the development of resistance. Patients with CAP should be treated for a minimum of 5 days, should be afebrile

for 48–72 hours, and should have no more than one CAP-associated sign of clinical instability (e.g., elevated heart rate and respiratory rate, hypotension) before discontinuing therapy. A longer duration may be needed if the initial therapy was not effective against the identified pathogen or if an extrapulmonary complication is present (e.g., meningitis).

S. pneumoniae has shown increasing resistance to beta-lactams (antimicrobials containing the beta-lactam ring, including penicillins and cephalosporins), macrolides (an antimicrobial class including erythromycin, clarithromycin, and azithromycin), and tetracyclines (an antimicrobial class including tetracycline, doxycycline, and minocycline); strains with these resistance characteristics are known as drug-resistant *S. pneumoniae* (DRSP) or, less commonly, multidrug-resistant *S. pneumoniae* (MDRSP). The mechanism of resistance of DRSP is a result of an alteration in intracellular protein-binding sites, rendering formerly effective antimicrobials incapable of destroying the pathogen. Risk factors for DRSP include systemic antimicrobial therapy in the previous 3 months, exposure to children in day care, age older than 65 years, alcohol abuse, multiple comorbidities (e.g., COPD, coronary heart disease, diabetes mellitus), and immunosuppressive state including use of corticosteroids and other immunosuppressing medications and chronic illness.

Respiratory fluoroquinolones (e.g., levofloxacin [Levaquin], gemifloxacin [Factive], moxifloxacin [Avelox]) provide enhanced activity against DRSP and atypical organism coverage and stability in the presence of beta-lactamase. High-dose amoxicillin (≥3 g/d) and certain cephalosporins, such as cefuroxime, are additional treatment options. Macrolides (erythromycin, azithromycin [Zithromax, Zmax], clarithromycin [Biaxin]) and tetracyclines (tetracycline, minocycline [Minocin], doxycycline) do not exhibit activity against DRSP; use of these products could result in treatment failure in the presence of DRSP risk.

H. influenzae has the capacity to produce beta-lactamase, rendering penicillins ineffective; this varies regionally, but averages approximately 30% nationwide. Antimicrobials stable in the presence of beta-lactamase include macrolides, respiratory fluoroquinolones, and cephalosporins; adding clavulanate to amoxicillin (Augmentin) inactivates beta-lactamase and provides effective activity against H. influenzae.

Because atypical pathogens (*M. pneumoniae, C. pneumoniae, Legionella*) do not have a cell wall, beta-lactams are ineffective against these organisms. Macrolides, tetracyclines, and respiratory fluoroquinolones provide activity against these pathogens. When considering the use of macrolides, it is important to note that these agents are associated with QTc interval prolongation and risk for torsades de pointes. This is a result of a metabolic interaction potential (drug-drug interactions) as well as an intrinsic arrhythmogenic capability of these agents. With a growing number of medications available associated with QTc prolongation, NPs should be aware of concomitant use of multiple QTc-prolonging agents that can put the patient at risk for cardiovascular events. Additionally, the use of clarithromycin or erythromycin, potent cytochrome P450 3A4 inhibitors, concomitantly with select calcium channel blockers has been associated with an increased risk for profound hypotension. Clarithromycin's use with select statins (lova-, simva- and atorvastatin, all CYP3A4 substrates) can dramatically increase the risk of myositis and rhabdomyolysis.

The American Thoracic Society and the Infectious Disease Society of America offer guidelines for CAP assessment and

intervention. Factors influencing the choice of antimicrobial agent include patient comorbidity and risk if treatment fails. All treatment options offer activity against *S. pneumoniae*, *H. influenzae*, and atypical pathogens, the most common organisms implicated in CAP; consideration also needs to be given for DRSP risk (Tables 6–14 and 6–15).

TABLE 6-14

Community-acquired Pneumonia: Likely Causative Pathogens, Characteristics, and Effective Antimicrobials

Pathogen	Description	Antimicrobial Resistance	Comment
S. pneumoniae	Gram-positive diplococci	Via altered protein binding sites in bacterial cell (~25% nationwide) DRSP risk: Recent antimicrobial use (within past 3 mo), age ≥65 yr, exposure to a child in day care, alcohol abuse, medical comorbidities, immunosuppressive therapy or illness Effective antimicrobials for nonresistant *S. pneumoniae*: Macrolides (azithromycin, clarithromycin, erythromycin), standard-dose amoxicillin (1.5–2.5 g/d), select cephalosporins, tetracyclines including doxycycline Preferred antimicrobials for DRSP: High-dose (3–4 g/d) amoxicillin, telithromycin* (Ketek), respiratory fluoroquinolones (moxifloxacin, levofloxacin, gemifloxacin)	Most common cause of fatal community-acquired pneumonia
M. pneumoniae *C. pneumoniae*	Not revealed by Gram stain	Effective antimicrobials: Macrolides, respiratory fluoroquinolones, tetracyclines including doxycycline Ineffective antimicrobials: Beta-lactams (cephalosporins, penicillins)	Largely transmitted by cough, often seen in people who have recently spent extended time in close proximity (closed communities such as correctional facilities, college dormitories, long-term care facilities)
H. influenzae	Gram-negative bacillus	Beta-lactamase production (~40% nationwide) Effective antimicrobials: Agents with activity against gram-negative organisms and stable in presence of or active against beta-lactamase—macrolides, cephalosporins, amoxicillin-clavulanate, respiratory fluoroquinolones, tetracyclines including doxycycline	Common respiratory pathogen with tobacco-related lung disease
Legionella spp.	Not revealed by Gram stain	Effective antimicrobials: Macrolides, respiratory fluoroquinolones, tetracyclines, including doxycycline Ineffective antimicrobials: Beta-lactams (cephalosporins, penicillins)	Usually contracted by inhaling mist or aspirating liquid that comes from a water source contaminated with *Legionella*. No evidence for person-to-person spread of the disease

DRSP, drug-resistant *S. pneumoniae*.
Source: Gilbert DN, Moellering RC, Eliopoulos GM, Chambers HF, Saag MS. *The Sanford Guide to Antimicrobial Therapy*, 43rd ed. Sperryville, VA: Antimicrobial Therapy, Inc., 2013.
*Per FDA Advisory, health-care providers should monitor patients taking telithromycin for signs or symptoms of liver problems and the drug promptly discontinued if this occurs. Visit www.fda.gov for the latest FDA telithromycin advisory information.

TABLE 6-15

Infectious Disease Society of America/American Thoracic Society (IDSA/ATS) Community-acquired Pneumonia Classification and Recommended Treatment

IDSA/ATS Classification	Likely Causative Pathogens	Recommended Treatment	Comment
Previously healthy No recent (within 3 mo) antimicrobial use	S. pneumoniae (gram-positive) with low DRSP risk Atypical pathogens (M. pneumoniae, C. pneumoniae, Legionella) Respiratory virus	**Strong recommendation** Macrolide such as azithromycin, clarithromycin, or erythromycin **Or** **Weak recommendation** Doxycycline	Erythromycin: Limited gram-negative coverage Erythromycin, clarithromycin: CYP3A4 inhibitors
Comorbidities including COPD, diabetes, renal or congestive heart failure, asplenia, alcoholism, immunosuppressing conditions or use of immunosuppressing medications, malignancy, or use of an antimicrobial in past 3 mo	S. pneumoniae (gram-positive) with DRSP risk H. influenzae (gram-negative) Atypical pathogens (M. pneumoniae, C. pneumoniae) Respiratory virus	Respiratory fluoroquinolone (levofloxacin,* moxifloxacin or gemifloxacin) **Or** Advanced macrolide plus beta-lactam such as high-dose amoxicillin (3–4 g/d), high-dose amoxicillin-clavulanate (4 g/d), ceftriaxone (Rocephin), cefpodoxime (Vantin), cefuroxime (Ceftin) Alternative to macrolide: Doxycycline	Recent antimicrobial use increases risk of infection with DRSP. Given comorbidity, risk of poor outcome if treatment failure Recent use of fluoroquinolone should dictate selection of a nonfluoroquinolone regimen, and vice versa

*With levofloxacin use, the 750 mg dose × 5 days regimen is recommended.
COPD, chronic obstructive pulmonary disease; DRSP, drug-resistant S. pneumoniae.
Source: Mandell L, Wunderink RG, Anzueto A, Bartlett JG, Campbell GD, Dean NC, Dowell SF, File TM Jr, Musher DM, Niederman MS, Torres A, Whitney CG. Infectious Diseases Society of America; American Thoracic Society. Infectious Disease Society of America/American Thoracic Society consensus guidelines on the management of community-acquired pneumonia in adults. *Clin Infect Dis* 44(Suppl 2):S27–S72, 2007. Available at http://cid.oxfordjournals.org/content/44/Supplement_2/S27.full.pdf+html, accessed 12/2/13.

NPs are ideally positioned to help minimize risk for pneumonia through immunization and hygienic measures. Nearly two-thirds of all fatal cases of pneumonia are caused by S. pneumoniae, the pneumococcal organism. Although available for decades, antipneumococcal vaccine (e.g., Pneumovax, Prevnar) continues to be underused. Pneumovax is a 23-valent polysaccharide vaccine that protects against 23 pneumococcal serotypes and is recommended for adults 65 years and older, as well as younger adults at high risk for disease. PCV13 or Prevnar 13 is a pneumococcal conjugate vaccine that is approved for adults 50 years and older and protects against 13 serotypes. The use of influenza vaccine can help minimize the risk of postinfluenza pneumonia, an often debilitating and potentially fatal condition. Both vaccines can be given together and in the presence of moderately severe illness. Ensuring adequate ventilation, reinforcing cough hygiene, and proper hand washing can help minimize pneumonia risk.

DISCUSSION SOURCES

Gilbert DN, Moellering RC, Eliopoulos GM, Chambers HF, Saag MS. *The Sanford Guide to Antimicrobial Therapy*, 44th ed. Sperryville, VA: Antimicrobial Therapy, Inc., 2014, pp. 39–41.

Mandell L, Wunderink RG, Anzueto A, Bartlett JG, Campbell GD, Dean NC, Dowell SF, File TM Jr, Musher DM, Niederman MS, Torres A, Whitney CG. Infectious Diseases Society of America; American Thoracic Society. Infectious Disease Society of America/American Thoracic Society consensus guidelines on the management of community-acquired pneumonia in adults. *Clin Infect Dis* 44(Suppl 2):S27–S72, 2007. http://cid.oxfordjournals.org/content/44/Supplement_2/S27.full.pdf+html

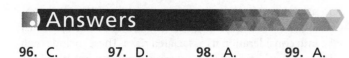
Acute Bronchitis

96. Cough associated with acute bronchitis can typically last up to:
 A. 1 week.
 B. 2 weeks.
 C. 3 weeks.
 D. 3 months.

97. Approximately _____ of acute bronchitis cases are caused by a viral infection.
 A. 15%
 B. 30%
 C. 65%
 D. 90%

98. Bacterial pathogens implicated in causing acute bronchitis include all of the following except:
 A. *S. pneumoniae.*
 B. *M. pneumoniae.*
 C. *C. pneumoniae.*
 D. *B. pertussis.*

99. A 34-year-old woman presents with a 7-day history of cough with no fever or difficulty breathing. She is otherwise healthy. She is producing small amounts of yellow-tinged sputum. As part of her treatment, you recommend:
 A. an antitussive.
 B. an antihistamine.
 C. a macrolide antimicrobial.
 D. a beta-lactam antimicrobial.

Answers

96. C.   **97.** D.   **98.** A.   **99.** A.

Persistent cough is one of the most common reasons for healthcare provider office visits and acute bronchitis is usually the diagnosis for these patients. Acute bronchitis is a self-limited infection that can persist for approximately 3 weeks, though occasionally persisting as long as 4-6 weeks. The diagnosis is usually limited to those without chronic airway disease (e.g., asthma or COPD). Acute bronchitis can be differentiated from the common cold (which lasts approximately 7 to 10 days, frequently with nasal congestion and rhinorrhea) or pneumonia (presence of fever, tachypnea, tachycardia, clinical lung findings).

Though rarely identified in clinical practice, the causative pathogen for acute bronchitis is viral in more than 90% of cases. These include adenovirus, coronavirus, influenza A or B, respiratory syncytial virus, and rhinovirus. When a bacterial infection is implicated in acute bronchitis, the most common species are *Bordetella pertussis, Chlamydophila pneumoniae,* and *Mycoplasma pneumoniae.* Sputum culture is not recommended given the high prevalence of viral infections and the low yield of viral cultures. However, testing for select organisms may be helpful during outbreaks of acute bronchitis in select scenarios, especially when a bacterial pathogen is suspected (e.g., pertussis outbreak). Sputum characteristics (e.g., clear, yellow, or green color) are not reliable indicators to differentiate between a viral or bacterial infection.

Treatment of acute bronchitis should focus on symptom management. Guidelines from the American College of Chest Physicians (ACCP) suggest that the use of antitussives (e.g., dextromethorphan) is a reasonable choice despite a lack of consistent evidence supporting their use. However, antitussives should not be used in children younger than 8 years because of a lack of effectiveness and risk of adverse effects. The use of expectorants and inhaler medications are not recommended for routine use in patients with acute bronchitis. However, patients with wheezing have shown some response with the use of beta2-agonist inhalers. For severe persistent cough, a short course of a systemic corticosteroid such as prednisone 40 mg daily for 3 to 5 days can offer significant symptom relief.

Routine use of antimicrobial therapy is not recommended for the treatment of acute bronchitis. Historically, the overuse of antimicrobials to treat viral infections has contributed to the rising prevalence of antimicrobial resistance in the community and, potentially, the growing number of cases of community-associated *Clostridium difficile* infection. Clinical studies demonstrate that antimicrobial therapy does not significantly change the course of acute bronchitis and only provides minimal benefit compared with the risks associated with their use. ACCP does not recommend the routine use of antimicrobials for acute bronchitis and suggests that healthcare providers take some time to explain the reasoning to patients who are typically expecting a prescription. Antimicrobials can be considered in certain situations, such as if pertussis, which can be treated with a macrolide, is suspected; with suspected pertussis, appropriate testing and health authority notification should take place. Antiviral medications can also be considered during influenza season for high-risk patients who present within 36 hours of symptom onset.

DISCUSSION SOURCES

Albert RH. Diagnosis and treatment of acute bronchitis. *Am Fam Physician* 82:1345–1350, 2010.

Braman SS. Chronic cough due to acute bronchitis: ACCP evidence-based clinical practice guidelines. *Chest* 129(1 Suppl):95S–103S, 2006.

Lung Cancer

100. Lung cancer ranks number ____ as a cause of cancer-related death in men and women.
 A. 1
 B. 2
 C. 3
 D. 4

101. Symptoms of lung cancer caused by a primary tumor include all of the following except:
A. chest discomfort.
B. dyspnea.
C. hoarseness.
D. hemoptysis.

102. According to ACCP guidelines, annual screening for lung cancer should occur in 55- to 74-year-old smokers with a smoking history of at least ___ pack-years.
A. 15
B. 30
C. 50
D. 70

103. Guidelines from the National Comprehensive Cancer Network (NCCN) recommend screening high-risk smokers beginning at age:
A. 40 years.
B. 45 years.
C. 50 years.
D. 55 years.

104. When compared with screening for breast cancer, screening for lung cancer results in:
A. a lower number needed to screen to prevent one death.
B. approximately the same number needed to screen to prevent one death.
C. a higher number needed to screen to prevent one death.
D. a higher percentage of patients identified where cancer can be prevented.

105. Current limitations of screening smokers with CT scan include all of the following except:
A. a high false-positive rate.
B. low sensitivity.
C. radiation exposure from multiple CT scans.
D. patient anxiety.

Answers

100. A.	102. B.	104. A.
101. C.	103. C.	105. B.

In the United States, lung cancer is the leading cause of cancer-related death in both men and women, accounting for nearly 160,000 deaths in 2013. This is more than the expected number of deaths from breast, colon, prostate, and pancreatic cancer combined. Early detection is essential since early-stage lung cancers are more likely to respond to treatment, such as surgery. The 5-year survival rate for localized stage lung cancer is 52% versus 16% for all stages combined. Currently, however, only 15% of lung cancers are diagnosed at the localized stage.

Typical presentation occurs at late-stage disease when patients become symptomatic. Patients may present with nonspecific systemic symptoms of fatigue, anorexia, and weight loss. A primary tumor may be associated with chest discomfort, cough, dyspnea, and hemoptysis. Forty percent of patients diagnosed with lung cancer initially present with signs and symptoms of intrathoracic spread. This can be associated with hoarseness (from laryngeal nerve paralysis), phrenic nerve paralysis, a superior pulmonary sulcus tumor (Pancoast tumor) with Horner syndrome, and/or chest wall invasion with persistent, pleuritic pain. Nearly one-third of patients present with extrathoracic spread, including spread to the bones, liver, adrenal glands, lymph nodes, brain, and spinal cord.

Guidelines from the American College of Chest Physicians (ACCP) recommend that patients at significant risk for lung cancer be offered annual screening with low-dose computed tomography (LDCT). High-risk patients include current smokers aged 55 to 74 years with a smoking history of at least 30 pack-years as well as former smokers of the same age who have quit within the past 15 years but have the same smoking history. Guidelines from the NCCN differ on who should be screened. NCCN recommends annual CT screening for younger patients (50 years or older) with a less extensive smoking history (at least 20 pack-years) who have one additional risk factor, such as a history of cancer or lung disease, family history of lung cancer, radon exposure, or occupational exposure. Screening of high-risk smokers is predicted to prevent one death from lung cancer for every 320 screened. In comparison, breast cancer screening with mammograms prevents one death for every 780 screened.

Although screening certain high-risk patients offers the potential to reduce lung cancer mortality, the decision-making process concerning whether to offer screening must take into consideration its associated risks. These include high false-positive rates, radiation exposure from multiple CT scans, patient anxiety, and unnecessary invasive procedures. Clinicians can mitigate these risks by offering screening only to those patients who fall within the parameters outlined in the ACCP or NCCN guidelines.

DISCUSSION SOURCES

Detterbeck FC, Mazzone PJ, Naidich DP, Bach PB. Screening for lung cancer: Diagnosis and management of lung cancer, 3rd ed: American College of Chest Physicians evidence-based clinical practice guidelines. *Chest* 143(5 suppl):e78S–92S, 2013.

National Lung Screening Trial Research Team, Aberle DR, Adams AM, Berg CD, et al. Reduced lung-cancer mortality with low-dose computed tomographic screening. *N Engl J Med* 365(5): 395–409, 2011.

American Cancer Society. Cancer Facts and Figures. 2013. Available at www.cancer.org/acs/groups/content/@epidemiologysurveilance/documents/document/acspc-036845.pdf

Gastrointestinal Disorders

7

Anal Fissure

1. The most common anal fissure location is:
   A. posterior midline of the anus.
   B. anterior anal midline.
   C. anterior and posterior anal midline.
   D. transversely across the anal mucosa.

2. Rectal bleeding associated with anal fissure is usually described by the patient as:
   A. drops of blood noticed when wiping.
   B. dark brown to black in color and mixed in with normal-appearing stool.
   C. a large amount of brisk red bleeding.
   D. significant blood clots and mucus mixed with stool.

3. A 62-year-old woman who reports frequent constipation is diagnosed with an anal fissure. First-line therapy includes all of the following except:
   A. stool-bulking supplements.
   B. high fiber diet.
   C. intraanal corticosteroids.
   D. the periodic use of oral mineral oil.

4. A 54-year-old man with an anal fissure responds inadequately to dietary intervention and standard therapy during the past 2 weeks. Additional treatment options include all of the following except:
   A. intraanal nitroglycerine ointment.
   B. botulinum toxicum injection to the internal anal sphincter.
   C. surgical sphincterotomy.
   D. rubber band ligation of the lesion.

5. In a patient who presents with a history consistent with anal fissure but with notation of an atypical anal lesion, alternative diagnoses to consider include all of the following except:
   A. condyloma acuminata.
   B. Crohn's disease.
   C. anal squamous cell carcinoma.
   D. *C. difficile* colitis.

6. Which of the following is the most likely patient report with anal fissure?
   A. "I have anal pain that is relieved with having a bowel movement."
   B. "Even after having a bowel movement, I feel like I still need to 'go' more."
   C. "I have anal pain for up to 1–2 hours after I have a bowel movement."
   D. "I itch down there almost all the time."

7. Long term, recurrent high-dose oral use of mineral oil can lead to deficiency in:
   A. iron.
   B. vitamin A.
   C. vitamin C.
   D. vitamin B_{12}.

Answers

1. A.	4. D.	7. B.
2. A.	5. D.	
3. C.	6. C.	

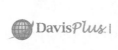 See full color images of this topic on DavisPlus at
http://davisplus.fadavis.com |
Keyword: Fitzgerald

In anal fissure, there is an ulcer or tear of the margin of the anus; most fissures occur posteriorly. The most common patient report is one of severe anal pain during a bowel movement, with the pain lasting several minutes to hours afterward. The pain recurs with every bowel movement, and the patient commonly becomes afraid or unwilling to have a bowel movement, leading to a cycle of worsening constipation, harder stools, and more anal pain. If rectal bleeding is noted with anal fissure, this is usually limited to drops of blood noted when wiping, not protracted bleeding.

Anal fissure risk factors include a history of recent or recurrent constipation (most potent risk factor), recurrent or recent severe diarrhea, recent childbirth, and anal intercourse or other anal insertion practices. The best treatment for anal fissure is avoidance of the trigger condition or activity that triggers or contributes to the condition.

Given that constipation is the most common anal fissure risk factor, the primary treatment goal is to prevent constipation and, therefore, break the cycle that contributes to the condition. First-line therapies include increased dietary fiber and fiber supplementation and stool softener. These interventions alone are often not sufficient to facilitate stool passing and a laxative needs to be added. Mineral oil helps lubricate the stool and renders defecation more comfortable and minimizes anal mucosal damage; long-term use is discouraged due to its potential to attenuate the absorption of the fat soluble vitamins A D, E, and K, and essential fatty acids when used consistently in large amounts. Local measures such as sitz baths and cool compresses can provide additional relief. With this approach, the majority of anal fissures will heal within a few weeks. Relapse is common and is usually noted when recommended therapy is abandoned and constipation recurs.

If symptoms persist with the above-mentioned therapies or are particularly severe, intraanal application of 0.4% nitroglycerin (NTG) can be applied directly to the internal sphincter. NTG is believed to relax the internal sphincter and increase blood flow to the anal mucosa. This can provide pain relief. Adverse effects are identical to what is reported with other NTG forms and include headache and dizziness; this significantly limits the use of the product. An additional option, available through specialty consultation, is the use of botulinum toxin (Botox) into the anal sphincter; spasm at this point is thought to be the cause of particularly painful anal fissure. Botulinum injections provide relief for approximately 3 months during which time the hope is that the fissure will heal. Surgical sphincterotomy is an option in the most recalcitrant of cases.

A number of other conditions can present similar to anal fissure. If the fissure is off the midline, transverse or irregular, another diagnosis should be considered. These include Crohn's disease, anal squamous cell cancer, and anal condyloma acuminata, among others.

DISCUSSION SOURCE

Poritz L., Geibel J. Anal Fissure. http://emedicine.medscape.com/article/196297

◖Hemorrhoids

8. Rectal bleeding associated with hemorrhoids is usually described as:
   A. streaks of bright red blood on the stool.
   B. dark brown to black in color and mixed in with normal-appearing stool.
   C. a large amount of brisk red bleeding.
   D. significant blood clots and mucus mixed with stool.

9. Therapy for hemorrhoids includes all of the following except:
   A. weight control.
   B. low-fat diet.
   C. topical corticosteroids.
   D. the use of a stool softener.

10. The NP is advising a 58-year-old woman about the benefits of a high-fiber diet. Which of the following foods provides the highest fiber content?
    A. a small banana
    B. 1 cup of cooked oatmeal
    C. a ½ cup serving of brown rice
    D. a medium-size blueberry muffin

11. A 62-year-old man presents with a 2-month history of noting a "bit of dark blood mixed in with my stool most days." Physical examination reveals external hemorrhoids, no rectal mass, and a small amount of dark brown stool on the examining digit. In-office fecal occult blood test is positive, and hemogram reveals a microcytic hypochromic anemia. The next best step in his care is to:
    A. perform in-office anoscopy.
    B. advise the patient use sitz baths post bowel movement.
    C. refer to gastroenterology practice for colonoscopy.
    D. order a double contrast barium enema.

12. Risk factors for the development of hemorrhoidal symptoms include all of the following except:
    A. prolonged sitting.
    B. insertive partner in anal intercourse.
    C. chronic diarrhea.
    D. excessive alcohol use.

13. Which of the following best describes Grade III internal hemorrhoids?
    A. The hemorrhoids do not prolapse.
    B. The hemorrhoids prolapse upon defecation but reduce spontaneously.
    C. The hemorrhoids prolapse upon defecation and must be reduced manually.
    D. The hemorrhoids are prolapsed and cannot be reduced manually.

14. Which of the following patients should be evaluated for possible surgical intervention for hemorrhoids?
    A. a 28-year-old woman with symptomatic external hemorrhoids who gave birth 6 days ago
    B. a 48-year-old man with Grade II internal hemorrhoids and improvement with standard medical therapy
    C. a 44-year-old woman who has internal and external hemorrhoids with recurrent prolapse
    D. a 58-year-old man who has Grade I internal hemorrhoids and improvement with psyllium supplements

Answers

8. A.	11. C.	14. C.
9. B.	12. B.	
10. B.	13. C.	

The superior hemorrhoidal veins form internal hemorrhoids, whereas the inferior hemorrhoidal veins form external hemorrhoids. Both forms are normal anatomical findings but cause discomfort when there is an increase in the venous pressure and resulting dilation and inflammation. Contrary to common thought, hemorrhoids do not represent varicosities. Internal hemorrhoids are graded on a scale of I–IV as follows: Grade I—the hemorrhoids do not prolapse; Grade II—the hemorrhoids prolapse upon defecation but reduce spontaneously; Grade III—the hemorrhoids prolapse upon defecation and must be reduced manually; and Grade IV—the hemorrhoids are prolapsed and cannot be reduced manually. External hemorrhoids are not graded.

In many cases, the cause for hemorrhoids is unknown. At the same time, a number of clinical conditions and activities increase the risk for development of hemorrhoids, including excessive alcohol use, chronic diarrhea or constipation, obesity, high fat/low fiber diet, prolonged sitting, sedentary lifestyle, receptive partner in anal intercourse, and loss of pelvic floor muscle tone. Over time, tissue and vessel redundancy develop, resulting in rectal protrusion and increased risk for bleeding. The rectal bleeding associated with hemorrhoids is usually minor and typically described as a red streak on the stool. Reports of persistent bleeding, dark blood mixed with stool, or development of anemia related to rectal bleeding warrants prompt referral for colonoscopy for evaluation for colorectal cancer or alternative diagnosis. With chronically protruding or prolapsing hemorrhoids, the patient often reports itch, mucous leaking, and staining of undergarments with streaks of stool. Manual reduction of the protruding hemorrhoid after evacuation can be helpful.

As with anal fissure, prevention of hemorrhoidal engorgement and inflammation is the best treatment. Strategies include weight control, high-fiber diet, fiber supplements, regular aerobic physical activity, and increased fluid intake. The average adult should strive for a minimum of 20 to 30 grams of fiber per day, preferably through eating high-fiber foods. Examples of fiber foods include dry beans, peas, oat products and most, but not all, whole fruits and vegetables. Treatment for acute hemorrhoid flare-ups includes the use of astringents and topical corticosteroids, sitz baths, and analgesics.

Surgical intervention is warranted when more conservative therapy fails to yield clinical improvement. Rubber band ligation is often the surgical intervention of choice for lower grade (I and II) internal hemorrhoids and a single Grade III or IV hemorrhoid; this procedure is done in office, usually in a surgical practice. Surgical hemorrhoidectomy is recommended with multiple hemorrhoid columns, especially Grade III and IV, as well as extensive external and internal hemorrhoids.

Thrombosed external hemorrhoids can cause sudden-onset excruciating anal pain; the patient with this condition often reports to the emergency room for care. On physical examination, a deep purple-blue, exquisitely tender anal lesion is visible. Surgical excision of the skin overlying the thrombosed hemorrhoid provides rapid symptomatic relief. If this intervention is not available or declined by the patient, conservative therapy with cool compresses, sitz baths, stool softener, and analgesics can be used. The thrombus will resolve in 1 to 2 weeks without surgical intervention.

DISCUSSION SOURCE

American Gastroenterological Association medical position statement: Diagnosis and treatment of hemorrhoids. www.gastrojournal.org/article/S0016-5085(04)00354-3/abstract

Acute Appendicitis

15. All of the following are typically noted in a young adult with the diagnosis of acute appendicitis except:
A. epigastric pain.
B. positive obturator sign.
C. rebound tenderness.
D. marked febrile response.

16. A 26-year-old man presents with acute abdominal pain. As part of the evaluation for acute appendicitis, you order a white blood cell (WBC) count with differential and anticipate the following results:
A. total WBCs, 4500 mm³; neutrophils, 35%; bands, 2%; lymphocytes, 45%.
B. total WBCs, 14,000 mm³; neutrophils, 55%; bands, 3%; lymphocytes, 38%.
C. total WBCs, 16,500 mm³; neutrophils, 66%; bands, 8%; lymphocytes, 22%.
D. total WBCs, 18,100 mm³; neutrophils, 55%; bands, 3%; lymphocytes, 28%.

17. You see a 72-year-old woman who reports vomiting and abdominal cramping occurring over the past 24 hours. In evaluating a patient with suspected appendicitis, the clinician considers that:
A. the presentation can differ according to the anatomical location of the appendix.
B. this is a common reason for acute abdominal pain in elderly patients.
C. vomiting before onset of abdominal pain is often seen.
D. the presentation is markedly different from the presentation of pelvic inflammatory disease.

18. The psoas sign can be best described as abdominal pain elicited by:
A. passive extension of the hip.
B. passive flexion and internal rotation of the hip.
C. deep palpation.
D. asking the patient to cough.

19. The obturator sign can be best described as abdominal pain elicited by:
   A. passive extension of the hip.
   B. passive flexion and internal rotation of the hip.
   C. deep palpation.
   D. asking the patient to cough.

20. An 18-year-old man presents with periumbilical pain, vomiting, and abdominal cramping over the past 48 hours. Physical examination reveals rebound tenderness, and laboratory analysis shows the presence of bandemia and a total WBC of 28,000 mm³. To support the diagnosis of acute appendicitis with suspected appendiceal rupture, you consider obtaining the following abdominal imaging study:
   A. magnetic resonance image (MRI).
   B. computed tomography (CT) scan.
   C. ultrasound.
   D. flat plate.

21. Which of the following WBC forms is an ominous finding in the presence of severe bacterial infection?
   A. neutrophil
   B. lymphocyte
   C. basophil
   D. metamyelocyte

22. Which of the following best represents the peak ages for occurrence of acute appendicitis?
   A. 1 to 20 years
   B. 20 to 40 years
   C. 10 to 30 years
   D. 30 to 50 years

23. Clinical findings most consistent with appendiceal rupture include all of the following except:
   A. abdominal discomfort less than 48 hours in duration.
   B. fever greater than 102°F (>38°C).
   C. palpable abdominal mass.
   D. marked leukocytosis with total WBC greater than 20,000/mm³.

24. Which of the following imaging studies potentially exposes the patient being evaluated for abdominal pain to the lowest ionizing radiation burden?
   A. ultrasound
   B. barium enema
   C. CT scan
   D. abdominal flat plate

25. Commonly encountered diagnoses other than acute appendicitis can include which of the following in a 28-year-old with a 2-day history of lower abdominal pain and with right-sided pain slightly worse than left? (More than one can apply.)
   A. constipation
   B. pelvic inflammatory disease
   C. ectopic pregnancy
   D. splenetic infarct

26. Rebound tenderness is best described as abdominal pain that worsens with:
   A. light palpation at the site of the discomfort.
   B. release of deep palpation at the site of the discomfort.
   C. palpation on the contralateral side of the abdomen.
   D. deep palpation at the site of the discomfort.

27. Abdominal palpation that yields rebound tenderness is also known as a positive _____ sign.
   A. Markel's
   B. Murphy's
   C. Blumberg's
   D. Nikolsky's

28. Which of the following findings would you expect to encounter in a 33-year-old man with appendiceal abscess?
   A. leukopenia with lymphocytosis
   B. positive Cullen's sign
   C. protracted nausea and vomiting
   D. dullness to percussion in the abdominal right lower quadrant

▶ Answers

15. D.	20. B.	25. A, B, C
16. C.	21. D.	26. B.
17. A.	22. C.	27. C.
18. A.	23. A.	28. D.
19. B.	24. A.	

Acute appendicitis is an inflammatory disease of the vermiform appendix caused by infection or obstruction. The peak age of patients with acute appendicitis is 10 to 30 years; this condition is uncommon in infants and elderly adults. At either end of the life span, a delay in diagnosis of appendicitis commonly occurs because providers do not consider appendicitis a possibility.

There is no true classic presentation of acute appendicitis. Vague epigastric or periumbilical pain often heralds its beginning, with the discomfort shifting to the right lower quadrant over the next 12 hours. Pain is often aggravated by walking or coughing. Nausea and vomiting are late symptoms that invariably occur a number of hours after the onset of pain; this late onset helps to differentiate appendicitis from gastroenteritis, in which vomiting usually precedes abdominal cramping. The presentation of appendicitis also differs significantly according to the anatomical position of the appendix, with pain being reported in the epigastrium, flank, or groin. The obturator and psoas signs indicate inflammation of the respective muscles and strongly suggest peritoneal irritation and the diagnosis of appendicitis; these signs are also known as obturator muscle and iliopsoas muscle signs. Rebound tenderness, which is abdominal pain that worsens with release of deep palpation, indicates the likelihood of peritoneal irritation and helps with the diagnosis of acute appendicitis. The presence of rebound tenderness is also known as a positive Blumberg's sign.

A total WBC count and differential are obtained as part of the evaluation of patients with suspected appendicitis. The most typical WBC count pattern found in this situation is the "left shift." A "left shift", a colloquial term, is usually seen in the presence of severe bacterial infection, such as acute appendicitis, bacterial pneumonia, and pyelonephritis. The following are typically noted in the "left shift":

- Leukocytosis: An elevation in the total WBC.
- Neutrophilia: An elevation in the number of neutrophils in circulation. Neutrophilia is defined as an absolute neutrophil count (ANC) of greater than 7000 neutrophils/mm³. The ANC is calculated by multiplying the percentage of neutrophils by the total WBC in mm³. A total WBC (TWBC) of 12,000 mm³ x 70% neutrophils yields an ANC of 8300 neutrophils/mm³. Neutrophils are also known as "polys" or "segs," both referring to the polymorph shape of the segment nucleus of this WBC.
- Bandemia: An elevation in the number of bands or young neutrophils in circulation. Usually less than 4% of the total WBCs in circulation are bands. When this percentage is exceeded, and the absolute band count (ABC) is greater than 500 mm³, bandemia is present. A TWBC of 12,000 mm³ with 8% bands yields an ABC of 860/mm³. The presence of bandemia indicates that the body has called up as many mature neutrophils as were available in the storage pool and is now accessing less mature forms. The presence of bandemia further reinforces the seriousness of the infection. An increase in circulating bands also occurs in pneumonia, meningitis, septicemia, pyelonephritis, and tonsillitis when caused by bacterial infection.

Although additional neutrophil forms exist, these do not belong in circulation even with severe infection. Myelocytes and metamyelocytes are immature neutrophil forms that are typically found in only the granulopoiesis pool. The presence of these cells is an ominous marker of life-threatening infection, and these are occasionally found in the presence of appendiceal rupture.

Given that appendicitis is an inflammatory disease, adding a test to detect inflammation, such as the C-reactive protein (CRP), is also an option. An elevated CRP provides a degree of support for the diagnosis whereas a normal value helps to rule out the condition. For women of childbearing age, pregnancy should be ruled out via urinary beta-human chorionic gonadotropin (beta-hCG); the presentations of acute appendicitis and early ectopic pregnancy have many features in common.

Abdominal computerized tomography (CT) of the abdomen is generally considered the imaging of choice in suspected appendicitis; its ability to define better the anatomical abnormality associated with appendicitis is superior to other imaging options. Abdominal CT is the preferred diagnostic procedure when there is a suspicion of appendiceal perforation because this study reveals periappendiceal abscess formation or when an atypical presentation raises the issue of another possible diagnosis. Because of concerns about patient exposure to radiation during a CT scan, abdominal or pelvic ultrasonography (US) can be considered as a safer primary diagnostic modality for appendicitis. With abnormality noted on ultrasound, including inability to clearly visualize the appendix, CT is then used to further help with the diagnostic process. In particular, this is an appealing option to minimize radiation exposure in children and women of reproductive age. MRI has limited use in the evaluation of suspected appendicitis. Due to its lack of ionizing radiation, this is an option when evaluating a pregnant woman with suspected appendicitis; unfortunately, the normative changes noted during pregnancy render abdominal ultrasound of limited use for evaluation of a pregnant woman with abdominal pain.

Given the variety of imaging modalities available and the frequency of their use, the ionizing radiation burden of a study should be considered prior to ordering. (See Table 7–9, Radiation Doses from Common Imaging Studies). The long time risk of excessive ionizing radiation is presumed to include carcinogenesis; children and women of reproductive age are considered to be particularly vulnerable.

Appendiceal perforation, commonly referred to as a ruptured or burst appendix, is usually associated with a marked leukocytosis with total WBC count often exceeding 20,000 mm³ to 30,000 mm³, fever greater than 102°F (greater than 38°C), peritoneal inflammation findings, and symptoms lasting longer than 48 hours. An ill-defined right lower quadrant abdominal mass, usually dull to percussion with or without a degree of rebound tenderness, in a person with a presentation consistent with appendiceal perforation is suggestive of abscess formation. Surgical removal of an inflamed appendix via laparoscopy or laparotomy is indicated. If there is evidence of rupture with localized abscess and peritonitis, CT-directed abscess aspiration may be indicated first, with an appendectomy performed after appropriate antimicrobial therapy.

DISCUSSION SOURCES

Craig S, Brenner B. Appendicitis. http://emedicine.medscape.com/article/773895,

Ferri F. Appendicitis. In: *Ferri's Best Test: A Practical Guide to Clinical Laboratory Medicine and Diagnostic Imaging,* 2nd ed. Philadelphia, PA: Elsevier Mosby, 2009, p. 190.

Gallstones

29. A 43-year-old woman has a 12-hour history of sudden onset of right upper quadrant abdominal pain with radiation to the shoulder, fever, and chills. She has had similar, milder episodes in the past. Examination reveals marked tenderness to right upper quadrant abdominal palpation. Her most likely diagnosis is:
    A. hepatoma.
    B. acute cholecystitis.
    C. acute hepatitis.
    D. cholelithiasis.

30. Which of the following is usually not seen in the diagnosis of acute cholecystitis?
A. elevated serum creatinine
B. increased alkaline phosphatase level
C. leukocytosis
D. elevated aspartate aminotransferase (AST) level

31. Murphy's sign can be best described as abdominal pain elicited by:
A. right upper quadrant abdominal palpation.
B. asking the patient to stand on tiptoes and then letting body weight fall quickly onto the heels.
C. asking the patient to cough.
D. percussion.

32. Which of the following is the most common serious complication of cholecystitis?
A. adenocarcinoma of the gallbladder
B. gallbladder empyema
C. hepatic failure
D. pancreatitis

33. A 58-year-old man reports intermittent right upper quadrant abdominal pain. He is obese and being actively treated for hyperlipidemia. Imaging in a patient with suspected symptomatic cholelithiasis usually includes obtaining an abdominal:
A. magnetic resonance image (MRI).
B. CT scan.
C. ultrasound of the right upper quadrant.
D. flat plate.

34. Which of the following is most likely to be found in a person with acute cholecystitis?
A. fever
B. vomiting
C. jaundice
D. palpable gallbladder

35. Risk factors for the development of cholelithiasis include all of the following except:
A. rapid weight loss.
B. male gender.
C. obesity.
D. Native American ancestry.

36. A gallstone that is not visualized on standard x-ray is said to be:
A. radiopaque.
B. radiolucent.
C. calcified.
D. unclassified.

◗ Answers

29. B.	**32.** D.	**35.** B.
30. A.	**33.** C.	**36.** B.
31. A.	**34.** B.	

Gallstone formation occurs when substances in bile are present in high concentration; the bile becomes supersaturated and the substance precipitates out into a microscopic crystal. The crystals are trapped in the gallbladder mucosa, with resulting formation of sludge. Over time, more substance precipitates out and the crystals grow, forming macroscopic stones. Duct occlusion by stones or sludge causes the majority of the symptoms and clinical problems with gallstone disease. The most common form of stones is cholesterol or cholesterol-dominant (80% to 85%).

Major risk factors for gallstone formation include age older than 50 years, female gender, obesity, hyperlipidemia, rapid weight loss (including patients who have undergone bariatric surgery), pregnancy, genetic factors, European or Native American ancestry, and ingestion of a diet with a high glycemic index.

Cholelithiasis is defined as a condition in which there is the formation of calculi or gallstones, but without the presence of gallbladder or associated structure. About 75% of all patients with cholelithiasis have no symptoms and become aware of the condition only when it is found during evaluation for another health problem. About 10% to 25% of individuals initially without symptoms become symptomatic over the next decade. In the absence of symptoms, prophylactic cholecystectomy is not usually indicated.

Many patients with gallstones have intermittent discomfort as a result of this condition. The pain is described as being of sudden onset, usually post prandial, particularly within 1 hour of a fatty meal, in the abdominal right upper quadrant or epigastrium, occasionally radiating to the tip of the right scapula; the presence of radiating pain is known as Collins' sign. Episodes of discomfort typically last 1 to 5 hours, with a pattern of increasing then decreasing discomfort as the gallbladder contracts and the stone position shifts. Nausea and vomiting are common during painful episodes. Indeed, vomiting often provides significant pain relief. Biliary colic is a term used to describe these acutely painful paroxysms.

Acute cholecystitis results from an acute inflammation of the gallbladder, nearly always caused by gallstones. Right upper quadrant or epigastric pain and tenderness are present along with vomiting (70% or more) and occasional fever (33%); vomiting often affords temporary symptom relief. Tenderness on palpating the right upper quadrant of the abdomen significant enough to cause inspiratory arrest (Murphy's sign) is nearly always present. A palpable gallbladder is rarely noted. Approximately 25% to 50% of those affected have some degree of jaundice. Leukocytosis is usually present, with a typical total WBC count of 12,000 mm^3 to 20,000 mm^3, and elevated levels of the hepatic enzymes (Table 7–1).

Combined with the health history, physical examination findings, and laboratory testing, imaging results help to support the diagnosis of cholecystitis. Right upper quadrant abdominal ultrasound usually reveals stones and is considered the diagnostic test of choice; given the lack of

TABLE 7-1
Hepatic Enzyme Elevations and Their Significance

Enzyme Elevation	Comment, Associated Conditions	Example
Alanine aminotransferase (ALT, formerly known as SGPT)	Measure of hepatic cellular enzymes found in circulation, elevated when hepatocellular damage is present. Highly liver specific. This enzyme has circulatory half-life of 37–57 hr; levels increase relatively slowly in response to hepatic damage and clear gradually after damage ceases. See AST for contrast in this rise and fall pattern In hepatitis A, B, C, D, or E, or drug-associated or industrial chemical–associated hepatitis, ALT usually increases higher than AST, with enzyme increases ≥10 times ULN In nonalcoholic fatty liver steatohepatitis (NASH, also known as nonalcoholic fatty liver disease [NAFLD]), ALT usually increases higher than AST, with enzyme increases usually within 3 times ULN	A 22 y.o. woman with acute hepatitis A AST 678 U/L (normal 0–31 U/L) ALT 828 U/L (normal 0–31 U/L) ALT:AST ratio ≥1 A 66 y.o. woman with obesity, type 2 diabetes mellitus, and nonalcoholic fatty liver disease AST 44 U/L ALT 78 U/L ALT:AST ratio >1
Aspartate aminotransferase (AST, formerly known as SGOT)	Measure of hepatic cellular enzymes found in circulation, elevated when hepatocellular damage is present. Enzyme also present in lesser amounts in skeletal muscle and myocardium AST has circulatory half-life of ~12–24 hr; levels increase in response to hepatic damage and clear quickly after damage ceases In alcohol-related hepatic injury AST usually increases higher than ALT In acetaminophen overdose, massive increases in AST and ALT are often noted, ≥20 times ULN	A 38 y.o. man with a 10-yr history of increasingly heavy alcohol use AST 83 U/L (normal 0–31 U/L) ALT 50 U/L (normal 0–31 U/L) AST:ALT ratio ≥1 A 26 y.o. man with intentional acetaminophen overdose AST 15,083 U/L (normal 0–31 U/L) ALT 10,347 U/L (normal 0–31 U/L)
Alkaline phosphatase (ALP)	Enzyme found in rapidly dividing or metabolically active tissue, such as liver, bone, intestine, placenta. Elevated levels can reflect damage or accelerated cellular division in any of these areas. Most in circulation is of hepatic origin. Levels increase in response to biliary obstruction and are a sensitive indicator of intrahepatic or extrahepatic cholestasis	A 40 y.o. woman with acute cholecystitis AST 45 U/L (0–31) ALT 55 U/L (0–31) ALP 225 U/L (0–125)
Gamma glutamyl transferase (GGT)	Enzyme involved in the transfer of amino acids across cell membranes. Found primarily in the liver and kidney In liver disease, usually parallels changes in alkaline phosphatase Marked elevation often noted in obstructive jaundice, hepatic metastasis, intrahepatic cholestasis	A 40 y.o. woman with acute cholecystitis AST 45 U/L (0–31) ALT 55 U/L (0–31) ALP 225 U/L (0–125) GGT 245 U/L (0–45)

ULN, upper limits of normal.
Source: Ferri F. *Ferri's Best Test: A Practical Guide to Clinical Laboratory Medicine and Diagnostic Imaging,* 2nd ed. Philadelphia, PA: Elsevier Mosby, 2009.

ionizing radiation with ultrasound, this is also a test that can be used during pregnancy. Abdominal CT is less helpful in the diagnosis when compared to US but can assist in ruling out other GI pathology. A hepatoiminodiacetic acid (HIDA) scan is more sensitive and specific at revealing an obstructed cystic duct. Most gallstones are radiolucent—that is, unable to be visualized on standard x-ray. As a result, an abdominal flat plate is of limited value. Abdominal MRI seldom plays a role in diagnosing gallstone disease. A variety of percutaneous and endoscopic diagnostic procedures are utilized in complicated or uncertain scenarios.

Acute cholecystitis symptoms usually subside with conservative therapy, such as a low-fat diet of clear liquids and analgesics. Antimicrobial therapy is occasionally indicated with evidence of infection. Cholecystectomy, usually performed via laparoscope, should be considered because of the likelihood of recurrence.

Complications of gallstone disease include pancreatitis and sepsis; both are most common in elders who develop the condition. In a person who is seriously ill with other health problems and considered too high a risk to undergo cholecystectomy, ultrasound-guided gallbladder aspiration or percutaneous cholecystectomy can delay or occasionally eliminate the need for further surgical intervention. Stone-dissolving medications, such as ursodeoxycholic acid, are available but can take 2 years to dissolve stones. Approximately 50% of patients treated with stone-dissolving medications have a return of stones within 5 years; consequently, the use of this therapy has largely fallen out of favor.

DISCUSSION SOURCE

Bloom A, Katz, J. Cholecystitis. http://emedicine.medscape.com/article/175667

Colorectal Cancer

37. Which of the following is true concerning colorectal cancer?
    A. Most colorectal cancers are found during rectal examination.
    B. Rectal carcinoma is more common than cancers involving the colon.
    C. Early manifestations include abdominal pain and cramping.
    D. Later disease presentation often includes iron-deficiency anemia.

38. According to the American Cancer Society recommendations, which of the following is the preferred method for annual colorectal cancer screening in a 51-year-old man?
    A. digital rectal examination
    B. fecal occult blood test
    C. colonoscopy
    D. barium enema study

39. Which of the following is most likely to be noted in a person with colorectal cancer?
    A. gross rectal bleeding
    B. weight loss
    C. few symptoms
    D. nausea and vomiting

40. Which of the following does not increase a patient's risk of developing colorectal cancer?
    A. family history of colorectal cancer
    B. familial polyposis
    C. personal history of neoplasm
    D. long-term aspirin therapy

41. According to current American Cancer Society data, colorectal cancer is the number _____ cause of cancer death in men and women.
    A. 1
    B. 3
    C. 5
    D. 7

Answers

37. D.	39. C.	41. B.
38. B.	40. D.	

Colorectal cancer is the third leading cause of cancer death in both genders in the United States, with approximately 5% of the population developing the disease. Only lung cancer (both genders), prostate cancer (men), and breast cancer (women) exceed this disease in cancer-related mortality. Most colorectal malignancies prove to be adenocarcinomas, with about 70% found in the colon and 30% found in the rectum. Risk factors include a history of inflammatory bowel disease (ulcerative colitis [UC] and Crohn's disease), personal history of neoplasia, age older than 50 years, a family history of colorectal cancer, and familial polyposis syndrome. In addition, an autosomal dominant condition known as hereditary nonpolyposis colorectal cancer (HNPCC) has been identified. Although this condition accounts for only about 3% of all colorectal cancers, persons with this risk factor tend to develop disease earlier and have a 70% likelihood of colon cancer by age 65 years. A thorough family history is important in assessing an individual's risk of colorectal cancer. A diet high in fat, high in red meat, and low in calcium has also been implicated as a contributing factor. The use of antioxidants, calcium supplements, and low-dose aspirin has been shown in limited study to reduce colorectal cancer rates.

A person presenting with colorectal cancer is usually asymptomatic until disease is quite advanced. At that time, vague abdominal complaints coupled with iron-deficiency anemia (as a result of chronic low-volume blood loss) is often noted. The mass is most often beyond the examining digit. As a result, digital rectal examination is an ineffective method of colorectal cancer screening. In addition, the American Cancer Society colorectal cancer screening guidelines do not recommend the use of the fecal occult blood test (FOBT) obtained via the digital rectal examination in the provider's office, which is not an adequate substitute for the recommended at-home procedure of collecting two samples from three consecutive specimens. Toilet-bowl FOBT tests also are not recommended. Compared with guaiac-based tests for the detection of occult blood, immunochemical tests are more patient-friendly and are likely to be equal or better in sensitivity and specificity. There is no justification for repeating FOBT in response to an initial positive finding. Colonoscopy should be done if test results are positive.

The most commonly recommended colorectal cancer screening method in adults is a colonoscopy at 10-year intervals, starting at age 50 years. Alterative testing methods and schedules include flexible sigmoidoscopy, double-contrast barium enema, and CT colonography (virtual colonoscopy) every 5 years starting at age 50 years.

Alternative screening schedules, usually including more frequent testing or earlier testing or both, are considered when colorectal cancer risk factors are increased. These risk factors include a personal history of colorectal cancer or adenomatous polyps, Crohn's disease or UC, a strong family history (first-degree relative [parent, sibling, or child] younger than 60 years or two or more first-degree relatives of any age) of colorectal cancer or polyps, or a known family history of hereditary colorectal cancer syndromes such as familial adenomatous polyposis or HNPCC. These alternative schedules should be pursued in conjunction with expert consultation.

Treatment of colorectal cancer usually includes surgery combined with chemotherapy and radiation. Long-term survival depends on many factors, including the size and depth of the tumor, the presence of positive nodes, and the overall health of the patient.

DISCUSSION SOURCES

Albo D. Tumors of the colon and rectum. In: Rakel R, Bope E, (eds). *Conn's Current Therapy*. Philadelphia, PA: Saunders Elsevier; 2013, pp. 558–563.

Rex D, Johnson D, Anderson J, Schoenfield P, Burke C, Inadomi J. American College of Gastroenterology Guidelines for Colorectal Cancer Screening. *Am J Gastroenterol* 104:739–750, 2009. http://gi.org/guideline/colorectal-cancer-screening/

Colonic Diverticulosis

42. Colonic diverticulosis most commonly occurs in the walls of the:
A. ascending colon.
B. descending colon.
C. transverse colon.
D. sigmoid colon.

43. Approximately what percent of the population will develop diverticulosis by the time they reach 50 years of age?
A. 10%
B. 20%
C. 33%
D. 50%

44. Which of the following is most consistent with the presentation of a patient with colonic diverticulosis?
A. diarrhea and leukocytosis
B. constipation and fever
C. few or no symptoms
D. frank blood in the stool with reduced stool caliber

45. Which of the following is most consistent with the presentation of a patient with acute colonic diverticulitis?
A. cramping, diarrhea, and leukocytosis
B. constipation and fever
C. right-sided abdominal pain
D. frank blood in the stool with reduced stool caliber

46. Major risk factors for diverticulosis include all of the following except:
A. low-fiber diet.
B. family history of the condition.
C. older age.
D. select connective tissue disorders (e.g., Marfan syndrome).

47. To avoid the development of acute diverticulitis, treatment of diverticulosis can include:
A. avoiding foods with seeds.
B. the use of fiber supplements.
C. ceasing cigarette smoking.
D. limiting alcohol intake.

48. The location of discomfort with acute diverticulitis is usually in which of the following areas of the abdomen?
A. epigastrium
B. left lower quadrant
C. right lower quadrant
D. suprapubic

49. Which of the following best describes colonic diverticulosis?
A. bulging pockets in the intestinal wall
B. poorly contracting intestinal walls
C. strictures of the intestinal lumen
D. flaccidity of the small intestine

50. You are seeing Mr. Lopez, a 68-year-old man with suspected acute colonic diverticulitis. In choosing an appropriate imaging study to support this diagnosis, which of the following abdominal imaging studies is most appropriate?
A. flat plate
B. ultrasound
C. CT scan with contrast
D. barium enema

51. In the evaluation of acute diverticulitis, the most appropriate diagnostic approach to rule out free air in the abdomen includes:
    A. barium enema.
    B. plain abdominal film.
    C. abdominal ultrasound.
    D. lower endoscopy.

52. A 56-year-old woman is diagnosed with mild diverticulitis. In addition to counseling her about increased fluid intake and adequate rest, you recommend antimicrobial treatment with:
    A. amoxicillin with clarithromycin.
    B. linezolid with daptomycin.
    C. ciprofloxacin with metronidazole.
    D. nitrofurantoin with doxycycline.

53. Lower gastrointestinal (GI) hemorrhage associated with diverticular disease usually manifests as:
    A. a painless event.
    B. a condition noted to be found with a marked febrile response.
    C. a condition accompanied by severe cramp-like abdominal pain.
    D. a common chronic condition.

54. Measures to prevent colonic diverticulosis and diverticulitis include all of the following except:
    A. increased whole grain intake.
    B. regular aerobic exercise.
    C. adequate hydration.
    D. refraining from excessive alcohol intake.

Answers

42. D.	47. B.	52. C.
43. C.	48. B.	53. A.
44. C.	49. A.	54. D.
45. A.	50. C.	
46. A.	51. B.	

In colonic diverticulosis, bulging pockets are present in the intestinal wall, most commonly in the wall of the sigmoid colon, though the abnormality can occur in any part of the large intestine. In the United States, approximately one-third of the population will develop diverticulosis by age 50 years and approximately two-thirds by age 80 years. Inflammation is not present, however, and the patient is usually asymptomatic; diverticulosis is often found during studies done for other reasons, such as colorectal cancer screening. Historically, a major risk factor for the condition was thought to be long-term low-fiber diet, since the condition is more common in developed countries in which a diet focused on high levels of processed foods is the normal. However, more recent studies fail to support this as a cause. Major risk factors are considered to be aging, family history of the disease, and select connective tissue disorders, including Marfan syndrome.

When symptoms are present in diverticulosis, left-sided abdominal cramping, increased flatus, and a pattern of constipation alternating with diarrhea are often reported. Intervention includes a high-fiber diet, along with the use of fiber supplements such as bran, psyllium, and methylcellulose. The goal of treatment is to minimize the risk of complications such as diverticulitis. Although avoidance of seeds and other similar food products has been recommended in the past as a way to avoid acute diverticulitis, few studies exist to support this dietary change.

In acute colonic diverticulitis, the diverticula are inflamed, causing fever, leukocytosis, diarrhea, and left lower quadrant abdominal pain. Intestinal perforation is the likely origin of the condition, with the perforation ranging from pinpoint lesions that cause local infection and respond to conservative management to major tears, which necessitate surgical repair and are often complicated by intra-abdominal abscess or peritonitis. Imaging is often obtained to support the diagnosis and assess disease severity or complications. An abdominal CT scan with contrast is helpful in identifying findings consistent with the condition inducing bowel wall thickening; complications including abscess and fistulas can also be identified with this diagnostic modality. A plain abdominal film is often normal in milder disease but can be helpful in identifying free air, indicated diverticular perforation, or altered bowel air patterns consistent with obstruction. Because of the potential risk of complication, a barium enema should not be obtained during an acute episode of diverticular disease. Abdominal ultrasound is not helpful in this condition. Endoscopic evaluation of the colon is contraindicated in acute diverticulitis, as insufflation of air can result in or exacerbate free perforation and peritonitis.

Occasionally, diverticular hemorrhage, caused by an erosion of a vessel by a fecalith held in a diverticular sac, can occur. The condition usually manifests with painless lower GI bleeding. The management is usually directed by the clinical presentation and usually includes fluid and blood replacement; surgical intervention is often required.

In mild cases of diverticulitis, conservative management is adequate, including a liquid diet to ensure gut rest, with an emphasis on an adequate hydration, for the duration of the illness and antimicrobial therapy. Because of its strong activity against anaerobic organisms implicated in the conditions, metronidazole is an antibiotic of choice. Since the infection is often polymicrobial, a second agent should be added that exhibits activity against the gram-negative organisms that are implicated, such as E. coli. These antimicrobials include ciprofloxacin, levofloxacin, moxifloxacin, tigecycline, or trimethoprim-sulfamethoxazole (TMP-SMX) (Table 7–2). If the patient fails to respond within 2 to 3 days or becomes significantly worse during that time, particularly if peritoneal signs develop, an abdominal CT scan and specialty surgical consultation should be obtained. With recurrent diverticulitis episodes, particularly with a complicated course, surgical intervention with partial colectomy is an option.

Measures to prevent colonic diverticulosis and diverticulitis include regular aerobic exercise, adequate hydration,

TABLE 7-2

Antimicrobial Treatment Options in Acute Diverticulitis

Causative Organisms	Primary Oral Treatment Regimen When Suitable for Outpatient Therapy	Alternative Oral Treatment Regimen When Suitable for Outpatient Therapy
Enterobacteriaceae, *P. aeruginosa, Bacteroides* spp., enterococci	TMP-SMX-DS bid or ciprofloxacin 750 mg bid or levofloxacin 750 mg qd plus metronidazole 500 mg q 6 hr, all for 7–10 days	Amoxicillin-clavulanate ER 1000/62.5 mg 2 tabs bid for 7–10 days *or* Moxifloxacin 400 mg q 24 hr for 7–10 days

TMP-SMX, trimethoprim-sulfamethoxazole.
Source: Gilbert D, Moellering R, Eliopoulos G, Chambers HF, Saag MS. *The Sanford Guide to Antimicrobial Therapy*. 44th ed. Sperryville, VA: Antimicrobial Therapy, Inc., 2014.

and a high-fiber diet. All of these measures help increase bowel motility and tone.

DISCUSSION SOURCES

Ferri F. Diverticular disease. In: *Ferri's Fast Facts*. Philadelphia, PA: Elsevier Mosby; 2005, p. 1156.
Wilkins T, Embry K, George R. Diagnosis and management of acute diverticulitis. *Am Fam Physician* 87:612–620, 2013.
Gilbert D, Moellering R, Eliopoulos G, Chambers HF, Saag MS. *The Sanford Guide to Antimicrobial Therapy*, 44th ed. Sperryville, VA: Antimicrobial Therapy, Inc., 2014.

Peptic Ulcer Disease

55. The gastric parietal cells produce:
    A. hydrochloric acid.
    B. a protective mucosal layer.
    C. prostaglandins.
    D. prokinetic hormones.

56. Antiprostaglandin drugs cause stomach mucosal injury primarily by:
    A. a direct irritative effect.
    B. altering the thickness of the protective mucosal layer.
    C. decreasing peristalsis.
    D. modifying stomach pH level.

57. A 24-year-old man presents with a 3-month history of upper abdominal pain. He describes it as an intermittent, centrally located "burning" feeling in his upper abdomen, most often occurring 2 to 3 hours after meals. His presentation is most consistent with the clinical presentation of:
    A. acute gastritis.
    B. gastric ulcer.
    C. duodenal ulcer.
    D. cholecystitis.

58. When choosing pharmacological intervention to prevent recurrence of duodenal ulcer in a middle-aged man, you prescribe:
    A. a proton pump inhibitor (PPI).
    B. timed antacid use.
    C. antimicrobial therapy.
    D. a histamine$_2$-receptor antagonist (H$_2$RA).

59. The H$_2$RA most likely to cause drug interactions with phenytoin and theophylline is:
    A. cimetidine.
    B. famotidine.
    C. nizatidine.
    D. ranitidine.

60. Which of the following is least likely to be found in a patient with gastric ulcer?
    A. history of long-term naproxen use
    B. age younger than 50 years
    C. previous use of H$_2$RA or antacids
    D. cigarette smoking

61. Nonsteroidal antiinflammatory drug (NSAID)-induced peptic ulcer can be best limited by the use of:
    A. timed antacid doses.
    B. an H$_2$RA.
    C. an appropriate antimicrobial.
    D. misoprostol.

62. Cyclooxygenase-1 (COX-1) contributes to:
    A. the inflammatory response.
    B. pain transmission.
    C. maintenance of gastric protective mucosal layer.
    D. renal arteriole constriction.

63. Cyclooxygenase-2 (COX-2) contributes to:
    A. the inflammatory response.
    B. pain transmission inhibition.
    C. maintenance of gastric protective mucosal layer.
    D. renal arteriole dilation.

64. You see a 48-year-old woman who has been taking a cyclooxygenase-2 (COX-2) inhibitor for the past 3 years. In counseling her, you mention that long-term use of COX-2 inhibitors is associated with all of the following except:
    A. hepatic dysfunction.
    B. gastropathy.
    C. cardiovascular events.
    D. cerebrovascular events.

65. A 64-year-old woman presents with a 3-month history of upper abdominal pain. She describes the discomfort as an intermittent, centrally located "burning" feeling in the upper abdomen, most often with meals and often accompanied by mild nausea. Use of an over-the-counter H₂RA affords partial symptom relief. She also uses diclofenac on a regular basis for the control of osteoarthritis pain. Her clinical presentation is most consistent with:
    A. acute gastroenteritis.
    B. gastric ulcer.
    C. duodenal ulcer.
    D. chronic cholecystitis.

66. Which of the following statements about *Helicobacter. pylori* is false?
    A. *H. pylori* is a gram-negative, spiral-shaped bacterium.
    B. Infection with *H. pylori* is the most potent risk factor for duodenal ulcer.
    C. The organism is often resistant due to the production of beta-lactamase.
    D. *H. pylori* is transmitted via the oral-fecal or oral-oral route.

67. The most sensitive and specific test for *H. pylori* infection from the following list is:
    A. stool Gram stain, looking for the offending organism.
    B. serological testing for antigen related to the infection.
    C. organism-specific stool antigen testing.
    D. fecal DNA testing.

68. Which of the following medications is a PPI?
    A. loperamide
    B. metoclopramide
    C. nizatidine
    D. lansoprazole

69. Peptic ulcer disease can occur in any of the following locations except:
    A. duodenum.
    B. stomach.
    C. esophagus.
    D. large intestine.

70. An ulcer that is noted to be located in the region below the lower esophageal sphincter and before the pylorus is usually referred to as a(n) _____ ulcer.
    A. duodenal
    B. esophageal
    C. gastric
    D. stomach

71. A 56-year-old man with a 60 pack-year cigarette smoking history, recent 5-lb unintended weight loss, and a 3-month history of new-onset symptoms of peptic disease presents for care. He is taking no medications on a regular basis and reports drinking approximately six 12-oz beers per week with no more than 3 beers per day. Physical examination is unremarkable except for mild pharyngeal erythema and moderate epigastric tenderness without rebound. The most helpful diagnostic test at this point in his evaluation is a:
    A. upper endoscopy.
    B. barium swallow.
    C. evaluation of *H. pylori* status.
    D. esophageal pH monitoring.

72. Which of the following medications is a prostaglandin analog?
    A. sucralfate
    B. misoprostol
    C. esomeprazole
    D. metoclopramide

73. Long-term PPI use is associated with all of the following except:
    A. increased risk of pneumonia in hospitalized patients.
    B. increased risk of *C. difficile* colitis in hospitalized patients.
    C. reduced absorption of calcium and magnesium.
    D. reduced absorption of dietary carbohydrates.

74. To avoid rebound gastric hyperacidity following discontinuation of long-term PPI use, all of the following methods can be used except:
    A. gradually tapering the PPI dose with supplemental antacid.
    B. switch to every-other-day dosing of PPI with supplemental antacid.
    C. switch to a low-dose H₂RA therapy with supplemental antacid.
    D. empiric *H. pylori* therapy.

Answers

55. A.	62. C.	69. D.
56. B.	63. A.	70. C.
57. C.	64. A.	71. A.
58. C.	65. B.	72. B.
59. A.	66. C.	73. D.
60. B.	67. C.	74. D.
61. D.	68. D.	

GI irritation and ulcer occur when there is an imbalance between gastric protective mechanisms and irritating factors such as hydrochloric acid and other digestive juices. Gastric parietal cells secrete hydrochloric acid, mediated by histamine₂-receptor sites.

In a resting state, the stomach's pH in health is about 2, which kills many swallowed potentially harmful bacteria and viruses. Gastric acid production is about 1 to 2 mEq/hr in a resting, empty stomach and increases to 30 to 50 mEq/hr after a meal. The stomach is protected by numerous mechanisms, including a mucus coat with a gel layer. This layer provides mechanical protection from shearing as a result of ingestion of rough substances. In addition, bicarbonate is held within the protective layer and helps maintain pH to protect the mucosa from stomach acidity. Endogenous prostaglandins stimulate and thicken the mucus layer, enhance bicarbonate secretion, and promote cell renewal and blood flow. Endogenous prostaglandin levels normally decrease with age, which places older adults at increased risk for gastric damage. As part of the stress response, there is an increase in endogenous gastric acid and pepsin production and the potential for gastric mucosa injury and gastritis. Exogenous reasons for damage to the stomach's protective mechanism include the use of standard NSAIDs, such as ibuprofen and naproxen.

A significant amount of peptic ulcer disease, particularly gastric ulcer, acute gastritis, and NSAID-induced gastropathy, is caused by use of NSAIDs and the use of systemic corticosteroids. This is partly because of the action of these products against cyclooxygenase. Cyclooxygenase-1 (COX-1) is an enzyme found in gastric mucosa, small and large intestine mucosa, kidneys, platelets, and vascular epithelium. COX-1 contributes to the health of these organs through numerous mechanisms, including the maintenance of the protective gastric mucosal layer and proper renal perfusion. Cyclooxygenase-2 (COX-2) is an enzyme that produces prostaglandins important in the inflammatory cascade and pain transmission. The standard NSAIDs and systemic corticosteroids inhibit the synthesis of COX-1 and COX-2, controlling pain and inflammation, but producing gastric and renal complications. NSAIDs, such as celecoxib (Celebrex®), spare COX-1 and are more COX-2-selective and afford pain and inflammatory control. Although short-term studies supported lower rates of gastropathy with COX-2-selective NSAIDS (COX-2 inhibitors), this effect usually attenuates with long-term use and is absent with concomitant aspirin use. In addition, use of COX-2 inhibitors is associated with increased risk for cardiovascular and cerebrovascular events. Besides the use of NSAIDs and systemic corticosteroid use, major risk factors for gastric ulcer include age older than 60 years, history of peptic ulcer disease (especially gastric ulcer), and previous use of H_2RA or antacids for the treatment of GI symptoms. Additional, less potent risk factors include: cigarette smoking, cardiac disease, and alcohol use; taking more than one NSAID; and the concurrent use of NSAIDs and anticoagulants.

Peptic ulcer disease is located in areas, such as the duodenum, stomach, esophagus, and small intestine that are exposed to peptic juices such as acid and pepsin. Clinically, the description of the resulting disease includes a notation of where the ulcer is—for example, duodenal ulcer, gastric (stomach) ulcer, or esophageal ulcer. Peptic ulcer disease usually includes loss of mucosal surface, extending to muscularis mucosae, that is at least 5 mm in diameter, with most losses two to five times this size.

The clinical presentation of peptic ulcer disease (PUD) differs according to the location of the lesion. Symptoms associated with acute gastritis and gastric ulcer often become worse with eating because of the increase in irritating stomach acid production on top of the lesion. The symptoms often lessen within an hour as food buffers the acid. In contrast, duodenal ulcer symptoms often worsen as the stomach pH decreases when emptying after a meal, resulting in a sensation of stomach burning about 2 hours after a meal. However, significant variation in clinical presentation is common and the exact diagnosis of PUD location cannot be made by history and presentation alone.

Duodenal ulcer is more common than gastric ulcer. The most potent risk factor for this condition is most likely infection with H. pylori, a gram-negative, spiral-shaped organism with sheathed flagella found in at least 90% of patients with duodenal ulcer. The pathogen is also found in about 40% to 70% of individuals with gastric ulcer. Infection with H. pylori is transmitted via the oral-fecal and oral-oral route, and rates of infection approach 100% in developing nations with impure water supplies. In developed nations with pure water supplies, at least 75% of the population older than 50 years has been infected at some time. Eradication of the organism dramatically alters the risk of relapse. Numerous antimicrobial combinations are effective in treating symptomatic H. pylori infection (Table 7-3).

In the past, the adage "no stress, no extra acid, no ulcer" was often quoted. Treatment for peptic ulcer disease often included the use of psychotropic medications for relief of stress, according to the hypothesis that this would reduce the acid production. In reality, only 30% to 40% of persons with duodenal ulcer have higher than average acid secretion rates. In addition, coffee drinking and occasional alcohol use are not risk factors for peptic ulcer disease. Alcohol abuse with cirrhosis remains a risk factor, however. H. pylori is also found in individuals with asymptomatic gastritis and dyspepsia without ulceration; eradication of the organism does not seem to make a difference in symptoms in patients with these conditions.

A variety of diagnostic measures are available when confirmation of the lesion(s)'s location is required. An upper GI series identifies more than 80% of all ulcers larger than 0.5 cm, whereas upper GI endoscopy identifies nearly all such ulcers. In particular, upper endoscopy should be considered as a first-line diagnostic test in adults older than 50 years of age who present with new-onset PUD symptoms, as this modality also allows for ruling out gastric ulcer or gastric cancer. (See Table 7-4 for further information on diagnostic testing in PUD.)

Stool antigen testing is the most cost-effective method of diagnosing H. pylori infection, particularly when coupled with a clinical presentation consistent with peptic ulcer disease. Serological testing is also available, with the limitation that titers can take years to decline after effective treatment; however, 50% of patients have undetectable

TABLE 7-3

Treatment Options in *Helicobacter pylori* Infection Associated With Duodenal/Gastric Ulcer

Antimicrobials and Acid-Suppressing Medication	Usual Duration of Therapy	Comments
Sequential therapy with rabeprazole 20 mg bid plus amoxicillin 1 g bid x 5 days then rabeprazole 20 mg bid plus clarithromycin 500 mg plus tinidazole 500 mg bid x additional 5 days	10 days total	Generally well tolerated. Helpful when a shorter course of therapy is desirable.
Bismuth salicylate 2 tabs qid plus metronidazole 500 mg qid plus tetracycline 500 mg qid plus omeprazole 20 mg bid	10–14 days	With 10 days of quadruple therapy, eradication rates were 93% in a per protocol population. Exercise caution regarding potential interactions with other medications, contraindications in pregnancy, and warnings for other special populations.

Source: Gilbert D, Moellering R, Eliopoulos G, Chambers H, Saag M. *The Sanford Guide to Antimicrobial Therapy*. 44th ed. Sperryville, VA: Antimicrobial Therapy, Inc., 2014

TABLE 7-4

Assessing a Patient With Peptic Ulcer Disease

Location and Type of Peptic Ulcer Disease	Risk and Contributing Factors	Presenting Signs and Symptoms	Diagnostic Testing
Duodenal ulcer	*Helicobacter pylori* infection (most common), NSAID use, corticosteroid use (much less common)	Epigastric burning, gnawing pain about 2–3 hr after meals; relief with foods, antacids. Clusters of symptoms with periods of feeling well; awakening at 1–2 a.m. with symptoms common, morning waking pain rare. Tender at the epigastrium, left upper quadrant abdomen; slightly hyperactive bowel sounds	Stool antigen testing ≥90% sensitive and specific. If *H. pylori* stool antigen test is positive and PUD history, assume active infection and treat because cost of treatment less than that of confirmatory endoscopy. Repeat stool antigen test ≥8 wk posttreatment. *H. pylori* testing; serological testing for anti-*H. pylori* antibodies positive with acute infection but can take decades post infection to decline. A less sensitive and specific option when compared with stool antigen testing. Urea breath test establishes presence of acute infection. Endoscopy with biopsy and urease testing of biopsy specimen or staining, looking for *H. pylori* organisms, is diagnostic gold standard
Gastric ulcer	NSAID and corticosteroid use (potent risk factor). Cigarette smoking. Male:female ratio equal	Pain often reported with or immediately after meals. Nausea, vomiting, weight loss common	Difficulty distinguishing gastric ulcer from stomach cancer through UGI imaging. UGI endoscopy with biopsy vital to rule out gastric malignancy.

TABLE 7-4

Assessing a Patient With Peptic Ulcer Disease—cont'd

Location and Type of Peptic Ulcer Disease	Risk and Contributing Factors	Presenting Signs and Symptoms	Diagnostic Testing
	Peak incidence in fifth and sixth decades of life; nearly all found in patients without *H. pylori* infection are a result of chronic NSAID or long term systemic corticosteroid use		Need confirmation of presence of *H. pylori* before treatment, as is present in some of cases
Nonerosive gastritis, chronic type B (antral) gastritis	Most likely caused by *H. pylori* infection	Nausea Burning and pain limited to upper abdomen without reflux symptoms	Upper GI endoscopy is helpful diagnostic test, likely with *H. pylori* testing
Erosive gastritis	Usually secondary to alcohol and NSAID use, ASA use, stress *H. pylori* infection usually not a factor	Nausea Burning and pain limited to upper abdomen without reflux symptoms; bleeding common	Upper GI endoscopy is helpful diagnostic test, likely with *H. pylori* testing

ASA—acetylsalicylic acid; NSAID—nonsteroidal anti-inflammatory drug; PUD—peptic ulcer disease; UGI—upper gastrointestinal.

titers 12 to 18 months after therapy. The organism produces urease, which breaks down urea into ammonia and CO_2; this allows the organism to control pH in its local environment in the stomach by neutralizing H^+ ions in gastric acid. As a result, urea breath testing is also a helpful diagnostic procedure when attempting to establish the presence of *H. pylori* infection, although it is usually more expensive than the stool antigen test.

Suppression or neutralization of gastric acid is a critical part of peptic ulcer disease therapy. H_2RAs (whose names have the "-tidine" suffix, such as ranitidine [Zantac®], famotidine [Pepcid®], and cimetidine [Tagamet®]) competitively block the binding of histamine to the H_2-receptor site, reducing the secretion of gastric acid. In prescription dosages, these products suppress approximately 90% of hydrochloric acid production, whereas over-the-counter dosages suppress about 80%. These products are generally well tolerated. Cimetidine is the only H_2RA that significantly inhibits cytochrome P-450, slowing metabolism of many drugs. As a result, drug interactions between cimetidine and warfarin, diazepam, phenytoin, quinidine, carbamazepine, theophylline, imipramine, and other medications can occur; these interactions are not noted with the use of the other H_2RAs.

Proton pump inhibitors (PPIs) include omeprazole (Prilosec®), esomeprazole (Nexium®), and lansoprazole (Prevacid®). These drugs inhibit gastric acid secretion by inhibiting the final step in acid secretion by altering the activity of the "proton pump" (H^+,K^+-ATPase). As a result, there is a virtual cessation of stomach hydrochloric acid production, particularly owing to its significant action against the postprandial acid surge. PPI use is indicated in the treatment of peptic ulcer disease and gastroesophageal reflux disease (GERD) when an H_2RA is ineffective, and in refractory erosive esophagitis and Zollinger-Ellison syndrome. With many of the PPIs, clinical efficacy is improved when the medication is taken on an empty stomach one-half hour prior to breakfast. Protracted PPI use had been associated with reduced absorption of iron, vitamin B_{12}, and other micronutrients. An increase in fracture risk of the hip, spine, wrist, and forearm has also been noted with long-term PPI use; this risk is possibly associated with the decreased absorption of calcium and magnesium during PPI use. In particular, individuals with multiple health problems when hospitalized or in long-term care who are on chronic PPI therapy have an increased risk of contracting pneumonia and of developing *C. difficile* colitis. As a result, PPI use should not extend beyond the period of time needed for the clinical condition.

Often patients report an increase in upper GI distress when discontinuing long-term PPI use. The likely cause is rebound gastric hyperacidity; this problem can be minimized by gradually tapering the PPI dose (if possible) or trying every-other-day dosing with a supplemental dose of an antacid when symptoms flare. An alternative is to try low-dose H₂RA therapy with supplemental antacid use as needed. This gap therapy is usually continued for approximately 1 month.

H₂RAs likely offer protection against NSAID-induced duodenal ulcer and perhaps gastritis, but not against gastric ulcer. PPIs afford better protection against peptic ulcer disease. A prostaglandin analogue, misoprostol (Cytotec®), is a drug specifically designed for gastric protection with NSAID; the use of this medication is possibly helpful in minimizing renal injury secondary to NSAID use.

DISCUSSION SOURCES

Abraham N. Proton Pump Inhibitors: Potential Adverse Effects, *Curr Opin Gastroenterol* 28(6):615–620, 2012.

Ferri F. Peptic ulcer disease. In: *Ferri's Fast Facts*. Philadelphia, PA: Elsevier Mosby; 2005, pp. 324–326.

Gilbert D, Moellering R, Eliopoulos G, Chambers H, Saag M. *The Sanford Guide to Antimicrobial Therapy*. 44th ed. Sperryville, VA: Antimicrobial Therapy, Inc., 2014. , p.

Kenthu S, Moss S. Gastritis and peptic ulcer disease. In: Rakel R, Bope E (eds). *Conn's Current Therapy*. Philadelphia, PA: Saunders Elsevier; 2013, pp. 527–533.

❯ GERD

75. A 35-year-old woman complains of a 6-month history of periodic "heartburn" primarily after eating tomato-based sauces. Her weight is unchanged and examination reveals a single altered finding of epigastric tenderness without rebound. As first-line therapy, you advise:
   A. avoiding trigger foods.
   B. the use of a prokinetic agent.
   C. addition of sucralfate with meals.
   D. increased fluid intake with food intake.

76. You see a 62-year-old man diagnosed with esophageal columnar epithelial metaplasia. You realize he is at increased risk for:
   A. esophageal stricture.
   B. esophageal adenocarcinoma.
   C. gastroesophageal reflux.
   D. *H. pylori* colonization.

77. In caring for a patient with symptomatic gastroesophageal reflux, you prescribe a PPI to:
   A. enhance motility.
   B. increase the pH of the stomach.
   C. reduce lower esophageal pressure.
   D. help limit *H. pylori* growth.

78. A 38-year-old nonsmoking man presents with signs and symptoms consistent of GERD. He has self-treated with over-the-counter antacids and acid suppression therapy with effect. His weight is stable, and he denies nausea, vomiting, diarrhea, or melena. Which of the following represents the most appropriate diagnostic plan for this patient?
   A. fecal testing for *H. pylori* antigen
   B. upper GI endoscopy
   C. barium swallow
   D. no specific diagnostic testing is needed

79. Which of the following is most likely to be found in a 50-year-old woman with new-onset reflux esophagitis?
   A. recent initiation of estrogen-progestin hormonal therapy
   B. recent weight loss
   C. report of melena
   D. evidence of *H. pylori* infection

80. Which of the following is likely to be reported in a patient with persistent GERD?
   A. hematemesis
   B. chronic sore throat
   C. diarrhea
   D. melena

81. A 58-year-old man recently began taking an antihypertensive medication and reports that his "heartburn" has become much worse. He is most likely taking:
   A. atenolol.
   B. trandolapril.
   C. amlodipine.
   D. losartan.

82. You prescribe a fluoroquinolone antibiotic to a 54-year-old woman who has occasional GERD symptoms that she treats with an antacid. When discussing appropriate medication use, you advise that she should take the antimicrobial:
   A. with the antacid.
   B. separated from the antacid use by 2 to 4 hours before or 4 to 6 hours after taking the fluoroquinolone.
   C. without regard to antacid use.
   D. apart from the antacid by about 1 hour on either side of the fluoroquinolone dose.

83. A 48-year-old man with obesity and a 1-year history of classic GERD symptoms has been on the consistent use of a therapeutic dose of a PPI for the past 6 months. He states he is "really no better with the medicine and I have cut out most of the food that bothers my stomach. I even cut out all alcohol and soda." Physical examination reveals stable weight, mildly erythematous pharynx, and epigastric tenderness without rebound. Next step options include:
   A. obtaining an upper GI series.
   B. referral for GERD surgery.
   C. further evaluation with upper GI endoscopy.
   D. obtaining FOBT testing.

84. Which of the following is not an "alarm" finding in the person with GERD symptoms?
    A. weight gain
    B. dysphagia
    C. odynophagia
    D. iron-deficiency anemia

85. Risk factors for Barrett esophagus include all of the following except:
    A. history of cigarette smoking.
    B. older than 50 years of age.
    C. male gender.
    D. African American ethnicity.

86. A 57-year-old male is in need of evaluation for Barrett esophagus. You recommend:
    A. *H. pylori* testing.
    B. CT scan.
    C. upper GI endoscopy with biopsy.
    D. barium swallow.

87. A 64-year-old male with diagnosed Barrett esophagus has shown no sign of dysplasia in two consecutive evaluations within the past year. You recommend additional surveillance testing should be conducted every:
    A. 6 months.
    B. 12 months.
    C. 2 years.
    D. 3 years.

88. The most common form of esophageal cancer in the United States is:
    A. squamous cell cancer.
    B. adenocarcinoma.
    C. basal cell carcinoma.
    D. melanoma.

89. Esophageal adenocarcinoma is usually located:
    A. in the upper esophagus.
    B. near the upper esophageal sphincter.
    C. at the junction of the esophagus and stomach.
    D. in the lower esophagus.

90. Esophageal squamous cell cancer is usually located:
    A. in the upper esophagus.
    B. near the upper esophageal sphincter.
    C. at the junction of the esophagus and stomach.
    D. in the lower esophagus.

91. Which of the following is at greatest risk of esophageal cancer?
    A. 34-year-old male who eats a high-fat diet
    B. 76-year-old male who stopped smoking 15 years ago
    C. 45-year-old woman with a history of 6 full-term pregnancies
    D. 58-year-old female vegetarian

92. The presence of esophageal cancer is commonly associated with:
    A. renal impairment.
    B. chronic bronchitis.
    C. iron-deficiency anemia.
    D. unexplained weight gain.

Answers

75. A.	81. C.	87. D.
76. B.	82. B.	88. B.
77. B.	83. C.	89. C.
78. D.	84. A.	90. A.
79. A.	85. D.	91. B.
80. B.	86. C.	92. C.

GERD (gastroesophageal reflux disease) is a common but troublesome condition. Reflux of stomach contents occurs regularly. Most reflux is asymptomatic with no resulting esophageal injury. GERD is present when there are symptoms or evidence of tissue damage. The most common GERD presentation includes dyspepsia, chest pain at rest, and postprandial fullness. In addition, non-GI symptoms, including chronic hoarseness, sore throat, nocturnal cough, and wheezing, are often reported, occasionally in the absence of more classic GERD symptoms, and particularly when the condition is chronic. (For additional information on diagnosing GERD, see Table 7–5.)

Decreased lower esophageal sphincter tone and the resulting reflux of gastric contents cause GERD. Esophageal mucosal irritation results from exposure to hydrochloric acid and pepsin.

The use of certain medications including estrogen, progesterone/progestins, theophylline, calcium channel blockers, and nicotine; can result in a decrease in lower esophageal sphincter pressure and worsen GERD, these medications should be discontinued if clinically possible. Initial therapy for patients with GERD includes identifying trigger foods and reducing their intake. Most commonly mentioned food includes alcohol, tomato-based products, chocolate, peppermint, colas, citrus juices, and food high in fat content. Behavioral intervention includes avoiding or minimizing conditions or situations that encourage esophageal reflux: remaining upright and avoiding assuming the supine position within 3 hours of a meal, eating smaller meals, and eliminating occasions of overeating. Because abdominal obesity contributes to GERD, weight loss can also be helpful. Elevation of the head of the bed on 4-inch blocks can also offer some relief; propping the head and upper thorax on pillows is not effective. (For additional information on managing GERD, see Table 7–5.) In patients with classic GI and extra-GI symptoms, the diagnosis of GERD is usually made clinically with no specific diagnostic testing performed, particularly when clinical response is noted with standard therapy.

The use of antacids after meals and at bedtime is often sufficient to control milder, particularly intermittent, GERD

TABLE 7-5
Diagnosis and Management of GERD

ESTABLISHING THE DIAGNOSIS OF GERD
- A presumptive diagnosis of GERD can be established in the setting of typical symptoms of heartburn and regurgitation. Empiric medical therapy with a proton pump inhibitor (PPI) is recommended in this setting.
- Screening for *Helicobacter pylori* infection is not recommended in GERD patients. Treatment of *H. pylori* infection is not routinely required as part of antireflux therapy.
- Upper endoscopy is not required in the presence of typical GERD symptoms. Endoscopy is recommended in the presence of alarm symptoms and for screening of patients at high risk for complications. Repeat endoscopy is not indicated in patients without Barrett's esophagus in the absence of new symptoms.
- Routine biopsies from the distal esophagus are not recommended specifically to diagnose GERD
- Barium radiographs should not be performed to diagnose GERD.
- Esophageal manometry plays no role in the diagnosis of GERD. If GERD surgical intervention is being considered, esophageal manometry is recommended for preoperative evaluation.
- Ambulatory esophageal reflux monitoring is indicated before consideration of endoscopic or surgical therapy in patients with non-erosive disease, as part of the evaluation of patients refractory to PPI therapy, and in situations when the diagnosis of GERD is in question. Ambulatory reflux monitoring is the only test that can assess reflux symptom association.

MANAGEMENT OF GERD
- An 8-week course of PPIs is the therapy of choice for symptom relief and healing of erosive esophagitis.
- PPI therapy should be initiated at once a day dosing, before the first meal of the day. For patients with partial response to once daily therapy, tailored therapy with adjustment of dose timing and/or twice daily dosing should be considered in patients with night-time symptoms, variable schedules, and/or sleep disturbance. Switching to another PPI is also an option though there are no major differences in efficacy between the different PPIs.
- Traditional delayed release PPIs such as omeprazole should be administered 30–60 min before a meal for maximal pH control.
- Maintenance PPI therapy should be administered for GERD patients who continue to have symptoms after PPI is discontinued and in patients with complications including erosive esophagitis and Barrett's esophagus.
- Patients who do not respond to PPI should be referred for evaluation.
- Routine global elimination of food that can trigger reflux (including chocolate, caffeine, alcohol, acidic foods) is not recommended in the treatment of GERD. At the same time, foods that are known to trigger symptoms should be eliminated or minimized.
- Weight loss is recommended for GERD patients who are overweight, obese, or have had recent weight gain.
- Head of bed elevation and avoidance of meals 2–3 h before bedtime should be recommended for patients with nocturnal GERD.
- For patients who require long-term PPI therapy, the medication should be administered in the lowest effective dose, including on demand or intermittent therapy. H_2-receptor antagonist (H_2RA) therapy can be used as a maintenance option in patients without erosive disease if patients experience heartburn relief.
- Sucralfate and prokinetic agents do not play a role in the treatment of GERD.

Source: American College of Gastroenterology: Diagnosis and Management of Gastroesophageal Reflux Disease. Available at http://gi.org/guideline/diagnosis-and-managemen-of-gastroesophageal-reflux-disease

symptoms. Antacids neutralize secreted acids and inactivate pepsin and bile salts. These medications are most effective when used 1 to 3 hours after meals and at bedtime. Antacids interact with many other medications and should be used at least 2 hours apart; with the use of a fluoroquinolone such as ciprofloxacin, antacid use should be 2 to 4 hours before or 4 to 6 hours after the fluoroquinolone.

If the use of antacids and lifestyle modification are inadequate to control milder, intermittent GERD symptoms, an H_2RA at full prescription strength bid should be added. If there is no improvement in 6 weeks, longer term H_2RA therapy is

unlikely to be helpful. With moderate to severe symptoms that do not respond to a prescription dosage of H_2RA, a PPI such as omeprazole (Prilosec) or lansoprazole (Prevacid) should be prescribed; an alternative is to simply start therapy with a PPI. Compared with H_2RAs, PPIs have superior postprandial and nocturnal acid suppression. An 8-week course of PPI therapy is usually adequate to heal acute esophageal inflammation noted with ongoing GERD. If symptoms do not resolve with this PPI course, referral to gastroenterology for further evaluation, including upper GI endoscopy, is warranted. In the past, sucralfate and prokinetic agents were considered to be treatment options for GERD; little evidence supports the use of these medications and these medications are no longer considered therapeutic option in this condition.

The course of GERD is usually straightforward. However, "alarm" symptoms in GERD that warrant further evaluation include dysphagia (difficulty swallowing), odynophagia (painful swallowing), gastrointestinal bleeding, unexplained weight loss, and persistent chest pain. The development of iron-deficiency anemia as a result of chronic low volume GI blood loss in the presence of GERD symptoms is a rare but worrisome finding. A component of the additional evaluation is referral to gastroenterology for upper endoscopy. These alarm findings can be indicative of erosive esophagitis or esophageal cancer; upper endoscopy can clarify the diagnosis and provide, if required, a vehicle of esophageal biopsy.

Surgical intervention in GERD is a treatment option usually limited to patients with the most severe symptoms that are not improved by the use of standard treatment. As additional endoscopic interventions become available, with evidence of the long-term efficacy and safety of the procedures, this option is likely to increase in utility. Obese patients contemplating surgical therapy for GERD should be considered first for bariatric surgery. Gastric bypass would be the preferred operation in these patients; restrictive bariatric surgery will likely contribute to GERD symptoms.

Reflux-induced esophageal injury, also known as reflux esophagitis, is present in 40% of patients with GERD. Erosions and ulcerations in squamous epithelium of the esophagus are present and are most common in elderly patients and individuals with longstanding GERD history. Complications of reflux esophagitis include esophageal stricture and columnar epithelial metaplasia, also known as Barrett esophagus (BE), which typically involves the distal esophagus. In patients at risk for BE, an upper GI endoscopy should be performed and appropriate biopsy specimens taken. Although BE has long been mentioned as a potent risk factor for esophageal adenocarcinoma, this risk is not thought to be as significant as in the past. Risk factors for BE include GERD of long duration, certain ethnicity (i.e., white, Hispanic), male gender, advancing age (older than 50 years of age), tobacco use, and obesity. Intervention in BE is based on aggressive acid suppression, with the anticipated end product of minimizing further esophageal damage. For patients with established BE of any length and with no dysplasia after two consecutive examinations within 1 year, an acceptable interval for additional surveillance is every 3 years. The clinician should remain aware of the latest recommendations on BE intervention and surveillance.

Esophageal cancer can be found in a variety of forms. Squamous cell cancer, usually found in the upper part of the esophagus, represents approximately 90% to 95% of all esophageal cancer worldwide. Adenocarcinoma, usually located at the junction of the esophagus and stomach, comprises more than 50% of all esophageal cancer in the United States. As with BE, esophageal cancer is more common in men, with a male to female ratio of approximately 3:1. The disease is most often diagnosed in the sixth and seventh decades of life.

In early esophageal cancer, regardless of etiology, the patient is usually without symptoms. In later disease, dysphagia—particularly difficulty swallowing solid foods—and weight loss are among the most commonly reported findings. Less commonly reported symptoms are epigastric or retrosternal pain, persistent hoarseness, and cough, though these are also common to GERD. Due to chronic low volume bleeding from the esophageal tumor, iron-deficiency anemia often develops. Often, esophageal cancer is not detected until advanced. Prognosis is dependent on the extent of the disease. When esophageal cancer is suspected, esophagogastroduodenoscopy (upper GI endoscopy) with appropriate biopsies is the preferred method of initial diagnostic testing. Additional testing is based on initial findings.

DISCUSSION SOURCES

American Gastroenterological Association Medical Position Statement on the Management of Barrett's Esophagus. Available at www.gastrojournal.org/article/S0016-5085(11)00084-9/fulltext

American College of Gastroenterology, Diagnosis and Management of Gastroesophageal Reflux Disease. Available at http://gi.org/guideline/diagnosis-and-management-of-gastroesophageal-reflux-disease

Baldwin K, Espat J. Esophageal Cancer. Available at http://emedicine.medscape.com/article/277930

Viral Hepatitis

93. A 36-year-old man complains of nausea, fever, malaise, and abdominal pain. He shows signs of jaundice and reports darkly-colored urine. Diagnostic results show elevated serum aminotransferase less than 10 times upper limits of normal (ULN). His most likely diagnosis is:
    A. GERD.
    B. viral hepatitis.
    C. Crohn's disease.
    D. Barrett esophagus.

94. A serological marker for acute hepatitis A virus (HAV) infection is:
    A. HAV IgM.
    B. HAV viral RNA.
    C. TNF-α.
    D. IL-10.

95. You are caring for a 45-year-old woman from a developing country. She reports that she had "yellow jaundice" as a young child. Her physical examination is unremarkable. Her laboratory studies are as follows: AST, 22 U/L (normal, 0 to 31 U/L); alanine aminotransferase (ALT), 25 U/L (normal, 0 to 40 U/L); hepatitis A virus immunoglobulin G (HAV IgG) positive. Laboratory testing reveals:
    A. chronic hepatitis A.
    B. no evidence of prior or current hepatitis A infection.
    C. resolved hepatitis A infection.
    D. prodromal hepatitis A.

96. The most common source of hepatitis A infection is:
A. sharing intravenous drug equipment.
B. cooked seafood.
C. contaminated water supplies.
D. sexual contact.

97. In addition to the laboratory work described, results reveal the following for the above-mentioned patient: hepatitis B surface antigen (HBsAg) positive. These findings are most consistent with:
A. no evidence of hepatitis B infection.
B. resolved hepatitis B infection.
C. chronic hepatitis B.
D. evidence of effective hepatitis B immunization.

98. The average incubation time for HAV is approximately:
A. 10 days.
B. 28 days.
C. 60 days.
D. 6 months.

99. Current vaccine guidelines recommend administering the immunization against HAV to:
A. those living in or traveling to areas endemic for the disease.
B. food handlers and day-care providers.
C. military personnel.
D. any person who wishes to receive the vaccine.

100. All of the following are effective methods to kill the hepatitis A virus except:
A. heating food to more than 185°F (85°C) for at least 1 minute.
B. adequately chlorinating water.
C. cleaning surfaces with a 1:100 bleach solution.
D. freezing food for at least 1 hour.

101. You see a 27-year-old man who says he ate at a restaurant last week that was later reported to have a worker identified with hepatitis A. He is healthy and shows no sign of infection but is concerned about contracting HAV infection. You recommend:
A. HAV vaccine.
B. HAV immune globulin.
C. HAV vaccine plus immune globulin.
D. no intervention at this time and wait until symptoms manifest.

102. A 54-year-old man has been recently diagnosed with HAV infection. You recommend all of the following except:
A. eating smaller, more frequent meals to help combat nausea.
B. avoiding consumption of any alcohol.
C. reviewing current medication use for consideration of discontinuation.
D. taking daily acetaminophen to alleviate joint pains.

103. A 38-year-old man with a recent history of injection drug use presents with malaise, nausea, fatigue, and "yellow eyes" for the past week. After ordering diagnostic tests, you confirm the diagnosis of acute hepatitis B. Anticipated laboratory results include:
A. the presence of hepatitis B surface antibody (HBsAb).
B. neutrophilia.
C. thrombocytosis.
D. the presence of HBsAg.

104. Clinical findings in patients with acute hepatitis B likely include all of the following except:
A. abdominal rebound tenderness.
B. scleral icterus.
C. a smooth, tender, palpable hepatic border.
D. report of myalgia.

105. Risk factors for hepatitis B virus (HBV) infection include all of the following except:
A. having multiple sexual partners.
B. having an occupation that exposes you to human blood.
C. injection drug user.
D. eating food prepared by a person with an HBV infection.

106. You see a woman who has been sexually involved without condom use with a man newly diagnosed with acute hepatitis B. She has not received hepatitis B immunization. You advise her to:
A. start hepatitis B immunization series.
B. limit the number of sexual partners.
C. be tested for HBsAb.
D. receive hepatitis B immune globulin and start hepatitis B immunization series.

107. The HBV vaccine should not be offered to individuals who have a history of anaphylactic reaction to:
A. eggs.
B. Baker's yeast.
C. peanuts.
D. shellfish.

108. Which of the following groups should be screened for hepatitis B surface antigen (HBsAg)?
A. pregnant women with no history of receiving HBV vaccine
B. pregnant women with documented prior HBV infection
C. all pregnant women regardless of HBV vaccine history
D. all newborn infants born to mothers with chronic HBV infection

109. Routine testing for the presence of HBsAb after immunization with the HBV vaccine is recommended for all of the following except:
    A. healthcare providers.
    B. immunocompromised patients.
    C. restaurant workers.
    D. dialysis patients.

110. A 26-year-old male reports that he has shared a needle with a friend during injection drug use. He is certain that his friend has chronic hepatitis B infection and is uncertain about his own immunization history. You recommend:
    A. starting the HBV vaccine series.
    B. administering hepatitis B immune globulin.
    C. starting the HBV vaccine series and administering hepatitis B immune globulin.
    D. waiting until the HBsAg results before administering hepatitis B immune globulin.

111. You see a 22-year-old male who is an injection drug user who has recently been diagnosed with chronic HBV infection. You recommend additional testing for all of the following except:
    A. Lyme disease.
    B. HIV.
    C. HAV.
    D. HCV.

112. Antiviral treatment for chronic HBV infection includes all of the following except:
    A. entecavir.
    B. tenofovir.
    C. lamivudine.
    D. fidaxomicin.

113. Which of the following statements is true concerning hepatitis C infection?
    A. It usually manifests with jaundice, fever, and significant hepatomegaly.
    B. Among health-care workers, it is most commonly found in nurses.
    C. At least than 50% of persons with acute hepatitis C go on to develop chronic infection.
    D. Interferon therapy is consistently curative.

114. Which of the following characteristics is predictive of severity of chronic liver disease in a patient with chronic hepatitis C?
    A. female gender, age younger than 30
    B. co-infection with hepatitis B, daily alcohol use
    C. acquisition of virus through intravenous drug use, history of hepatitis A infection
    D. frequent use of aspirin, nutritional status

115. When answering questions about hepatitis A vaccine, you consider that all of the following are true except:
    A. it does not contain live virus.
    B. it should be offered to individuals who frequently travel to developing countries.
    C. it is a recommended immunization for healthcare workers.
    D. it is given as a single dose.

116. To prevent an outbreak of hepatitis D infection, a NP plans to:
    A. promote a campaign for clean food supplies.
    B. immunize the population against hepatitis B.
    C. offer antiviral prophylaxis against the agent.
    D. encourage frequent hand washing.

117. Which of the following is true concerning hepatitis B vaccine?
    A. The vaccine contains live hepatitis B virus.
    B. Most individuals born since 1986 in the United States who have been fully immunized have received vaccine against HBV.
    C. The vaccine is contraindicated in the presence of HIV infection.
    D. Postvaccination arthralgias are often reported.

118. Hyperbilirubinemia can cause all of the following except:
    A. potential displacement of highly protein-bound drugs.
    B. scleral icterus.
    C. cola-colored urine.
    D. reduction in urobilinogen.

119. Monitoring for hepatoma in a patient with chronic hepatitis B or C often includes periodic evaluation of:
    A. erythrocyte sedimentation rate.
    B. HBsAb.
    C. alpha-fetoprotein.
    D. bilirubin.

120. Which of the following is an expected laboratory result in a patient with acute hepatitis A infection (normal values: AST, 0 to 31 U/L; ALT, 0 to 40 U/L)?
    A. AST, 55 U/L; ALT, 50 U/L
    B. AST, 320 U/L; ALT, 190 U/L
    C. AST, 320 U/L; ALT, 300 U/L
    D. AST, 640 U/L; ALT, 870 U/L

121. Which of the following is most likely to be reported in a patient on long-term use of a 3-hydroxy-3-methylglutaryl–coenzyme A (HMG-CoA) reductase inhibitor (statin)?
    A. AST, 22 U/L; ALT, 28 U/L
    B. AST, 320 U/L; ALT, 190 U/L
    C. AST, 32 U/L; ALT, 120 U/L
    D. AST, 440 U/L; ALT, 670 U/L

122. When discussing the use of immunoglobulin (IG) with a 60-year-old woman who was recently exposed to the hepatitis A virus, you consider that:
    A. IG is derived from pooled donated blood.
    B. the product must be used within 1 week of exposure to provide protection.
    C. its use in this situation constitutes an example of active immunization.
    D. a short, intense flu-like illness often occurs after its use.

123. You see a 48-year-old woman with nonalcoholic fatty liver disease. Evaluation of infectious hepatitis includes the following:
    Anti-HAV IgG—negative
    Anti-HBs—negative
    Anti-HCV—negative
    When considering her overall health status, you advise receiving which of the following vaccines?
    A. immunization against hepatitis A and B as based on her lifestyle risk factors
    B. immunization against hepatitis B and C
    C. immunization against hepatitis A and B
    D. immunization against hepatitis A, B, and C

124. Which of the following hepatitis forms is most effectively transmitted from the man to the woman via heterosexual vaginal intercourse?
    A. hepatitis A
    B. hepatitis B
    C. hepatitis C
    D. hepatitis D

Answers

93. B.	104. A.	115. D.
94. A.	105. D.	116. B.
95. C.	106. D.	117. B.
96. C.	107. B.	118. D.
97. C.	108. C.	119. C.
98. B.	109. C.	120. D.
99. D.	110. C.	121. A.
100. D.	111 A.	122. A.
101. A.	112. D.	123. C.
102. D.	113. C.	124. B.
103. D.	114. B.	

Numerous infective agents cause viral hepatitis (Table 7–5). Hepatitis A infection is caused by hepatitis A virus (HAV), a small RNA virus. Transmitted primarily by fecal-contaminated drinking water and food supplies, hepatitis A is typically a self-limiting infection with a very low mortality rate. Fecal-contaminated water supplies are the most common source of infection, although eating raw shellfish that grew in impure water can be problematic. In developing countries with limited pure water, most children contract this disease by age 5 years. In North America, adults 20 to 39 years old account for nearly 50% of the reported cases, though overall reported cases have decreased in the last decade. Due to the risk to a given population, the local public health department should be consulted for advice when an outbreak of hepatitis A infection occurs.

The clinical presentation of all forms of acute viral hepatitis typically includes nausea, anorexia, fever, malaise, abdominal pain, and jaundice. Clay-colored stools, dark-colored urine, and joint pains are commonly reported. Laboratory findings include elevated serum aminotransferase (hepatic enzyme) levels, most often 20 or more times the upper limits of normal. Since the clinical presentation is the same for all types of acute viral hepatitis, the diagnosis must be confirmed by a positive serological test for the specific hepatitis. In hepatitis A, immunoglobulin M (IgM) antibody to hepatitis A virus develops (HAV) (see Table 7–6). The onset of symptoms in hepatitis A usually occurs about 15 to 50 days after the organism is contracted; the average incubation period for the virus is about 28 days, with a range of 15 to 50 days. The majority (more than 70%) of children less than age 6 years will have few or no symptoms during infection with the HAV.

All children and select other groups should be immunized against HAV. Candidates for immunization include individuals who reside in or travel to areas in which the disease is endemic, food handlers, sewage workers, animal handlers, day-care attendees and workers, long-term care residents and workers, military personnel, and health-care workers. Injection drug users also benefit from the vaccine. HAV is rarely transmitted sexually or from needle sharing; rather, injection drug users often live in conditions that facilitate the oral-fecal transmission of HAV. In addition, co-infection with hepatitis A and C, co-infection with hepatitis A and B, or acute hepatitis A in addition to chronic liver disease can lead to a rapid deterioration in hepatic function. Persons with chronic hepatitis B or C or both or any chronic liver disease should be immunized against hepatitis A. Persons who have clotting factor disorders and are receiving clotting factor concentrates who have not had hepatitis A should also be immunized. Currently, hepatitis A vaccine guidelines have been expanded to include all individuals who would like to be immunized against the condition.

HAV is a heat-sensitive virus that can be killed by heating food to higher than 185°F (higher than 85°C) for one minute. Adequate chlorination of water, as recommended in the United States, kills HAV that enters the water supply. The virus is capable of surviving on select surfaces for many weeks. Proper hand hygiene and cleaning environmental surfaces with a 1:100 bleach solution are measures that can help minimize the spread of this infection.

Two doses of HAV vaccine are usually given 6 to 12 months apart to ensure an enhanced immunological response; an alternative accelerated dosing schedule is also licensed for use with a combined hepatitis A and B vaccine. Hepatitis A vaccine, which does not contain live virus, is usually well tolerated without systemic reaction. Postvaccine HAV immunity typically lasts at least 15 to 25 years. Postexposure prophylaxis against hepatitis A is also available; IG and HAV vaccine are

TABLE 7-6

Infectious Hepatitis: Key Features to Transmission and Diagnosis

Type	Route of Transmission	IZ available? Postexposure prophylaxis?	Sequelae	Disease Marker
HEPATITIS A	Fecal-oral	IZ=Yes Postexposure prophylaxis with IZ and/or IG for close contacts	None, survive or die (low mortality rate)	*Acute disease marker* • HAV IgM (M=miserable) • Elevated hepatic enzymes≥10 x ULN *Chronic disease marker* • None, as chronic hepatitis A does not exist *Disease in past, Hx IZ=* • Anti-HAV (total of HAV IgM and HAV IgG [G=gone]) present • Hepatic enzymes normalize *Still susceptible to hepatitis A infection* • Anti-HAV negative (Negative="Never had")

HEPATITIS B	Blood, body fluids	IZ=Yes Postexposure prophylaxis with IZ and/or HBIG for blood, body fluid contacts	Chronic hepatitis B, hepatocellular carcinoma (HCC, primary liver cancer, hepatoma), hepatic failure	*Acute disease markers*
				• HBsAg=Always growing
				• HBeAg=Extra contagious, extra growing
				• Elevated hepatic enzymes≥10 x ULN
				Chronic disease marker
				• Patient without symptoms
				• NL or slight elevated hepatic enzymes
				• HBsAg (Ag=Always growing)
				  • Only present if HBV on board
				  • Surrogate marker for HBV
				Hepatitis B in past, Hx IZ
				• HBsAb (Anti-HBs)
				  • B=Bye, as no HBV on board
				  • A protective antibody, unable to get HBV in the future
				• Hepatic enzyme normalized
				Still susceptible to hepatitis B infection
				• HBsAg negative
				• Anti-HBc negative
				• HBsAb (Anti-HBs) negative

HEPATITIS C	Blood, body fluids	No No	Chronic hepatitis C, hepatocellular carcinoma (HCC, primary liver cancer, hepatoma), hepatic failure	*Acute disease marker* • Anti-HCV present • HCV viral RNA • Elevated hepatic enzymes *Chronic disease marker* • Anti-HCV present • HCV viral RNA • Normal to slightly elevated hepatic enzymes *Disease in the past* • Anti-HCV present (nonprotective antibody) • HCV RNA absent • Normalized hepatic enzymes

Continued

TABLE 7-6
Infectious Hepatitis: Key Features to Transmission and Diagnosis—cont'd

Type	Route of Transmission	IZ available? Postexposure prophylaxis?	Sequelae	Disease Marker
HEPATITIS D	Blood, body fluids	No, but prevent B and you can prevent D	Severe infection, hepatic failure, death	*Acute or chronic* hepatitis B (HBsAg) markers *plus* hepatitis D IgM. Usually with markedly elevated hepatic enzymes.

NB: The content of this table is not meant to be a comprehensive guide for the diagnosis of infectious hepatitis but rather an overview. For additional information, see Ferri F. *Ferri's Best Test: A Practical Guide to Clinical Laboratory Medicine and Diagnostic Imaging*, 2nd Ed. St. Louis: Elsevier Health Sciences, 2009; and Desai S. *Clinician's Guide to Laboratory Medicine*. Houston, TX, Pocket, 2009, MD2B.

used for this purpose. For healthy persons 12 months to 40 years old, a dose of hepatitis A vaccine at the age-appropriate dose is preferred to IG because of vaccine advantages that include long-term protection and ease of administration. For persons older than 40 years, IG is preferred because of the lack of information regarding vaccine performance and the more severe manifestations of hepatitis A in this age group; vaccine can be used if IG cannot be obtained. IG, a form of passive immunity, is highly effective in preventing HAV infection if given within 2 weeks of exposure. IG is a product derived from pooled blood that contains preformed antibodies against the virus and has an outstanding safety profile. HAV vaccine should be encouraged with IG use.

There is no specific treatment for HAV infection as the body will clear the virus on its own, with the liver typically healing itself within a month or two. Treatment primarily focuses on alleviating the signs and symptoms of the infection. Patients may feel tired and have less energy, and thus should rest when needed. To combat nausea, patients can try to eat small snacks rather than 3 large meals, and choose higher-calorie foods over lower-calorie foods if the patient is having trouble eating enough calories. Finally, any insult to the liver should be avoided during HAV infection. If possible, any medications processed by the liver, including acetaminophen, should be stopped or changed, and alcohol consumption should be avoided while signs and symptoms persist.

Hepatitis B is caused by a small double-stranded DNA virus that contains an inner core protein of hepatitis B core antigen and an outer surface of HBsAg. Hepatitis B virus (HBV) is usually transmitted through an exchange of blood and body fluids. Risk factors for HBV infection include having sex with more than one partner, men who have sexual contact with other men, sharing needles during injection drug use, having a job with exposure to human blood, or traveling to areas with high infection rates of HBV (such as Africa, Central and Southeast Asia, and Central Europe). The predominant mode of transmission of the HBV virus is through sexual activity and injection

drug use. HBV is also a major occupational hazard of health workers. HBV cannot be spread by contaminated food or water, nor can it be spread casually in the workplace. The virus can be killed with a 1:10 dilution of bleach to clean up blood spills. Gloves and eye protection should be worn when cleaning up blood spills.

Acute hepatitis B is a serious illness that can lead to hepatic failure. Approximately 5% of individuals with acute hepatitis B go on to develop chronic hepatitis B; chronic hepatitis B is a potent risk factor for hematoma or primary hepatocellular carcinoma and hepatic cirrhosis. A person with chronic hepatitis B continues to be able to transmit the virus, although the person appears clinically well.

Hepatitis B infection can be prevented by limiting exposure to blood and body fluids and through immunization. Recombinant hepatitis B vaccine, which does not contain live virus, is well-tolerated; one contraindication to receiving the vaccine is a personal history of anaphylaxis to baker's yeast. In the United States, this vaccine has been routinely used in children since 1986; as a result, most of the population born during or after 1986 has been immunized. The vaccine should be offered to adults born before 1986 and to all who have not been immunized, particularly persons at highest risk for contracting the virus. Nonimmunized individuals being treated for other sexually transmitted infections should be encouraged to receive protection against HBV. Refer to the latest immunization guidelines for further information on this important public health issue.

Infants who become infected perinatally with HBV have an estimated 25% lifetime chance of developing hepatocellular carcinoma or cirrhosis. As a result, all pregnant women should be screened for HBsAg at the first prenatal visit, regardless of HBV vaccine history. Because the HBV vaccine is not 100% effective and perinatal transmission is possible, a woman could have carried HBV before becoming pregnant. About 90% to 95% of individuals who receive the vaccine develop HBsAb (anti-HBs) after three doses, implying protection from the virus. Routine testing for the presence of HBsAb after immunization is not recommended. HBsAb testing should be considered, however, to confirm the development of HBV protection in persons with high risk for infection (e.g., certain healthcare workers who have risk for frequent and high-volume blood exposures, injection drug users, sex workers) and persons at risk for a poor immune response (e.g., dialysis patients, patients with immunosuppression).

Booster doses of hepatitis B vaccine are recommended only in certain circumstances. For hemodialysis patients, the need for booster doses should be assessed by annual testing for antibody to hepatitis B surface antigen (anti-HBs). A booster dose should be administered when anti-HBs levels decline to less than 10 mIU/mL. For other immunocompromised persons (e.g., HIV-infected persons, hematopoietic stem-cell transplant recipients, and persons receiving chemotherapy), the need for booster doses has not been determined. When anti-HBs levels decline to less than 10 mIU/mL, annual anti-HBs testing and booster doses should be considered for persons with an ongoing risk for exposure. Ongoing serological surveillance in immunocompetent persons is not recommended.

Postexposure prophylaxis is effective in preventing HBV infection. In a person who has written documentation of a complete hepatitis B vaccine series and who did not receive postvaccination testing, a single vaccine booster dose should be given with a nonoccupational known HBsAg-positive exposure source. A person who is in the process of being vaccinated, but who has not completed the vaccine series, should receive the appropriate dose of hepatitis B immunoglobulin (HBIG) and should complete the vaccine series. Unvaccinated persons should receive HBIG and hepatitis B vaccine as soon as possible, preferably within 24 hours, after exposure. Testing for HIV, other sexually transmitted infections, and hepatitis A and C should also be offered, and postexposure prophylaxis and immunization should be offered when applicable. Owing to the complexity of care, intervention for a person with occupational exposure should be done with expert consultation in this area.

Currently, treatment with pegylated interferon and an antiviral such as entecavir, adefovir, and lamivudine has shown clinical utility in inducing remission in some patients with chronic hepatitis B. Additional options include telbivudine and tenofovir. Because of the rapid advances being made in this area, the NP and patient must be aware of the most up-to-date treatment options.

Hepatitis C infection is transmitted through the exchange of blood and body fluids. A single-strain RNA virus causes the infection. Although this is the most frequent cause of blood transfusion-associated hepatitis, less than 4% of all cases of hepatitis C can be attributed to this cause. Since the advent of screening of the blood supply for hepatitis C virus (HCV), the risk of transfusion-associated hepatitis C has decreased from 10% in the early 1980s to 0.1% or less today. More than 50% of cases of HCV infection are caused by injection drug use with needle sharing. Other risk behaviors include tattooing, branding, piercing, or other similar practices when shared or poorly sanitized equipment is used. Transmission through sexual contact is possible, but this risk seems to be relatively low. Maternal-fetal transmission is also uncommon and is usually limited to women with high circulating HCV levels. Transmission through breastfeeding has not been reported.

The HCV incubation period is about 6 to 7 weeks, and the infection rarely causes a serious acute illness. Diagnosis is made by the presence of anti-HCV, an antibody that persists in the presence of the virus and is not protective. At least 50% to 80% of individuals with hepatitis C go on to develop chronic infection and exhibit anti-HCV along with a positive hepatitis C viral load. Progression to cirrhosis occurs in about 20% of people infected with chronic hepatitis C after 20 years of disease. HCV-related cirrhosis risk is increased in men, with disease acquisition after age 40 years, and in people who drink the equivalent of 50 g or more of alcohol per day (15 g alcohol = 12 oz beer, 5 oz wine, 1.5 oz 80 proof whiskey). If anti-HCV persists in the absence of a positive hepatitis C viral load, this suggests that active infection is not present.

Because of the significant potential sequelae of chronic hepatitis C infection, expert consultation should be obtained so that the patient and primary care provider are well versed on the latest evaluation, monitoring, and treatment options. Currently, treatment with pegylated interferon with or without select antivirals has shown clinical utility in inducing remission in some patients with chronic hepatitis C; response depends on many factors, including other health problems, viral genotype, and viral load. Because of the rapid advances being made in this area, the clinician and patient must be aware of the most up-to-date treatment options.

Because the hepatitis D virus is an RNA virus that can occur only concurrently in the presence of HBV, it is found only in persons with acute or chronic hepatitis B. A patient with hepatitis B and D acute coinfection has a course of illness similar to that in a patient with only hepatitis B infection. If a patient with chronic hepatitis B becomes superinfected with hepatitis D virus, a fulminant or severe acute hepatitis often results. Prevention of hepatitis B through immunization also prevents hepatitis D.

The presentation of viral hepatitis, most commonly with acute HAV and HBV infection, usually includes malaise, myalgia, fatigue, nausea, and anorexia. Aversion to cigarette smoke exposure is often reported. Occasionally, arthritis-like symptoms and skin rash are also noted. Mild fever occasionally occurs. Hepatomegaly with usually mild right upper quadrant abdominal tenderness without rebound is found in about 50% of patients, with splenomegaly in about 15%. Jaundice typically occurs about 1 week after the onset of symptoms. Jaundice is not found in most cases, however. The course of the illness is typically 2 to 3 weeks. During this period, a gradual increase in energy, appetite, and well-being is reported.

Laboratory findings common to all forms of viral hepatitis include leukopenia with lymphocytosis. Atypical lymphocytes are often found. Bilirubin in the urine is usually found in the absence of icterus. Hepatic enzyme elevation is universal. Serological findings help with the diagnosis of the type of hepatitis. Knowledge of measures to prevent hepatitis or minimize its acquisition after exposure is important to safe, effective practice (see Table 7–6).

The test of liver enzymes is an evaluation of the degree of hepatic inflammation. Hepatic enzymes are found in the circulation because of hepatic growth and repair. The aspartate aminotransferase (AST) level increases in response to hepatocyte injury, as often occurs in alcohol abuse, acetaminophen misuse or overdose, and quite rarely the therapeutic use of HMG-CoA reductase inhibitors (lipid-lowering drugs whose names have the "-statin" suffix, such as simvastatin). This enzyme is also found in skeletal muscle, myocardium, brain, and kidneys in smaller amounts, and so damage to these areas may also cause an increase in AST.

AST (formerly known as serum glutamic oxaloacetic transaminase [SGOT]) is a hepatic enzyme with a circulatory half-life of approximately 12 to 24 hours; levels increase in response to hepatic damage and clear quickly after damage ceases. AST elevation is generally found in only about 10% of problem drinkers. If the AST level is elevated with normal alanine aminotransferase (ALT) level and mild macrocytosis (mean corpuscular volume 100 fL or greater, seen in about 30% to 60% of men who drink five or more drinks per day and in women who drink three or more drinks per day), long-standing alcohol abuse is the likely cause.

ALT (formerly known as serum glutamate pyruvate transaminase [SGPT]) is more specific to the liver, having limited concentration in other organs. This enzyme has a longer half-life, 37 to 57 hours, than AST. Elevation of ALT levels persists longer after hepatic damage has ceased. The greatest elevation of this enzyme is likely seen in hepatitis caused by infection or inflammation, with a lesser degree of elevation noted in the presence of alcohol abuse. When evaluating a patient with suspected substance abuse causing hepatic dysfunction, the NP must note the degree of AST or ALT elevation.

An increase in bilirubin level is typically found in patients with viral hepatitis. Clinical jaundice is found when the total bilirubin level exceeds 2.5 mg. Bilirubin is the degradation product of heme, with 85% to 90% arising from hemoglobin and a smaller percentage arising from myoglobin. Bilirubin is produced at a rate of about 4 mg/kg/d in healthy individuals. Because the rate of excretion usually matches the rate of production, the levels remain low and stable. Reticuloendothelial cells take in haptoglobin, a protein that binds with hemoglobin from aged red blood cells (RBCs). The reticuloendothelial cells remove the iron from hemoglobin for recycling. The remaining substances are degraded to bilirubin in its unconjugated, or indirect, form. This form is not water soluble.

When unconjugated bilirubin is released into the circulation, it binds to albumin and is transported to the liver. When unconjugated bilirubin arrives at the liver, hepatocytes detach bilirubin from the albumin. It is then in a water-soluble form, also known as conjugated, or direct, bilirubin. Conjugated bilirubin loosely attaches to albumin and is easily detached in the kidney. The passing of small amounts of conjugated bilirubin through the kidney gives urine its characteristic yellow color. Conjugated bilirubin not excreted by the kidney is reabsorbed by the small intestine and converted to urobilinogen by bacterial action in the gut. This urobilinogen can be reabsorbed into the circulation, and excess amounts can appear in the urine. Small amounts of urobilinogen may also be found in a fecally contaminated urine sample because urobilinogen is normally found in the large intestine.

When there is an excess of urinary excretion of bilirubin, as found in patients with viral hepatitis, urine develops a characteristic brown color, often described by a patient as looking like cola or dark tea. Also, excess bilirubin could displace drugs with a high propensity for protein (albumin) binding, increasing free drug and possibly causing drug toxicity.

Treatment of acute viral hepatitis is largely supportive. Corticosteroids, antiviral agents, and interferon are used occasionally. Because of the seriousness of hepatitis B and C sequelae and risk of the development of chronic infection, considerable research is under way to develop effective, well-tolerated therapies. Chronic hepatitis B and C are potent risk factors for hematoma or primary hepatocellular carcinoma. Periodic monitoring for alpha-fetoprotein is often used to look for an increase in the level that indicates hepatic tumor growth, usually coupled with imaging such as abdominal ultrasound or CT. Consultation with a hepatitis specialist and awareness of the latest recommendations for ongoing monitoring are critical.

DISCUSSION SOURCES

Centers for Disease Control and Prevention: Hepatitis A FAQs for Health Professionals. Available at www.cdc.gov/hepatitis/hav/havfaq.htm
Centers for Disease Control and Prevention: Hepatitis B Information for Health Professionals. Available at www.cdc.gov/hepatitis/hbv

IBS and IBD

125. In a 28-year-old man who presents with a 6-month history of involuntary weight loss, recurrent abdominal cramping, loose stools, and anterior and posterior anal fissure, which of the following diagnoses should be considered?
    A. ulcerative colitis
    B. Crohn's disease
    C. *C. difficile* colitis
    D. condyloma acuminata

126. Which of the following patient complaints should be evaluated further in making a differential of irritable bowel syndrome (IBS)?
    A. a 52-year-old female with a first degree family history of colorectal cancer, recent constipation, and abdominal pain
    B. a middle-aged adult with low albumin and leukocytosis
    C. both patients outlined in responses A and B
    D. a 16-year-old female with chronic, alternating constipation and diarrhea when she is studying for high school exams and worrying about her parents' impending divorce

127. The pathophysiology of IBS can be best described as:
    A. shares the same pathophysiology as inflammatory bowel disease.
    B. a patchy inflammatory process in the small bowel that most adolescents will outgrow with vigorous exercise and a low residue diet.
    C. a condition that is the result of abnormal gut motor/sensory activity
    D. an overstimulation of pancreatic beta cell production.

128. Diagnostic criteria for irritable bowel syndrome include abdominal pain that is associated with all of the following except:
    A. improvement with defecation.
    B. a change in frequency of stool.
    C. a change of stool form.
    D. unexplained weight loss.

129. When considering an IBS diagnosis, the NP should be aware that:
    A. diagnosis is largely based on clinical presentation and application of the Rome III Criteria.
    B. a colonoscopy should be done routinely when the diagnosis is suspected.
    C. CBC, ESR, CRP and serum albumin should be the initial labs for an IBS workup.
    D. once an IBS diagnosis has been confirmed, you can assure the patient that treatment is generally curative.

130. Altering the gut pain threshold in IBS is a possible therapeutic outcome with the use of:
    A. loperamide (Imodium®).
    B. dicyclomine (Bentyl®).
    C. bismuth subsalicylate (Pepto-Bismol®).
    D. amitriptyline (Elavil®).

131. Tenesmus is defined as which of the following?
    A. rectal burning with defecation
    B. a sensation of incomplete bowel emptying that is distressing and sometimes painful
    C. weight loss that accompanies many bowel diseases
    D. appearance of frank blood in the stool

132. Concerning IBS, which of the following statements is most accurate?
    A. Patients most often report chronic diarrhea as the most distressing part of the problems.
    B. Weight gain is often reported.
    C. Patients can present with bowel issues ranging from diarrhea to constipation.
    D. The condition is associated with a strongly increased risk of colorectal cancer.

133. An example of a medication with prokinetic activity is:
    A. dicyclomine (Bentyl).
    B. metoclopramide (Reglan®).
    C. loperamide (Imodium).
    D. psyllium (Metamucil®).

134. Diagnostic testing in IBS often reveals:
    A. evidence of underlying inflammation.
    B. anemia of chronic disease.
    C. normal results on most testing.
    D. mucosal thickening on abdominal radiological imaging.

135. Which of the following is an appropriate treatment for IBS?
    A. high fat, low residue diet.
    B. high fiber, low fat diet and stress modification.
    C. antispasmotics and loperamide for diarrhea predominance.
    D. tricyclic antidepressants for constipation predominance.

136. The clinical indication for the use of lubiprostone (Amitiza®) is for:
    A. the treatment of constipation that is not amenable to standard therapies.
    B. intervention in intractable diarrhea.
    C. control of intestinal inflammation.
    D. the relief of intestinal spasms.

137. Irritable bowel syndrome is characterized by all of the following except:
    A. weight loss and malnutrition.
    B. abdominal pain or discomfort (hypersensitivity) at least three times per month for a 6-month period.
    C. ltered bowel pattern in the absence of detected structural abnormalities.
    D. occurs two to three times more often in women than men.

138. Diagnostic testing in inflammatory bowel disease (IBD) often reveals:
    A. evidence of underlying inflammation.
    B. notation of intestinal parasites.
    C. normal results on most testing.
    D. a characteristic intraabdominal mass on radiological imaging.

139. Laboratory evaluation during an IBD flare will reveal elevated levels of all of the following except:
A. CRP.
B. SeCr.
C. ESR.
D. WBC.

140. IBD is associated with all of the following types of anemia except:
A. anemia of chronic disease.
B. iron-deficiency anemia.
C. megaloblastic anemia.
D. anemia associated with acute blood loss.

141. Which of the following best describes the hemogram results in a person with anemia of chronic disease that often accompanies IBD?
A. microcytic, hypochromic
B. macrocytic, normochromic
C. normocytic, normochromic
D. hyperproliferative

142. IBD is a term usually used to describe:
A. ulcerative colitis and irritable bowel syndrome.
B. *C. difficile* colitis and Crohn's disease.
C. Crohn's disease and ulcerative colitis.
D. inflammatory colitis and ileitis.

143. "Skip lesions" are usually reported during colonoscopy in:
A. irritable bowel syndrome.
B. ulcerative colitis.
C. Crohn's disease.
D. *C. difficile* colitis.

144. First-line therapy for Crohn's disease or ulcerative colitis is:
A. oral aminosalicylates.
B. parenteral corticosteroids.
C. antibiotics.
D. immune modulators.

145. Immune modulators are often used for intervention in:
A. ulcerative colitis.
B. irritable bowel syndrome.
C. Crohn's disease.
D. ulcerative colitis and Crohn's disease.

146. After a decade of disease, a person with ulcerative colitis is at increased risk of malignancy involving the:
A. small bowel.
B. large intestine.
C. duodenum.
D. stomach.

147. Crohn's disease is associated with increased risk of malignancy involving the:
A. small bowel.
B. large intestine.
C. duodenum.
D. stomach.

148 to 158. Which of the following statements is most consistent with IBD, IBS, or both conditions?

_____ **148.** Onset of symptoms is before age 30 to 40 years in most cases.

_____ **149.** The patient population is predominately female.

_____ **150.** The condition is often referred to as spastic colon by the general population.

_____ **151.** Extraintestinal manifestations occasionally include nondestructive arthritis and renal calculi.

_____ **152.** This is a potentially life-threatening condition.

_____ **153.** The etiology likely involves an autoimmune response to the GI tract.

_____ **154.** Patients should be advised to avoid trigger foods.

_____ **155.** Involvement can be limited to intestinal mucosa only, or the full thickness of the intestinal wall can be involved.

_____ **156.** The etiology is considered to be an alteration in small and large bowel motility.

_____ **157.** Potential complications include fistula formation and perineal disease.

_____ **158.** Potential complications include increased risk for colonic malignancy.

● Answers

125. B.	**137.** A.	**149.** IBS
126. C.	**138.** A.	**150.** IBS
127. C.	**139.** B.	**151.** IBD
128. D.	**140.** C.	**152.** IBD
129. A.	**141.** C.	**153.** IBD
130. D.	**142.** C.	**154.** Both
131. B.	**143.** C.	**155.** IBD
132. C.	**144.** A.	**156.** IBS
133. B.	**145.** D.	**157.** IBD
134. C.	**146.** B.	**158.** IBD
135. C.	**147.** A.	
136. A.	**148.** Both	

Irritable bowel syndrome (IBS) is a functional bowel disorder characterized by abdominal pain or discomfort and altered bowel habits in the absence of detectable structural abnormalities. This condition is sometimes called spastic colon, irritable colon, or nervous colon. Around the world, 10% to 20% of adults and adolescents have symptoms consistent with IBS and most studies show a female predominance. IBS affects all ages but most have their first symptoms before age 45. Women are diagnosed two to three times as often as men and make up 80% of the population with severe IBS. IBS symptoms tend to come and go over time and often overlap with other functional disorders such as fibromyalgia, headache, backache, and genitourinary symptoms. Severity of symptoms varies and can significantly impact quality of life and drive up healthcare costs.

Diagnosis of the condition is usually made via careful history and clinical presentation, with a focus on excluding other conditions as there are no clear diagnostic markers. The Rome III criteria for the diagnosis of IBS require that patients must have recurrent abdominal pain or discomfort (uncomfortable sensation not described as pain) at least 3 days/month in the last 3 months associated with two or more of the following: discomfort relieved by defecation, symptom onset associated with a change in stool frequency, or symptom onset associated with a change in stool form or appearance. Abdominal pain/discomfort is highly variable in its intensity and location. Often it is episodic and crampy, may be mild, or it may interfere with activities of daily living (ADLs). Additional symptoms usually include altered stool frequency, form, or passage (or a combination of two or all three), usually accompanied by mucorrhea and abdominal bloating or the sensation of distention or both. Malnutrition is rare and sleep deprivation is infrequent except for those with severe IBS; nocturnal pain is a poor discriminator of organic versus functional bowel disease. Bleeding is not a feature of IBS unless hemorrhoids are present. Malabsorption and weight loss does not occur.

People with IBS often present with one of four typical bowel patterns:

- IBS, diarrhea prominent (IBS-D): small volumes of loose stools, volumes less than 200 ml without nocturnal diarrhea. Is often aggravated by emotional stress or eating, with passage of large amounts of mucous,
- IBS, constipation predominant (IBS-C): can be first episodic then become intractable to laxatives with hard, narrowed stool caliber and a sense of incomplete evacuation for weeks or months interrupted with brief periods of diarrhea,
- IBS, diarrhea and constipation alternating (IBS-A): eventually one becoming more predominant or a mixed stool pattern,
- IBS, mixed diarrhea and constipation (IBS-M).

Also, gut dysfunction occurs along a continuum, with most patients moving from type to type. Usually the patient reports that these symptoms have been present for many years before care was sought. Patients frequently complain of abdominal distension, increased belching or flatulence, which they contribute to increased gas. Most IBS patients have normal amounts of intestinal gas, but have impaired transit and tolerance to the intestinal gas loads. Belching may be explained by reflux gas from the distal to more proximal intestine. Approximately 25% to 50% of patients complain of upper GI symptoms, including dyspepsia, heartburn, nausea, and vomiting.

Women are diagnosed with the condition more often. Most individuals with the condition have onset of symptoms before age 35 years, often reporting problems since childhood. Although IBS onset can occur after age 40 years, an alternative GI diagnosis, including malignancy, becomes more likely and should be carefully considered.

Advances in research and science have demonstrated that the etiology of IBS may be multifactorial, with proposed mechanisms involving abnormal gut motor/sensory activity, central neural dysfunction, psychological disturbances, mucosal inflammation, stress, and luminal factors. Although the mood component of the disease has often been attributed to the resulting disease-induced suffering, in reality, anxiety or depression or both often predate IBS onset.

Unstimulated colonic myoelectric and motor activity studies have not shown consistent abnormalities in IBS. Patients frequently exhibit exaggerated sensory responses to visceral stimulation. Central nervous system factors are strongly suggested by clinical associations of emotional disorders and stress that affect the mid-cingulate cortex— the brain region concerned with attention processes and response selection—showing greater activation in response to distal colonic stimulation. The risk of developing IBS increases after an episode of acute gastroenteritis. Additionally, a high prevalence of small intestinal bacterial overgrowth detected by positive lactulose hydrogen breath testing has been seen. Probiotic use is an emerging treatment option that likely helps to normalize the possibly altered gut flora. A small subset of IBS-D patients also have elevated serotonin (5HT)-containing enterochromaffin cells in the colon as a contributing factor to their disease.

Due to the nonspecific GI symptoms of IBS, several other diagnoses must be considered, including inflammatory bowel disease (IBD), colonic neoplasia, Celiac disease, lactase deficiency, endometriosis, depression and anxiety, sexual and physical abuse, and small bowel bacterial overgrowth. On physical presentation, a person with IBS usually has tenderness in the sigmoid region; the remainder of the examination is usually normal. Diagnostic testing is not required initially in patients whose symptoms are compatible with IBS. However, further tests are warranted in those who do not improve in 2 to 4 weeks of empiric therapy. Laboratory analysis is usually directed at ruling out another cause for the condition and typically reveals a normal hemogram, a normal erythrocyte sedimentation rate, and a negative test for fecal occult blood. Glucose or lactulose breath tests are used to rule out small bowel bacterial overgrowth. Stool analysis for ova, parasite, enteric pathogens, leukocytes, and *Clostridium difficile* toxin are negative. If imaging studies, such as GI barium study, ultrasound, or abdominal CT or endoscopy, are indicated by clinical presentation, the results are usually normal. Referral to a gastroenterology specialist should be considered, particularly if the diagnosis is in question; a gastroenterology specialist also can provide input to the treatment plan.

Intervention in IBS involves patient support and education about the nature of the condition, including information that life expectancy is not affected, the condition is usually chronic with periodic exacerbations, and stress is a common trigger. Nutritional intervention can be helpful, with adequate hydration, addition of dietary fiber (at least 25 to 35 grams daily with at least four to six glasses of water), avoidance of trigger foods, and moderation of caffeine intake often reported as being helpful. Common triggers to aggravate IBS symptoms include coffee, disaccharides, legumes, cabbage, a high carbohydrate diet, and excessive fructose and artificial sweeteners, such as sorbitol or mannitol. Fiber supplementation is often helpful with diarrhea and constipation; polycarbophil-based products, such as FiberCon®, offer a potential advantage over psyllium by causing less flatulence. Although some patients report improvement with avoidance of lactose or fructose, others do not.

Intervention with medications is usually aimed at treating the predominant symptom (Table 7–7). Loperamide (Imodium) and anticholinergics/antispasmodics such as dicyclomine (Bentyl) are prescribed to treat diarrhea; the use of these medications can result in constipation. Low-dose tricyclic antidepressant or selective serotonin reuptake inhibitor use can be helpful in altering the gut pain threshold, resulting in less abdominal pain; the anticholinergic effects of the tricyclic antidepressants can help with limiting stool frequency, but also worsen constipation. Prokinetic or promotility agents have been used for patients with constipation-dominant symptoms. Because of safety issues, many of these products have significant use limitations; some have been withdrawn from the market. Other prokinetics, such as metoclopramide (Reglan) and erythromycin, have not yielded consistent benefits in patients with IBS. Lubiprostone (Amitiza), approved for the treatment of constipation that is not amenable to standard therapies, promotes fluid secretion into the intestinal lumen and is a helpful option in constipation-dominant IBS.

Inflammatory bowel disease (IBD) is a disease of unclear etiology, but likely involves an autoimmune response to the

TABLE 7-7
Treatment Medication Classifications for IBD

ANTISPASMODICS (ANTICHOLINERGIC) AGENTS:
Dicyclomine, hyoscyamine, methscopolamine

ANTIDIARRHEAL AGENTS:
Loperamide

OSMOTIC LAXATIVES:
Miralax®
Milk of magnesia
Lubiprostone

TRICYCLIC AND RELATED ANTIDEPRESSANTS (NOT RECOMMENDED WITH PATIENTS WITH PREDOMINANT CONSTIPATION):
Nortriptyline, desipramine, or imipramine

SEROTONIN REUPTAKE INHIBITORS (NOT RECOMMENDED FOR PATIENTS WITH PREDOMINANT DIARRHEA):
Sertraline, Fluoxetine, Citalopram, Paroxetine

GI tract. This condition has a genetic component; whether this is a predisposition or susceptibility is unclear. The two major types of IBD are ulcerative colitis (UC), in which the pathological changes are limited to the colon, and Crohn's disease, in which the changes can involve any part of the GI tract. In contrast to IBS, the male-to-female ratio is approximately equal for UC and Crohn's disease. Similar to IBS, IBD is most often diagnosed in late adolescence to early adulthood, with most individuals who develop the disease showing symptoms by their late 20s. Less commonly, new-onset IBD is diagnosed in a child or adult.

The diagnosis of IBD is usually made through a combination of careful health history, physical examination, and appropriate diagnostic investigations, including radiography, endoscopy, and biopsy. The manifestations of IBD generally depend on the area of the intestinal tract involved. Patients with UC or Crohn's disease frequently have bloody diarrhea, occasionally with tenesmus. Patients with Crohn's disease involving the small intestine frequently have abdominal pain, involuntary weight loss, diarrhea, and occasionally they have symptoms of intestinal obstruction. The presence of anterior and posterior anal fissures should raise suspicion for Crohn's disease. A cobblestone mucosal pattern is often identified on endoscopy or contrast radiography in Crohn's disease. "Skip lesions," areas of affected mucosal tissue alternating with normal tissue, are common; the rectum is often spared with the terminal ileum and right colon involved in most cases. In UC, inflammation is limited to the mucosa, whereas in Crohn's disease, the entire intestinal wall is involved.

During an IBD flare, serological markers of inflammation, including C-reactive protein (CRP) and erythrocyte sedimentation rate (ESR or sed rate) are usually elevated. Leukocytosis is often present. In Crohn's disease, fistulas and perianal disease are often noted. Toxic colitis, characterized by nonobstructive colonic dilation with signs of systemic toxicity, can occur as a potentially life-threatening complication of either condition; this condition is usually infectious in origin, with *C. difficile* often implicated.

Anemia is a common problem in IBD; its etiology is often from multiple causes. Iron-deficiency anemia, manifesting as a microcytic, hypochromic anemia, occurs as a result of chronic blood loss. Anemia of chronic disease, a normocytic, normochromic anemia, is a result of inflammation of IBD, whereas anemia associated with acute blood loss can occur as a result of GI hemorrhage during a flare. Vitamin B_{12} deficiency, manifesting as a macrocytic, normochromic anemia, can also result in Crohn's disease, usually in the presence of significant terminal ileum disease. Because of the difficulty with micronutrient absorption, including iron and vitamin B_{12}, with Crohn's disease, parenteral replacement therapy is often preferred over the oral route. Additional extraintestinal manifestations in IBD include a nondestructive axial or peripheral arthritis in 15% of cases. Renal calculi are often found with Crohn's disease.

The care for a person with IBD is usually a combination of lifestyle support, medication, and occasionally surgery. A person with IBD should be counseled to keep track of dietary triggers. Lactose intolerance is common in Crohn's disease, but no more common than in the general population in people with UC. Tobacco use is associated with greater Crohn's disease, but not UC, activity. Smoking cessation should be encouraged for this and its numerous additional health benefits. Gut rest is often used during treatment of Crohn's disease, but not UC flares. Although IBD is likely genetic, not psychological, in origin, mental health and social support are important treatment components as the patient and family cope with this chronic, life-altering, and potentially life-threatening disease.

Medication therapy in IBD is usually initiated at the time of a flare, often the most common point of disease diagnosis. In Crohn's disease and UC, oral aminosalicylates, including sulfasalazine (Azulfidine®) and mesalamine (Apriso®), are usually the first-line therapy and are equally effective. Mesalamine is usually better tolerated and can be used in the presence of sulfa allergy. In UC, when disease is limited to the distal colon, mesalamine and corticosteroids can be administered rectally. Oral or parenteral corticosteroid use can provide rapid symptom relief because of potent anti-inflammatory effects. In Crohn's disease, metronidazole and ciprofloxacin are used when perineal disease or an inflammatory mass is noted; antibiotic use in UC is discouraged because of the increased risk of *C. difficile* infection. Immune modulators including 6-mercaptopurine and azathioprine are often prescribed to provide long-term disease control. A monoclonal antibody against tumor necrosis factor-alpha, infliximab (Remicade®), is also a potentially helpful, although costly, treatment option, assisting in remission in about 80% of individuals with Crohn's disease and about 50% of

individuals with UC. Additional biologicals approved for the treatment of IBD include adalimumab (Humira®, monoclonal antibody against TNF-α), certolizumab (Cimzia®, monoclonal antibody against TNF-α), and natalizumab (Tysabri®, monoclonal antibody against alpha-4 integrin). Other immune modulators such as methotrexate and cyclosporine have been used with some success. Probiotic therapy is an emerging option, used to help normalize gut flora.

The course of IBD is quite variable. A person with UC has approximately a 50% chance of having a flare in 2 years after achieving disease remission; this number is lower, about 40%, for a person with Crohn's disease. With UC, colorectal cancer risk is greatly increased after about a decade of disease; as a result, surveillance colonoscopy is recommended every 2 years after 8 to 10 years of disease. In contrast, with Crohn's disease, there is an increased risk for small bowel malignancy. At present, no effective screening is available for IBD. Given the complexities in diagnosis and treatment for a person with IBD, expert consultation should be sought.

Table 7–8 compares IBS and IBD.

DISCUSSION SOURCES

Lehrer J, Lichtenstein G. http://emedicine.medscape.com/article/180389, eMedicine: Irritable bowel syndrome
Rowe W. Inflammatory bowel disease. http://emedicine.medscape.com/article/179037, eMedicine
Harrison's Principles of Internal Medicine, 18th Edition Textbook. Accessed from: www.harrisonsim.com.
Quick Answers to Medical Diagnosis and Treatment: Lange Medical Books. Accessed from: www.accessmedicine.com/content.aspx?aID=3267440&searchStr=irritable+bowel+syndrome.

TABLE 7-8
Irritable Bowel Syndrome (IBS) versus Inflammatory Bowel Disease (IBD)

WHAT THESE HAVE IN COMMON: HISTORY
Chronically recurring symptoms of abdominal pain, discomfort (urgency and bloating), and alterations in bowel habits

WHAT ARE THEIR DIFFERENCES?

IBS	IBD (Ulcerative Colitis, Crohn's Disease)
No detectable structural abnormalities	Intestinal ulceration, inflammation
Absence of rectal bleeding, fever, weight loss, elevated CRP, ESR	• Crohn's: Mouth to anus
Intervention	• UC: Colon only
• Lifestyle modification such as diet, fiber, fluids, exercise	Rectal bleeding, diarrhea, fever, weight loss, elevated CRP, ESR, leukocytosis, especially during flares
• Medications as indicated by symptoms (antidiarrheals or promotility agents)	Intervention
	• Lifestyle modification such as diet, fluids, exercise
	• Immune modulators
	• Anti-inflammatory medications as indicated by clinical presentation and response
	• Surgical intervention often needed and careful ongoing monitoring for gastrointestinal malignancy

CRP—C-reactive protein; ESR—erythrocyte sedimentation rate.

Celiac Disease

159. Celiac disease is also called all of the following except:
A. gluten-induced enteropathy
B. celiac sprue
C. sprue
D. small bowel malabsorption syndrome

160. All of the following characterize celiac disease except:
A. temporary immunological gluten disorder.
B. affects more often people of Northern European ancestry.
C. causes diffuse damage to the proximal small intestinal mucosa with malabsorption of nutrients.
D. often misdiagnosed as irritable bowel disease.

161. Celiac disease's classic presentation can include all of the following except:
A. weight loss, chronic diarrhea, and muscle wasting.
B. flatulence and abdominal distension.
C. as growth restriction when diagnosed in children less than 2 years old.
D. reported egg intolerance.

162. The most accurate serological markers to diagnose celiac sprue are:
A. ESR and CRP.
B. IgA endomysial and IgA tTG antibodies.
C. mucosal biopsies of the terminal ileum.
D. *H. pylori* IgG antibodies.

163. Patients with celiac disease present with similar signs and symptoms of all of the following conditions except:
A. acute appendicitis.
B. bacterial overgrowth.
C. cow's milk intolerance.
D. tropical sprue.

164. Which of the following would be an acceptable food choice for a person with celiac disease?
A. beer and popcorn
B. vegetarian pizza
C. steak with mashed potatoes
D. chicken nuggets

165. An 8-year-old girl is diagnosed with celiac disease. When counseling her parents, you advise that the child should:
A. consume whole grains, especially wheat, oats and barley.
B. carefully plan exercise to minimize symptoms.
C. avoid intake of semolina, spelt, and rye.
D. avoid birthday parties or other gatherings that may expose the child to offending foods.

Answers

159. D.	**162.** B.	**165.** C.
160. A.	**163.** A.	
161. D.	**164.** C.	

Celiac disease (also called sprue, celiac sprue, and gluten enteropathy) is a permanent dietary disorder caused by an immunological response to gluten, a storage protein found in certain grains that results in diffuse damage to the proximal small intestinal mucosa with malabsorption of nutrients. Although symptoms may manifest between 6 months and 24 months of age after the introduction of weaning foods, the majority of cases present in childhood or adulthood. Population screening with serological testing suggests that the disease is present in 1:100 whites of Northern European ancestry. A clinical diagnosis is only made in about 10% of individuals and most cases tend to be undiagnosed or asymptomatic.

Although the precise pathogenesis is unclear, celiac disease arises in a small subset of genetically susceptible (-DQ2 or -DQ8) individuals when dietary gluten stimulates an inappropriate immunological response. Glutens are partially digested in the intestinal lumen into glutamine-rich peptides. Some of the glutamines are deamidated by the enzyme tTG, generating negatively charged glutamic acid residues. If these peptides are able to bind to HLA-DQ2 or -DQ8 molecules on antigen-presenting cells, they may stimulate an inappropriate T cell–mediated activation in the intestinal submucosa that results in destruction of mucosal enterocytes as well as a humoral immune response that results in antibodies to gluten, tTG, and other autoantigens.

Clinical presentation in adults may be confused with other diseases because of overlapping signs and symptoms. Symptoms are typically present for at least ten years before a correct diagnosis is made and often depend on the patient's age and extent of small bowel disease.

Many patients with chronic diarrhea and flatulence can be misdiagnosed as having irritable bowel syndrome. Celiac sprue must be distinguished from other causes of malabsorption. Severe pan-malabsorption of multiple nutrients almost always implies mucosal disease. Other causes such as tropical sprue, bacterial overgrowth, cow's milk intolerance, viral gastroenteritis, eosinophilic gastroenteritis, and acid hypersecretion from gastrinoma need to be ruled out.

Treatment is focused on a number of factors including the following:
- A gluten-free diet is essential (all wheat, rye, and barley must be eliminated). Examples of gluten substitutes are rice, corn, millet, potato, buckwheat, and soybeans. Refer to a knowledgeable dietician and encourage a lay support group.
- Avoidance of dairy products temporarily or permanently if necessary until intestinal symptoms resolve.
- Dietary supplements repletion until intestinal symptoms has resolved (folate, iron, calcium, and vitamins A, B_{12}, D, and E). Vitamin and mineral levels should be checked periodically to prevent deficiencies.

DISCUSSION SOURCES

Celiac Disease Foundation, 13251 Ventura Blvd, Suite #1, Studio City, CA 91604-1838. www.celiac.org.

Katz KD, et al. Screening for celiac disease in a North American population: Sequential serology and gastrointestinal symptoms. *Am J Gastroenterol* 106(7):1333–1339, 2011. [PMID: 21364545]

Papdakis MA, McPhee SJ, Rabow MW. *Current Medical Diagnosis & Treatment 2013.* CMDT Online 2013. The McGraw-Hill Companies.

Ionizing Radiation

Match the imaging study with the equivalent amount of background radiation: (An answer can be used more than once.)

166. Abdominal CT scan.

167. Abdominal MRI.

168. Abdominal ultrasound.

169. Abdominal X-ray.
A. No radiation
B. 62 to 88 days
C. 3 years

Answers

166. C.   **167.** A.   **168.** A.   **169.** B.

The use of radiography can be an essential tool in clinical evaluation and diagnosis. However, the rapid growth in the use of these procedures, such as CT scans, has led to concern about low-dose ionizing radiation doses. The primary concern with radiation exposure is an increased risk for developing a malignancy. Other adverse effects of exposure to low-dose ionizing radiation have also been suspected, such as an increased risk for the development of cataracts following repeated head CT scans that include the lens of the eye. Appropriate use of these techniques requires understanding the balance of long-term risks inherent with radiation exposure with the necessity of utilizing these imaging studies.

The amount of radiation exposure can vary significantly depending on the type of imaging study being conducted. It is important to remember that all of us are exposed to radiation on a daily basis, mainly from the sun and soil. The entire body is exposed to this background radiation, compared with only certain parts of the body when conducting medical imaging studies. A comparison of the radiation doses from various types of imaging studies is shown in Table 7-9.

Minimizing exposure to radiation depends on good methodology and quality control. Using the lowest possible dose should be desired, with consideration of first using non-ionizing radiation examinations, such as MRI or ultrasound, if possible. Repeating radiological examinations should be avoided at other clinics or sites.

DISCUSSION SOURCE

Coakley F, Gould R, Yeh B, Arenson R. CT Radiation Dose: What Can You Do Right Now in Your Practice? *AJR* 196:619–625, 2077. Available at: www.ajronline.org/content/196/3/619.full.pdf+html

Pancreatitis and Pancreatic Cancer

170. Risk factors for acute pancreatitis include all of the following except:
A. hypothyroidism.
B. dyslipidemia.
C. abdominal trauma.
D. thiazide diuretic use.

TABLE 7-9
Radiation Doses from Common Imaging Studies*

Test	Dose (mSv)	Equivalent Period of Background Radiation
Chest x-ray (standard two views)	0.06–0.1	8–12 days
Abdomen x-ray	0.5–0.7	62–88 days
Abdomen and pelvis CT*	10.0	3 years
Virtual colonoscopy	10.2	3 years
Whole-body PET/low dose CT	8.5–10.3	3 years
Whole-body PET/full dose CT	23.7–26.4	8–9 years
Abdominal ultrasound	No ionizing radiation exposure	Not applicable
Abdominal MRI	No ionizing radiation exposure	Not applicable

*The ionizing radiation doses mentioned here represent an average for the study.
Source: Coakley F, Gould R, Yeh B, Arenson R. CT Radiation Dose: What Can You Do Right Now in Your
   Practice? www.ajronline.org/content/196/3/619.full.pdf+html

171. Ms. Lane, a 38-year-old woman with a long-standing history of alcohol abuse, presents with a 4-day history of a midabdominal ache that radiates through to the back, remains relatively constant, and has been accompanied by nausea and three episodes of vomiting. She has tried taking antacids without relief. Her skin is cool and moist with a blood pressure of 90/72 mm Hg, pulse rate of 120 bpm, and respiratory rate of 24/min. Findings that would support a diagnosis of acute pancreatitis include all of the following except:
    A. elevated serum amylase level.
    B. elevated lipase level.
    C. jaundice.
    D. upper abdominal tenderness without localization or rebound.

172. Your next best action in caring for Ms. Lane in the previous question is to:
    A. refer to the acute care hospital for admission.
    B. attempt office hydration after administration of an analgesic agent.
    C. initiate therapy with ranitidine (Zantac) and an antacid.
    D. obtain serum electrolyte levels.

173. Other than the pancreas, other sources of amylase include all of the following except:
    A. salivary glands.
    B. lung cancer.
    C. ovarian cyst.
    D. adipose tissue.

174. Elevated lipase levels can be a result of all of the following conditions except:
    A. hepatic failure.
    B. renal failure.
    C. perforated duodenal ulcer.
    D. bowel obstruction or infarction.

175. Which of the following statements is true when evaluating a patient with acute pancreatitis?
    A. Diagnosis can be made by clinical assessment alone.
    B. The pancreas can be clearly visualized by abdominal ultrasound.
    C. Measuring serum lipase level along with amylase level increases diagnostic specificity in acute pancreatitis.
    D. Hypocalcemia is a nearly universal finding.

176. When using the Ranson criteria to evaluate the severity of acute pancreatitis, a severe clinical course is predicted with a score of:
    A. less than 2.
    B. 3 or greater.
    C. 6 or greater.
    D. 8 or greater.

177. Common signs and symptoms of a pancreatic pseudocyst include all of the following except:
    A. abdominal pain that radiates to the back.
    B. nausea and vomiting.
    C. jaundice.
    D. a mass that can be felt in the upper abdomen.

178. Which of the following diagnostic tests is most effective in determining if a pseudocyst is benign?
    A. CT scan
    B. MRI scan
    C. analysis of cyst fluid
    D. serum amylase and lipase levels

179. A 56-year-old man with a history of colon cancer undergoes a follow-up abdominal MRI scan. A small mass is identified on the pancreas that is later diagnosed as a benign pseudocyst. The pseudocyst is not causing any symptoms and measures 8 mm in diameter. You consider:
    A. repeating the scan in 1 year to check for any changes.
    B. draining the pseudocyst.
    C. surgical removal of the pseudocyst.
    D. initiating a regimen of antiinflammatory medication to decrease the size of the pseudocyst.

180. Risk factors for pancreatic cancer include all of the following except:
    A. hypertension.
    B. history of chronic pancreatitis.
    C. tobacco use.
    D. diabetes mellitus.

181. In assessing a person with suspected pancreatic cancer, the nurse practitioner anticipates which of the following findings?
    A. palpable midline abdominal mass
    B. midepigastric pain that radiates to the midback or lower back region
    C. presence of Cullen sign
    D. positive obturator and psoas signs

182. All of the following laboratory findings are expected in a patient with pancreatic cancer except:
    A. elevated total bilirubin.
    B. diminished platelet count.
    C. elevated alkaline phosphatase.
    D. elevated direct bilirubin.

183. The clinical presentation of pancreatic cancer involving the head of the pancreas usually includes:
    A. painless jaundice.
    B. polycythemia.
    C. hematuria.
    D. hyperkalemia.

184. Which of the following is least likely to be found in a person with pancreatic cancer?
A. history of chronic pancreatitis
B. lesion identified on abdominal CT
C. normocytic, normochromic anemia
D. elevation of amylase level

Answers

170. A.	175. C.	180. A.
171. C.	176. B.	181. B.
172. A.	177. C.	182. B.
173. D.	178. C.	183. A.
174. A.	179. A.	184. D.

Pancreatitis, characterized by an acute or chronic inflammation of the organ, is a potentially life-threatening condition. The most common risks for pancreatitis are biliary tract disease including gallstones (45%), excessive alcohol use (35%), and elevated triglyceride levels and idiopathic causes (20% combined). Although alcohol abuse is commonly thought of as being one of the most common contributing factors for the disease, a small percentage of people who are problem drinkers develop the condition; likely the etiology of pancreatitis is multifactorial. Binge drinkers are at risk; most alcohol-related acute pancreatitis occurs in people with a minimum of 5 to 7 years of heavy ethanol ingestion, with binge drinkers having much lower risk. Less common risk factors are use of opioids, corticosteroid use, and thiazide diuretics, viral infection, and blunt abdominal trauma.

In a patient with acute pancreatitis, serum amylase level is typically elevated. Because elevated amylase level is often found in many other conditions, including perforated duodenal ulcer and other surgical abdominal emergencies, concurrently measuring serum lipase level increases diagnostic specificity (Table 7–10). If amylase and lipase levels are initially three times the upper limit of normal and gut perforation and infarction have been ruled out, these lab values clinch the diagnosis of pancreatitis. Abdominal ultrasound can assist in diagnosing contributing gallbladder disease; this study does not typically help with diagnosing acute or chronic pancreatitis because of limited views of the organ. Abdominal computed tomography (CT) scan usually provides a diagnostic view of the inflamed pancreas. Guidelines from the American College of Gastroenterology state that at least two of the following three criteria should be present to diagnose acute pancreatitis: 1) characteristic (severe) abdominal pain; 2) serum amylase and/or lipase exceeding 3 times the upper limit of normal; and/or 3) characteristic abdominal imaging findings. With expert consultation, additional studies are occasionally obtained if the diagnosis is unclear.

Significant pain and volume constriction are common in patients with acute pancreatitis. Intervention includes parenteral hydration and analgesia and gut rest. Treatment of the underlying cause, such as gallbladder disease or hypertriglyceridemia, or discontinuation of the causative agent, such as alcohol, corticosteroids, or thiazide diuretics, is also indicated. The clinical course of pancreatitis can range from a self-limiting condition to life-threatening illness. The Ranson criteria (Table 7–11) are usually used in assessing severity of pancreatitis. When three or more criteria are found on clinical presentation, a severe clinical course can be predicted with significant risk for pancreatic necrosis.

Persons with pancreatic cancer most commonly present with abdominal pain, weight loss, anorexia, nausea, and vomiting. The pain is generally abrupt in onset, steady, boring, and severe, often made worse with walking and lying supine

TABLE 7-10
Lipase and Amylase Evaluation in Acute Pancreatitis

Amylase	Lipase
• In pancreatitis • Appears 2–12 hr after symptom onset • Back to normal within 7 days of pancreatitis resolution	• In pancreatitis • Appears 4–8 hr after symptom onset • Peaks at 24 hr, decreases 8–14 days after pancreatitis resolution
• Amylase level >1000 U/L • 80% cholelithiasis diagnosis • 6% alcoholic pancreatitis diagnosis	
• Nonpancreatic amylase sources • Salivary glands • Ovarian cysts • Ovarian tumors • Tubo-ovarian abscess • Ruptured ectopic pregnancy • Lung cancer	• Nonpancreatic reasons for elevated lipase • Renal failure • Perforated duodenal ulcer • Bowel obstruction • Bowel infarction

TABLE 7-11
Ranson Criteria of Severity of Acute Pancreatitis

At Time of Patient Presentation	Development of the Following Within First 48 Hours Indicative of Worsening Prognosis
Age >55 years	Hematocrit decrease >10%
WBC >16,000 mm^3	Arterial PO_2 <60 mm Hg
Blood glucose >200 mg/dL (>11.1 mol/L)	Serum Ca^{++} <8 mg/dL
AST >250 U/L	Base deficit >4 mEq/L
LDH >350 IU/L	Estimate fluid sequestration of >6 L
	BUN increase >5 mg/dL over admission value

NO. CRITERIA	MORTALITY RATE PER RANSON CRITERIA
0–2	1%
3–4	15%
5–6	40%
>6	100%

AST—aspartate aminotransferase; BUN—blood urea nitrogen; LDH—lactate dehydrogenase; WBC—white blood cell count.

Sources: Ranson's criteria for pancreatitis mortality prediction. www.anzjsurg.com/view/0/ransonsCriteria.html, accessed 9/25/13.

Carroll JK, Herrick B, Gipson T, Lee SP. Acute pancreatitis: Diagnosis, prognosis, and treatment. *Am Fam Physician* 75:1513–1520, 2007.

and improved with sitting and leaning forward. Nausea and vomiting are typically present. Weakness, sweating, and anxiety are often present in severe attacks. There may be a history of alcohol ingestion or a heavy meal immediately preceding the attack. The upper abdomen is usually tender without guarding, rigidity or guarding with abdominal distension and absence of bowel sounds if ileus is present. Fever (38.4°C to 39.0°C [101.1°F to 102.2°F]), tachycardia, hypotension (even shock), pallor, cool, clammy skin, and mild jaundice may be noted. Occasionally, an upper abdominal mass is palpable due to an inflamed pancreas or the presence of a pancreatic pseudocyst. Acute renal injury may be seen in the early course of acute pancreatitis. In addition, when the disease involves the head of the pancreas, jaundice is often present, but usually without localized right upper quadrant abdominal tenderness seen in hepatic and biliary disorders such as cholecystitis and acute hepatitis.

Pancreatic pseudocysts consist of benign pockets of fluid lined with scar or inflammatory tissue. Though pseudocysts are often asymptomatic, signs and symptoms can include persistent abdominal pain that may radiate to the back, a mass that can be felt in the upper abdomen, and nausea and vomiting. A ruptured pseudocyst can be life-threatening as fluid released can damage nearby blood vessels and cause massive bleeding. In addition, infection can occur in the abdominal cavity. Often, pancreatic pseudocysts are identified during abdominal scans for other medical issues. MRI and CT scans are used to help differentiate a pseudocyst from cancer, but may require additional testing for a conclusive diagnosis. Fluid collected from the pseudocyst can be used to test for signs of cancer.

Pseudocysts that are not causing any signs or symptoms can be left alone but monitored. Cysts smaller than 10 mm can be imaged by CT scan after 1 year and then less frequently if they remain stable. Cysts larger than 10 mm usually require an endoscopic ultrasound to search for features of concern. A pseudocyst that is causing bothersome symptoms or growing larger must be drained. This is usually performed via endoscopic ultrasound-guided fine needle aspiration. Surgery may be needed to remove an enlarged pseudocyst.

Pancreatic cancer has high mortality rates because clinical presentation usually occurs with late disease and the spread of the cancer. Risk factors for pancreatic cancer include a history of chronic pancreatitis, tobacco use, and DM. About 5% of the time, a genetic factor contributes to the disease. About 40% of cases occur sporadically with no identifiable risk factors.

Abdominal CT scan is helpful in identifying pancreatic cancer. The usefulness of abdominal ultrasound is limited by the presence of intestinal gas. Normochromic, normocytic anemia is a common finding, as is elevated total and direct bilirubin and alkaline phosphatase. An elevation in amylase is an uncommon finding, unless concomitant pancreatitis is present.

DISCUSSION SOURCES

Erickson R, Larson C, Shabahang C. eMedicine. Pancreatic cancer. http://emedicine.medscape.com/article/280605,

Gardner TB, Katz J, Berk BS. Acute pancreatitis. http://emedicine.medscape.com/article/181364-overview,

Papadakis MA, McPhee SJ, Rabow MW. *Current Medical Diagnosis & Treatment 2013*, 52nd ed. The McGraw-Hill Companies, Inc., 2013.

Male Genitourinary System

8

Benign Prostatic Hyperplasia

1. Which of the following is inconsistent with the description of benign prostatic hyperplasia (BPH)?
   A. obliterated median sulcus
   B. size larger than 2.5 cm × 3 cm
   C. sensation of incomplete emptying
   D. boggy gland

2. When prescribing antihypertensive therapy for a man with BPH and hypertension, the NP considers that:
   A. loop diuretics are the treatment of choice.
   B. an $alpha_1$ antagonist should not be used as a solo or first-line therapeutic agent.
   C. angiotensin receptor antagonist use is contraindicated.
   D. beta-adrenergic antagonist use often enhances urinary flow.

3. When assessing a 78-year-old man with suspected BPH, the NP considers that:
   A. prostate size does not correlate well with severity of symptoms.
   B. BPH affects less than 50% of men of this age.
   C. he is at increased risk for prostate cancer.
   D. limiting fluids is a helpful method of relieving severe symptoms.

4. Which of the following medications can contribute to the development of acute urinary retention in an older man with BPH?
   A. amitriptyline
   B. loratadine
   C. enalapril
   D. lorazepam

5. A 78-year-old man presents with a 3-day history of new-onset fatigue and difficulty with bladder emptying. Examination reveals a distended bladder but is otherwise unremarkable. Blood urea nitrogen level is 88 mg/dL (31.4 mmol/L); creatinine level is 2.8 mg/dL (247.5 μmol/L). The most likely diagnosis is:
   A. prerenal azotemia.
   B. acute glomerulonephritis.
   C. tubular necrosis.
   D. postrenal azotemia.

6. Surgical intervention in BPH should be considered with all of the following except:
   A. recurrent urinary tract infection.
   B. bladder stones.
   C. persistent obstruction despite medical therapy.
   D. acute tubular necrosis.

7. Finasteride (Proscar, Propecia) and dutasteride (Avodart) are helpful in the treatment of BPH because of their effect on:
   A. bladder contractility.
   B. prostate size.
   C. activity at select bladder receptor sites.
   D. bladder pressure.

8. Tamsulosin (Flomax) is helpful in the treatment of BPH because of its effect on:
   A. bladder contractility.
   B. prostate size.
   C. activity at select bladder receptor sites.
   D. bladder pressure.

9. Concerning BPH, which of the following statements is true?

A. Digital rectal examination is accurate in diagnosing the condition.

B. The use of a validated patient symptom tool is an important part of diagnosing the condition.

C. Prostate size directly correlates with symptoms and bladder emptying.

D. Bladder distention is usually present in early disease.

10. Concerning herbal and nutritional therapies for BPH treatment, which of the following statements is false?

A. The mechanism of action of the most effective and best studied products is similar to prescription medications for this condition.

B. These therapies are currently considered emerging therapy by the American Urological Association.

C. Major areas of concern with use of these therapies include issues of product purity and quality control.

D. These therapies are safest and most effective when used with prescription medications.

Answers

1.	D.	5.	D.	9.	B.
2.	B.	6.	D.	10.	D.
3.	A.	7.	B.		
4.	A.	8.	C.		

Benign prostatic hyperplasia (BPH) is a common disorder in older men. Based on autopsy studies, the prevalence of BPH increases from approximately 8% in men 31 to 40 years old to approximately 50% in men 51 to 60 years old and to more than 80% in men 80 years old and older. Far fewer men have clinically symptomatic disease. This enlargement of the prostate, not associated with or a precursor to malignancy, can lead to bladder outlet obstruction, likely as a result of an enlargement in prostatic connective tissue and an increase in the number of epithelial and smooth muscle cells. To empty the bladder effectively in the face of increasing outflow tract obstruction, bladder detrusor hypertrophy occurs with occasional notation of subsequent diverticula. Chronic incomplete bladder emptying causes stasis and predisposes to calculus formation and infection with secondary inflammatory changes, including prostatitis and urinary tract infection. The cause of BPH is not fully understood, but it seems to be at least partly a response to androgenic hormones.

Diagnosis of BPH is based on numerous components of the evaluation. Digital rectal examination (DRE) is an integral part of the evaluation where prostate size and contour can be assessed, nodules can be evaluated, and areas suggestive of malignancy can be detected. On rectal examination, the prostate usually is enlarged, has a rubbery consistency, and in many cases has lost the median sulcus or furrow. DRE of prostate size is often misleading, however; a prostate that is apparently small on digital rectal examination can cause significant symptoms. The use of a validated tool such as the American Urological Association Symptom Score for Benign Prostatic Hyperplasia (available at http://www.auanet.org/common/pdf/education/clinical-guidance/Benign-Prostatic-Hyperplasia.pdf [see Appendix 6 of document]) increases the likelihood of an accurate diagnosis. Other tests can be used to rule out infection or other conditions that can cause similar symptoms. These include a urinalysis (to assess for presence of blood, leukocytes, bacteria, protein, or glucose), and/or urine culture. Additional diagnostic procedures used to confirm that an enlarged prostate is causing the symptoms include urinary flow test, postvoid residual volume test, transrectal ultrasound, and a prostate biopsy. A systematic evaluation for prostate cancer must be done on any man who has an abnormal prostate examination with or without urinary symptoms.

BPH can lead to bladder outlet obstruction from urethral narrowing. As a result, men with BPH develop symptoms of increased frequency of urination, decreased force of urinary stream, nocturia, and the sensation of incomplete emptying. Other symptoms can include urinary urgency, hesitancy (i.e., difficulty initiating the urinary stream; interrupted, weak stream), and a need to strain or push to initiate or maintain urination to more fully empty the bladder. Prolonged obstruction can lead to hydronephrosis and compromised renal function; this is the etiology of postrenal azotemia, a potentially life-threatening condition. Postrenal azotemia accounts for about 5% of all renal failure. It is characterized by urea nitrogen and creatinine elevation and evidence of urinary retention and outflow tract obstruction; other reasons for renal failure have been ruled out. Intervention in postrenal azotemia is focused on relieving the urinary outflow tract obstruction. When postrenal azotemia is promptly detected, renal function returns to baseline after treatment.

Patient education about BPH should include information on measures to avoid making symptoms worse. Drugs with anticholinergic effect, such as tricyclic antidepressants and first-generation antihistamines (e.g., diphenhydramine [Benadryl], chlorpheniramine [Chlor-Trimeton]), can cause acute urinary retention in men with BPH; opioid use and inactivity also increase the risk of urinary retention. In addition, urinary frequency occasionally becomes worse with ingestion of certain bladder irritants, such as caffeine, alcohol, and artificial sweeteners. Although men with BPH are often tempted to limit fluid intake to minimize urinary frequency, this can yield more concentrated and perhaps irritating urine, possibly leading to increased symptoms.

The prostate and bladder base contain numerous alpha$_1$ receptor sites. When these receptor sites are stimulated, the prostate contracts, increasing outflow tract obstruction. As a result, treatment with alpha$_1$ receptor antagonists (alpha blockers) including tamsulosin (Flomax) can be helpful in improving the symptoms of BPH. The use of alpha blockers as a solo or first-line antihypertensive agent has been associated with higher than expected rates of stroke and heart failure. Alpha blockers should be considered as a desirable agent in treating a man with hypertension and BPH but only as medication added on to existing therapy; an alpha blocker that is specifically indicated for BPH therapy only, such as tamsulosin, has minimal effect on blood pressure. The use of finasteride (Proscar) and dutasteride (Avodart), 5-alpha-reductase inhibitors that block the conversion of testosterone to dihydrotestosterone, helps to reduce the size of the prostate and ameliorate symptoms. Tadalafil (Cialis), a phosphodiesterase inhibitor, is also approved for the treatment of BPH. However, this agent cannot be used in combination with alpha blockers or with patients taking nitrates.

Surgical intervention in BPH should be considered when medication and lifestyle modification therapy is ineffective and any of the following are present and clearly secondary to the condition: recurrent urinary tract infection, recurrent or persistent gross hematuria, bladder stones, or renal insufficiency. Surgeries can include transurethral resection of the prostate or open prostatectomy. A number of minimally invasive therapies, including thermal and laser interventions, are now available and offer an attractive alternative to more aggressive surgery, although less is known about long-term outcomes.

Herbal and nutritional therapies, including saw palmetto, rye, and pumpkin, are considered emerging therapies by the American Urological Association, pending further study. The observed effect of these plant-based therapies is usually attributed to a mechanism of action similar to approved prescription BPH therapies. As with other herbal and nutritional therapies available over-the-counter (OTC), issues of product purity and strength and potential interaction with prescription and other OTC products remain a concern.

DISCUSSION SOURCES

Deters LA, Costabile RA, Leveillee RJ, et al. Benign prostatic hypertrophy. http://emedicine.medscape.com/article/437359-overview
McVary KT, Roehrborn CG, Avins AL, et al. American Urological Association Guideline: Management of benign prostatic hyperplasia. http://www.auanet.org/education/guidelines/benign-prostatic-hyperplasia.cfm

Chancroid

11. You examine a 32-year-old man with chancroid and anticipate finding:
A. a verruciform lesion.
B. a painful ulcer.
C. a painless, crater-like lesion.
D. a plaquelike lesion.

12. All of the following are typical findings for a patient with chancroid except:
A. multiple lesions.
B. spontaneous rupture of affected nodes.
C. blood-tinged penile discharge.
D. dense, matted lymphadenopathy on the ipsilateral side of the lesion.

13. The causative organism of chancroid is:
A. *Ureaplasma* species.
B. *Chlamydia trachomatis.*
C. *Mycoplasma hominis.*
D. *Haemophilus ducreyi.*

14. Treatment options for chancroid include all of the following except:
A. azithromycin.
B. ciprofloxacin.
C. ceftriaxone.
D. amoxicillin.

15. When ordering laboratory tests to confirm chancroid, the NP considers that:
A. concomitant infection with herpes simplex is often found.
B. a disease-specific serum test is available.
C. a white blood cell count with differential is indicated.
D. dark-field examination is needed.

Answers

11. B.   **13.** D.   **15.** A.
12. C.   **14.** D.

The gram-negative bacillus *Haemophilus ducreyi* causes chancroid. The organism is most often contracted sexually (Table 8–1). Transmission to healthcare providers and other caregivers through direct contact with chancroid lesions has also been documented. The chancroid lesion is typically found at the site of inoculation with a vesicular-form to pustular-form lesion that creates a painful, soft ulcer with a necrotic base. Multiple lesions, acquired through autoinoculation, usually are found. A dense, matted lymphadenopathy can be found on the ipsilateral side of the lesion. The affected nodes often spontaneously rupture. A definitive diagnosis of chancroid involves identification of *H. ducreyi* on special culture media. However, diagnosis of the condition can be challenging because cultures often fail to reveal the offending organism (sensitivity is <80%). Although not FDA approved, polymerase chain reaction testing is 100% sensitive; drawbacks include the expense of the test. Treatment options include azithromycin, ciprofloxacin, and ceftriaxone.

As with all sexually transmitted infections (STIs), a critical part of care is discussion of preventive strategies, including using condoms and limiting the number of sexual partners. NPs should offer and encourage testing for other STIs, including HIV, hepatitis B, and syphilis. Consideration should also be given to offering testing for hepatitis C and human herpesvirus type 2 (herpes simplex type 2). Immunization that provides protection against hepatitis A, hepatitis B, and HPV should be offered as needed and appropriate.

TABLE 8-1

Sexually Transmitted Male Genitourinary Infections

Conditions	Causative Organism	Clinical Presentation	Treatment Options
Chancroid	*H. ducreyi*	Painful genital ulcer, multiple lesions common, inguinal lymphadenitis.	Primary: Azithromycin 1 g orally in a single dose, or ceftriaxone 250 mg intramuscularly (IM) in a single dose. Alternative: Ciprofloxacin 500 mg orally twice a day for 3 days, or erythromycin base 500 mg orally three times a day ×7 days.
Genital herpes	Human herpesvirus 2 (HHV-2) (also known as herpes simplex type 2) less common by HHV-1 (also known as herpes simplex type 1)	Common to be asymptomatic or have atypical symptoms; subclinical, asymptomatic transmission common. Classic presentation with painful ulcerated lesions, lymphadenopathy with initial lesions.	For primary infection (initial episode): Acyclovir (Zovirax®) 400 mg PO tid ×7–10 days or acyclovir 200 mg PO five times per day for 7–10 days or famciclovir (Famvir®) 250 mg PO tid ×7–10 days or valacyclovir (Valtrex®) 1 g PO bid ×7–10 days. For episodic recurrent infection: Acyclovir 800 mg tid ×2 days or 400 mg tid ×5 days or 800 mg bid ×5 days or famciclovir 1000 mg bid ×1 day or 125 mg bid ×5 days or 500 mg once followed by 250 mg bid ×2 days or valacyclovir 1 g PO qd ×5 days or 500 mg bid ×3 days. For suppression of recurrent infection: Acyclovir 400 mg PO bid or famciclovir 250 mg PO bid or valacyclovir 1g PO qd. For patient with ≤9 recurrences per year, another treatment option: Valacyclovir 500 mg qd with an increase to 1 g qd if breakthrough.
Lymphogranuloma venereum	Invasive serovar L1, L2, L3 of *C. trachomatis*	Vesicular or ulcerative lesion on external genitalia with inguinal lymphadenitis or buboes.	Primary therapy: Doxycycline 100 mg PO bid ×21 days. Alternative therapy: Erythromycin base 500 mg qid ×21 days.
Nongonococcal urethritis	*Chlamydia trachomatis, Ureaplasma urealyticum, Mycoplasma genitalium*	Irritative voiding symptoms, occasional mucopurulent penile discharge. In women: Often without symptoms. Microscopic examination of discharge: Large number of WBCs.	Primary therapy: Azithromycin 1 g PO as a single dose or doxycycline 100 mg PO bid ×7 days. Alternative therapy: Erythromycin base 500 mg PO qid ×7 days or erythromycin ethylsuccinate 800 mg PO qid ×7 days or ofloxacin 300 mg PO bid ×7 days or levofloxacin 500 mg PO qd ×7 days.

TABLE 8-1

Sexually Transmitted Male Genitourinary Infections—cont'd

Conditions	Causative Organism	Clinical Presentation	Treatment Options
Gonococcal urethritis	*N. gonorrhoeae*	Irritative voiding symptoms, occasional purulent discharge. Often without symptoms in either gender. Microscopic examination of discharge: Large number of WBCs.	Recommended therapy: Combination therapy for uncomplicated infection. Single dose ceftriaxone 250 mg IM plus either single dose azithromycin 1 g PO or doxycycline 100 mg PO bid ×7 days. Alternative: single dose cefixime 400 mg PO plus either single-dose azithromycin 1 g PO or doxycycline 100 mg PO bid × 7 days. Alternative therapy in the presence of severe beta-lactam allergy: Azithromycin 2 g PO as a single dose.
Genital warts (condyloma acuminata)	Human papillomavirus, most commonly HPV-6 or HPV-11, causing genital warts. (HPV-16, -18, -31, -33 are most commonly associated with GU malignancies. Infection with multiple HPV types is common.)	Verruca-form lesions, can be subclinical or unrecognized.	Location of lesion can guide choice of treatment. Patient-applied therapy: Podofilox 0.5% solution or gel or imiquimod 5% cream or sinecatechins 15% ointment. Provider-applied therapy: Liquid nitrogen or cryoprobe, trichloroacetic acid or bichloroacetic acid (80%–90%), podophyllin resin (10%–25% in a compound tincture of benzoin), or surgical removal.
Balanitis (inflammation of glans of penis)	*Candida* (40%), Group B streptococcus, *Gardnerella*	Occurs in about ¼ of all male sex partners of women with *Candida* vaginitis. Can also occur in presence of immuno-suppression systemic antimicrobial use, or DM.	Oral azole therapy: Single dose of metronidazole 2 g PO or single dose of fluconazole 150 mg PO or itraconazole 200 mg PO bid ×1 day.
Trichomoniasis	*Trichomonas vaginalis*	Males without symptoms, treatment usually triggered by female partner's diagnosis.	Oral metronidazole 2 g or tinidazole 2 g as a one-time dose. Alternative therapy: Oral metronidazole 500 mg bid ×7 days. Patients should be advised to avoid consuming alcohol during treatment with oral metronidazole or tinidazole. Abstinence from alcohol use should continue for 24 hours after completion of metronidazole or 72 hours after completion of tinidazole.

Continued

TABLE 8-1
Sexually Transmitted Male Genitourinary Infections—cont'd

Conditions	Causative Organism	Clinical Presentation	Treatment Options
Syphilis	*Treponema pallidum*	Primary stage: Chancre, a firm, round, painless genital and/or anal ulcer(s) with clean base and indurated margins, accompanied by localized lymphadenopathy, ~3 weeks duration, resolve without therapy. Secondary stage: Nonpruritic skin rash, often involving palms and soles, as well as mucous membrane lesions. Fever, lymphadenopathy, sore throat, patchy hair loss, headaches, weight loss, muscle aches, and fatigue commonly reported. Resolution without treatment possible. Latent stage: Presentation variable occurs when primary and secondary symptoms have resolved.	Antimicrobial therapy, with dose and length of therapy usually dictated by disease stage. Options include injectable penicillin (preferred), tetracycline or doxycycline used with beta-lactam allergy.

Sources: Gilbert D, Moellering RC, Eliopoulos GM, Chambers HF, Saag MS. *The Sanford Guide to Antimicrobial Therapy*, ed. 44th. Sperryville, VA: Antimicrobial Therapy, Inc., 2014, pp. 23–27.
Centers for Disease Control and Prevention. Sexually transmitted diseases treatment guidelines, 2010. *MMWR* 59(No. RR-12):1–116, 2010.

DISCUSSION SOURCES

Gilbert D, Moellering RC, Eliopoulos GM, Chambers HF, Saag MS. *The Sanford Guide to Antimicrobial Therapy*, ed. 44th. Sperryville, VA: Antimicrobial Therapy, Inc., 2014,
MMWR Centers for Disease Control and Prevention. Sexually transmitted diseases treatment guidelines, 2010. *MMWR* 59 (No. RR-12):1–116, 2010.

DavisPlus | See full color images of this topic on DavisPlus at **http://davisplus.fadavis.com** | Keyword: Fitzgerald

Lymphogranuloma Venereum

16. The most common causative organism of lymphogranuloma venereum is:
A. *Ureaplasma genitalium.*
B. *C. trachomatis* types 1 to 3.
C. *Neisseria gonorrhoeae.*
D. *H. ducreyi.*

17. Symptoms of lymphogranuloma venereum typically occur how long after contact with an infected host?
A. 5–7 days
B. 1–4 weeks
C. 4–6 weeks
D. 2–3 months

18. Physical examination findings in lymphogranuloma venereum include:
A. verruciform lesions.
B. lesions that fuse and create multiple draining sinuses.
C. a painless crater.
D. plaquelike lesions.

19. Treatment options for lymphogranuloma venereum include:
A. doxycycline.
B. penicillin.
C. ceftriaxone.
D. dapsone.

Answers

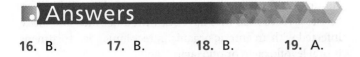

16. B.   17. B.   18. B.   19. A.

Lymphogranuloma venereum is an STI caused by *Chlamydia trachomatis* types L1 to L3. The clinical presentation, usually occurring approximately 1 to 4 weeks after contact with an infected host, consists of a vesicular or ulcerative lesion on the external genitalia, often not noted by the patient, which progresses to cause inguinal lymphadenitis or buboes. These can fuse and then drain, forming multiple sinus tracts with resultant scarring. Polymerase chain reaction assays have been used to aid in the diagnosis but have had availability limited to reference laboratories. Treatment options include doxycycline and erythromycin (see Table 8–1).

As with all STIs, a critical part of care is discussion of preventive strategies, including using condoms and limiting the number of sexual partners. NPs should offer and encourage testing for other STIs, including HIV, hepatitis B, and syphilis. Consideration should also be given to offering testing for hepatitis C and human herpes type 2 (herpes simplex type 2). Immunization that provides protection against hepatitis A, hepatitis B, and HPV should be offered as needed and appropriate.

DISCUSSION SOURCES

Gilbert D, Moellering RC, Eliopoulos GM, Chambers HF, Saag MS. *The Sanford Guide to Antimicrobial Therapy*, ed. 44th. Sperryville, VA: Antimicrobial Therapy, Inc., 23–27, 2014.

Centers for Disease Control and Prevention. Sexually transmitted diseases treatment guidelines, 2010. *MMWR* 59(No. RR-12):1–116, 2010.

Acute Epididymitis

20. The presentation of acute epididymitis in an otherwise-well 22-year-old man includes:
A. the presence of a positive Prehn sign.
B. low back pain.
C. absent cremasteric reflex.
D. diffuse abdominal pain.

21. The most likely causative pathogens in a 26-year-old man with acute epididymitis include:
A. *Escherichia coli.*
B. *Enterobacteriaceae.*
C. *C. trachomatis.*
D. *Pseudomonas* species.

22. A likely causative pathogens in a 25-year-old man with acute epididymitis who has sex with men is:
A. *Escherichia coli.*
B. *Mycoplasma* spp.
C. *Chlamydia trachomatis.*
D. *Acinetobacter baumannii.*

23. Which of the following is a reasonable treatment option for a 30-year-old man with acute epididymitis who presents without gastrointestinal upset and will be treated as an outpatient?
A. doxycycline with ceftriaxone
B. amoxicillin with clavulanate
C. metronidazole with linezolid
D. clindamycin with cefixime

24. Appropriate treatment of acute epididymitis for a 32-year-old man who has sex with other men is:
A. ceftriaxone.
B. azithromycin.
C. levofloxacin.
D. TMP-SMX.

25-30. Indicate whether each finding would be present in acute epididymitis (yes or no).

25. irritative voiding symptoms

26. penile discharge

27. ulcerative lesion

28. scrotal swelling

29. boggy prostate

30. epididymoorchitis in later stages of disease

Answers

20. A.	**24.** C.	**28.** yes
21. C.	**25.** yes	**29.** no
22. A.	**26.** yes	**30.** yes
23. A.	**27.** no	

Acute epididymitis is a male upper reproductive tract infectious disease caused by various pathogens. In men younger than age 35 years, it is usually caused by *C. trachomatis* or *N. gonorrhoeae*; the organism is acquired through sexual contact. In men older than age 35 years, acute epididymitis is often seen secondary to prostatitis and is typically caused by a gram-negative organism. In men who have sex with other men, sexually-transmitted acute epididymitis is more likely caused by enteric organisms (such as *Escherichia coli* and *Pseudomonas* spp.). This condition manifests with irritative voiding symptoms; fever; and an acutely painful, enlarged epididymis. Pain often radiates up the spermatic cord to the ipsilateral lower abdomen. The Prehn sign, a reduction in pain when the scrotum is elevated above the symphysis pubis, is usually noted. Urethritis, scrotal swelling, and penile discharge are often found. As the disease progresses, the ipsilateral testis may become involved, swelling so that the two testes cannot be distinguished; this is known as epididymo-orchitis.

Treatment options differ according to age and risk factors. In younger men with low risk for epididymo-orchitis as a complication of urinary tract infection, particularly with risk for STI, antimicrobials effective against gonorrhea and chlamydia such as ceftriaxone followed by doxycycline should be used (Table 8–2). In men at risk for epididymo-orchitis as a complication of urinary tract infection, the choice of antimicrobial agent should be directed by urine culture. A fluoroquinolone such as ciprofloxacin is likely to be effective. In men who have sex with other men and likely infected with an enteric organism, recommended treatment is oral levofloxacin or ofloxacin.

As with all STIs, a critical part of care is discussion of preventive strategies, including using condoms and limiting the number of sexual partners. NPs should offer and encourage testing for other STIs, including HIV, hepatitis B, and syphilis. Consideration should also be given to offering testing for hepatitis C and human herpes type 2 (herpes simplex type 2). Immunization that provides protection against

TABLE 8-2
Assessment and Treatment of Male Genitourinary Infections

Causative	Conditions/Organism	Clinical Presentation	Treatment Options
Epididymitis Epididymoorchitis Age ≤35 y.o.	N. gonorrhoeae, C. trachomatis	Irritative voiding symptoms, fever, and painful swelling of epididymis and scrotum	Primary: Ceftriaxone 250 mg intramuscularly (IM) as a single dose plus doxycycline 100 mg bid ×10 days. Advise scrotal elevation to help with symptom relief. Advise scrotal elevation to help with symptom relief.
Epididymitis Epididymoorchitis Age >35 y.o. or insertive partner in anal intercourse	Enterobacteriaceae (coliforms)	Irritative voiding symptoms, fever, and painful swelling of epididymis and scrotum	Primary: Ciprofloxacin 500 mg qd or levofloxacin 750 mg qd ×10–14 days. Alternative: Intravenous ampicillin with sulbactam, third-generation cephalosporin, other parenteral agents as indicated by severity of illness.
Acute bacterial prostatitis (≤35 y.o.)	N. gonorrhoeae, C. trachomatis	Irritative voiding symptoms, suprapubic, perineal pain, fever, tender, boggy prostate, leukocytosis	Primary: One-time dose of ceftriaxone 250 mg IM or cefixime 400 mg PO, then doxycycline 100 mg PO bid ×10 days.
Acute bacterial prostatitis (age 35 y.o. or older, or men who have sex with other men)	Enterobacteriaceae (coliforms)	Irritative voiding symptoms, suprapubic, perineal pain, fever, tender, boggy prostate, leukocytosis	Levofloxacin 500–750 mg IV/PO qd or ciprofloxacin 500 mg PO bid or 400 mg IV bid ×10–14 days
Chronic bacterial prostatitis	Enterobacteriaceae (coliforms) (80%), entero-cocci(15%), P. aeruginosa	Irritative voiding symptoms, dull, poorly localized, suprapubic, perineal pain	Ciprofloxacin 500 mg PO bid ×4–6 weeks or levofloxacin 750 mg PO qd ×4 weeks. Alternative: TMP-SMX DS 1 tab bid ×1–3 mo. With treatment failure, consider prostatic stones.

Sources: Gilbert D, Moellering RC, Eliopoulos GM, Chambers HF, Saag MS. *The Sanford Guide to Antimicrobial Therapy*, ed. 43. Sperryville, VA: Antimicrobial Therapy, Inc., 2013, pp. 23–27.
Centers for Disease Control and Prevention. Sexually transmitted diseases treatment guidelines, 2010. *MMWR* 59(No. RR-12):1–116, 2010.

hepatitis A, hepatitis B, and HPV should be offered as needed and appropriate.

DISCUSSION SOURCES

Gilbert D, Moellering RC, Eliopoulos GM, Chambers HF, Saag MS. *The Sanford Guide to Antimicrobial Therapy*, ed. 44th. Sperryville, VA: Antimicrobial Therapy, Inc., 2014, pp. 23–27.

Centers for Disease Control and Prevention. Sexually transmitted diseases treatment guidelines, 2010. *MMWR* 59(No. RR-12): 1–116, 2010.

Gonorrhea

31. *Neisseria gonorrhoeae* are best described as:
    A. gram-positive cocci.
    B. gram-positive rods.
    C. gram-negative diplococci.
    D. gram-negative bacilli.

32. The preferred treatment for uncomplicated gonococcal proctitis is:
    A. ceftriaxone 250 mg IM as a single dose plus a single dose of azithromycin 1 g po.
    B. oral erythromycin 500 mg bid for 7 days.
    C. oral norfloxacin 400 mg bid with metronidazole 500 mg bid for 3 days
    D. azithromycin 1 g po as a single dose plus single dose of injectable doxycycline 100 mg.

33. Which of the following is recommended by the Centers for Disease Control and Prevention as single-dose therapy for uncomplicated urethritis caused by *N. gonorrhoeae* when an oral product is the most appropriate option?
    A. cefixime
    B. metronidazole
    C. azithromycin
    D. amoxicillin

34. You see a 42-year-old man with uncomplicated urogenital gonorrhea. His medical records indicate a severe allergic reaction to penicillin that includes difficulty breathing and diffuse urticaria. You recommend treatment with:
    A. cefixime.
    B. levofloxacin.
    C. azithromycin.
    D. tigecycline.

35. In gonococcal infection, which of the following statements is true?
    A. Risk of transmission from an infected woman to a male sexual partner is about 20% to 30% with a single coital act.
    B. Most men have symptomatic infection.
    C. The incubation period is about 2 to 3 weeks.
    D. The organism rarely produces beta-lactamase.

36–39. Indicate whether each finding normally would be present in gonorrheal urethritis in an otherwise well 28-year-old man (yes or no).

36. dysuria

37. milky penile discharge

38. scrotal swelling

39. fever

Answers

31. C.	34. C.	37. yes
32. A.	35. A.	38. no
33. A and C	36. yes	39. no

Gonorrhea, caused by the gram-negative diplococcus *N. gonorrhoeae*, is one of the most common STIs. This pathogen has a short incubation period, 1 to 5 days, and is likely to cause infection in approximately 20% to 30% of men who have sexual contact with an infected woman and approximately 60% to 80% of women who have sexual contact with an infected man. Male-to-male and female-to-female rates of transmission are not as well documented.

In men, presentation typically includes dysuria with a milky, occasionally blood-tinged penile discharge. Most men are asymptomatic, however. With anal-insertive sex, rectal infection leading to proctitis is often seen. Gonorrheal infection is usually confirmed by amplification testing of the DNA present in the organism.

Because the organism frequently produces beta-lactamase, therapeutic agents should include those with beta-lactamase stability and a cephalosporin, such as injectable ceftriaxone or oral cefixime (see Table 8–1). Due to increasing rates of resistance where dual antimicrobial therapy is possibly helpful and there is the likelihood of coinfection with *C. trachomatis* or other similar organisms, current guidelines recommend the addition of either a single dose of azithromycin 1 g orally or doxycycline 100 mg orally twice daily for 7 days. Increasing prevalence of fluoroquinolone-resistant gonococcus limits the usefulness of these medications; fluoroquinolone is no longer recommended for gonorrheal infection. For those with a severe allergic reaction to cephalosporins, an alternative regimen is azithromycin 2 g orally in a single dose. For those treated with this alternative regimen, the patient should return in 1 week for a test-of-cure.

As with all STIs, a critical part of care is discussion of preventive strategies, including using condoms and limiting the number of sexual partners. NPs should offer and encourage testing for other STIs, including HIV, hepatitis B, and syphilis. Consideration should also be given to offering testing for hepatitis C and human herpes type 2 (herpes simplex type 2). Immunization that provides protection against hepatitis A, hepatitis B, and HPV should be offered as needed and appropriate. ■

DISCUSSION SOURCES

Gilbert D, Moellering RC, Eliopoulos GM, Chambers HF, Saag MS. *The Sanford Guide to Antimicrobial Therapy*, ed. 44th. Sperryville, VA: Antimicrobial Therapy, Inc., 2014, pp. 23–27.

Centers for Disease Control and Prevention. Sexually transmitted diseases treatment guidelines, 2010. *MMWR* 59(No. RR-12): 1–116, 2010.

●) Bacterial Prostatitis

40. Risk factors for acute bacterial prostatitis include all of the following except:
    A. having unprotected sex.
    B. use of a urinary catheter.
    C. prior bladder infection.
    D. age >70 years.

41. The most common causative organisms of acute bacterial prostatitis in men <35 years are:
    A. *E. coli* and *K. pneumoniae*.
    B. *N. gonorrhoeae* and *C. trachomatis*.
    C. *Pseudomonas* and *Acinetobacter* species.
    D. enterococci.

42. When choosing an antimicrobial agent for the treatment of chronic bacterial prostatitis, the NP considers that:
    A. gram-positive organisms are the most likely cause of infection.
    B. cephalosporins are the first-line choice of therapy.
    C. choosing an antibiotic with gram-negative coverage is critical.
    D. length of antimicrobial therapy is typically 5 days.

43. All of the following are likely to be reported by patients with acute bacterial prostatitis except:
    A. perineal pain.
    B. irritative voiding symptoms.
    C. penile discharge.
    D. fever.

44. During acute bacterial prostatitis, the digital rectal examination usually reveals a gland described as:
    A. boggy.
    B. smooth.
    C. irregular.
    D. cystic.

45. A 30-year-old man with prostatitis presents with a fever of 102.3° F (39.1° C). What would be the expected CBC findings from this patient?
    A. WBC = 15,000/mm³; neutrophils = 4000/mm³
    B. WBC = 18,000/mm³; neutrophils = 11,500/mm³
    C. WBC = 7200/mm³; neutrophils = 3200/mm³
    D. WBC = 4000/mm³; neutrophils=1200/mm³

46. Appropriate antimicrobial treatment for a 25-year-old man with acute bacterial prostatitis is:
    A. oral azithromycin.
    B. IM ceftriaxone followed by oral doxycycline.
    C. oral ofloxacin.
    D. oral amoxicillin-clavulanate.

47. Appropriate antimicrobial treatment for a 65-year-old man with acute bacterial prostatitis is:
    A. erythromycin.
    B. cefepime.
    C. TMP-SMX.
    D. ciprofloxacin.

48. Symptoms in chronic bacterial prostatitis often include:
    A. fever.
    B. gastrointestinal upset.
    C. low back pain.
    D. penile discharge.

49. The most common causative organisms in chronic bacterial prostatitis include:
    A. gram-negative rods.
    B. gram-positive cocci.
    C. gram-negative cocci.
    D. gram-positive coccobacilli.

50. Which of the following is the best choice of therapy in chronic bacterial prostatitis?
    A. oral trimethoprim-sulfamethoxazole for 2 weeks
    B. parenteral ampicillin for 4 weeks
    C. oral ciprofloxacin for 4 weeks
    D. injectable gentamicin for 2 weeks

51. The best diagnostic test to identify the offending organism in acute bacterial prostatitis is:
    A. a urine culture.
    B. a urethral culture.
    C. antibody testing.
    D. a urine Gram stain.

●) Answers

40. D	44. A	48. C
41. B	45. B	49. A
42. C	46. B	50. C
43. C	47. D	51. A

Infection with a gram-negative rod such as *E. coli* and *Pseudomonas* species usually causes acute bacterial prostatitis in older men. In younger men (<35 years) or men at risk for STIs, gonorrhea or chlamydia or both are most often implicated. Less often, gram-positive organisms such as enterococci are implicated. In older men (>35 years) or those who have sex with other men, Enterobacteriaceae (coliforms) are more commonly implicated. Other risk factors include having a past episode of prostatitis, history of bladder or urethral infection, pelvic trauma, dehydration, or use of a urinary catheter. Irritative voiding symptoms, suprapubic pain, and perineal pain are typically reported. Objective findings include fever; a tender, boggy prostate; leukocytosis with neutrophilia; and a urine culture positive for the causative organism. Urine Gram stain usually fails to identify the offending organism.

Treatment for acute bacterial prostatitis is similar to treatment for acute pyelonephritis—an antimicrobial agent with activity against gram-negative organisms and excellent tissue penetration. In men younger than 35 years, a single dose of ceftriaxone followed by doxycycline is recommended; causative organisms are usually the sexually transmitted organisms *C. trachomatis* and *N. gonorrhoeae*. Length of doxycycline therapy is usually 10 to 14 days. In men 35 years old and older or men who have sex with men, antimicrobial therapy with a higher-dose fluoroquinolone, such as ciprofloxacin or levofloxacin, for 10–14 days is advised.

In patients with chronic bacterial prostatitis, irritative voiding symptoms, low back and perineal pain, and a history of urinary tract infection are typically reported. Objective findings include a tender, boggy, or indurated prostate. Urinalysis results are usually normal from a freshly voided specimen. Urinalysis and culture after prostatic massage usually yields leukocytes and the causative organism; prostatic massage is not recommended if acute prostatitis is known to be present. Antimicrobial therapy for 4 to 12 weeks using a product with excellent tissue penetration and strong gram-negative coverage is usually required (see Table 8–2).

As with all STIs, a critical part of care is discussion of preventive strategies, including using condoms and limiting the number of sexual partners. NPs should offer and encourage testing for other STIs, including HIV, hepatitis B, and syphilis. Consideration should also be given to offering testing for hepatitis C and human herpes type 2 (herpes simplex type 2). Immunization that provides protection against hepatitis A, hepatitis B, and HPV should be offered as needed and appropriate.

DISCUSSION SOURCES

Gilbert D, Moellering RC, Eliopoulos GM, Chambers HF, Saag MS. *The Sanford Guide to Antimicrobial Therapy*, ed. 44th. Sperryville, VA: Antimicrobial Therapy, Inc., 2014, pp. 23–27.

Centers for Disease Control and Prevention. Sexually transmitted diseases treatment guidelines, 2010. *MMWR* 59(No. RR-12): 1–116, 2010.

Turek PJ, Hedayati T, Stehman CR. eMedicine. http://www.emedicine.com/emerg/topic488.htm, Prostatitis, 2013

Prostate Cancer

52. You perform a digital rectal examination (DRE) on a 72-year-old man and find a lesion suspicious for prostate cancer. The findings are described as:
    A. a rubbery, enlarged prostatic lobe.
    B. an area of prostatic induration.
    C. an indurated gland.
    D. prostatic tenderness.

53. Which part of the prostate is readily palpable during a DRE?
    A. anterior lobe
    B. median lobe
    C. lateral lobes
    D. posterior lobe

54. A 54-year-old white man with no obvious risk for prostate cancer opted to undergo PSA screening and DRE testing. The DRE findings are normal and his PSA is 3.7 ng/mL. You recommend:
    A. repeating the PSA test immediately.
    B. repeat screening in 1 year.
    C. repeat screening in 2 years.
    D. repeat screening in 5 years.

55. Risk factors for prostate cancer include all of the following except:
    A. African ancestry.
    B. history of genital trauma.
    C. family history of prostate cancer.
    D. high-fat diet.

56. The average American man has an approximately ___% lifetime risk of prostate cancer and an approximately ___% likelihood of clinical disease.
    A. 15, 5
    B. 25, 8
    C. 40, 10
    D. 60, 15

57. All of the following can cause an elevated PSA level except:
    A. prostate infection.
    B. cystoscopy.
    C. BPH.
    D. prostatectomy.

58. According to recent epidemiologic studies, prostate cancer is the number ___ cause of cancer death in men residing within the United States?
    A. 1
    B. 2
    C. 3
    D. 4

◼ Answers

52. B.	55. B.	58. B.
53. D.	56. C.	
54. B.	57. D.	

Prostate cancer is the most common noncutaneous cancer in men in the United States. Although clinically detectable prostate cancer is a cause of considerable mortality and morbidity, most cancers are likely occult and limited to the prostate with little risk of metastasis. Prostate cancer has been found on autopsy in two-thirds of men 80 to 89 years old. The average American man has a 40% lifetime risk of latent prostate cancer, an approximate 10% risk of clinically significant disease, and an approximate 3% risk of dying of prostate cancer; prostate cancer is the second cause of male cancer death in the United States, after lung cancer. Risk factors include older age, African American ancestry, a family history of prostate cancer, and obesity.

Most cases of prostate cancer are asymptomatic unless the disease is advanced. Consequently, a high level of vigilance for prostate cancer is important. Although periodic digital rectal examination (DRE) and prostate-specific antigen (PSA) testing are advised for some men, this screening protocol has limitations in the effectiveness. The prostatic DRE can reveal a discrete, painless lesion or area of induration in the posterior lobe of the prostate but is often normal until disease is advanced. PSA is a glycoprotein produced in benign and malignant prostate cells. Nearly two-thirds of men with PSA levels greater than 10 ng/mL (normal PSA <4 ng/mL in an older man, <2.5 ng/mL in a younger man) have prostate cancer, whereas about 25% of men with PSA values of 4 to 10 ng/mL have disease, and approximately the same percentage of men in the at-risk age group have evidence of prostate cancer with a normal PSA. Correlating an abnormal prostate examination finding with an abnormal PSA level increases the likelihood of a diagnosis of prostate cancer. PSA level can also be elevated transiently in conditions other than prostate cancer, including prostatitis or immediately after prostatic instrumentation such as cystoscopy. Levels often remain chronically elevated in patients with BPH. Serial increases even in the presence of a normal prostate examination should be evaluated further.

The American Cancer Society recommends that a discussion about screening should take place at age 50 for men who are at average risk of prostate cancer and expected to live at least 10 more years. For men at higher risk (such as African Americans and men who have a first-degree relative [father, brothers] diagnosed with prostate cancer at <65 years of age), the discussion should take place at age 45 years. Men at even higher risk because of multiple first-degree relatives affected at an early age should have the discussion at age 40 years. Following the discussion, those men who want to be screened should be tested with the PSA blood test. The DRE can also be done as part of screening. If no cancer is detected, the frequency of future screenings depends on the result of the PSA

test. If the PSA level was <2.5 ng/mL, retesting should occur every 2 years. If the PSA was ≥2.5 ng/mL, testing should be conducted annually.

Because of its low sensitivity and specificity, transrectal ultrasound should not be used as a first-line screening test for prostate cancer. This test can be helpful, however, when coupled with PSA and DRE findings and for guiding prostatic biopsy, the usual next step when a diagnosis of prostate cancer is considered. Pathology and disease staging guide prostate cancer treatment options. Watchful waiting is often a reasonable option for older men with local disease.

DISCUSSION SOURCES

American Cancer Society. http://www.cancer.org/cancer/prostatecancer/moreinformation/prostatecancerearlydetection/prostate-cancer-early-detection-acs-recommendations, American Cancer Society recommendations for prostate cancer early detection

American Urological Association. http://www.auanet.org/education/guidelines/prostate-cancer.cfm, Guideline for the management of clinically localized prostate cancer, 2007 (validity confirmed 2011)

◼ Testicular Torsion

59. A 24-year-old man presents with sudden onset of left-sided scrotal pain. He reports having intermittent unilateral testicular pain in the past but not as severe this current episode. Confirmation of testicular torsion would include all of the following findings except:
    A. unilateral loss of the cremasteric reflex.
    B. the affected testicle held higher in the scrotum.
    C. testicular swelling.
    D. relief of pain with scrotal elevation.

60. In assessing a man with testicular torsion, the NP is most likely to note:
    A. elevated PSA level.
    B. white blood cells reported in urinalysis.
    C. left testicle most often affected.
    D. increased testicular blood flow by color-flow Doppler ultrasound.

61. Anticipated organ survival exceeds 85% with testicular decompression within how many hours of torsion?
    A. 1
    B. 6
    C. 16
    D. 24

62. To prevent a recurrence of testicular torsion, which of the following is recommended?
    A. use of a scrotal support
    B. avoidance of testicular trauma
    C. orchiopexy
    D. limiting the number of sexual partners

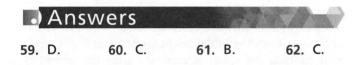 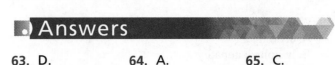

59. D.   **60.** C.   **61.** B.   **62.** C.

Testicular torsion is a urological emergency caused by a twisting of the testis and spermatic cord around a vertical axis; experimental modeling of the event reveals that a 720-degree twist is needed to occlude arterial and venous blood flow and cause the resulting testicular swelling and testicular tissue death. Findings include severe unilateral scrotal pain and swelling, the affected testicle held high in the scrotum, absent cremasteric reflex, and lack of pain relief with scrotal elevation. Approximately 50% of men presenting with torsion report intermittent unilateral testicular pain in the past, perhaps caused by partial, reversible torsion. The left testicle is most often affected. Radionuclide testicular scan and color-flow Doppler ultrasound usually show reduction of blood flow.

Prompt referral to a urological surgeon for detorsion of the organ and restoration of testicular blood flow is indicated. Testicular survival surpasses 85% if detorsion is accomplished within 6 hours. Manual manipulation of the testicle to unwind the torsion is occasionally helpful, although surgical intervention is more common. A bilateral orchiopexy, a procedure in which both testes are brought down and tacked lower in the scrotum, is usually performed to avoid subsequent torsion.

DISCUSSION SOURCE

Rupp T. eMedicine. http://www.emedicine.com/emerg/TOPIC573. HTM, Testicular torsion

Varicocele

63. A 23-year-old man has a nontender "bag of worms" mass within the left scrotum that disappears when he is in the supine position. He is diagnosed with a varicocele. What is a risk factor that may have contributed to this condition?
A. younger age
B. current cigarette smoker
C. multiple sexual partners
D. none of the above

64. Which of the following is a common finding in a man with varicocele?
A. lower sperm count with increased number of abnormal forms
B. increased rate of testicular cancer
C. recurrent scrotal pain
D. BPH

65. Treatment options for varicocele repair include all of the following except:
A. open surgery.
B. laparoscopic surgery.
C. treatment with a thrombolytic agent.
D. percutaneous embolization.

63. D.   **64.** A.   **65.** C.

A varicocele is an abnormally dilated spermatic vein within the scrotum. Typically described as a "bag of worms" lesion and most often found in the left scrotum, a varicocele is present while the man is standing and disappears in the supine position. A decreased sperm count with an increase in abnormal forms is noted in about two-thirds of men with the condition. Although varicocele is considered one of the most common correctable forms of male infertility, many men with the condition have normal fertility. Although there are no apparent significant risk factors for varicocele, being overweight may increase the risk.

Treatment of varicocele might not be necessary unless it causes pain, testicular atrophy, or infertility. Varicocele repair involves surgery that aims to seal off the affected vein to redirect blood flow into normal veins. Varicocele repair can involve open surgery, laparoscopic surgery, or percutaneous embolization (not as commonly used as surgery). A scrotal support can be helpful for relief of discomfort associated with varicocele. The impact of varicocele repair on infertility is unclear.

DISCUSSION SOURCE

Men's Health. http://www.mayoclinic.com/health/Varicocele/DS00618, Varicocele

Syphilis

66. How long after contact does the onset of clinical manifestations of syphilis typically occur?
A. less than 1 week
B. 1 to 3 weeks
C. 2 to 4 weeks
D. 4 to 6 weeks

67. Which of the following is not representative of the presentation of primary syphilis?
A. a painless ulcer
B. localized lymphadenopathy
C. flulike symptoms
D. a spontaneously healing lesion

68. Which of the following is representative of the presentation of secondary syphilis?
A. generalized rash
B. chancre
C. pupillary alterations
D. aortic regurgitation

69. Which of the following is found in tertiary syphilis?
    A. arthralgia
    B. lymphadenopathy
    C. maculopapular lesions involving the palms and soles
    D. gumma

70. Syphilis is most contagious at which of the following times?
    A. before onset of signs and symptoms
    B. during the primary stage
    C. during the secondary stage
    D. during the tertiary stage

71. First-line treatment options for primary syphilis include:
    A. penicillin.
    B. ciprofloxacin.
    C. erythromycin.
    D. ceftriaxone.

Caused by the spirochete *Treponema pallidum*, syphilis is a complex, multiorgan disease. Sexual contact is the usual route of transmission. The initial lesion forms about 2 to 4 weeks after contact; contagion is greatest during the secondary stage. Treatment is guided by the stage of disease and clinical manifestation (Table 8–3).

As with all STIs, a critical part of care is discussion of preventive strategies, including using condoms and limiting the number of sexual partners. NPs should offer and encourage testing for other STIs, including HIV, hepatitis B, and syphilis. Consideration should also be given to offering testing for hepatitis C and human herpes type 2 (herpes simplex type 2). Immunization that provides protection against hepatitis A, hepatitis B, and HPV should be offered as needed and appropriate.

DISCUSSION SOURCES

Gilbert D, Moellering RC, Eliopoulos GM, Chambers HF, Saag MS. *The Sanford Guide to Antimicrobial Therapy*, ed. 44th. Sperryville, VA: Antimicrobial Therapy, Inc., 2014, pp. 23–27.

See full color images of this topic on DavisPlus at http://davisplus.fadavis.com | Keyword: Fitzgerald

● Answers

66. C.	68. A.	70. C.
67. C.	69. D.	71. A.

TABLE 8-3

Stages of Syphilis, Clinical Manifestations, and Recommended Treatment

Stage of Syphilis	Clinical Manifestations	Treatment Options	Comment
Primary syphilis	Painless genital ulcer with clean base and indurated margins, localized lymphadenopathy	Recommended therapy: • Benzathine penicillin G 2.4 million U intramuscularly (IM) as a one-time dose Alternative therapy in penicillin allergy: • Doxycycline 100 mg PO bid ×2 weeks *or* Ceftriaxone 1 g IM or intravenously q24h ×8–10 days	Azithromycin 2 g as a one-time dose has been suggested, although issues of emerging resistance are concerning.
Secondary syphilis	Diffuse maculopapular rash involving palms and soles, generalized lymphadenopathy, low-grade fever, malaise, arthralgias and myalgia, headache	Recommended therapy: • Benzathine penicillin G 2.4 million U IM as a one-time dose Alternative therapy in penicillin allergy: • Doxycycline 100 mg PO bid ×2 weeks	Also treatment for latent syphilis of <1 year duration.
Late or tertiary syphilis	Gumma (granulomatous lesions involving skin, mucous membranes, bone), aortic insufficiency, aortic aneurysm, Argyll Robertson pupil, seizures	Recommended therapy: • Benzathine penicillin G 2.4 million U IM ×3 weekly doses Alternative therapy in penicillin allergy: • Doxycycline 100 mg PO bid ×4 weeks Expert consultation advisable, especially in the face of neurosyphilis.	Also treatment for latent syphilis of >1 year or unknown duration.

Source: Sexually Transmitted Diseases Treatment Guidelines, 2010. Centers for Disease Control and Prevention Website. http://www.cdc.gov/std/treatment/2010/STD-Treatment-2010-RR5912.pdf, accessed 8/13/13.

Centers for Disease Control and Prevention. Sexually transmitted diseases treatment guidelines, 2010. *MMWR* 59(No. RR-12): 1–116, 2010.

Human Papillomavirus

72. Sequelae of genital human papillomavirus (HPV) infection in a man can include:
    A. anorectal carcinoma.
    B. low sperm count.
    C. paraphimosis.
    D. Reiter syndrome.

73. Which of the following best describes the lesions associated with condyloma acuminatum?
    A. verruciform
    B. plaquelike
    C. vesicular
    D. bullous

74. Treatment options for patients with condyloma acuminatum include all of the following except:
    A. imiquimod.
    B. podofilox.
    C. topical acyclovir.
    D. cryotherapy.

75. Which HPV types are most likely to cause anorectal carcinoma?
    A. 1 and 3
    B. 6 and 11
    C. 16 and 18
    D. 72 and 81

76. Which HPV types are most likely to cause condyloma acuminatum?
    A. 1, 2, and 3
    B. 6 and 11
    C. 16 and 19
    D. 22 and 24

77. Routine anal Pap tests can be considered for all of the following patient populations except:
    A. men with HIV.
    B. men who have sex with men (MSM).
    C. women with a history of anogenital HPV infection.
    D. all males under age 25 years.

Answers

72. A.	**74.** C.	**76.** B.
73. A.	**75.** C.	**77.** D.

Condyloma acuminatum, the verruciform lesion seen in genital warts, is an STI. The causative agent is human papillomavirus (HPV), and multiple HPV types are usually seen with genital infection. Anal, penile, and cervical carcinoma can be consequences of HPV infection. Not all HPV types are correlated with malignancy, however. HPV types with a high-malignancy risk include types 16, 18, 31, 33, 35, 39, and 45, whereas low malignancy risk is seen with infection from types 6, 11, 40, 42, 43, 44, 54, 61, 70, 72, and 81. HPV types 6 and 11 most often cause genital warts.

About 50% of patients have a spontaneous regression of warts without intervention. The most common treatment options include podofilox, imiquimod, trichloroacetic acid, or cryotherapy. Patient-administered therapies such as imiquimod (Aldara) or podofilox save on the cost and inconvenience of office visits. Surgical intervention and laser ablation are typically reserved for complicated, recalcitrant lesions.

Screening for anal cancer is not routinely recommended for men, although some experts recommend anal cancer screening every 1-3 years via anal Pap tests for MSM and HIV-positive men. The rate of anal cancer among HIV-negative MSM is 20 times higher than the general population; among HIV-positive MSM the rate is 80 times higher. Anal Pap tests can also be considered for women with a history of anogenital HPV infection, anal-receptive intercourse, multiple sexual partners, and a history of sexually transmitted disease or anal condyloma.

Primary prevention of HPV disease is now available through immunization. As with all STIs, a critical part of care is discussion of preventive strategies, including using condoms and limiting the number of sexual partners. NPs should offer and encourage testing for other STIs, including HIV, hepatitis B, and syphilis. Consideration should also be given to offering testing for hepatitis C and human herpes type 2 (herpes simplex type 2). Immunization that provides protection against hepatitis A, hepatitis B, and HPV should be offered as needed and appropriate.

DISCUSSION SOURCES

Gilbert D, Moellering RC, Eliopoulos GM, Chambers HF, Saag MS. *The Sanford Guide to Antimicrobial Therapy*, ed. 44th. Sperryville, VA: Antimicrobial Therapy, Inc., 2014, pp. 23–27.
Centers for Disease Control and Prevention. Sexually transmitted diseases treatment guidelines, 2010. *MMWR* 59(No. RR-12): 1–116, 2010.

Genital Herpes

78. What approximately what percentage of sexually active adults has serological evidence of human herpesvirus 2 (HHV-2 or herpes simplex type 2)?
    A. 5
    B. 15
    C. 25
    D. 40

79. All of the following are likely reported in a man with an initial episode of genital HSV-2 (HHV-2) infection except:
    A. painful ulcer.
    B. inguinal lymphadenopathy.
    C. fever and body aches.
    D. pustular lesions.

80. In the person with HSV-2 infection, the virus can spread via contact through which of the following methods? More than one can apply.
   A. genital secretions.
   B. oral secretions.
   C. intact skin.

81. During asymptomatic HSV-2 infection, genital shedding of the virus occurs during approximately _____ of days.
   A. 10%
   B. 25%
   C. 50%
   D. 100%

82. Diagnostic testing of a person with primary HSV-2 infection would likely show:
   A. negative virologic and serologic test results.
   B. negative virologic test result and positive serologic test result.
   C. positive virologic test result and negative serologic test result.
   D. positive virologic and serologic test results.

83. Treatment options for HSV-2 genital infection include:
   A. ribavirin.
   B. indinavir.
   C. famciclovir.
   D. cyclosporine.

84. Suppressive therapy reduces the frequency of genital herpes recurrences by:
   A. 5%–10%.
   B. 20%–25%.
   C. 40%–50%.
   D. 70%–80%.

Answers

78. B.	81. A.	84. D.
79. D.	82. C.	
80. A, B, C	83. C.	

Genital herpes is a result of infection with a HHV (human herpesvirus, also known as herpes simplex virus [HSV]). Most often, HSV-2 is the causative organism; HSV-1, the virus form that causes cold sores (herpes labialis), is rarely implicated. HSV-2 can infect the perioral area, however. The clinical presentation usually includes a painful ulcerated genital lesion, often accompanied by inguinal lymphadenopathy. An initial outbreak can also be associated with flulike symptoms, including fever, body aches, and swollen glands.

HSV-2 can be spread through contact with lesions, mucosal surfaces, genital secretions, or oral secretions. The virus can also be shed from skin that is intact and appears normal. In those with asymptomatic infections, genital shedding of the virus occurs on 10% of days, even in the absence of any signs or symptoms. Transmission most commonly occurs from an infected partner who does not have a visible sore and may not know that he or she is infected.

Diagnosis can be performed through direct (virologic) or indirect (serologic) testing. Viral culture is the standard for diagnosing genital herpes, which requires a collection of a sample from a lesion. PCR can also be used to test for the presence of viral DNA or RNA and can allow for more rapid and accurate results. Serologic approaches can detect for the presence of antibodies in the blood. In symptomatic patients, the use of direct and indirect assays can differentiate between a new infection versus a newly recognized older infection. A positive virologic test with a negative serologic test would suggest a new infection. Positive results for both tests would indicate a recurrent infection. Approximately 15% of the adult population in the United States is seropositive for HHV-2; at the same time, only about 10-20% of the seropositive popluation have clinically evident disease in the form of genital herpes.

Although there is no curative treatment for herpes, antiviral therapy for recurrent outbreaks can be given as suppression therapy to reduce the frequency of recurrences or episodically to shorten the duration of lesions. Treatment with an antiviral such as acyclovir, famciclovir, or valacyclovir for acute infection, recurrence, or suppression is highly effective. Suppressive therapy reduces the frequency of genital herpes recurrences by 70%–80% in those who have frequent recurrences. Treatment is also effective in those who have less frequent recurrences. Suppression therapy also has the advantage of decreasing the risk for viral transmission to susceptible partners.

As with all STIs, a critical part of care is discussion of preventive strategies, including using condoms and limiting the number of sexual partners. NPs should offer and encourage testing for other STIs, including HIV, hepatitis B, and syphilis. Consideration should also be given to offering testing for hepatitis C. Immunization that provides protection against hepatitis A, hepatitis B, and HPV should be offered as needed and appropriate.

DISCUSSION SOURCES

2010 Sexually Transmitted Diseases Surveillance. Centers for Disease Control and Prevention Website. http://www.cdc.gov/std/stats10/other.htm#herpes

Genital Herpes—CDC Fact Sheet. Centers for Disease Control and Prevention Website. http://www.cdc.gov/std/herpes/STDFact-Herpes.htm

Erectile Dysfunction

85. Which of the following is not a common risk factor for erectile dysfunction (ED)?
   A. diabetes mellitus
   B. hypertension
   C. cigarette smoking
   D. testosterone deficiency

86. Patient education about the use of sildenafil (Viagra) includes the following:
- A. A spontaneous erection occurs about 1 hour after taking the medication.
- B. This medication helps regain erectile function in nearly all men who use it.
- C. With the use of the medication, sexual stimulation also is needed to achieve an erection.
- D. Nitrates can be safely used concurrently.

87. When discussing ED with a 70-year-old man, the NP considers that:
- A. it is a normal consequence of aging.
- B. most cases have an underlying contributing cause.
- C. although depression is common in older men, it is usually not correlated with increased rates of ED.
- D. treatment options for younger men are seldom effective in older men.

88. Which of the following medications for ED treatment has the longest half-life?
- A. sildenafil (Viagra)
- B. tadalafil (Cialis)
- C. vardenafil (Levitra)
- D. avanafil (Stendra)

89. When taking a PDE-5 inhibitor, concomitant use of which medication must be avoided?
- A. statins
- B. sulfonylurea
- C. ACE inhibitors
- D. nitrates

90. For patients with erectile dysfunction who fail therapy with a PDE-5 inhibitor, alternative approaches include all of the following except:
- A. alprostadil injection into the penis.
- B. mechanical vacuum devices.
- C. insertion of a nitroglycerin pellet in the urethra.
- D. implantation of a prosthetic device.

Answers

85. D.	87. B.	89. D.
86. C.	88. B.	90. C.

Erectile dysfunction (ED), also known as impotency, is defined as the repeated inability to get or keep a penile erection firm enough for sexual intercourse. The spectrum of ED includes the total inability to achieve erection, an inconsistent ability to do so, and a tendency to sustain only brief erections. Achieving and sustaining a penile erection requires a precise sequence of events that depends on healthy nervous system function (brain, spinal column, and penile innervation), appropriate muscle response, and intact blood flow via patent veins and arteries in and near the corpora cavernosa. Any disorder that causes injury to the nerves or impairs blood flow in the penis has the potential to cause ED. Diabetes mellitus,

kidney disease, chronic alcohol abuse, vascular disease, tobacco use, neuropathy, and urological surgery such as radical prostatectomy are implicated in at least 70% of cases of ED. Certain medications, such as antihypertensives, antidepressants, and cimetidine, can produce ED as an adverse effect. The presence of a mood disorder significantly contributes to the risk of ED. Hormonal disorders, particularly testosterone deficiency, pose a significant but uncommon ED risk.

The incidence of ED increases with age; it is found in about 5% of 40-year-old men and 15% to 25% of 65-year-old men. ED should not be thought to be an inevitable consequence of aging, however. Although most ED in older men has a physical cause, such as disease, injury, or adverse effects of drugs, treatment can often help the patient regain satisfactory sexual function.

Intervention in ED starts with treating or minimizing the underlying cause. With currently available therapies, effective treatment can be provided for most men with ED. Medications such as the phosphodiesterase-5 (PDE-5) inhibitors, sildenafil, vardenafil, avanafil, and tadalafil, work by enhancing the effects of nitric oxide, a chemical that relaxes smooth muscles in the penis during sexual stimulation and allows increased blood flow. Use of these agents does not trigger an automatic erection, and they should be taken about 1 hour before the anticipated onset of sexual activity. The half-life of sildenafil, avanafil vardenafil is approximately 4 to 5 hours, whereas tadalafil has a longer half-life of approximately 17 hours; as a result of its long T 1/2, tadalafil is the only ED medication recommended for lower dose daily use. The concomitant use of a drug such as sildenafil with a nitrate is contraindicated because of the risk of profound hypotension; the duration of an adverse effect of a PDE-5 inhibitor is likely to persist for a period related to the drug's duration of action and half-life.

Drugs injected directly into the penis, such as alprostadil (Caverject), cause vasodilation and are highly effective. An alprostadil pellet inserted into the urethra (Muse) can achieve the same effect. Mechanical vacuum devices cause erection by creating a partial vacuum, which draws blood into the penis, engorging and expanding it. An elastic band is placed around the base of the penis to maintain the erection after the cylinder is removed and during intercourse by preventing blood from flowing back into the body. This mechanical method of ED treatment is particularly helpful when other methods fail to achieve desired results. Surgical options include vessel repair to treat the underlying ED; it should be kept in mind, however, that atherosclerosis is a widespread disease, and outcomes are unpredictable. Implantation of devices such as prostheses or pumps is another option, albeit with the associated risks and costs of any surgical procedure.

DISCUSSION SOURCES

Grant P, Jackson G, Baig I, Quin J. Erectile dysfunction in general medicine. *Clin Med* 13:136–140, 2013.
Shamloul R, Ghanem H. Erectile dysfunction. *Lancet* 381:153–165, 2013.

Musculoskeletal Disorders

9

Bursitis

1. The most common cause of acute bursitis is:
   A. inactivity.
   B. joint overuse.
   C. fibromyalgia.
   D. bacterial infection.

2. First-line treatment options for bursitis usually include:
   A. corticosteroid bursal injection.
   B. heat to area.
   C. weight-bearing exercises.
   D. nonsteroidal anti-inflammatory drugs (NSAIDs).

3. Patients with olecranon bursitis typically present with:
   A. swelling and redness over the affected area.
   B. limited elbow range of motion (ROM).
   C. nerve impingement.
   D. destruction of the joint space.

4. Patients with subscapular bursitis typically present with:
   A. limited shoulder ROM.
   B. heat over affected area.
   C. localized tenderness under the superomedial angle of the scapula.
   D. cervical nerve root irritation.

5. Patients with gluteus medius or deep trochanteric bursitis typically present with:
   A. increased pain from resisted hip abduction.
   B. limited hip ROM.
   C. sciatic nerve pain.
   D. heat over the affected area.

6. Likely sequelae of intrabursal corticosteroid injection include:
   A. irreversible skin atrophy.
   B. infection.
   C. inflammatory reaction.
   D. soreness at the site of injection.

7. First-line therapy for prepatellar bursitis should include:
   A. bursal aspiration.
   B. intrabursal corticosteroid injection.
   C. acetaminophen.
   D. knee splinting.

8. Clinical conditions with a presentation similar to acute bursitis include: (More than one option can apply.)
   A. rheumatoid arthritis.
   B. septic arthritis.
   C. joint trauma.
   D. pseudogout.

Answers

1. B.	4. C.	7. A.
2. D.	5. A.	8. A, B, C, and D
3. A.	6. D.	

The human body contains more than 150 bursa. These fluid-filled sacs act as a cushion between tendons and bones. Bursitis develops when the synovial tissue that lines the sac becomes thickened and produces excessive fluid, leading to swelling and resulting pain. The bursae are lined by synovial tissue, which produces fluid that lubricates and reduces friction between these structures. The most commonly affected bursa are the subdeltoid, olecranon, ischial, trochanter, and prepatellar. In contrast to most forms of arthritis, bursitis typically presents with an abrupt onset with focal tenderness and swelling. The joint range of motion (ROM) is usually full but is often limited by pain (Table 9–1).

Risk factors for acute bursitis include joint overuse, trauma, infection, or arthritis conditions such as rheumatoid arthritis or osteoarthritis. Because recurrence is common, prevention of further joint overuse and trauma should be emphasized.

With prepatellar bursitis, bursal aspiration should be considered as a first-line therapy because this procedure affords significant pain relief and allows the bursa to reapproximate. In other sites, first-line therapy includes minimizing or eliminating the offending activity, applying ice

TABLE 9-1
Clinical Presentation of Bursitis

Location of Bursitis	Clinical Presentation	Comments
Prepatellar (knee)	Knee swelling and pain in the front of the knee, normal ROM	Risk factors include frequent kneeling (also known as housemaid's knee)
Olecranon (elbow)	Pain, swelling behind the elbow, swelling in same area, often described as ball or sac hanging from the elbow	Risk factors include prolonged pressure or trauma to the elbow (also known as draftsman's elbow)
Trochanter (hip)	Gait disturbance, local trochanter tenderness, pain on hip rotation, and resisted hip abduction with normal hip ROM	Risk factors include back disease, leg-length discrepancy, and leg problems that lead to altered gait OA seldom implicated
Subscapular (shoulder)	Local tenderness under superomedial angle of the scapula over the adjacent rib, normal shoulder ROM, no nerve root impingement	Risk factors include repeated back-and-forth motion Common in assembly-line workers
Pre-Achilles (heel)	Pain and localized swelling behind the heel, minimal pain with dorsiflexion, normal ankle ROM	Usually not disabling and does not contribute to tendon rupture Often confused with Achilles tendonitis
Retrocalcaneal (heel)	Pain behind ankle worsened by walking Patient often runs fingers along both sides of Achilles tendon	Risk factors include wearing high-heeled shoes and repetitive ankle motion such as stair-climbing, running, jogging, and walking

OA, osteoarthritis; ROM, range of motion.

Sources: Anderson B. *Office Orthopedics for Primary Care: Diagnosis* ed. 1. Philadelphia: Saunders, 2006.
Anderson B. *Office Orthopedics for Primary Care: Treatment*, ed. 3. Philadelphia: Saunders, 2006.

to the affected area for 15 minutes at least four times per day, and taking nonsteroidal anti-inflammatory drugs (NSAIDs). If these conservative measures have not worked after approximately 4 to 8 weeks, intrabursal corticosteroid injection should be performed. Before injection, patients should be informed of the risks of this procedure, especially the most common problem, soreness at the injection site. After corticosteroid injection, infection, tissue atrophy, and inflammatory reaction are possible, but rarely encountered, complications.

DISCUSSION SOURCES

Del Buono A, Franceschi F, Palumbo A, et al. Diagnosis and management of olecranon bursitis. *Surgeon* 10:297–300, 2012.
Lohr K, Gellman H. Bursitis. http://emedicine.medscape.com/article/2145588

◗ Epicondylitis

9. Patients with lateral epicondylitis typically present with:
   A. electric-like pain elicited by tapping over the median nerve.
   B. reduced joint ROM.
   C. pain that is worst with elbow flexion.
   D. decreased hand grip strength.

10. Risk factors for lateral epicondylitis include all of the following except:
    A. repetitive lifting.
    B. playing tennis.
    C. hammering.
    D. gout.

11. Up to what percent of patients with medial epicondylitis recover without surgery?
    A. 35%
    B. 50%
    C. 70%
    D. 95%

12. Initial treatment of lateral epicondylitis includes all of the following except:
    A. rest and activity modifications.
    B. corticosteroid injections.
    C. topical or oral NSAIDs,
    D. counterforce bracing.

13. Extracorporeal shock-wave therapy can be used in the treatment of epicondylitis as a means to:
    A. improve ROM.
    B. build forearm strength.
    C. promote the natural healing process.
    D. stretch the extensor tendon.

14. Patients with medial epicondylitis typically present with:
- A. forearm numbness.
- B. reduction in ROM.
- C. pain on elbow flexion.
- D. decreased grip strength.

15. Risk factors for medial epicondylitis include playing:
- A. tennis.
- B. golf.
- C. baseball.
- D. volleyball.

Answers

9. D.	**12.** B.	**15.** B.
10. D.	**13.** C.	
11. D.	**14.** D.	

The painful condition that arises as a result of injury to the extensor tendon at the lateral epicondyle is called tennis elbow or lateral epicondylitis. Patients usually give a history of an aggravating activity followed by forearm weakness and point to tenderness over the inner aspect of the humerus (Table 9–2). Medial epicondylitis, often called golfer's elbow, is similar to lateral epicondylitis but occurs on the inside of the elbow.

Approximately 80% to 95% of patients with epicondylitis can be successfully treated without surgery. Rest and avoidance of the precipitating activity for up to several weeks is the first course of treatment. NSAIDs (aspirin and ibuprofen) can be used to reduce pain and inflammation. For sports-related injuries, conducting an equipment check and working with an expert on proper form can reduce the risk of aggravating the injury. Physical therapy can be helpful in strengthening muscles in the arm or performing muscle-stimulating techniques to improve healing. For lateral epicondylitis, a counterforce brace centered over the back of the forearm can help relieve symptoms. Local corticosteroid injection can be helpful if symptoms persist beyond 6 to 8 weeks or are particularly severe. Extracorporeal shock-wave therapy can also be considered, which uses sound waves to create microtrauma to the elbow that promotes the body's natural healing process. The use of a tennis elbow band can help prevent recurrence.

DISCUSSION SOURCE

Lohr K, Gellman H. Bursitis, available at http://emedicine.medscape.com/article/2145588.

TABLE 9-2
Clinical Presentation of Epicondylitis

Condition	Presentation	Comments
Medial epicondylitis	Patient complains of pain over medial epicondyle or inner aspect of lower humerus. Pain worsens with wrist flexion and pronation activities. Local epicondylar tenderness, elbow pain, forearm weakness, pain aggravated by wrist flexion, and pronation activities with decreased grip strength and full ROM occur.	Often called golfer's elbow; results from repetitive activity such as lifting, use of certain tool, playing sports involving a tight grip. Prevent recurrence by using palm-up lifting, using a tennis elbow band, avoiding precipitating causes, ensuring proper use of tools, using proper body mechanics, and developing flexibility and strength of the involved musculature
Lateral epicondylitis	Patient complains of pain over lateral epicondyle or outer aspect of lower humerus, which increases with resisted wrist extension, especially with elbow. Hand grip is often weak on affected side. Elbow ROM usually is normal.	Often called tennis elbow; results from repetitive activity such as lifting, use of certain tools, playing sports involving a tight grip. Prevent recurrence by avoiding precipitating causes, ensuring proper use of tools, using proper body mechanics, and developing of flexibility and strength of the involved musculature

ROM, range of motion.
Sources: Gibbs SJ. eMedicine. http://emedicine.medscape.com/article/327860-overview, Physical medicine and rehabilitation for epicondylitis.
Walrod BJ. http://emedicine.medscape.com/article/96969-overview, Lateral epicondylitis.

Gouty Arthritis

16. Risk factors for acute gouty arthritis include:
    A. obesity.
    B. female gender.
    C. rheumatoid arthritis.
    D. joint trauma.

17. The use of all of the following medications can trigger gout except:
    A. aspirin.
    B. statins.
    C. diuretics.
    D. niacin.

18. Secondary gout can be caused by all of the following conditions except:
    A. psoriasis.
    B. hemolytic anemia.
    C. bacterial cellulitis.
    D. renal failure.

19. The clinical presentation of acute gouty arthritis affecting the base of the great toe includes:
    A. slow onset of discomfort over many days.
    B. greatest swelling and pain along the median aspect of the joint.
    C. improvement of symptoms with joint rest.
    D. fever.

20. The most helpful diagnostic test to perform during acute gouty arthritis is:
    A. measurement of erythrocyte sedimentation rate (ESR).
    B. measurement of serum uric acid.
    C. analysis of aspirate from the affected joint.
    D. joint radiography.

21. First-line therapy for treating patients with acute gouty arthritis usually includes:
    A. aspirin.
    B. naproxen sodium.
    C. allopurinol.
    D. probenecid.

22. Tophi are best described as:
    A. ulcerations originating on swollen joints.
    B. swollen lymph nodes.
    C. abscesses with one or more openings draining pus onto the skin.
    D. nontender, firm nodules located in soft tissue.

23. Which of the following patients with acute gouty arthritis is the best candidate for local corticosteroid injection?
    A. a 66-year-old patient with a gastric ulcer
    B. a 44-year-old patient taking a thiazide diuretic
    C. a 68-year-old patient with type 2 diabetes mellitus
    D. a 32-year-old patient who is a binge drinker

24. The most common locations for tophi include all of the following except:
    A. the auricles.
    B. the elbows.
    C. the extensor surfaces of the hands.
    D. the shoulders.

25. Dietary recommendations for a person with gouty arthritis include avoiding foods high in:
    A. artificial flavors and colors.
    B. purine.
    C. vitamin C.
    D. protein.

26. Which of the following dietary supplements is associated with increased risk for gout?
    A. vitamin A
    B. gingko biloba
    C. brewer's yeast
    D. glucosamine

27. Pseudogout is caused by the formation of what type of crystals in joints?
    A. uric acid
    B. calcium oxalate
    C. struvite
    D. calcium pyrophosphate dihydrate

28. Pseudogout has been linked with abnormal activity of the:
    A. liver.
    B. kidneys.
    C. parathyroid.
    D. adrenal gland.

29. Differentiation between gout and pseudogout can involve all of the following diagnostic approaches except:
    A. analysis of minerals in the blood.
    B. analysis of joint fluid.
    C. x-ray of the affected joint.
    D. measuring thyroid function.

30. Treatment of pseudogout can include all of the following except:
    A. NSAIDs.
    B. colchicine.
    C. allopurinol.
    D. oral corticosteroids.

Answers

16. A.	21. B.	26. C.
17. B.	22. D.	27. D.
18. C.	23. A.	28. C.
19. B.	24. D.	29. C.
20. C.	25. B.	30. C.

Gouty arthritis, often simply called gout, manifests as acute monoarticular arthritis, usually triggered by a disorder causing a decrease of uric acid excretion that allows an accumulation of urates in joints, bones, and subcutaneous tissues. Urate precipitates out of biological fluids when levels are elevated, a condition that usually follows the inability of the kidney to eliminate uric acid. About 90% of patients presenting with primary gout are men; the condition is rarely seen in women before menopause. Gout risk factors include obesity, diabetes mellitus, and a family history of the condition. Less often, acute gout is caused by excessive uric acid production, usually coupled with decreased urate excretion. The use of select medications, including thiazide diuretics, niacin, aspirin, and cyclosporine, can precipitate gout by causing hyperuricemia; alcohol use is also a possible precipitant. Other causes of secondary gout include conditions characterized by increased catabolism and purine turnover, such as psoriasis, myeloproliferative and lymphoproliferative diseases, and chronic hemolytic anemia, and conditions with decreased renal uric acid clearance, such as intrinsic kidney disease and renal failure.

This acutely painful condition typically affects the metacarpophalangeal joint of the great toe. The onset is sudden and is accompanied by significant distress. Although the disease manifests acutely, the metabolic disorder behind the problem is typically present for months to years before the clinical presentation. Patients report the inability to walk, move the joint, or even tolerate the weight of a bed sheet on the affected joint because of severe pain. The entire great toe is usually reddened and enlarged, with the greatest amount of swelling noted along the medial border of the joint; this usually is also the point of greatest discomfort. Although the clinical presentation of gout can mimic that of an acutely infected joint, gout is 100 times more common than monoarticular septic arthritis. With repeated episodes, nontender firm nodules known as tophi can develop in soft tissue. Because the gouty crystals that fill tophi precipitate more easily in cooler areas of the body, these lesions often develop in the external ear; less common locations include nasal cartilage, extensor surfaces of the hands and feet, and over the elbows.

The diagnosis of acute gouty arthritis is usually straightforward, particularly with repeated episodes. With the first episode, an initial uric acid level is obtained in most cases but is usually normal. Uric acid levels are often reduced during the acute phase, or the etiology of the attack is largely poor urate excretion. Analysis of joint aspirate for urate crystals is diagnostic; the erythrocyte sedimentation rate (ESR) or C-reactive protein (CRP) is usually high, but these findings are neither sensitive nor specific for gout and simply reflect the inflammation associated with the condition. Radiographs are not needed unless a concurrent history of trauma and risk of fracture are present.

The treatment of acute gouty arthritis should include minimizing or removing contributing factors, such as alcohol use or use of certain medications. Treatment should be aimed at reducing inflammation first and then treating hyperuricemia, trying to avoid a rapid reduction in serum uric acid, which can make the episode worse. A loading dose of an NSAID,

such as 750 mg of naproxen followed by lower doses, can be helpful. Because aspirin use can precipitate gout, its use in the presence of the condition is contraindicated. Colchicine can be used but is often poorly tolerated. Suggested dosing is 1.2 mg initially, then 0.6 mg 1 hour later followed by 0.6 mg once or twice daily (up to 2.4 mg total dose in 24 hours) or when gastrointestinal symptoms occur. A short course of a systemic corticosteroid, such as prednisone (0.5 mg/kg/day for 5–10 days, or 0.5 mg/kg/day for 2–5 days, then taper for 7–10 days), is a helpful alternative to colchicine. Local injection with corticosteroids can provide significant relief and offers a treatment alternative to NSAIDs, particularly in the presence of warfarin use, renal failure, or peptic ulcer disease.

Several medications are available to prevent gout attacks by blocking uric acid production or improving uric acid removal. Xanthin oxidase inhibitors (XOIs), including allopurinol (Aloprim, Lopurin, Zyloprim) or febuxostat (Uloric), limit the amount of uric acid the body produces. Common adverse effects of allopurinol include rash and low blood counts, whereas febuxostat is associated with rash, nausea, and reduced liver function. Probenecid (Probalan) improves the kidney's ability to remove uric acid from the body. Probenecid use leads to higher concentrations of uric acid in the urine, resulting in a greater risk of kidney stones. Other adverse effects include rash and abdominal pain.

Dietary modification to avoid foods with high purine content is an important and often overlooked intervention to minimize the risk of future gout episodes. Examples of high-purine foods include certain seafood (scallops, mussels), organ and game meats, beans, spinach, asparagus, oatmeal, and baker's and brewer's yeasts when taken as dietary supplements.

After the acute flare has subsided, a 24-hour urine collection for uric acid helps assess whether the patient overproduces or undersecretes uric acid. Long-term care to avoid future attacks is directed by the result; undersecretors benefit from probenecid, and overproducers benefit from allopurinol or febuxostat. Other medications not specifically designated for gout treatment, including fenofibrate and losartan, have been studied and found to be helpful with urate excretion and can be used as therapeutic adjuncts as part of a comprehensive uric acid–lowering strategy.

Pseudogout, also called calcium pyrophosphate deposition (CPPD) disease, presents similarly to gout but is caused by the presence of calcium pyrophosphate dehydrate crystals in the joint. The knees are most commonly affected but the wrists and ankles also can be involved, with symptoms of swollen, warm, and severely painful joints. Risk factors include older age, joint trauma, family history of the condition, and mineral imbalances (e.g., hemochromatosis, hypercalcemia, or hypomagnesemia). Pseudogout has also been associated with hypothyroidism or hyperparathyroidism.

Proper diagnosis of pseudogout involves detecting calcium pyrophosphate crystals in the affected joint. Blood tests can detect abnormal thyroid or parathyroid function and abnormal mineral levels linked to pseudogout. The goal of treatment is primarily to relieve pain and improve joint function and includes the use of NSAIDs, colchicine, and oral corticosteroids.

DISCUSSION SOURCES

Khanna D, Fitzgerald JD, Khanna PP, et al. 2012 American College of Rheumatology guidelines for management of gout. Part 1: Systematic nonpharmacologic and pharmacologic therapeutic approaches to hyperuricemia. *Arthritis Care Res (Hoboken)* 64:1431–1446, 2012.

Cassagnol M, Saad M. Pharmacologic management of gout. *US Pharmacist* 38:22–26, 2013, available at http://www.uspharmacist.com/content/d/feature/c/39863.

See full color images of this topic on DavisPlus at
**http://davisplus.fadavis.com |
Keyword: Fitzgerald**

⬤ Osteoarthritis

31. Which of the following joints is most likely to be affected by osteoarthritis (OA)?
A. wrists
B. elbows
C. metacarpophalangeal joint
D. distal interphalangeal joint

32. Changes to the joint during osteoarthritis can typically include all of the following except:
A. widening of the joint space.
B. articular cartilage wears away.
C. formation of bone spurs.
D. synovial membrane thickens.

33. Clinical findings of the knee in a patient with OA include all of the following except:
A. coarse crepitus.
B. joint effusion.
C. warm joint.
D. knee often locks or a pop is heard.

34. Radiographic findings of osteoarthritis of the knee often reveal:
A. microfractures.
B. decreased density of subchondral bone.
C. osteophytes.
D. no apparent changes to the joint structure.

35. Approximately what percent of patients with radiological findings of osteoarthritis of the knee will report having symptoms?
A. 25%
B. 50%
C. 70%
D. 95%

36. Deformity of the proximal interphalangeal joints found in an elderly patient with OA is known as:
A. Heberden nodes.
B. Bouchard nodes.
C. hallus valgus.
D. Dupuytren contracture.

37. Which of the following best describes the presentation of a patient with OA?
A. worst symptoms in weight-bearing joints later in the day
B. symmetrical early morning stiffness
C. sausage-shaped digits with associated skin lesions
D. back pain with rest and anterior uveitis

38. As part of the evaluation of patients with OA, the NP anticipates finding:
A. anemia of chronic disease.
B. elevated CRP level.
C. no disease-specific laboratory abnormalities.
D. elevated antinuclear antibody (ANA) titer.

39. First-line pharmacological intervention for milder OA should be a trial of:
A. acetaminophen.
B. tramadol.
C. celecoxib.
D. intraarticular corticosteroid injection.

40. In caring for a patient with OA of the knee, you advise that:
A. straight-leg raising should be avoided.
B. heat should be applied to painful joints after exercise.
C. quadriceps-strengthening exercises should be performed.
D. physical activity should be avoided.

41. The mechanism of action of glucosamine and chondroitin is:
A. via increased production of synovial fluid.
B. through improved cartilage repair.
C. via inhibition of the inflammatory response in the joint.
D. largely unknown.

42. An adverse effect associated with the use of glucosamine is:
A. elevated ALT and AST.
B. bronchospasm.
C. increased bleeding risk.
D. QT prolongation.

43. A 72-year-old man presents at an early stage of osteoarthritis in his left knee. He mentions that he heard about the benefits of using glucosamine and chondroitin for treating joint problems. In consulting the patient, you mention all of the following except:
A. any benefit can take at least 3 months of consistent use before observed.
B. glucosamine is not associated with any drug interactions.
C. clinical studies have consistently shown benefit of long-term use of glucosamine and chondroitin for treating OA of the knee.
D. chondroitin should be used with caution because of its antiplatelet effect.

44. The American Academy of Orthopaedic Surgeons (AAOS) favors all of the following in the management of symptomatic OA of the knee except:
A. low-impact aerobic exercises.
B. weight loss for those with a BMI ≥25 kg/m².
C. acupuncture.
D. strengthening exercises.

45. AAOS strongly recommends all of the following therapeutic agents for the management of symptomatic OA of the knee except:
A. oral NSAIDs.
B. topical NSAIDs.
C. tramadol.
D. opioids.

46. Among surgical and procedural interventions, AAOS strongly recommends the use of which of the following for the management of symptomatic OA of the knee?
A. intraarticular corticosteroid use
B. hyaluronic acid injections
C. arthroscopy with lavage and/or débridement
D. none of the above

47. Regarding the current scientific evidence on the use of glucosamine and chondroitin for the management of symptomatic OA of the knee, AAOS:
A. strongly favors their use.
B. provides a moderate-strength recommendation for their use.
C. cannot recommend for or against the use of these supplements (limited evidence).
D. cannot recommend the use of these supplements.

48. You see a 67-year-old woman who has been treated for pain due to OA of the hip for the past 6 months and who asks about hip replacement surgery. She complains of pain even at night when sleeping and avoids walking even moderate distances unless absolutely necessary. In counseling the patient, you mention all of the following except:
A. arthroplasty can be considered when pain is not adequately controlled.
B. arthroplasty is not needed if the patient can walk even short distances.
C. arthroplasty candidates must be able to tolerate a long surgical procedure.
D. rehabilitation following surgery is essential to achieve maximal function of the joint.

49. Recommended exercises for patients with OA of the knee include all of the following except:
A. squatting with light weights.
B. straight-leg raises without weights.
C. quadriceps sets.
D. limited weight-bearing aerobic exercises.

50. Recommended exercises for patients with OA of the hip include all of the following except:
A. stretching exercises of the gluteus muscles.
B. straight-leg raises without weights.
C. isometric exercises of the iliopsoas and gluteus muscles.
D. weight-bearing aerobic exercises.

Answers

31. D.	**38.** C.	**45.** D.
32. A.	**39.** A.	**46.** D.
33. C.	**40.** C.	**47.** D.
34. C.	**41.** D.	**48.** B.
35. B.	**42.** B.	**49.** A.
36. B.	**43.** C.	**50.** D.
37. A.	**44.** C.	

Osteoarthritis (OA) is the most common joint disease in North America; it is a degenerative condition that manifests without systemic manifestations or acute inflammation. Although the distal interphalangeal joint is the most common OA site, the most problematic joint involvement is in the hip and knee. Worst symptoms are reported with use of the joints. As a result, discomfort typically increases as the day progresses, and there is minimal morning stiffness; in contrast, with rheumatoid arthritis (RA), morning stiffness is usually most problematic. Risk factors for OA include a positive family history of the condition and contact sport participation. Obesity is likely the most common personal risk factor, especially with hip and knee involvement. In OA, the articular cartilage becomes rough and wears away. Bone spurs often form, and the synovial membrane thickens. Consequently, the joint space narrows. The clinical presentation in patients with OA includes an insidious onset of symptoms, including use-related joint pain that is relieved by rest and joint stiffness that occurs with rest but resolves with less than 15 minutes of activity. Physical examination usually reveals smooth, cool joints and coarse crepitus. Particularly when the knee is affected, joint effusion is common and can be minimal to severe with up to 20 mL of fluid. Patients cannot achieve full knee flexion in the effused joint. The knee often locks, or a pop is heard, which suggests a degenerative meniscal tear.

Radiological findings in patients with OA include narrowing of the joint space and increased density of subchondral bone. Bone cysts and osteophytes are often present, developed as part of the body's repair process; however, only about 50% of patients with radiological findings have symptoms. Because OA is typically a noninflammatory disease, ESR and CRP levels, both markers of inflammation, are typically normal. In contrast to RA and systemic lupus erythematosus (SLE), antinuclear antibodies (ANAs), rheumatoid factor, and other markers of systemic arthritis syndromes are absent from the serum unless there is concomitant disease.

Therapeutic goals for patients with OA include preventing further articular cartilage destruction, minimizing pain, and enhancing mobility. Therapies for symptom control include lifestyle modifications, such as weight loss and exercise with minimal weight-bearing, such as swimming or water-based activities, and exercise to maintain joint flexibility and enhance strength in the surrounding muscles (Table 9–3). Application of heat to minimize pain and stiffness in the morning before activity can be helpful, and applying ice to the joint after activity can minimize discomfort; the use of heat or ice should be directed by patient response. For OA of the knee, guidelines from the American Academy of Orthopaedic Surgeons (AAOS) recommend the use of NSAIDs (oral or topical) and tramadol (Ultram) for controlling pain. Although NSAIDs also have potential anti-inflammatory activity, this mechanism of drug action is seldom needed in OA therapy because inflammation is a minor contributor to symptoms. Tramadol, an opioid analgesic, is effective for treating moderate to moderately severe pain. Long-term use of this agent, however, can lead to physical or mental dependence and cause adverse effects when discontinued. Duloxetine (Cymbalta) has also been approved for the treatment of chronic osteoarthritis pain. AAOS does not recommend for or against the use of acetaminophen, other opioids, or pain patches for managing symptomatic OA of the knee. Because of the gastropathy potential associated with long-term use of NSAIDs, a trial of acetaminophen is warranted for symptom control in less severe cases of OA, recognizing that NSAIDs are usually associated with superior analgesic effect. Long-acting opioids are occasionally required if symptom control cannot be achieved. The risks versus benefits of opioid analgesia need to be carefully evaluated with each patient.

Glucosamine, an amino acid, is usually used as first-line treatment for OA in many European nations and is available as an over-the-counter nutritional supplement in the United States. The results of research studies have differed on the effectiveness of its use, with many reporting no improvement in arthritis symptoms and others reporting a reduction in pain, increased joint flexion, and increased articular function. If effective, glucosamine must be used consistently for a minimum of 2 weeks and likely 3 months before therapeutic effect is seen. Although no drug interactions or hepatotoxicity has been noted with its use, glucosamine should be used with caution because there is a risk of bronchospasm. Chondroitin is often used in conjunction with glucosamine because the two appear to have synergistic activity, although this has been disputed in limited studies. The mechanism of action of these products is not well understood. Although chondroitin is generally well tolerated, it should be used with caution because of a potential anticoagulant effect. As with all nutritional supplements, using a preparation that is supplied by a manufacturer with *United States Pharmacopeia* or other similar verification is advised. In particular, a 2-year study demonstrated no clinically significant change in pain or function as compared with placebo over 2 years with the use of glucosamine alone or in combination with chondroitin. AAOS does not recommend using glucosamine and chondroitin for patients with symptomatic OA of the knee.

Intraarticular corticosteroid joint injection is often recommended when conservative therapy has failed. AAOS, however, does not recommend for or against the use of intraarticular corticosteroid injections because of a lack of compelling evidence comparing the benefits with risks. AAOS also does not recommend using hyaluronic acid injections for treating symptomatic OA of the knee because of lack of efficacy observed in clinical trials.

Treatment of OA of the hip is similar to treating OA of the knee. Resting the hip, physical therapy to strengthen the muscles surrounding the hip, and decreasing body mass if overweight can be helpful. NSAIDs can be used to help

TABLE 9-3
Exercise Regimens in Osteoarthritis

Joint Condition	Exercise Regimen	Comments
Osteoarthritis in the knee	• Straight-leg raises without weights, advance to using weights as tolerated • Quadriceps sets • Non–weight-bearing or limited weight-bearing aerobic activity	Avoid squatting and kneeling, high-impact exercise
Osteoarthritis of the hip	• Straight-leg raises without weights, advance to using weights as tolerated • Stretching exercises of adductors, rotator, and gluteus muscles • Isometric exercises of iliopsoas and gluteus muscles • Non–weight-bearing or limited weight-bearing aerobic activity	Avoid high-impact exercise

manage pain. Hip injection of corticosteroids is a technically challenging procedure that can be done with fluoroscopic guidance. For advanced stages of OA, when pain occurs even when resting at night, and/or the hip is severely deformed, arthroplasty may be considered.

Knee and hip joint replacement should be considered when pain cannot be adequately controlled, when function is severely compromised, or when more than 80% of the articular cartilage is worn away. The ideal candidate for joint replacement is able to tolerate a surgical procedure that lasts for several hours, followed by an aggressive postoperative course of rehabilitation. Many patients with OA who have been debilitated by poor mobility have improved health when ambulation becomes possible after hip or knee replacement. Rehabilitation following joint replacement is critical to restore flexibility of the joint and strengthen muscles needed for normal functioning.

DISCUSSION SOURCES

Anderson B. *Office Orthopedics for Primary Care: Diagnosis*, ed. 1,. Philadelphia: Saunders Elsevier, 2006.

Anderson B. *Office Orthopedics for Primary Care: Treatment*, ed. 3. Philadelphia: Saunders Elsevier, 2006.

Glucosamine/Chondroitin Arthritis Intervention Trial (GAIT), available at http://nccam.nih.gov/research/results/gait.

AAOS. Treatment of osteoarthritis of the knee: Evidence-based practice guidelines, ed. 2, available at http://www.aaos.org/research/guidelines/TreatmentofOsteoarthritisoftheKneeGuideline.pdf.

Stone L. Aches, pains and osteoarthritis. *Aust Fam Physician* 37: 912–917, 2008.

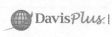 See full color images of this topic on DavisPlus at http://davisplus.fadavis.com | Keyword: Fitzgerald

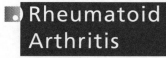

Rheumatoid Arthritis

51. Which of the following is not characteristic of rheumatoid arthritis (RA)?
    A. It is more common in women at a 3:1 ratio.
    B. Family history of autoimmune conditions often is reported.
    C. Peak age for disease onset in individuals is age 50 to 70 years.
    D. Wrists, ankles, and toes often are involved.

52. Which of the following best describes the presentation of a person with RA?
    A. worst symptoms in weight-bearing joints later in the day
    B. symmetrical early-morning stiffness
    C. sausage-shaped digits with characteristic skin lesions
    D. back pain with rest and anterior uveitis

53. NSAIDs cause gastric injury primarily by:
    A. direct irritative effect.
    B. slowing gastrointestinal motility.
    C. thinning of the protective gastrointestinal mucosa.
    D. enhancing prostaglandin synthesis.

54. Of the following individuals, who is at highest risk for NSAID-induced gastropathy?
    A. a 28-year-old man with an ankle sprain who has taken ibuprofen for the past week and who drinks four to six beers every weekend
    B. a 40-year-old woman who smokes and takes about six doses of naproxen sodium per month to control dysmenorrhea
    C. a 43-year-old man with dilated cardiomyopathy who uses ketoprofen one to two times per week for low back pain
    D. a 72-year-old man who takes aspirin four times a day for pain control of osteoarthritis

55. Which of the following is the preferred method of preventing NSAID-induced gastric ulcer?
    A. a high-dose histamine 2 receptor antagonist
    B. timed antacid use
    C. sucralfate (Carafate)
    D. misoprostol (Cytotec)

56. Taking a high dose of aspirin or ibuprofen causes:
    A. an increase in the drug's half-life.
    B. enhanced renal excretion of the drug.
    C. a change in the drug's mechanism of action.
    D. a reduction of antiprostaglandin effect.

57. Which of the following statements is most accurate concerning RA?
    A. Joint erosions are often evident on radiographs or MRI.
    B. RA is seldom associated with other autoimmune diseases.
    C. A butterfly-shaped facial rash is common.
    D. Parvovirus B$_{19}$ infection can contribute to its development.

58. Which of the following hemograms would be expected for a 46-year-old woman with poorly controlled RA?
    A. Hg = 11.1 g/dL (12–14 g/dL); MCV = 66 fL (80–96 fL); reticulocytes = 0.8% (1%–2%).
    B. Hg = 10.1 g/dL (12–14 g/dL); MCV = 103 fL (80–96 fL); reticulocytes = 1.2% (1%–2%).
    C. Hg = 9.7 g/dL (12–14 g/dL); MCV = 87 fL (80–96 fL); reticulocytes = 0.8% (1%–2%).
    D. Hg = 11.4 g/dL (12–14 g/dL); MCV = 84 fL (80–96 fL); reticulocytes = 2.3% (1%–2%).

59. X-rays will fail to show changes in affected joints in approximately what percent of patients with RA at disease onset?
A. 30%
B. 50%
C. 75%
D. 95%

60. RA disease progression is typically evaluated using all of the following approaches except:
A. x-ray.
B. MRI.
C. echosonography.
D. ultrasound.

61. Mrs. Sanchez is a 42-year-old mother of three who reports pain and stiffness in multiple joints that have lasted for more than 6 months. She is diagnosed with rheumatoid arthritis. She has no other clinical conditions of significance. You recommend which of the following treatments for first-line therapy?
A. topical analgesics and oral NSAIDs
B. methotrexate plus oral NSAIDs
C. acetaminophen plus leflunomide
D. anakinra and systemic corticosteroids

62. You see a 37-year-old man with rheumatoid arthritis who has been treated with hydroxychloroquine and oral NSAIDs for the past 3 months with little improvement in symptoms. Radiography indicates slight progression of RA in several major joints. You recommend:
A. maintaining the current regimen.
B. increasing the dose of NSAIDs.
C. adding methotrexate to his regimen.
D. switching from hydroxychloroquine to a biologic agent.

63. A significant adverse effect of biologic therapy for treating RA is:
A. myopathy.
B. infections.
C. renal impairment.
D. elevated liver enzymes.

64. Which of the following tests is most specific to the diagnosis of RA?
A. elevated levels of rheumatoid factor
B. abnormally high ESR
C. leukopenia
D. positive ANA titer

65. A positive ANA test is a sensitive marker for the presence of:
A. hyperparathyroidism.
B. systemic lupus erythematosus (SLE).
C. Kawasaki disease.
D. leukocytosis.

66. A 52-year-old woman has RA. She now presents with decreased tearing, "gritty"-feeling eyes, and a dry mouth. You consider a diagnosis of:
A. systemic lupus erythematosus.
B. vasculitis.
C. Sjögren syndrome.
D. scleroderma.

67. Cyclooxygenase-1 (COX-1) contributes to:
A. inflammatory response.
B. pain transmission.
C. maintenance of gastric protective mucosal layer.
D. renal arteriole function.

68. Cyclooxygenase-2 (COX-2) contributes to all of the following except:
A. inflammatory response.
B. pain transmission.
C. maintenance of gastric protective mucosal layer.
D. renal arteriole constriction.

69. Which of the following special examinations should be periodically obtained during hydroxychloroquine sulfate use?
A. dilated eye retinal examination
B. bone marrow biopsy
C. pulmonary function tests
D. exercise tolerance test

70. Common physical findings of SLE include all of the following except:
A. weight gain.
B. joint pain and swelling.
C. fatigue.
D. facial rash.

71. All of the following diagnostic findings are expected in a patient with SLE except:
A. elevated ESR.
B. anemia.
C. negative ANA test.
D. proteinuria.

72. First-line treatment of SLE in a patient with mild symptoms is:
A. systemic corticosteroids.
B. hydroxychloroquine plus NSAIDs.
C. anakinra.
D. methotrexate.

73. All of the following agents can be considered for the treatment of severe cases of SLE except:
A. leflunomide.
B. azathioprine.
C. rituximab.
D. belimumab.

74. You see a 26-year-old woman who has been recently diagnosed with SLE and has initiated therapy to control moderate symptoms of the disease, including fatigue and joint pain. She mentions that she and her husband are hoping to start a family soon. In counseling her about pregnancy, you consider that:
A. there is a low probability of conception during symptomatic flares of SLE.
B. most treatments for SLE must be discontinued once a woman becomes pregnant.
C. SLE is associated with a high risk of pregnancy loss.
D. there is a higher risk of gestational diabetes in women with SLE.

Answers

51. C.	59. A.	67. C.
52. B.	60. C.	68. C.
53. C.	61. B.	69. A.
54. D.	62. C.	70. A.
55. D.	63. B.	71. C.
56. A.	64. A.	72. B.
57. A.	65. B.	73. C.
58. C.	66. C.	74. C.

Rheumatoid arthritis (RA) is a disease that causes chronic systemic inflammation, including the synovial membranes of multiple joints. As with most autoimmune diseases, RA is more common in women (ratio approximately 3:1); RA is often seen in people with other autoimmune diseases. Although new-onset RA can occur at any age, peak age at onset is 20 to 40 years. A family history of rheumatoid arthritis and other autoimmune diseases is often noted. Initial presentation may be with acute polyarticular inflammation. A clinical picture of slowly progressive malaise, weight loss, and stiffness is more common, however. The stiffness is symmetrical, is typically worst on arising, lasts about 1 hour, involves at least three joint groups, and can recur after a period of inactivity or exercise. The hands (with sparing of the distal interphalangeal joints), wrists, ankles, and toes are most often involved. Soft tissue swelling or fluid is also present, as are subcutaneous nodules. The disease is characterized by periods of exacerbation and remission. A set of classification criteria was developed to help identify newly presenting patients with RA (Table 9–4). Although in the past RA was believed to be a debilitating condition with little impact on longevity, more recent research shows that RA is now known potentially to shorten the life span while producing considerable disability, particularly without optimal treatment (Table 9–5).

TABLE 9-4
American College of Rheumatology/European League Against Rheumatism Classification Criteria for Diagnosis of Rheumatoid Arthritis in Newly Presenting Patients

Criterion	Score
Test patients who:	
1) have at least 1 joint with definite clinical synovitis	
2) have synovitis not better explained by another disease	
A. Joint involvement:	
1 large joint	0
2–10 large joints	1
1–3 small joints (with or without involvement of large joints)	2
4–10 small joints (with or without involvement of large joints)	3
>10 joints (at least 1 small joint)	5
B. Serology (at least 1 test result is needed for classification):	
Negative RF and negative ACPA	0
Low-positive RF or low-positive ACPA	2
High-positive RF or high-positive ACPA	3
C. Acute-phase reactants (at least 1 test result is needed for classification):	
Normal CRP and normal ESR	0
Abnormal CRP or abnormal ESR	1
D. Duration of symptoms:	
<6 weeks	0
≥6 weeks	1

After adding scores from A–D, a score of ≥6/10 indicates RA.
RF, rheumatoid factor; ACPA, anti-citrullinated protein antibody; CRP, C-reactive protein; ESR, erythrocyte sedimentation rate.
Source: Adapted from American College of Rheumatology. 2010 Rheumatoid arthritis classification criteria. *Arthritis Rheum* 62:2569–2581, 2010.

TABLE 9-5

Treatment of Rheumatoid Arthritis

Medication	Examples
Antiinflammatory agents	NSAIDs, COX-2 inhibitors, corticosteroids
Analgesics	Oral—NSAIDs, COX-2 inhibitors, acetaminophen, opioids
	Topical agents—NSAIDs, lidocaine, capsaicin, salicylates, menthol, camphor
DMARDs	Traditional DMARDS—methotrexate, leflunomide, sulfasalazine, hydroxychloroquine, minocycline, others
	Biological response modifiers—
	Non-TNF: abatacept, rituximab, anakinra, tocilizumab, others
	Anti-TNF: infliximab, adalimumab, , etanercept, certolizumab, golimumab, others
	Oral JAK inhibitors: tofacitinib

NSAIDs, nonsteroidal anti-inflammatory drugs; COX-2, cyclooxygenase 2; DMARDs, disease-modifying anti-rheumatic drugs; TNF, tumor necrosis factor.

Source: Singh JA, Furst DE, Bharat A, et al. 2012 Update of the 2008 American College of Rheumatology recommendations for the use of disease-modifying antirheumatic drugs and biologic agents in the treatment of rheumatoid arthritis. *Arthritis Care Res* 64:625–639, 2012.

The diagnosis of RA can be made only when clinical features are supported by laboratory testing. Usually initial diagnostic tests include ANA, ESR, CRP, anti-citrullinated protein antibody (ACPA), and rheumatoid factor (RF) measurements and radiographs, with additional testing often ordered because of diagnostic uncertainty. When interpreting results, the NP should bear in mind the following:

- Radiographs typically reveal joint erosion and loss of normal joint space. X-rays can help in detecting RA but often do not show any signs at the early stages of disease. Classic radiographic changes are not present in about 30% at disease onset. Musculoskeletal ultrasound and joint magnetic resonance imaging (MRI) are helpful in revealing RA-associated erosions and determining the severity of disease. Radiographic imaging at the early stages of disease can be helpful in determining disease progression.
- ESR and CRP are nonspecific tests of inflammation. In general, the higher the values, the greater the degree and intensity of the inflammatory process. Although ESR and CRP are frequently elevated in patients with RA, abnormal results are diagnostic of this or other conditions. In addition, a single elevated ESR or CRP is seldom helpful; however, following trends during flare and regression of disease often aids in charting the therapeutic course and response.
- Rheumatoid factor, an immunoglobulin M antibody, is present in approximately 50% to 90% of patients with RA. The level of the titer often corresponds to the severity of disease.
- An antibody to cyclic citrullinated peptide (anti-CCP), a ring-form amino acid that is usually not measurable in health, is a more specific, although less sensitive, marker of RA.
- Hemogram usually reveals normocytic, normochromic, hypoproliferative anemia associated with chronic disease.

- ANAs are antibodies against cellular nuclear components that act as antigens. ANA is occasionally present in healthy adults, but it is usually found in individuals with systemic rheumatic or collagen vascular disease. ANA is the most sensitive laboratory marker for SLE, detected in approximately 95% of patients, but it is found in only 30% to 50% of patients with RA. Patterns of immunofluorescence vary and have been given misplaced credence as to type of disease. Following are some examples of ANA patterns:
  - Homogeneous, diffuse, or solid pattern to DNA: High titers strongly associated with SLE
  - Peripheral or rim pattern: Associated with anti–double-stranded DNA and strongly correlated with SLE
  - Nucleolar pattern: Associated with antiribonucleoprotein and strongly correlated with scleroderma or CREST syndrome
  - Speckled pattern: Further antigen testing should be ordered with this result.
  - Cytoplasmic pattern is often found in the presence of biliary cirrhosis.

The goal of treatment of patients with RA is to reduce inflammation and pain, while preserving function and preventing deformity. Behavioral management is important because physiological and psychological stress precipitates RA flares. Allowing for proper rest periods is critical. Physical therapists can help develop a reasonable activity plan. Maintenance of physical activity through appropriate exercise is of greatest importance. Water exercise in particular is helpful because it includes mild resistance and buoyancy. Splints may provide joint rest while maintaining function and preventing contracture.

As helpful as NSAIDs are in symptom control, these products do not alter the underlying disease process; joint destruction continues despite control of symptoms and reduction in swelling. Disease-modifying antirheumatic drugs (DMARDs) help minimize the risk of joint damage and disease progression and should be started as soon as the diagnosis of RA is made (see Table 9–4). As the number and types of DMARDs available increase, knowledge of current RA therapy is critical for providing optimal patient care.

If an adequate trial of a DMARD and an NSAID fails to achieve control of pain or symptoms, additional therapy should be added. One option is intra-articular corticosteroid injection. This therapy can be quite helpful but should be limited to not more than two to three injections per joint per year to minimize risk of joint deterioration. Systemic corticosteroids can be most helpful in relieving inflammation, but use should not exceed 2 to 8 weeks, if possible, because of adverse reactions associated with these agents. With more advanced disease or for patients who fail to respond adequately to DMARDs, biologics are increasingly being used to achieve disease remission. Biologics are now available in injection and oral formulations. However, a major adverse effect of biologics is an increased risk for infection with some dormant infections (such as tuberculosis) activating once treatment begins. Vaccinations should be considered for patients considering initiating biologic therapy.

NSAIDs have been the backbone of RA drug treatment for years. These medications are helpful in controlling inflammation and pain. Aspirin and ibuprofen are two more commonly used products. With many of the NSAIDs, the half-life of the drug is increased as the dose is increased.

A significant amount of peptic ulcer disease, particularly gastric ulcer and gastritis, is caused by NSAID use. NSAIDs inhibit synthesis of prostaglandins from arachidonic acid, yielding an anti-inflammatory effect. This effect is caused in part by the action of these products against cyclooxygenase (COX). COX-1 is an enzyme found in gastric mucosa, small and large intestine mucosa, kidneys, platelets, and vascular epithelium. This enzyme contributes to the health of these organs through numerous mechanisms, including the maintenance of the protective gastric mucosal layer and proper perfusion of the kidneys. COX-2 is an enzyme that produces prostaglandins important in the inflammatory cascade and pain transmission. The standard NSAIDs and corticosteroids inhibit the synthesis of COX-1 and COX-2, controlling pain and inflammation, but with gastric and renal complications. NSAIDs such as celecoxib (Celebrex) that spare COX-1 and are more COX-2-selective afford control of the potential for arthritis symptoms. The gastrointestinal benefit of the COX-2 inhibitors is likely attenuated with long-term use, whereas the cardiovascular risk associated with their use is increased.

Sjögren syndrome is an autoimmune disease that usually occurs in conjunction with another chronic inflammatory condition, such as RA or SLE. Complaints usually concern problems related to decreased oral and ocular secretions. In addition, mouth ulcers and dental caries are common, and ESR is elevated in more than 90% of patients. A salivary gland biopsy for the presence of mononuclear cell infiltration is useful. Intervention for patients with Sjögren syndrome includes management of presenting symptoms with appropriate lubricants. Treating the underlying disease is critical.

SLE is a chronic autoimmune disease that can affect any organ system, including joints, skin, kidneys, blood cells, brain, heart, and lungs. Diagnosis can be difficult because signs and symptoms often mimic other conditions. Symptoms of SLE are highly variable and can include malar rash (covering the cheeks and nasal bridge but sparing the nasolabial folds); fever; fatigue; headaches; weight loss; and joint pain, stiffness, and swelling. Complications associated with SLE vary depending on the organ system that is affected. For pregnant women, SLE is a major risk factor for miscarriage; the condition increases the risk of preeclampsia and preterm birth. If possible, pregnancy should be delayed until SLE is under control for at least 6 months.

Diagnosis of SLE depends on findings from multiple laboratory and radiographic tests. Common findings include anemia, elevated ESR, proteinuria, and a positive ANA test. A chest x-ray may reveal inflammation in the lungs, whereas an echocardiogram will detect any changes to the heart. A kidney biopsy can be used to detect damage to these organs.

Treatment of SLE will depend on the manifestation of the disease. The antimalarial drug hydroxychloroquine has been shown to be effective for the long-term treatment of SLE. Mild disease that waxes and wanes is often controlled with oral NSAIDs. Systemic corticosteroids are used to counter the inflammation caused by SLE, although long-term use of these agents should be done with caution because of their potential adverse effects. For more severe cases or those that do not respond to initial therapy, immune suppressants can be beneficial. These include cyclophosphamide (Cytoxan), azathioprine (Imuran), mycophenolate (Cellcept), leflunomide (Arava), and methotrexate (Trexall). These agents are associated with increased risk of infection, liver damage, decreased fertility, and increased risk of cancer. Belimumab (Benlysta), a B-lymphocyte stimulator-specific inhibitor, is the first biologic agent approved for adults with SLE and may provide added benefits when added to current treatments.

DISCUSSION SOURCES

American College of Rheumatology. http://www.rheumatology.org/public/factsheets/diseases_and_conditions/ra.asp?aud=pat, Fact sheet on rheumatoid arthritis, update August 2012.

Ferri, FF. Ferri's Best Test: A Practical Guide to Laboratory Medicine and Diagnostic Imaging, ed. 3. Philadelphia: Mosby Elsevier, 2014.

Singh JA, Furst DE, Bharat A, et al. 2012 Update of the 2008 American College of Rheumatology recommendations for the use of disease-modifying antirheumatic drugs and biologic agents in the treatment of rheumatoid arthritis. Arthritis Care Res 64:625–639, 2012.

Bartels CM. Systemic lupus erythematosus (SLE). http://emedicine.medscape.com/article/332244-overview.

See full color images of this topic on DavisPlus at http://davisplus.fadavis.com | Keyword: Fitzgerald

Meniscal Tears

75. To confirm the results of a McMurray test, you ask the patient to:
- A. squat.
- B. walk.
- C. flex the knee.
- D. rotate the ankle.

76. The most common type of injury causing a sport-related meniscal tear involves:
- A. twisting of the knee.
- B. hyperextension of the knee.
- C. repetitive hard impact on the knee (i.e., running on hard surface).
- D. an unknown origin in most cases.

77. Which of the following best describes the presentation of a patient with complete medial meniscus tear?
- A. joint effusion
- B. heat over the knee
- C. inability to kneel
- D. loss of smooth joint movement

78. To help prevent meniscal tear, you advise:
- A. limiting participation in sports.
- B. quadriceps-strengthening exercises.
- C. using a knee brace.
- D. applying ice to the knee before exercise.

79. Initial treatment for meniscal tear includes all of the following except:
- A. NSAID use.
- B. applying ice to the affected area.
- C. elevation of the affected limb.
- D. joint aspiration of the affected knee.

Answers

75. A.	**77.** C.	**79.** D.
76. A.	**78.** B.	

A meniscal tear results from a disruption of the meniscus, the C-shaped fibrocartilage pad located between the femoral condyles and the tibial plateaus. This injury is often seen in athletes because of a twist-type injury to the knee. This condition can also be found in older, sedentary adults; in this case, the injury is usually because of degenerative changes. Because the purpose of the fibrocartilage pad is shock absorption and smooth joint mobility, patients with larger tears often report that the knee locks, makes a popping sound, or "gives out." Effusion is also common, with the patient reporting a sensation of knee tightness and stiffness. With certain positions, there is often sudden-onset, sharp, localized pain, usually on the medial aspect of the knee. Over time, premature OA is often seen as the normal joint space is compromised.

Meniscal tears are typically classified as complex or partial; traumatic or degenerative; lateral, posterior, horizontal, or vertical; and radial, parrot-beak, or bucket-handle. Patients

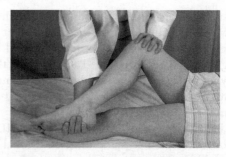

Figure 9-1 McMurray's test assesses the menisci. The medial meniscus is tested with the hip flexed and the knee externally rotated as the examiner moves the knee from full flexion to extension. To test the lateral meniscus, the knee is internally rotated during the procedure. A snap heard or felt during this maneuver suggests a tear of the tested meniscus. (From Goolsby, *Advanced Assessment*, 3rd ed. Philadelphia, PA: FA Davis; 2014.)

with partial, horizontal, and anterior tears often have relatively normal examination findings because the knee's mechanics are relatively unchanged even though these patients continue to have knee locking and pain with certain positions. The McMurray test, a palpable popping on the joint line, is highly specific but poorly sensitive for a meniscal tear; the Apley grinding test gives similar results. Squatting or kneeling is nearly impossible for patients with a large, complete, or bucket-handle meniscal tear. Joint effusion is typical, with ROM being limited by discomfort.

Knee radiographs, which can reveal osteoarthritic changes, foreign bodies, or other injuries, are reasonable as initial evaluation. Because the meniscus does not contain calcium, the structure is not visible on a plain film. MRI can identify the type and extent of the tear and should be considered if milder symptoms do not resolve within 2 to 4 weeks or if severe symptoms do not resolve earlier.

Initial treatment includes rest, elevation, ice application, and analgesia. Because joint effusion is nearly always present but is relatively mild, aspiration should be considered only if there is no improvement after 2 to 4 weeks of conservative therapy. Crutch walking should be encouraged, and a patellar stabilizer may be needed when significant knee instability is present. Straight-leg–raising exercises help strengthen the quadriceps and stabilize the joint. Arthroscopy, which provides the most accurate diagnosis with the possibility of concurrent treatment through débridement and repair, should be considered at 4 to 6 weeks if there is no improvement and earlier if joint locking, giving out, and effusion are particularly problematic.

DISCUSSION SOURCES

Achar S, Espinoza A. Common sports injuries. In: Rakel R, Bope E, eds. *Conn's Current Therapy 2013*. Philadelphia: Saunders Elsevier, 2013.

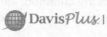 See full color images of this topic on DavisPlus at
http://davisplus.fadavis.com |
Keyword: Fitzgerald

Anderson B. *Office Orthopedics for Primary Care: Diagnosis*, ed. 1. Philadelphia: Saunders Elsevier, 2006.

Anderson B. *Office Orthopedics for Primary Care: Treatment*, ed. 3. Philadelphia: Saunders Elsevier, 2006.

Carpal Tunnel Syndrome

80. The Phalen test is described as:
    A. reproduction of symptoms with forced flexion of the wrists.
    B. abnormal tingling when the median nerve is tapped.
    C. pain on internal rotation.
    D. palmar atrophy.

81. The Tinel test is best described as:
    A. reproduction of symptoms with forced flexion of the wrists.
    B. abnormal tingling when the median nerve is tapped.
    C. pain on internal rotation.
    D. palmar atrophy.

82. All of the following statements about electromyography (EMG) are true except:
    A. EMG measures electrical impulses caused by muscles.
    B. diagnosis of carpal tunnel syndrome involves comparing EMG results of the muscles at rest versus contraction.
    C. EMG can detect muscle damage.
    D. EMG involves sending a small electrical impulse through the muscle tissue.

83. Results of a nerve conduction study in a person with carpal tunnel syndrome (CTS) would reveal:
    A. erratic nerve impulses during forearm muscle contraction.
    B. a lack of nerve impulses in the carpal tunnel.
    C. continued firing of the median nerve while the forearm muscles are at rest.
    D. a slowing of nerve impulses in the carpal tunnel.

84. Risk factors for CTS include all of the following except:
    A. pregnancy.
    B. untreated hypothyroidism.
    C. repetitive motion.
    D. multiple sclerosis.

85. Which of the following is least likely to be reported by patients with CTS?
    A. worst symptoms during the day
    B. burning sensation in the affected hand
    C. tingling pain that radiates to the forearm
    D. nocturnal numbness

86. Acroparesthesia, frequently reported in patients with CTS, is best described as:
    A. constant pain radiating from the elbow.
    B. a transient inability to move the fingers.
    C. waking up at night with numbness and burning pain in the fingers.
    D. muscle spasms that cause fist clenching.

87. Initial therapy for patients with CTS includes:
    A. intra-articular injection.
    B. joint splinting.
    C. systemic corticosteroids.
    D. referral for surgery.

88. Patients whose CTS fails to respond to conservative treatment measures should be considered for:
    A. systemic corticosteroid use.
    B. low-dose opioids.
    C. surgery.
    D. vitamin B_6 injections in the carpal tunnel.

89. Primary prevention of CTS includes:
    A. screening for thyroid dysfunction.
    B. treatment of concomitant arthritis forms.
    C. stretching and toning exercises.
    D. wrist splinting.

Answers

80. A.	84. D.	88. C.
81. B.	85. A.	89. C.
82. D.	86. C.	
83. D.	87. B.	

Carpal tunnel syndrome (CTS) is a painful condition caused by compression of the median nerve between the carpal ligament and other structures within the carpal tunnel. This compression leads to an entrapment neuropathy, causing symptoms in the distribution of the median nerve. The resulting symptoms are likely because of nerve ischemia rather than nerve damage.

The most common risk factor is repetitive motion; the condition is common with protracted computer keyboard use and in workers such as cake decorators and soldiers, who must consistently grasp a small object. CTS can also be part of the manifestation of a systemic disease, such as RA and sarcoidosis. Primary prevention of CTS includes limiting time spent in these activities, ensuring proper work breaks, and encouraging toning and stretching exercises.

Patients with CTS, the most commonly encountered peripheral compression neuropathy, usually report a burning, aching, or tingling pain radiating to the forearm in the distribution of the median nerve and occasionally to the shoulder, neck, and chest. Symptoms are often worst at night. A classic finding is the report of acroparesthesia, awakening at night with numbness and burning pain in the fingers. Physical examination findings occasionally include positive Tinel and Phalen tests, although the carpal compression test, in which symptoms are induced by direct application of pressure over the carpal tunnel, is likely a more sensitive and specific test. In later disease, muscle weakness and thenar atrophy are often noted.

Diagnostic tests for patients suspected to have CTS include electromyography (EMG) and nerve conduction studies that can confirm the median neuropathy. EMG is used to measure the electrical discharges produced by the muscles. Electrodes are used to measure the electrical activity of the muscles at rest and during contraction and will indicate if muscle damage is present. In a nerve conduction study, electrodes are taped to the skin and a small shock is passed through the medial nerve to assess if electrical impulses are slowed in the carpal tunnel, indicating damage to the nerve. Although plain x-rays are of little diagnostic value, MRI and high-resolution ultrasound results often support the diagnosis and can eliminate other causes of wrist pain, such as arthritis or a fracture.

Treatment of patients with CTS includes limiting the activity that caused the condition and elevating the affected extremity; application of a volar splint in a neutral position helps relieve the increase in intracanal pressure caused by wrist flexion and extension. NSAIDs and acetaminophen provide pain relief. Corticosteroid injection into the carpal tunnel at 6-week intervals can help reduce swelling and symptoms but should be performed only by a skilled practitioner. Surgery to release the transverse carpal ligament provides symptom relief in most patients whose CTS does not respond to conservative therapy. About 10% do not respond, however, because of nerve damage or new pressure within the carpal tunnel that results from recurrent compression caused by scar formation. Diuretics, vitamin B_6, and other nutraceutical therapies have been reported as helpful in minimizing CTS symptoms, although clinical studies have shown these agents to be no more effective than placebo.

CTS is often noted transiently at the end of pregnancy and in patients with untreated hypothyroidism. Pregnancy-induced CTS usually resolves quickly after the woman gives birth, and thyroxine supplements quickly ameliorate CTS caused by hypothyroidism. In the interim, splinting and analgesia can be helpful.

DISCUSSION SOURCES

Anderson B. *Office Orthopedics for Primary Care: Diagnosis*, ed. 1. Philadelphia: Saunders Elsevier, 2006.

Anderson B. *Office Orthopedics for Primary Care: Treatment*, ed. 3. Philadelphia: Saunders Elsevier, 2006.

Turner S. Musculoskeletal system. In: Goolsby M, Grubbs L, eds. *Advanced Assessment: Interpreting Findings and Formulating Differential Diagnosis*, ed. 2. Philadelphia: FA Davis, 2011, pp. 321–353.

LeBlanc KE, Cestia W. Carpal tunnel syndrome. *Am Fam Physician* 83:952–958, 2011.

Sarcoidosis

90. A risk factor for sarcoidosis is:
    A. male gender.
    B. African American race.
    C. age older than 60 years.
    D. type 2 diabetes mellitus.

91. Common symptoms of a patient with sarcoidosis include all of the following except:
    A. arthralgia.
    B. dyspnea upon exertion.
    C. blurred vision.
    D. cardiac palpitations.

92. A laboratory finding commonly observed in patients with sarcoidosis is:
    A. hyponatremia.
    B. hypercalcemia.
    C. hypokalemia.
    D. hyperkalemia.

93. Which of the following diagnostic approaches is used for confirmation of sarcoidosis?
    A. chest x-ray
    B. high-resolution CT scan
    C. biopsy
    D. ANA fluorescent staining

94. The primary treatment option for sarcoidosis is the use of:
    A. parenteral methotrexate.
    B. systemic corticosteroids.
    C. oral acetaminophen.
    D. oral hydroxychloroquine.

95. You see a 42-year-old woman recently diagnosed with sarcoidosis. She is reluctant to use any first-line medications for the condition because of severe adverse effects experienced previously. You consider prescribing all of the following alternatives except:
    A. hydroxychloroquine.
    B. tofacitinib.
    C. infliximab.
    D. azathioprine.

96. Evaluation for disease progression is a patient with sarcoidosis can involve:
    A. pulmonary function test and carbon monoxide capacity test.
    B. skin biopsy.
    C. check for WBCs in the urine.
    D. the Phalen test.

Answers

90. B.	93. C.	96. A.
91. D.	94. B.	
92. B.	95. B.	

Sarcoidosis is an inflammatory condition that results in the production of noncaseating granulomas in various sites of the body, predominantly in the lungs, lymph nodes, eyes, and skin. Although the exact cause of sarcoidosis is unknown, this disease is likely the result of an exaggerated immune response to an unidentified antigen, possibly inhaled from the air. The condition often occurs in adults between the ages of 20 and 40 years, with a slightly higher incidence in women than men. Individuals of African ancestry are also more likely to have the disease than white Americans and tend to have more severe disease that can cause pulmonary issues. A family history of the disease is also a risk factor.

Symptoms depend on the organs involved and severity of the disease. Sarcoidosis can develop gradually with symptoms that last for years, whereas others can have more rapid progression and resolution of the disease. Systemic symptoms include fever, fatigue, anorexia, and arthralgias, whereas pulmonary complaints include dyspnea on exertion, cough, and chest pain. Dermatologic signs include rash, lesions, color change, and nodule formations just under the skin. Ocular symptoms include blurred vision, eye pain, severe redness, and sensitivity to light.

Diagnosis sarcoidosis can be difficult because there can be few signs and symptoms in early disease and the symptoms can mimic several other disorders. The diagnostic process aims to exclude other disorders while also determining which organ systems are affected by the disease. Some serological markers have also been associated with sarcoidosis, including serum amyloid A (SAA), soluble interleukin-2 receptor, angiotensin-converting enzyme (ACE), and the glycoprotein KL-6. Patients with sarcoidosis are also more likely to present with hypercalcemia and hypercalciuria. Imaging studies are a key component of diagnosis. Chest x-ray can be used to check for lung damage or enlarged lymph nodes in the chest. High-resolution CT scanning of the chest can detect the presence of alveolitis or fibrosis. PET or MRI can detect if the disease is affecting the heart or central nervous system. Pulmonary function tests and carbon monoxide capacity tests are used in evaluation and follow-up to gauge pulmonary involvement and progression of the disease. Confirmation of the disease typically requires biopsy to check for the presence of noncaseating granulomas. This can involve a transbronchial biopsy (which gives a high diagnostic yield regardless of disease stage) or can occur from affected skin or the outer membrane of the eye.

Sarcoidosis is often self-limiting. Mild disease can be treated with NSAIDs to help relieve symptoms of arthralgias and other rheumatic complaints. Corticosteroids are the mainstay of treatment and can be taken orally, as a cream to affected skin, or inhaled for those with endobronchial disease. Optimal dosing for the treatment of sarcoidosis is unclear; some suggest using a low dose (10–40 mg daily) that is tapered to every other day over several weeks to months. Other agents used in the treatment of sarcoidosis include the antimalarial drug hydroxychloroquine and immune-suppressing medications used to treat rheumatoid arthritis (e.g., methotrexate, azathioprine, and tumor necrosis factor inhibitors [e.g., infliximab]). Other agents include chlorambucil, cyclophosphamide, and cyclosporine. For patients with extensive pulmonary damage resulting from the disease, lung transplantation may be a viable option.

DISCUSSION SOURCE

Kamangar N. Sarcoidosis. http://emedicine.medscape.com/article/301914-overview.

Low Back Pain

97. Approximately what percent of patients experiencing low back pain will have the symptoms resolve within 1 month without specific therapy?
    A. 33%
    B. 57%
    C. 78%
    D. 90%

98. Risk factors for the development of low back pain include all of the following except:
    A. older age.
    B. carpal tunnel syndrome.
    C. scoliosis.
    D. spinal stenosis.

99. Most episodes of low back pain are caused by:
    A. an acute precipitating event.
    B. disk herniation.
    C. muscle or ligamentous strain.
    D. nerve impingement.

100. With the straight-leg–raising test, the NP is evaluating tension on which of the following nerve roots?
    A. L1 and L2
    B. L3 and L4
    C. L5 and S1
    D. S2 and S3

101. A patient with a lumbosacral strain will typically report:
    A. numbness in the extremities.
    B. stiffness, spasm, and reduced ROM.
    C. "electric" sensation running down one or both legs.
    D. pain at its worst when in sitting position.

102. You see a 54-year-old man complaining of low back pain and is diagnosed with acute lumbosacral strain. Which of the following is the best advice to give about exercising?
    A. You should not exercise until you are free of pain.
    B. Back-strengthening exercises can cause mild muscle soreness.
    C. Electric-like pain in response to exercise is to be expected.
    D. Conditioning exercises should be started immediately.

103. Risk factors for lumbar radiculopathy include all of the following except:
    A. male gender.
    B. age <50 years.
    C. overweight.
    D. cigarette smoking.

104. A patient with sciatica will typically report:
    A. loss of bladder control.
    B. stiffness, spasm, and reduced ROM.
    C. shooting pain that starts at the hip and radiates to the foot.
    D. pain at its worst when lying down.

105. Early neurological changes in patients with lumbar radiculopathy include:
    A. loss of deep tendon reflexes.
    B. poor two-point discrimination.
    C. reduced muscle strength.
    D. footdrop.

106. Common causes of sciatica include all of the following except:
    A. herniated disk.
    B. spinal stenosis.
    C. compression fracture.
    D. soft tissue abnormality.

107. You see a 48-year-old woman who reports low back pain. During the evaluation, she mentions new-onset loss of bowel and bladder control. This most likely indicates:
    A. cauda equina syndrome.
    B. muscular spasm.
    C. vertebral fracture.
    D. sciatic nerve entrapment.

108. Loss of posterior tibial reflex often indicates a lesion at:
    A. L3.
    B. L4.
    C. L5.
    D. S1.

109. Loss of Achilles tendon reflex most likely indicates a lesion at:
    A. L1 to L2.
    B. L3 to L4.
    C. L5 to S1.
    D. S2 to S3.

110. Which test is demonstrated when the examiner applies pressure to the top of the head with the neck bending forward, producing pain or numbness in the upper extremities?
    A. Spurling
    B. McMurray
    C. Lachman
    D. Newman

111. Immediate diagnostic imaging for low back pain should be reserved for all of the following except:
    A. presence of signs of the cauda equina syndrome.
    B. presence of severe neurologic deficits.
    C. presence of risk factors for cancer.
    D. presence of moderate pain lasting at least 2 weeks.

112. Which of the following tests yields the greatest amount of clinical information in a patient with acute lumbar radiculopathy?
    A. lumbosacral radiograph series
    B. ESR measurement
    C. MRI
    D. bone scan

113. The most common site for cervical radiculopathy is:
    A. C3 to C4.
    B. C4 to C5.
    C. C5 to C6.
    D. C6 to C7

114. The most common sites for lumbar disk herniation are:
    A. L1 to L2 and L2 to L3.
    B. L2 to L3 and L4 to L5.
    C. L4 to L5 and L5 to S1.
    D. L5 to S1 and S1 to S2.

115. You see a 37-year-old man complaining of low back pain consisting of stiffness and spasms but without any sign of neurologic involvement. You recommend all of the following interventions except:
    A. application of cold packs for 20 minutes 3–4 times a day.
    B. use of NSAIDs or acetaminophen for pain control.
    C. initiation of aerobic and toning exercises.
    D. bed rest for at least 5 days.

Answers

97. D.	104. C.	111. D.
98. B.	105. A.	112. C.
99. C.	106. D.	113. D.
100. C.	107. A.	114. C.
101. B.	108. C.	115. D.
102. B.	109. C.	
103. B.	110. A.	

Low back pain is at least an occasional problem for nearly all adults, with a lifetime prevalence of 60% to 90%. In about 90% of patients with low back pain, symptoms are short-lived and resolve within 1 month without specific therapy. A few individuals have recurrent or chronic low back pain, however, and significant disability. Risk factors for low back pain include older age, overactivity, overweight or obesity and certain physiologic and degenerative disorders (e.g., spinal stenosis, degenerative spondylolisthesis, and scoliosis).

Lumbosacral strain or disk herniation and resulting lumbar radiculopathy and sciatica can cause musculoskeletal low back pain. Most often, contributing factors include muscle or ligamentous strain, degenerative joint disease, or a combination of these factors. Lumbosacral strain is the most common reason for a patient to present to the primary care practitioner with acute low back pain. In the typical scenario, the patient complains of stiffness, spasm, and reduced ROM. The erector spinae muscle is most often implicated. Sitting usually aggravates the pain, but there may be some relief if the patient lies supine on a firm surface. A precipitating event is reported by only a few patients because lumbosacral strain is usually the culmination of many events, including repeated use of improperly stretched muscles in patients with overall poor conditioning. In addition, poor posture, scoliosis, and spinal stenosis can be predisposing factors. The physical examination usually reveals a straightening of the lumbosacral curve, paraspinal muscle tenderness, spasm worst at the level of L3 to L4, and decreased lumbosacral flexion and lateral bending. The neurological examination findings are typically normal in lumbar sacral strain; if there is a neurological abnormality demonstrated on a well-performed clinical examination on a person presenting with low back pain, then the diagnosis of lumbar radiculopathy needs to be considered.

Diagnostic tests in lumbosacral strain vary according to the length and severity of symptoms. Radiographs are helpful only if there is a high degree of suspicion for spondylolisthesis, scoliosis, cancer, or fracture (Table 9–6). In the absence of these conditions, little is likely to be revealed. Radiography is likely to reveal the presence of lumbar arthritis, which has been observed in more than 90% of adults older than 40 years of age, although most do not report low back pain. Lumbosacral radiographs should not be routinely obtained. Computed tomography (CT) scanning or MRI should be considered if radiculopathy is present and clinical presentation does not improve after a reasonable trial of conservative therapy because these studies might reveal contributing factors, such as spinal stenosis and disk herniation. MRI is a superior study for revealing soft tissue problems, whereas CT provides superior information on bony structures.

Lumbosacral disk herniation usually occurs after years of episodes of back pain caused by repeated damage to the annular fibers of the disk and is less common than lumbosacral strain as a cause of low back pain. Risk factors for lumbar radiculopathy include smoking, diabetes, spinal infection, overweight or obesity, male gender, and older age. Lumbar disk herniation often leads to sciatica, neurological changes, and significant distress. Because the intravertebral disks contain less water and are more fibrous, the risk of disk rupture decreases after age 50 years. The most common sites of lumbosacral disk herniation are L4 to L5 and L5 to S1, with the posterolateral aspect of the disk protruding.

Neuralgia along the course of the sciatic nerve is known as sciatica. The cause of sciatica is usually pressure on lumbosacral nerve roots from a herniated disk, spinal stenosis, or a compression fracture. Occasionally, sciatica can be

TABLE 9-6
Diagnostic Imaging for Low Back Pain

Immediate Action	Suggestions for Initial Imaging
IMMEDIATE IMAGING Radiography plus ESR*, MRI	Major risk factors for cancer Risk factors for spinal infection Consider MRI if risk factors for or signs of the cauda equine syndrome; severe neurologic deficits, particularly if sudden onset
DEFER IMAGING AFTER A TRIAL OF STANDARD THERAPY Radiography ± ESR	Weaker risk factors for cancer; risk factors for or signs of ankylosing spondylitis; risk factors for vertebral compression fracture
MRI	Signs and symptoms of radiculopathy in patients who are candidates for surgery or epidural steroid injection; risk factors for or symptoms of spinal stenosis in patients who are candidates for surgery
NO IMAGING	No criteria for immediate imaging and back pain improved or resolved after at least 1-month trial of therapy; previous spinal imaging with no change in clinical status

*Consider MRI if the initial imaging result is negative but a high degree of clinical suspicion for cancer remains.
ESR, erythrocyte sedimentation rate.
Source: Chou, R., et al. Diagnostic imaging for low back pain: Advice for high-value health care from the American College of Physicians. *Ann Intern Med* 154:181–189, 2011, http://annals.org/article.aspx?articleid=746774.

caused by external pressure on the sciatic nerve, such as that often found in people who carry a wallet in a rear pants pocket and develop symptoms after prolonged sitting. Patients with sciatica complain of shooting pain that starts over the hip and radiates to the foot, often accompanied by leg numbness and weakness. The degree of pain can vary according to the degree of nerve involvement; it ranges from mildly bothersome and occasionally reported to be more itchy than painful to incapacitating pain.

Neck pain, a common clinical complaint, can result from abnormalities in the soft tissues, such as muscles, ligaments, and nerves, and in bones and joints of the spine. The most common causes of neck pain are soft tissue abnormalities caused by injury, poor posture, or prolonged wear and tear; rare causes of neck pain include infection and tumors. The most common site for a cervical disk lesion is C6 to C7. Cervical vertebral sprains is a frequent injury observed in athletes and victims of motor vehicle accidents and can include acute strains and sprains of neck muscles as well as soft-tissue contusions. Pain and stiffness are the chief complaints. An acute cervical sprain can be associated with a jammed-neck sensation with localized pain. After the injury, pain, swelling, and tenderness can become evident as local bleeding occurs in the muscle fibers. Neck motion can become painful, with peak pain occurring several hours later or the next day. However, the patient should have no radiation of pain to the extremities.

In patients who have herniated disks, whether in the neck or back, the degree of neurological involvement ranges from more minor symptoms of numbness to loss of extremity function. Deep tendon reflexes are usually absent. In cervical radiculopathy, the patient presents with neck and arm discomfort that can range from a dull ache to severe burning pain. The pain is commonly referred to the medial border of the scapula, and the chief complaint is shoulder pain. With progression, the pain can radiate to the upper and lower arm and into the hand. Lumbar radiculopathy is associated with pain that moves from the lower back to the buttocks, groin, and back of the leg. The pain often travels below the knee and can worsen when the patient coughs, sneezes, stands, or sits. Numbness, weakness, or tingling in the back of the legs is common. With cauda equina involvement, there is compression of the lower portion of the nerve root inferior to the spinal cord, usually secondary to disk herniation. This compression can lead to rectal or perineal pain and disturbance in bowel and bladder function. Signs of lumbosacral strain are present, and the straight-leg–raising maneuver reproduces pain.

Management of patients with low back pain differs according to presentation. In most patients with acute low back pain and intact neurological examination, treatment is aimed at maintaining function and minimizing symptoms. Longer periods of immobilization can contribute to deconditioning and are potentially harmful. Intervention for acute neck pain is similar. Application of cold packs for 20 minutes three to four times a day can help with pain control, and heat applications may help before gentle stretching exercise. NSAIDs or acetaminophen should be prescribed for pain control. Muscle relaxants have been shown to be helpful in some patients. These medications are usually sedating, however, and need to be used with caution; occasionally, these are used as drugs of abuse. Treatment should also include initiating aerobic and toning exercises and teaching the patient to minimize back stress through appropriate use of body mechanics.

Prompt referral to specialty care is needed when there is limb, bowel, or bladder dysfunction. Surgery is usually considered only if severe radiculopathy symptoms persist beyond 3 months. In addition, early referral is indicated in certain conditions that are particularly worrisome (Table 9–7).

DISCUSSION SOURCES

Chou R, Qaseem A, Snow V, Casey V, Cross JT, Shekelle P, Owens D; Clinical Efficacy Assessment Subcommittee of the American College of Physicians and the American College of Physicians/American Pain Society Low Back Pain Guidelines Panel. http://www.annals.org/cgi/content/full/147/7/478, Diagnosis and treatment of low back pain: a joint clinical practice guideline from the American College of Physicians and the American Pain Society, 2007.

TABLE 9-7
Low Back Pain: "Red Flags" for a Potentially Serious Underlying Cause

Possible Fracture	Possible Tumor or Infection	Cauda Equina Syndrome
History of recent trauma, particularly fall from significant height or motor vehicle accident	Age <20 y.o. or >50 y.o.	Bladder dysfunction, perineal sensory loss, or anal laxity
In person with or at risk for osteoporosis, minor trauma, or strenuous lifting	Constitutional symptoms such as unexplained weight loss, fever	Neurological deficit in lower extremities
	Recent bacterial infection, injection drug use, immunosuppression	Lower extremity motor weakness
	Increased pain with rest	
	History of cancer	

Source.annals.org/cgi/content/full/147/7/478.
Chou, R., et al. Diagnostic imaging for low back pain: Advice for high-value health care from the American College of Physicians. *Ann Intern Med* 154:181–189, 2011, http://annals.org/article.aspx?articleid=746774.

Chou, R., et al. Diagnostic imaging for low back pain: Advice for high-value health care from the American College of Physicians. *Ann Intern Med* 154:181–189, 2011, available at http://annals.org/article.aspx?articleid=746774.

Reactive Arthritis

116. A 22-year-old man presents with new onset of pain and swelling in his feet and ankles, conjunctivitis, oral lesions, and dysuria. To help confirm a diagnosis of reactive arthritis, the most important test to obtain is:
A. ANA analysis.
B. ESR measurement.
C. rubella titer measurement.
D. urethral cultures.

117. Symptoms commonly associated with reactive arthritis include all of the following except:
A. dactylitis.
B. bursitis.
C. enthesitis.
D. cervicitis.

118. Treatment for reactive arthritis (also known as Reiter syndrome) in a sexually active man usually includes:
A. antimicrobial therapy.
B. corticosteroid therapy.
C. antirheumatic medications.
D. immunosuppressive drugs.

119. In reference to reactive arthritis (also known as Reiter syndrome), which of the following statements is false?
A. When the disease is associated with urethritis, the male:female ratio is about 9:1.
B. When the disease is associated with infectious diarrhea, the male and female incidences are approximately equal.
C. ANA analysis reveals a speckled pattern.
D. Results of joint aspirate culture are usually unremarkable.

120. In men with reactive arthritis and associated urethritis, a common finding is:
A. ANA positive.
B. HLA-B27 positive.
C. RF positive.
D. ACPA positive.

121. You see a 33-year-old man diagnosed with reactive arthritis and urethritis. You recommend antimicrobial treatment with:
A. amoxicillin.
B. doxycycline.
C. TMP-SMX.
D. nitrofurantoin.

Answers

116. D.	**118.** A.	**120.** B.
117. B.	**119.** C.	**121.** B.

Reactive arthritis, formally known as Reiter syndrome, refers to acute nonpurulent arthritis complicating an infection elsewhere in the body. Two or more of the following findings are required to make the diagnosis, with at least one musculoskeletal finding needed: asymmetrical oligoarthritis, predominantly of the lower extremity; sausage-shaped finger (dactylitis); toe or heel pain or other enthesitis; cervicitis, prostatitis, or acute diarrhea within 1 month of onset of the arthritis; conjunctivitis or uveitis; and genital ulceration or urethritis. Joint pain, especially in the knees, ankles, and feet, is often involved; sacroiliitis is less common.

This condition is typically seen many days to weeks after an episode of acute bacterial diarrhea caused by *Shigella* species, *Salmonella* species, *Campylobacter* species, or a sexually transmitted infection such as *Chlamydia trachomatis* or *Ureaplasma urealyticum*. When seen with infectious diarrhea, the disease is found equally in both genders. When this condition is seen with urethritis, there is a male predominance of 9:1, with most being HLA-B27 positive (a human leukocyte antigen located on the surface of white blood cells). Cultures of joint aspirates in reactive arthritis typically have negative results. Diagnostic testing is aimed at finding the underlying cause, such as urethral or stool cultures. Because this is an inflammatory condition, ESR is elevated, but this is not particularly sensitive or specific for the condition. Laboratory tests for rheumatic disease, such as ANA and rheumatoid factor analyses, are not affected by the disease; checking these laboratory markers is not needed unless the diagnosis of RA or SLE is in question.

Treatment includes the use of anti-inflammatory drugs such as NSAIDs, systemic corticosteroids, or tumor necrosis factor blockers (e.g., etanercept or infliximab). Corticosteroid injections in the affected joints can be considered to reduce inflammation. Because reactive arthritis occurs weeks after infection, especially when associated with infectious diarrhea, antimicrobial therapy is is of limited benefit. However, when reactive arthritis occurs with urethritis, the use of an antibiotic can shorten the duration of symptoms. Urethritis can be treated with doxycycline for 7 days or a single dose of azithromycin. Alternative treatments include 7 days of erythromycin, ofloxacin, or levofloxacin. Early antimicrobial treatment of infectious urethritis seems to limit a patient's risk of developing reactive arthritis. No change in symptoms is usually seen with antibiotic use if infectious diarrhea was the precipitating event.

DISCUSSION SOURCE

Sarani N. eMedicine. http://emedicine.medscape.com/article/808833-overview, Reactive arthritis in emergency medicine.

Sports Participation Evaluation

122. A preparticipation physical screening examination should include:
    A. CBC.
    B. urinalysis.
    C. blood pressure measurement.
    D. radiograph of the spine.

123. Among individuals younger than 35 years, the most common cause of sudden cardiac death is:
    A. non-ST-segment myocardial infarction.
    B. ST-segment myocardial infarction.
    C. a congenital cardiac malformation.
    D. aortic stenosis.

124. During a preparticipation cardiovascular history, all of the following questions should be included except:
    A. past detection of a heart murmur.
    B. excessive, unexplained, and unexpected shortness of breath.
    C. prior occurrence of exertional chest pain/discomfort.
    D. prior use of NSAID use.

125. During a preparticipation sports examination, you hear a grade 2/6 early- to mid-systolic ejection murmur, heard best at the second intercostal space of the left sternal border, in an asymptomatic young adult. The murmur disappears with position change from supine to stand position change. This most likely represents:
    A. an innocent flow murmur.
    B. mitral valve incompetency.
    C. aortic regurgitation.
    D. mitral valve prolapse (MVP).

126. You see a 28-year-old Italian-American man who participates in recreational basketball and has mild hypertension. In considering treatment, you consider all of the following as viable options except:
    A. calcium channel blocker.
    B. angiotensin converting enzyme inhibitors.
    C. angiotensin receptor antagonists.
    D. beta-adrenergic antagonists.

127. You are examining an 18-year-old man who is seeking a sports clearance physical examination. You note a mid-systolic murmur that gets louder when he stands. This most likely represents:
    A. aortic stenosis.
    B. hypertrophic cardiomyopathy.
    C. a physiologic murmur.
    D. a Still murmur.

128. A Still murmur:
    A. is an indication to restrict sports participation selectively.
    B. has a buzzing quality.
    C. is usually heard in patients who experience dizziness when exercising.
    D. is a sign of cardiac structural abnormality.

129. Common signs of high-grade aortic stenosis in an individual during exercise include all of the following except:
    A. dyspnea.
    B. angina.
    C. seizure.
    D. syncope.

130. Risk factors for mitral regurgitation include a prior diagnosis of all of the following except:
    A. rheumatic heart disease.
    B. scarlet fever.
    C. endocarditis.
    D. calcific annulus.

131. You are examining a 19-year-old man who is diagnosed with a murmur of mitral regurgitation. When he asks about participation in sports activities, you counsel that:
    A. participation in sports activities should not be affected by his condition.
    B. he should refrain from any activities requiring physical exertion.
    C. participation will depend on the degree of atrial atrophy.
    D. participation will depend on the degree of ventricular enlargement.

132. A 23-year-old woman presents with mild mitral stenosis and is without symptoms. Which of the following is correct concerning sports participation?
    A. Full activity is likely acceptable.
    B. Prolonged aerobic exercise is discouraged.
    C. An ACE inhibitor should be prescribed prior to participation.
    D. Sports participation should be limited to noncontact sports.

133. A 22-year-old woman wants to know whether she can start a walking program. She has a diagnosis of MVP, with echocardiogram revealing trace mitral regurgitation. You respond that:
    A. she should have an exercise tolerance test.
    B. an ECG should be obtained.
    C. she may proceed in the absence of symptoms of activity intolerance.
    D. running should be avoided.

134. You hear a fixed split second heart sound (S_2) in a 28-year-old woman who wants to start an exercise program and consider that it is:
    A. a normal finding in a younger adult.
    B. occasionally found in uncorrected atrial septal defect.
    C. the result of valvular sclerosis.
    D. often found in patients with right bundle branch block.

135. Which of the following characteristics about atrial septic defect is false?
    A. It is more common in boys than girls.
    B. Child presentation can range from entirely well to heart failure.
    C. Full sports participation is typically acceptable with correction.
    D. Easy fatigability is a sign of atrial septic defect.

136. A 19-year-old man presents with Stage 1 hypertension. Which of the following statements is correct concerning sports participation?
    A. Full activity should be encouraged.
    B. Weight lifting is contraindicated.
    C. An exercise tolerance test is advisable.
    D. A beta-adrenergic antagonist should be prescribed.

137. A 25-year-old woman presents with sinus arrhythmia. Which of the following statements is correct concerning sports participation?
    A. Full activity should be encouraged.
    B. Weight lifting is contraindicated.
    C. An exercise tolerance test is advisable.
    D. A calcium channel antagonist should be prescribed.

138. Among young adults with an implantable cardioverter defibrillator (ICD), participation in sports should be:
    A. generally cautioned against.
    B. limited to noncontact sports.
    C. limited to anaerobic activities.
    D. determined on an individual basis.

139. Initial preparticipation screening of athletes should include:
    A. a resting 12-lead ECG.
    B. echocardiogram.
    C. both a resting 12-lead ECG and echocardiogram.
    D. neither a resting 12-lead ECG nor echocardiogram.

A preparticipation sports screening examination is an important step toward safe involvement in organized sports. The purpose of these screening exams is to maintain the health and safety of the athlete, not simply as a means to disqualify or exclude athletes from participating in sports. The screening process should involve multiple steps, including patient and family history, physical examination, and cardiovascular exam (Table 9–8). Urinalysis, CBC, and radiographic imaging of the spine are generally not recommended for individuals with an unremarkable medical history because these are not helpful screening tools.

Cardiovascular evaluation is an important component of the sports participation evaluation. Reducing the risk of exercised-induced sudden cardiac death and the progression or deterioration of cardiovascular function caused by exercise are the primary goals of preparticipation evaluation. The precise conditions responsible for athletic field deaths differ considerably according to age. In victims younger than 35 years, most sudden deaths are caused by cardiac malformations. Hypertrophic cardiomyopathy is the predominant abnormality in about one-third of cases, and congenital coronary anomalies rank as the second most common etiology. Most of these deaths occur while the victims are playing team sports. In athletes 35 years or older, most deaths are caused by atherosclerotic coronary artery disease, usually while the victims are participating in an individual endeavor such as long-distance running.

The preparticipation cardiovascular history should include questions about the following:
- Prior occurrence of exertional chest pain/discomfort or syncope/near syncope
- Excessive, unexpected, and unexplained shortness of breath or fatigue associated with exercise
- Past detection of a heart murmur or high blood pressure
- Family history of the following: premature death (sudden or otherwise), significant disability from cardiovascular disease in one or more close relatives younger than age 50 years, or specific knowledge of the occurrence of certain conditions (hypertrophic cardiomyopathy, dilated cardiomyopathy, long QT syndrome, Marfan syndrome, or clinically important dysrhythmias)

The cardiovascular physical examination should include the following:
- Precordial auscultation in the supine and standing positions to identify heart murmurs consistent with dynamic left ventricular outflow obstruction
- Assessment of the femoral artery pulses to exclude coarctation of the aorta
- Recognition of the physical stigmata of Marfan syndrome
- Blood pressure measurement in the sitting and standing positions

If any abnormalities in the history or physical examination are revealed, further evaluation or appropriate referral should follow. The ability to participate in athletic activities is determined by the results of these studies.

Answers

122. C.	128. B.	134. B.
123. C.	129. C.	135. A.
124. D.	130. B.	136. A.
125. A.	131. D.	137. A.
126. D.	132. A.	138. D.
127. B.	133. C.	139. D.

TABLE 9-8
Preparticipation Physical Examination Components

History/Exam	Components
Past medical history	• Allergies, asthma, birth defects, chickenpox, diabetes, eating disorders, glasses/contacts, heart murmurs, heart problems, hepatitis, hernia, high blood pressure, kidney disease, measles, medications, menstrual history, mental disorders, mononucleosis, pneumonia, rheumatic fever, seizures, sickle cell trait or disease, tuberculosis
Sports-specific history	• Orthopedic injuries (sprains, fractures, dislocations) or surgeries • Back or neck injuries • Dental trauma • Chest pain with exercise • Feeling faint or having passed out with exercise • "Burners" or "stinger" caused by contact that produces burning pain that moves into the extremity • Withholding from participating in a sport for medical reason
Family history	• Heart disease or high blood pressure • Diabetes • Unexpected death before the age of 50 years
Physical exam	• Pulse rate • Blood pressure rate • Height and weight • Vision and hearing
Exam by healthcare provider	• Head—eyes, ears, throat, teeth, neck • Thorax—heart, lungs, chest wall • Abdomen—liver, spleen kidney, intestines • Genitalia—sexual maturity, testicles, hernias • Neurological—reflexes, strength, coordination • Orthopedic—joints, spine, ligaments, tendons, bones (pain, range of motion, strength)

Source: American College of Sports Medicine. Pre-Participation physical examinations, http://www.acsm.org/docs/brochures/pre-participation-physical-examinations.pdf.

Hypertension is a common clinical problem. Because of the cardiovascular benefit of exercise, activity restriction is usually not advisable unless severely elevated hypertension or target organ damage is present. Certain antihypertensive agents may influence exercise tolerance. Generally, the use of angiotensin-converting enzyme inhibitors, angiotensin receptor blockers, and calcium channel antagonists has little to no impact on exercise tolerance. Use of a beta-adrenergic antagonist can reduce the ability to exercise, however, because of its ability to blunt the normal increase in heart rate in response to exercise. Diuretic use should be avoided if possible because of increased risk of dehydration and hypokalemia.

Cardiac rhythm disturbances are common and are usually benign. In particular, the presence of sinus arrhythmia in a younger adult is a normal finding and is not an indication for curtailing activity. Dysrhythmias associated with ischemic heart disease and certain supraventricular and ventricular rhythms can preclude sports participation.

A systolic cardiac murmur is often benign. The examiner simply hears the blood flowing through the heart, but no cardiac structural abnormality exists. Certain cardiac structural problems, such as valvular and myocardial disorders, can contribute to the development of a murmur, however (Table 9–9).

Normal heart valves allow one-way, unimpeded forward blood flow through the heart. The entire stroke output is able to pass freely during one phase of the cardiac cycle (diastole with the atrioventricular valves, systole with the others), and there is no backward flow of blood. When a heart valve fails to open to its normal size, it is stenotic. When it fails to close appropriately, the valve is incompetent, causing regurgitation of blood to the previous chamber or vessel. Both of these events place patients at significant risk for embolic disease.

Physiologic murmurs, also known as functional or innocent flow murmurs, are present in the absence of cardiac pathology. There is no obstruction to flow, and there is a normal gradient across the valve. This type of murmur can be heard in 80% of thin adults or children if the cardiac examination is performed in a soundproof booth, and it is best heard at the left sternal border. It occurs in early to middle

TABLE 9-9

Cardiac Conditions: Findings and Impact on Sports Participation

Cardiac Condition	Important Examination Findings	Additional Findings	Impact on Sports Participation
Hypertension	Elevated BP	With target organ damage: S_3, S_4 heart sounds; PMI displacement; hypertensive retinopathy	With all but markedly elevated BP or evidence of target organ damage, full participation should be encouraged because of cardiovascular benefit of exercise.
Physiologic murmur (also called innocent or functional murmur)	Grade 1–3/6 early to mid-systolic murmur, heard best at LSB, but usually audible over precordium	No radiation beyond precordium Softens or disappears with standing, increases in intensity with activity, fever, anemia S_1, S_2 intact, normal PMI	Full participation Patient should be asymptomatic, with no report of chest pain, HF symptoms, palpitations, syncope, and activity intolerance.
Aortic stenosis (AS)	Grade 1–4/6 harsh systolic murmur, usually crescendo-decrescendo pattern, heard best at second RICS, base	Radiates to carotids; may have diminished S_2, slow filling carotid pulse, narrow pulse pressure, loud S_4 Softens with standing The greater the degree of stenosis, the later the peak of murmur.	Impact in participation varies with degree of stenosis. Mild: Full participation Moderate: Selected participation Severe: No participation In younger adults, usually congenital bicuspid valve In older adults, usually calcific, rheumatic in nature Dizziness and syncope are ominous signs, pointing to severely decreased cardiac output.
Mitral stenosis (MS)	Grade 1–3/4 low-pitched late diastolic murmur heard best at the apex, localized Short crescendo-decrescendo rumble, similar to a bowling ball rolling down an alley or distant thunder	Often with opening snap, accentuated S_1 in the mitral area Enhanced by left lateral decubitus position, squat, cough, immediately after Valsalva maneuver	Impact on participation varies with degree of stenosis. Mild: Full participation Moderate: Selected participation Mild with atrial fibrillation: Selected participation Severe: No participation Nearly all cases rheumatic in origin Protracted latency period, then gradual decrease in exercise tolerance, leading to rapid downhill course as a result of low cardiac output Atrial fibrillation common

Continued

TABLE 9-9

Cardiac Conditions: Findings and Impact on Sports Participation—cont'd

Cardiac Condition	Important Examination Findings	Additional Findings	Impact on Sports Participation
Mitral regurgitation (MR)	Grade 1–4/6 high-pitched blowing systolic murmur, often extending beyond S_2 Sounds like long "haaa," "hooo" Heard best at RLSB	Radiates to axilla, often with laterally displaced PMI Decreased with standing, Valsalva maneuver Increased by squat, hand grip	Impact in participation varies with ventricular size and function. MR with normal LV size and function: Full participation MR with mild LV enlargement but normal function at rest: Selected participation MR with LV enlargement or any LV dysfunction at rest: No participation Origin: Rheumatic, ischemic heart disease, endocarditis Often with other valve abnormalities (AS, MS, AR)
Aortic regurgitation (AR)	Grade 1–3/4 high-pitched blowing diastolic murmur heard best at third LICS	May be enhanced by forced expiration, leaning forward Usually with S_3, wide pulse pressure, sustained thrusting apical impulse	Impact in participation varies with ventricular size, function, and dysrhythmias. AR with normal or mildly increased LV size and function: Full participation AR with moderate LV enlargement, premature ventricular contractions at rest and with exercise: Selected participation Mild to moderate AR with symptoms, severe AR, AR with progressive LVH: No participation More common in men, usually caused by rheumatic heart disease but occasionally by tertiary syphilis
Mitral valve prolapse (MVP)	Grade 1–3/6 late systolic crescendo murmur with honking quality, heard best at apex Murmur follows mid-systolic click	With Valsalva maneuver or standing, click moves forward into earlier systole, resulting in a longer sounding murmur With hand grasp or squat, click moves back further into systole, resulting in a shorter murmur	Impact on participation varies with ventricular function and dysrhythmia. MVP alone: Full participation MVP with mild to moderate regurgitation, dysrhythmias such as repetitive supraventricular tachycardia, complex ventricular dysrhythmias: Selected participation

TABLE 9-9

Cardiac Conditions: Findings and Impact on Sports Participation—cont'd

Cardiac Condition	Important Examination Findings	Additional Findings	Impact on Sports Participation
			Often seen with minor thoracic deformities such as pectus excavatum, straight back, and shallow anteroposterior diameter
Hypertrophic cardiomyopathy	Harsh mid-systolic crescendo-decrescendo murmur heard best at LLSB or at the apex	Murmur may increase with standing, squat, or Valsalva maneuver. Triple apical impulse, loud S_4, bisferiens carotid pulse	Dyspnea, chest pain, postexertional syncope often are reported. Sports participation should be determined on an individual basis according to degree of ventricular function and symptoms.
Still murmur (also called vibratory innocent murmur)	Grade 1–3/6 early systolic ejection, musical or vibratory, short, often buzzing, heard best midway between apex and LLSB	Softens or disappears when sitting or standing or with Valsalva maneuver Usual onset, 2–6 y.o.; may persist through adolescence Benign condition	Benign finding No limitation on sports participation
Atrial septal defect (without surgical intervention)	Grade 1–3/6 systolic ejection murmur heard best at ULSB with widely split fixed S_2 May be accompanied by a mid-diastolic murmur heard at the fourth ICS LSB common, caused by increased flow across tricuspid valve	Twice as common in girls Child may be entirely well or present with HF Often missed in the first few months of life or even entire childhood Watch for child with easy fatigability	With correction, full sports participation is typical. Without correction, sports participation should be determined on an individual basis according to degree of pulmonary hypertension, right-to-left shunt, and symptoms.
Ventricular septal defect (without surgical intervention)	Grade 2–5/6 regurgitant systolic murmur heard best at LLSB Occasionally holosystolic, usually localized	Usually without cyanosis With small to moderate-sized left-to-right shunt and without pulmonary hypertension, likely to have minimal symptoms Larger shunts may result in HF with onset in infancy	With correction, full sports participation is typical. Without correction, sports participation should be determined on an individual basis according to degree of pulmonary hypertension, right-to-left shunt, and symptoms.

BP, blood pressure; PMI, point of maximal impulse; LSB, left sternal border; S_1, S_2, S_3, and S_4, first to fourth heart sounds; HF, heart failure; RICS, right intercostal space; RLSB, right lower sternal border; LV, left ventricular; LICS, left intercostal space; LVH, left ventricular hypertrophy; LLSB, lower left sternal border; ULSB, upper left sternal border; ICS, intercostal space.

systole, leaving the two heart sounds intact. In addition, patients with a benign systolic ejection murmur deny having cardiac symptoms and have otherwise normal cardiac examination results, including an appropriately located point of maximal impulse and full pulses. Because no cardiac pathology is present in patients with a physiologic murmur, full activity should be encouraged.

Aortic stenosis is the inability of the aortic valves to open to optimal size. The aortic valve normally opens to 3 cm²; aortic stenosis usually does not cause significant symptoms until the valvular orifice is limited to 0.8 cm². In children and younger adults, aortic stenosis is occasionally found, usually caused by a congenital bicuspid (rather than tricuspid) valve or by a three-cusp valve with leaflet fusion. This defect is most often found in boys and men and is commonly accompanied by a long-standing history of becoming excessively short of breath with increased activity such as running. Other symptoms commonly experienced by athletes include angina or chest tightness, syncope or near syncope, fatigue during exercise, heart palpitations, and heart murmur. The physical examination results are usually normal except for the murmur. The ability to participate in sports or other vigorous activity is dictated by the degree of aortic stenosis and patient symptoms (see Table 9–9).

In older adults, calcification aortic stenosis leading to the inability of the valve to open to its normal size is usually the problem. In middle-aged adults without congenital aortic stenosis, the disease is usually sequelae of rheumatic fever, representing about 30% of cases of valvular dysfunction seen in patients with rheumatic heart disease. As with patients who have congenital aortic stenosis, the ability to participate in sports or an exercise program is dictated by the degree of valvular dysfunction, ventricular enlargement, and patient symptoms.

The murmur of mitral regurgitation arises from mitral valve incompetency, or the inability of the mitral valve to close properly. This incompetency allows a retrograde flow from a high-pressure area (left ventricle) to an area of lower pressure (left atrium). Mitral regurgitation is most often caused by the degeneration of the mitral valve, most commonly by rheumatic fever, endocarditis, calcific annulus, rheumatic heart disease, ruptured chordae, or papillary muscle dysfunction. In mitral regurgitation from rheumatic heart disease, some mitral stenosis is usually present. After a patient becomes symptomatic, without intervention the disease progresses in a downhill course of chronic heart failure over the next decade. Sports or other vigorous activity participation is dictated by the degree of mitral regurgitation and ventricular chamber enlargement.

Mitral valve prolapse (MVP) is likely the most common valvular heart problem; the condition is present in perhaps 10% of the general population. Most patients with MVP have a benign condition in which one of the valve leaflets is unusually long and buckles or prolapses into the left atrium, usually in mid systole. At that time, a click occurs, followed by a short murmur caused by regurgitation of blood into the atrium. Cardiac output is usually not compromised, and the event goes unnoticed by patients. Echocardiography fails to reveal any abnormality, simply noting the valve buckling, followed by a small-volume or trace mitral regurgitation. If there are no cardiac complaints and the rest of the cardiac examination, including ECG, is normal, no further evaluation is needed. One way of describing this variation from the norm is to inform patients that one leaflet of the mitral valve is a bit longer than usual. The "holder" (valve orifice) is of average size, however. This variation causes the valve to buckle a bit, just as a person's foot would if forced into a shoe that is one or two sizes too small. The heart makes an extra set of sounds (click and murmur) but is not diseased or damaged.

MVP is often found in people with minor thoracic deformities, such as pectus excavatum, a dish-shaped concave area at T1, and scoliosis. The second and much smaller group with MVP has systolic displacement of one or more of the mitral leaflets into the left atrium along with valve thickening and redundancy, usually accompanied by mild to moderate mitral regurgitation. These people typically have additional health problems, such as Marfan syndrome or other connective tissue disease. Because structural cardiac abnormality is present in these people, there is increased risk of bacterial endocarditis.

Barring other health problems, patients with MVP usually have normal cardiac output and tolerate a program of aerobic exercise well. Regular aerobic activity should be encouraged to promote health and well-being. Maintaining a high level of fluid intake should be encouraged in patients with MVP because the mitral valve prolapses more, increasing the murmur, when circulating volume is low. Treatment with beta-adrenergic agonists (beta blockers) is indicated only when symptomatic recurrent tachycardia or palpitations are an issue. Although this degree of distress (i.e., chest pain, dyspnea) may depend in part on the degree of mitral regurgitation, some studies have failed to reveal any difference in the rates of chest pain in patients with or without MVP. The potentially biggest threat is the rupture of chordae, which is usually seen only in individuals with connective tissue diseases (especially Marfan syndrome).

Hypertrophic cardiomyopathy is a disease of the cardiac muscle. The ventricular septum is thick and asymmetrical, leading to potential outflow tract blockade. Patients with hypertrophic cardiomyopathy often exhibit symptoms of cardiac outflow tract blockage with activity because the hypertrophic ventricular walls better approximate with the increased force of myocardial contraction associated with exercise. The presentation of hypertrophic cardiomyopathy is occasionally sudden cardiac death. Idiopathic hypertrophic subaortic stenosis is a type of cardiomyopathy. A strong family history is often present in individuals who have this autosomal-dominant disorder. The typical patient is a young adult with a history of dyspnea with activity, but those with hypertrophic cardiomyopathy may also be asymptomatic.

There are a growing number of teenagers and young adults susceptible to arrhythmias who are receiving implantable cardioverter defibrillators (ICDs). These devices detect the problematic dysrhythmia and automatically provide an electrical shock that restores a normal heartbeat. Consensus statements offer a note of caution about participation in sports by individuals with ICDs. These recommendations are largely based on postulated risks of failure to defibrillate, potential injury resulting from loss of control caused by dysrhythmia-related syncope, and damage to the ICD system itself during contact sports. However, study indicates that athletes with ICDs can engage in vigorous and competitive sports without physical injury or failure by the ICD to terminate the dysrhythmia. This was despite the occurrence of both appropriate and inappropriate electrical shocks. Patients with ICDs should be aware of the benefits and risks of sports participation, and the decision to participate should be made on an individual basis.

In individuals with congenital heart disease such as atrial or ventricular septal defect, recommendations for sports participation vary according to patient presentation and surgical intervention. Most often, if the defect has been surgically repaired with little residual dysfunction, full sports participation is allowed. If the defect is uncorrected, or if there is significant alteration in cardiac function despite repair, the degree of participation should be assessed on an individual basis with expert consultation.

Routine use of the resting 12-lead ECG or echocardiogram is not recommended to screen individuals during a preparticipation evaluation. However, the use of these tools can be considered when initial screening raises suspicion of the presence of a cardiovascular condition that needs further evaluation.

DISCUSSION SOURCES

American Heart Association Council on Nutrition, Physical Activity, and Metabolism. http://circ.ahajournals.org/cgi/content/full/115/12/1643, Recommendations and considerations related to preparticipation screening for cardiovascular abnormalities in competitive athletes: 2007 update.

American Heart Association. Preparticipation cardiovascular screening of young competitive athletes. Policy guidance (June 2012). http://www.heart.org/idc/groups/ahaecc-public/@wcm/@adv/documents/downloadable/ucm_443945.pdf.

American College of Sports Medicine. Pre-participation physical examinations. http://www.acsm.org/docs/brochures/pre-participation-physical-examinations.pdf.

Osteoporosis

140. All of the following are common sites of fracture in patients with osteoporosis except:
    A. the proximal femur.
    B. the distal forearm.
    C. the vertebrae.
    D. the clavicle.

141. Osteoporosis is more common in individuals:
    A. with type 2 diabetes mellitus.
    B. on long-term systemic corticosteroid therapy.
    C. who are obese.
    D. of African ancestry.

142. Clinical disorders that increase the risk for osteoporosis include all of the following except:
    A. rheumatoid arthritis.
    B. celiac disease.
    C. hyperlipidemia.
    D. hyperprolactinemia.

143. Osteoporosis is defined as having a bone density more than _____ standard deviation(s) below the average bone mass for women younger than 35 years old.
    A. 1
    B. 1.5
    C. 2.5
    D. 4

144. The preferred screening test for osteoporosis is:
    A. quantitative ultrasound measurement.
    B. dual-energy x-ray absorptiometry.
    C. qualitative CT.
    D. wrist, spine, and hip radiographs.

145. Osteoporosis prevention measures include all of the following except:
    A. calcium supplementation.
    B. selective estrogen receptor modulator use.
    C. vitamin B_6 supplementation.
    D. weight-bearing and muscle-strengthening exercises.

146. All of the following are common signs of osteoporosis except:
    A. gradual loss of height with stooped posture.
    B. hip or wrist fracture.
    C. increase in waist circumference.
    D. patient report of back pain.

147. How much daily calcium is recommended for women older than 50 years of age?
    A. 800 mg
    B. 1000 mg
    C. 1200 mg
    D. 1500 mg

148. Nondairy sources of calcium include all of the following except:
    A. tofu.
    B. spinach.
    C. brown rice.
    D. sardines.

149. Long-term bisphosphonate treatment (i.e., >5 years) has been associated with:
    A. atypical fractures.
    B. hyperprolactinemia.
    C. osteoarthritis.
    D. bone marrow suppression.

150. The use of calcitonin to treat osteoporosis has been associated with an increased risk of:
    A. type 2 diabetes.
    B. rheumatoid arthritis.
    C. malignancy.
    D. systemic lupus erythematosus.

151. Which of the following patients would be an appropriate candidate for treatment with teriparatide (Forteo)?
    A. a 54-year-old woman with osteopenia
    B. a 64-year-old woman with BMD T-score of -2.5 and prior hip fracture
    C. a 67-year-old man with a BMD T-score of -1
    D. a 72-year-old woman who has a stable BMD T-score of -1.5 with bisphosphonate treatment for the past 3 years

152. The bisphosphonate therapy given as an annual infusion is:
   A. risedronate.
   B. zoledronic acid.
   C. ibandronate.
   D. denosumab.

153. In counseling a postmenopausal woman, you advise her that systemic estrogen therapy users can possibly experience:
   A. an increase in breast cancer rates with long-term use.
   B. reduction in high-density lipoprotein cholesterol.
   C. a 10% increase in bone mass.
   D. no change in the occurrence of osteoporosis.

154. When counseling a patient taking a bisphosphonate such as alendronate (Fosamax), you advise that the medication should be taken with:
   A. a bedtime snack.
   B. a meal.
   C. other medications.
   D. a large glass of water.

❚) Answers

140.	D.	145.	C.	150.	C.
141.	B.	146.	C.	151.	B.
142.	C.	147.	C.	152.	B.
143.	C.	148.	C.	153.	A.
144.	B.	149.	A.	154.	D.

Osteoporosis is a disorder of bone thinning in which bone absorption exceeds bone formation to the degree that bone density is insufficient to meet skeletal needs. Osteoporosis is also defined as bone density more than 2.5 standard deviations below the average bone mass for women who are younger than 35 years old. For every reduction of bone mass by 1 standard deviation, the relative risk of fracture rises by 1.5-fold to 3-fold.

Estrogen deficiency is a potent risk factor, and osteoporosis is most common in postmenopausal women; by age 80 years, the average woman has lost more than 30% of her premenopausal bone density. Men appear to be at significantly less risk; this is partly because of inherently greater bone density. Body habitus and ethnicity can influence the risk of osteoporosis; the condition is most common in small-framed women of Asian and European ancestry, who usually have lower bone density in adulthood. At the same time, all ethnic groups are at risk. Obesity appears to minimize osteoporosis risk, in part because of high endogenous estrogen production by fatty tissue and increased bone weight-bearing. Additional risk factors for osteoporosis include select disorders involving the endocrine, gastrointestinal and central nervous systems as well as rheumatologic, autoimmune, and hematologic diseases; inactivity; and prolonged therapy with certain medications, including some anticonvulsants, thyroid hormones, and systemic corticosteroids (Table 9–11).

In patients with osteoporosis, hip, wrist, and spinal fractures most commonly occur, but all bones are at risk. Early disease usually does not have symptoms, but backache is commonly reported. Although hip fracture is often the first clinical

---

TABLE 9-10
Ligamentous Sprains: Grading, Presentation, and Intervention

Grade of Injury	Pathology and Presentation	Intervention
Grade I	Slight stretching or microscopic tear No instability	RICE (rest, ice, compression, elevation) Immobilizer Limit weight-bearing Analgesia Length of disability usually limited to a few days
Grade II	Partial ligamentous tear Moderate joint instability Moderate swelling Mild to moderate ecchymosis	Rest, ice, compression, elevation (RICE) Immobilizer Limit weight-bearing Analgesia Length of disability usually several weeks to a few months Orthopedic referral
Grade III	Complete ligamentous tear Complete ankle instability Significant swelling Moderate to severe ecchymosis	RICE Immobilizer Limit weight-bearing Analgesia Length of disability may be many months

Sources: Anderson B. *Office Orthopedics for Primary Care: Diagnosis*, ed. 1. Philadelphia: Saunders, 2006.
Anderson B. *Office Orthopedics for Primary Care: Treatment*, ed. 3. Philadelphia: Saunders, 2006.
Turner S. Musculoskeletal system. In: Goolsby M, Grubbs L, eds. *Advanced Assessment: Interpreting Findings and Formulating Differential Diagnosis*, ed. 2. Philadelphia: FA Davis, 2011, pp. 411-449.

manifestation of osteoporosis, it usually indicates advanced disease, as does loss of terminal adult height.

In patients with osteoporosis, the bone lost is from the baseline bone density. A small amount of loss can be of great significance against poor bone density, but of little consequence with greater density. Primary prevention of osteoporosis includes ensuring the development of maximal adult bone density. Because maximal bone density is achieved in the early adult years, encouraging adequate calcium intake and weight-bearing exercise throughout the teen and adult years is important. According to the latest recommendations from the National Osteoporosis Foundation (NOF), the calcium intake goal should be the equivalent of 1000 mg/d for men between 50 to 70 years of age, and the dose should be 1200 mg/day for women 51 years and older and men older than age 70 years. Vitamin D (minimal dose 800 to 1000 IU daily) is recommended for all adults older than age 50 years, with higher doses needed for those with vitamin D deficiency.

Foods should be one source of this important micronutrient, although few foods are abundant vitamin D sources. Exposing the skin to sunlight is the most important vitamin D source because the body readily synthesizes this nutrient in response to sunlight. Dietary calcium should be the primary source of calcium from dairy and nondairy options (e.g., spinach, sardines, tofu, select nuts, others). Given current lifestyles and dietary habits, supplements are often needed to meet recommended requirements.

Many tests are available to evaluate osteoporosis risk or detect progression of the disease (Table 9–11). Dual-energy x-ray absorptiometry is considered a reliable measure. Qualitative CT is precise but uses more radiation than dual-energy x-ray absorptiometry. Quantitative ultrasound is relatively inexpensive and can be performed with portable equipment. Plain radiographic films should not be used for screening or evaluation of osteoporosis because disease cannot be detected until 40% to 50% of bone mass is lost.

TABLE 9-11
Osteoporosis: Risks, Screening Guidelines, and Treatment

RISK FACTORS FOR OSTEOPOROSIS

Lifestyle factors (e.g., physical inactivity, low calcium intake, alcohol abuse)

Genetic factors (e.g., cystic fibrosis, Gaucher disease)

Hypogonadal states (e.g., androgen insensitivity, hyperprolactinemia)

Endocrine disorders (e.g., diabetes mellitus, adrenal insufficiency)

Gastrointestinal disorders (e.g., celiac disease, inflammatory bowel disease)

Hematologic disorders (e.g., multiple myeloma, leukemia)

Rheumatologic and autoimmune disorders (e.g., rheumatoid arthritis, lupus)

Central nervous system disorders (e.g., epilepsy, multiple sclerosis)

- Miscellaneous other conditions and diseases (e.g., AIDS/HIV, congestive heart failure)
- Use of certain medications (e.g., long-term corticosteroid medications, some anticonvulsants, thyroid hormones)

RECOMMENDATIONS FOR OSTEOPOROSIS SCREENING

- Women age 65 and older and men age 70 and older, regardless of risk factors
- Younger postmenopausal women, women in the menopausal transition, and men age 50 to 69 with clinical risk factors for fracture
- A woman or man after age 50 who has broken a bone
- Adults with a condition (e.g., rheumatoid arthritis) or taking a medication (e.g., long-term glucocorticoid) associated with low bone mass or bone loss

AVAILABLE SCREENING TESTS FOR OSTEOPOROSIS

Dual-energy x-ray absorptiometry (DXA) of the hip and spine. Using DXA to measure bone density of the hand, wrist, forearm, and heel also seems to detect women who are at increased risk for fracture

- Other tests to measure bone mineral density: Ultrasound, radiographic absorptiometry, single-energy x-ray, absorptiometry, peripheral DXA, and peripheral quantitative computed tomography

OSTEOPOROSIS TREATMENT

All to be used with appropriate calcium and vitamin D supplementation

- Bisphosphonates, such as alendronate, ibandronate, risedronate, and zoledronic acid
- Other antiresorptive medications including selective estrogen receptor modulators (SERMs), such as raloxifene, calcitonin, estrogen, and RANK ligand inhibitor (denosumab)
- Bone-forming (anabolic) medications such as teriparatide (parathyroid hormone)

Source: National Osteoporosis Foundation. http://nof.org/hcp/clinicians-guide, 2013 Clinician's Guide to Prevention and Treatment of Osteoporosis.

When taken with calcium supplements, postmenopausal hormone therapy (estrogen supplementation with or without a progestin) can help reduce the risk of postmenopausal fracture by up to 34% by minimizing further bone loss; the benefit must be balanced against the noted increased risk of breast cancer and other problems with short-term and long-term use. A selective estrogen receptor modulator such as raloxifene (Evista) helps preserve bone density. Because raloxifene does not attach to estrogen receptor sites in the breast or uterus, a selective estrogen receptor modulator is often considered an alternative to hormone therapy. The parathyroid hormone teriparatide (Forteo) is an anabolic agent that can reduce the risk of vertebral fractures by 65% in patients with osteoporosis. This treatment is typically reserved for women with very low bone density or who have had a prior fracture. Treatment with teriparatide should be limited to a 2-year duration because of a potentially increased risk of osteosarcoma.

Bisphosphonates such as alendronate (Fosamax), ibandronate (Boniva), risedronate (Actonel), and zoledronic acid (Reclast) inhibit the resorptive activity of osteoclasts, can help modestly increase bone mass, and can significantly reduce fracture risk. To minimize the risk of drug-induced esophagitis, patients taking an oral bisphosphonate should be cautioned to take the medication in the morning with a full glass of water. At least 30 minutes must elapse before food, other liquids, or medications are ingested. In addition, patients should remain upright for at least 1 hour. Zoledronic acid is administered as an IV infusion once a year to treat osteoporosis or every 2 years to prevent osteoporosis. In rare cases, low trauma atypical femoral fractures have been associated with long-term use of bisphosphonates (i.e., >5 years). Pain in the thigh or groin area often precedes these fractures. Because the most robust effects of bisphosphonates occur during the first 5 years of treatment and these agents provide some antifracture reduction benefits even when treatment is discontinued, some recommend a drug holiday after 5 to 10 years of therapy. The duration of therapy and the drug holiday should be based on fracture risk, with low-risk patients considering stopping treatment after 5 years and remaining off treatment as long as BMD is stable. Higher-risk patients can be treated for 10 years and have a drug holiday of no more than 1 to 2 years with consideration of a nonbisphosphonate treatment during that time.

Calcitonin (Miacalcin or Fortical) is another antiresorptive medication that is most helpful in building vertebral bone. The FDA advises that the risks associated with calcitonin use outweigh the benefits in treating osteoporosis, largely based on two large studies indicating slightly higher rates of malignancy among patients taking this agent. The FDA supports the continued use of these agents because these medications provide an important option for patients who do not tolerate other treatments. Denosumab (Prolia) is a receptor activator of nuclear factor kappa-B ligand (RANKL) inhibitor that reduces the incidence of vertebral fractures by about 68% in patients with osteoporosis. It is given as a subcutaneous injection every 6 months. With all therapies, calcium supplementation should be continued, and vitamin D deficiency should be appropriately treated.

DISCUSSION SOURCES

National Osteoporosis Foundation. http://www.nof.org/professionals/NOF_Clinicians_Guide.pdf, Clinician's guide to prevention and treatment of osteoporosis.

Watts NB, Diab DL. Long-term use of bisphosphonates in osteoporosis. *J Clin Endocrin Metab* 95:1555–1565, 2010o, http://jcem.endojournals.org/content/95/4/1555.full.

See full color images of this topic on DavisPlus at http://davisplus.fadavis.com | Keyword: Fitzgerald

Sprains

155. The most common site of sprain is the:
A. wrist.
B. shoulder.
C. ankle.
D. knee.

156. Risk factors for ankle sprain include all of the following except:
A. poor conditioning.
B. running on paved surfaces.
C. inappropriate footwear.
D. lack of a warm-up period prior to exercising.

157. A Grade II ankle sprain is best described as:
A. minor swelling and minimal joint instability.
B. moderate joint instability without swelling or ecchymosis.
C. moderate swelling, mild to moderate ecchymosis, and moderate joint instability.
D. complete ankle instability, significant swelling, and moderate to severe ecchymosis.

158. A person with a Grade III ankle sprain presents with:
A. minor swelling and minimal joint instability.
B. moderate joint instability without swelling or ecchymosis.
C. moderate swelling, mild to moderate ecchymosis, and moderate joint instability.
D. complete ankle instability, significant swelling, and moderate to severe ecchymosis.

159. Patients with a Grade III ankle sprain should be advised that full recovery is likely to take:
A. a few days.
B. 2 to 3 weeks.
C. 4 to 6 weeks.
D. many months.

160. Which of the following is usually not part of treatment of a sprain?
A. immobilization
B. applying ice to the area
C. joint rest
D. local corticosteroid injection

161. For a Grade I ankle sprain, weight-bearing should be avoided for at least:
  A. 24 hours.
  B. 72 hours.
  C. 1 week.
  D. until full ROM is restored.

162. A short leg cast is often needed for what type of ankle sprain?
  A. grade I
  B. grade II
  C. grade III
  D. grade IV

Answers

155. C.	158. D.	161. A.
156. B.	159. D.	162. C.
157. C.	160. D.	

A sprain is a partial or complete injury of a ligament either within the ligament body or at its site of attachment to the bone. Inversion injuries of the ankle cause about 85% of all sprains and are the most common injury sustained while jumping or running. Sprains can also involve the wrist, elbow, and knee. Wearing appropriate footwear, improved conditioning, pre-exercise warm-up exercises, and taping can be helpful in avoiding sprains.

Ankle sprains are often graded according to presentation and proposed underlying degree of ligamentous injury (see Table 9–10). The ankle anterior drawer test is used to assess for excessive laxity of the tibiotarsal joint. Excessive anterior motion is usually seen with a Grade III sprain. Immobilization is important in helping appropriate healing and minimizing sequelae. Grade II and III injuries are occasionally associated with persistent joint laxity and a risk of future sprain. The injured ankle should not bear weight for the first 24 hours after the sprain and even longer depending on the severity of the sprain. Grade II sprains may require an immobilizer or splint, whereas a Grade III sprain may require a short leg cast or a cast-brace for 2 to 3 weeks. Although rarely needed, surgical reconstruction is possible for Grade III sprains.

DISCUSSION SOURCES

Anderson B. *Office Orthopedics for Primary Care: Diagnosis*, ed. 1. Philadelphia: Saunders Elsevier, 2006.

Anderson B. *Office Orthopedics for Primary Care: Treatment*, 3rd ed. Philadelphia: Saunders Elsevier, 2006.

Turner S. Musculoskeletal system. In: Goolsby M, Grubbs L, eds. *Advanced Assessment: Interpreting Findings and Formulating Differential Diagnosis*, ed. 2. Philadelphia: FA Davis, 2011, pp. 411-449.

Tendonitis

163. Which of the following statements about tendonitis is false?
  A. Tendonitis is typically the result of overuse.
  B. Tendonitis is the result of a macroscopic or partial tear of the tendon.
  C. Acute pain results when firm pressure is applied to the tendon.
  D. Signs of tendonitis include reduced ROM caused by stiffness and discomfort.

164. Activities that commonly contribute to the development of rotator cuff tendonitis include all of the following except:
  A. swimming.
  B. throwing a football.
  C. bowling.
  D. pitching a baseball.

165. All of the following are common symptoms of wrist tendonitis except:
  A. muscle cramping.
  B. reduced ROM.
  C. swelling of the wrist.
  D. muscle weakness.

166. With initial presentation, the diagnosis of tendonitis is usually made from:
  A. clinical presentation.
  B. plain radiographic films.
  C. CT scan of the area.
  D. laboratory diagnosis.

167. Complications of Achilles tendonitis include:
  A. tendon rupture.
  B. neurological sequelae.
  C. stress fracture.
  D. bursitis.

168. Which of the following is often found with rotator cuff tendonitis?
  A. osteoarthritis
  B. tendon rupture
  C. bursitis
  D. joint effusion

169. First-line therapy for biceps tendonitis usually includes:
  A. applying ice to the area.
  B. local corticosteroid injection.
  C. orthopedic referral.
  D. nerve block.

170. A 36-year-old man has experienced shoulder pain associated with tendonitis for the past 4 weeks despite the use of ice and analgesics (NSAIDs) and undergoing physical therapy. An appropriate next step would include:
A. systemic corticosteroid use.
B. x-ray of the shoulder.
C. MRI of the shoulder.
D. use of an upper arm sling.

Answers

163. B.	**166.** A.	**169.** A.
164. C.	**167.** A.	**170.** C.
165. A.	**168.** C.	

The most common sites for tendonitis are the rotator cuff, elbow, biceps (shoulder), wrist, and heel. In most cases, a microscopic tear causes tendon inflammation; the resulting swelling and inflammation in the tendon are a result of overuse. The clinical presentation usually includes a report of reduced ROM caused by joint stiffness and discomfort and a dull, aching pain over the affected tendon, especially with joint use. This pain can become sharp and acute when the tendon is squeezed.

Rotator cuff tendonitis is often associated with repetitive overhead activities, such as throwing, raking, or washing cars or windows, or it can be the result of injury. Symptoms include a dull pain radiating from the outer arm to several inches below the top of the shoulder. With rotator cuff involvement, abduction and elevation of the shoulder joint worsen symptoms. A clicking in the shoulder can occur when raising the arm above the head.

In the elbow region, tendonitis can occur as either biceps tendinitis or triceps tendinitis. Biceps tendonitis occurs through repetitive overhead activity, including throwing a baseball, swimming, or playing tennis or golf. Symptoms include pain when the arm is overhead or bent and localized tenderness where the tendon passes over the groove in the upper arm bone.

Wrist tendonitis, or tenosynovitis, typically occurs at points where the tendons cross each other or pass over a bony prominence. The condition is caused by overuse, such as repetitive motions during sports or work-related activities (e.g., writing, typing, and assembly-line work). Wrist tendonitis is associated with pain over the area of inflammation with swelling of the surrounding soft tissue. Reduced ROM and muscle weakness are also common.

With initial presentation, the diagnosis of tendonitis is usually straightforward, with no special studies required. If these signs and symptoms occur with a history of recent trauma, plain radiographic films of the affected area occasionally reveal calcium deposits on the tendon. Because bursitis and tendonitis often occur concurrently, assessment often reveals both conditions. MRI is generally not recommended for routine diagnosis of tendonitis. However, if there is a question about accompanying soft tissue injury or suspected tendon tear, or for chronic tendonitis sufferers even after rehabilitation, MRI can be helpful in detecting damage to the tendon.

Treatment of tendonitis includes limiting or discontinuing the contributing activity. Applying ice to the region is helpful. NSAIDs can be used to reduce pain. When the hand or wrist is affected, splinting can be beneficial. Achilles tendonitis often necessitates treatment with a posterior splint to immobilize the heel and heel cord stretching and orthotics after the acute phase to prevent recurrence. There is a 10% risk of tendon rupture with recurrent Achilles tendonitis; the risk can exceed 12% with biceps tendonitis. With rotator cuff involvement, the likelihood of concurrent bursitis is high; treatment includes limiting overhead movement and intrabursal corticosteroid injection.

DISCUSSION SOURCES

Anderson B. *Office Orthopedics for Primary Care: Diagnosis*, ed. 1. Philadelphia: Saunders Elsevier, 2006.

Anderson B. *Office Orthopedics for Primary Care: Treatment*, ed. 3. Philadelphia: Saunders Elsevier, 2006.

Turner S. Musculoskeletal system. In: Goolsby M, Grubbs L, eds. *Advanced Assessment: Interpreting Findings and Formulating Differential Diagnosis*, ed. 2. Philadelphia: FA Davis, 2011, pp. 411-449.

Fibromyalgia

171. Fibromyalgia is caused by:
A. increased production of serotonin.
B. an autoimmune reaction following infection.
C. a genetic autoimmune disorder that targets neuronal axons.
D. a largely unknown mechanism.

172. Which of the following statements is most consistent with fibromyalgia?
A. It is predominantly diagnosed in African Americans.
B. It affects less than 1% of the general population.
C. It is four to seven times more common in women than in men.
D. It is most often initially diagnosed in adults younger than 20 years old and older than 55 years old.

173. Fibromyalgia is more common in patients with:
A. type 2 diabetes.
B. rheumatoid arthritis and systemic lupus erythematosus.
C. migraine headaches.
D. COPD.

174. Which of the following is inconsistent with the clinical presentation of fibromyalgia?
A. widespread body aches
B. joint swelling
C. fatigue
D. cognitive changes

175. The diagnosis of fibromyalgia involves:
A. a CT scan of the head.
B. MRI of various joints throughout the body.
C. identifying multiple tender points throughout the body.
D. a positive ANA or RF test result.

176. When examining a patient with fibromyalgia, tender points:
A. are located only above the waist.
B. can be identified by applying enough pressure to blanch the nail bed of the examiner.
C. are easily identified through radiography.
D. can wax and wane throughout the day.

177. A diagnosis of fibromyalgia requires detecting at least how many tender points?
A. 4
B. 7
C. 11
D. 18

178. When discussing physical activity with a 40-year-old woman with fibromyalgia, you advise that:
A. limiting exercise is an important component of symptom management.
B. weight-bearing exercise would be most helpful.
C. physical activity aimed at increasing flexibility is an important part of treatment.
D. although possibly helpful in minimizing pain, physical activity usually significantly worsens fatigue.

179. Analgesic approaches used in the management of fibromyalgia include all of the following except:
A. acetaminophen.
B. NSAIDs.
C. fentanyl patch.
D. topical capsaicin.

180. Drug classes used in the treatment of fibromyalgia include all of the following except:
A. tricyclic antidepressants.
B. antiepileptics.
C. SSRIs.
D. opioids.

181. Which of the following medications is approved by the U.S. Food and Drug Administration (FDA) for pain management in a person with fibromyalgia?
A. trazodone
B. nortriptyline
C. pregabalin
D. gabapentin

182. Patients with fibromyalgia should be encouraged to all of the following except
A. consider adopting a high-intensity aerobic activity such as jogging.
B. limit caffeine use.
C. utilize stress management techniques.
D. participate in a program of exercise focused on maintaining flexibility.

Answers

171. D.	175. C.	179. C.
172. C.	176. B.	180. D.
173. B.	177. C.	181. C.
174. B.	178. C.	182. A.

Fibromyalgia is a common, complex disorder composed of a specific set of signs and symptoms that likely affects at least 2% of the general population; the condition is one of the most common central pain-related syndromes. Although its etiology is not fully understood, central nervous system dysfunction and central sensitization are likely the source of the multiple clinical findings associated with this condition. Biochemical changes noted in the central nervous system in a person with fibromyalgia include low serotonin levels, elevated levels of substance P, and other biological markers; these changes likely contribute to the diffuse hypersensitivity to pain signals in the brain. Symptoms sometimes begin after a physical trauma, surgery, infection, or significant psychological stress. In other cases, symptoms can gradually develop over time with no apparent triggering event. Genetic factors may also play a role.

Fibromyalgia is four to seven times more common in women than in men; the reason for this finding is not understood. Symptom onset is usually between ages 20 and 55 years. Fibromyalgia is found in all ethnic groups. The presence of rheumatoid arthritis or lupus increases the risk for fibromyalgia.

No particular test is diagnostic for fibromyalgia. The diagnosis is made after careful consideration of the patient's health history and physical examination. The patient usually presents with a complaint of persistent fatigue combined with nonrefreshing sleep. Chronic, often migratory, pain, usually described as burning, aching, soreness, or feeling bruised (without objective evidence of bruising), is usually reported. Fibromyalgia is characterized by additional pain when pressure is applied to specific tender points in certain parts of the body. Many with fibromyalgia also have tension headaches, temporomandibular joint disorder, irritable bowel syndrome, anxiety, and/or depression.

According to the American College of Rheumatology criteria, the diagnosis of fibromyalgia is supported by the presence of tender points in specific locations; the tenderness is triggered at the area where pressure, enough to cause the examiner's nail bed to blanch, or about 4 kg. pressure, is applied, and there is no referred pain. The locations of the tender points are as follows: on the anterior body, usually bilaterally, at the fifth through seventh intertransverse spaces of the cervical spine, in the pectoral muscle at the second costochondral junctions, approximately three finger breadths (2 cm) below the lateral epicondyle, and at the medial fat pad proximal to the joint line. Posteriorly, bilateral findings are as follows: tenderness at the upper border of the shoulder in the trapezius muscle midway from the neck to the shoulder joint, the craniomedial border of the scapula at the origin of the supraspinatus, in the upper outer quadrant of the gluteus medius, and just posterior to the prominence of the greater trochanter at the piriformis insertion. The diagnostic is supported by the presence of pain in all four quadrants of the body and in the axial skeleton for 3 or more months and is noted in 11 or more of 18 anatomically specific tender points. Additional patient symptoms often include chronic gastrointestinal problems, including intermittent diarrhea and constipation, cognitive changes, and/or altered mood.

Intervention in fibromyalgia is complex and requires a comprehensive, interdisciplinary approach; simply attempting to treat the pain associated with the condition is inadequate. Patient education should include information about the need for physical activity, such as flexibility exercises, progressive stretching, and low-impact activities such as aquatic exercise, which has been shown to reduce pain and increase function. Exercise programs that involve high intensity and high impact such as running or jogging, while not contraindicated, are generally poorly tolerated by the person with fibromyalgia. Stress management techniques can be helpful, and getting sufficient sleep is essential for those with fibromyalgia. Those with fibromyalgia should be encouraged to maintain a healthy lifestyle, including eating healthy foods, limiting caffeine intake, and participating in enjoyable and fulfilling activities each day.

Pharmacotherapy can be used to reduce pain and improve sleep. Trigger point injection has been noted to be helpful in certain patients. Acetaminophen and NSAIDs can be used to alleviate pain, although their effectiveness varies. Medications such as trazodone can be helpful in improving sleep latency and duration. Antidepressants (such as nortriptyline, duloxetine [Cymbalta], or milnacipran [Savella]) and antiepileptics (including gabapentin [Neurontin] and pregabalin [Lyrica]) have been shown to minimize symptoms in fibromyalgia and numerous other chronic pain conditions; these medications can be helpful in treating the concomitant altered mood that often accompanies, but is not the cause of, fibromyalgia. Some of these medications, particularly the tricyclic antidepressants, help promote sleep. Pregabalin and duloxetine are approved by the FDA for pain reduction in fibromyalgia. Consistant use of topical treatments such as capsaicin are often helpful treatment adjuncts.

DISCUSSION SOURCES

American College of Rheumatology. http://www.rheumatology.org/practice/clinical/classification/fibromyalgia/fibro_2010.asp.

Mayo Clinic. Fibromyalgia. http://www.mayoclinic.com/health/fibromyalgia/DS00079.

Gilliland R. eMedicine. http://emedicine.medscape.com/article/312778-overview, Rehabilitation and fibromyalgia.

Vitamin D Deficiency

183. Which of the following statements regarding vitamin D is false?
    A. diminishes secretion of insulin.
    B. inhibits abnormal cellular growth.
    C. encourages the absorption and metabolism of calcium and phosphorus.
    D. reduces inflammation.

184. Which of the following provides the most abundant source of vitamin D?
    A. fortified dairy products
    B. fatty fish
    C. exposure of the skin to the sun
    D. leafy green vegetables

185. Which of the following statements is false regarding sunlight exposure and vitamin D production?
    A. In the continental United States, summertime exposure to sunlight can produce the majority of the body's requirement for vitamin D.
    B. One glass of fortified milk has an equivalent amount of vitamin D as what is produced after 10 minutes of exposure to summer sunlight in a healthy young individual.
    C. Use of sunscreen can block the majority of solar-induced vitamin D production.
    D. A person with a darker skin tone produces less vitamin D with sun exposure compared with a person with a lighter skin tone.

186. The vitamin D needs for a 36-year-old person who is taking phenytoin are best described as:
    A. easily met by a well-balanced diet.
    B. equivalent to what is required by other adults in this age group.
    C. markedly increased by twofold to fivefold from the age norm.
    D. reduced from baseline because of the drug's vitamin D–preserving qualities.

187. Clinical manifestations of vitamin D deficiency include all of the following except:
    A. rickets.
    B. osteomalacia.
    C. antigravity muscle weakness.
    D. azotemia.

188. Which precursor of vitamin D is the form that is commonly measured in laboratory tests to determine vitamin D status?
A. vitamin D_2
B. 25-hydroxyvitamin D
C. vitamin D_3
D. 1,25-dihydroxyvitamin D

189. Which of the following provides the least amount of vitamin D?
A. fortified milk (8 oz.)
B. fortified orange juice (8 oz.)
C. 1 egg yolk
D. infant formula (8 oz.)

190. Which of the following servings of fish (3.5 oz.) contains the greatest amount of vitamin D?
A. fresh wild salmon
B. fresh farmed salmon
C. canned tuna
D. canned mackerel

191. A child must consume ___ oz. of fortified milk each day to receive the recommended 400 IU daily of vitamin D.
A. 8
B. 16
C. 32
D. 48

192. For adults 70 years and younger, what is the recommended daily intake of vitamin D?
A. 200 IU
B. 400 IU
C. 600 IU
D. 1000 IU

193. The daily amount of vitamin D_3 recommended for pregnant or lactating women is:
A. 300 IU.
B. 600 IU.
C. 1000 IU.
D. 1200 IU.

194. You see a 46-year-old woman diagnosed with vitamin D deficiency with a 25(OH)D level of 18 ng/mL. Treatment should be initiated with which of the following vitamin D dosing regimens?
A. 400 IU twice a day
B. 1000 IU daily
C. 10,000 IU twice a week
D. 50,000 IU weekly

Answers

183. A.	187. D.	191. C.
184. C.	188. B.	192. C.
185. B.	189. C.	193. B.
186. C.	190. A.	194. D.

Vitamin D has long been recognized as essential for the efficient utilization of dietary calcium and for bone and muscle health. Recent studies have highlighted this important micronutrient's multiple roles. As an inhibitor of abnormal cellular growth, vitamin D is needed to help with cell differentiation and minimizing abnormal cell proliferation, a key step in cancer development. A stimulator of insulin secretion in response to increased insulin demands, vitamin D plays a role in the maintenance of normoglycemia, possibly minimizing the risk of type 2 diabetes mellitus development. Because vitamin D receptors (VDR) are expressed by most cells of the immune system, the micronutrient plays an important role as an immunomodulator. When vitamin D is available in physiologic amounts, this micronutrient acts as a renin producer, therefore contributing to blood pressure control.

Vitamin D deficiency is a common problem, with studies finding this problem in 36% of healthy adults aged 18 to 29 in Boston by winter's end and in 27% of otherwise healthy Asian children in the United Kingdom. Additional studies revealed vitamin D deficiency in 57% of patients on a hospital medical ward and in 93% of patients with nonspecific musculoskeletal pain at a Minneapolis pain clinic. Considering this, vitamin D deficiency is a common problem in the healthy and the sick.

A combination of dietary intake of foods rich in vitamin D in addition to regular periods of skin exposure to the sun should provide the body with an adequate supply of this important micronutrient (Table 9–12). However, with little time spent outdoors and diets replete with highly processed foods, seldom is vitamin D intake and synthesis sufficient to avoid deficiency. Fatty fish and vitamin D–enriched dairy products can supply a small amount of the estimated 3000 to 5000 IU/d of vitamin D the body needs; the average U.S. dietary intake is typically less than 5% of the body's requirement. Vitamin D intake recommendations from the Institute of Medicine suggest 400 IU/day for infants (0–12 months), 600 IU/day for individuals 1–70 years old, and 800 IU/day for those older than 70 years of age. Pregnant and lactating women should intake 600 IU/day.

Skin exposure to the sun's rays should supply ≥95% of the daily requirements by triggering the body's natural ability to synthesize this vitamin. The ability of the body's uninduced vitamin D synthesis is determined by a number of factors, including the skin's melanin pigmentation. A person with a darker skin tone will synthesize less vitamin D with sun exposure when compared with a person with a lighter skin tone. The use of sunscreen, although helpful in minimizing the risk of certain skin cancers and other solar damage, likely increases the risk of vitamin D deficiency because application of a sunscreen with sun protection factor 8 reduces the capacity of the skin to produce vitamin D by as much as 95%. Obviously, individuals who spend little time outdoors have a significant vitamin D deficiency risk. The time of year and place of residence also influence sun-induced vitamin D synthesis, with winter sun and northern latitudes providing the weakest effect. Even people who are

TABLE 9-12

Dietary and Supplemental Sources of Vitamin D

Source	Vitamin D Content
Sunlight exposure	~3000 IU of vitamin D_3 after 5–10 minutes exposure to arms and legs (dependent on latitude)
Fortified milk	~100 IU/8 oz., usually vitamin D_3
Fortified orange juice	~100 IU/8 oz., vitamin D_3
Infant formulas	~100 IU/8 oz., vitamin D_3
Fortified yogurts	~100 IU/8 oz., usually vitamin D_3
Fortified breakfast cereals	~100 IU per serving, usually vitamin D_3
Salmon	
Fresh, wild (3.5 oz.)	~600-1000 IU of vitamin D_3
Fresh, farmed (3.5 oz.)	~100–250 IU of vitamin D_3 or D_2
Tuna, canned (3.6 oz.)	~230 IU of vitamin D_3
Mackerel, canned (3.5 oz.)	~250 IU of vitamin D_3
Cod liver oil (1 tsp.)	~400–1000 IU of vitamin D_3
Shitake mushrooms	
Fresh (3.5 oz.)	~100 IU of vitamin D_2
Sun-dried (3.5 oz.)	~1600 IU of vitamin D_2
Egg yolk	~20 IU of vitamin D_3 or D_2

regularly involved in outdoor activities that facilitate exposure to sunshine can have vitamin D deficiency if little skin is exposed to the sun. Exposing the hands, face, arms, or legs daily for about 5 to15 minutes of sun between the hours of 11AM and 2PM at a strength found in northern latitudes such as Boston will help provide an adequate amount of vitamin D synthesis. This level of sun exposure is unlikely to induce sunburn or increase skin cancer risk. The use of certain medications, including phenytoin (Dilantin) and phenobarbital, is potentially vitamin D depleting; as a result, patients taking these medications require two to five times the recommended daily amount of vitamin D. Vitamin D deficiency is also common in the presence of hepatic or renal disease after gastric bypass.

In infants and children, severe vitamin D deficiency results in the failure of growing bone to mineralize. The resulting condition is rickets. In contrast, adult bones are no longer growing but are in a state of constant cell renewal and therefore susceptible to problems related to vitamin D deficiency including persistent, nonspecific musculoskeletal pain. To appreciate this, consider some of the clinical effects of vitamin D deficiency.

Without sufficient amounts of vitamin D, intestinal calcium absorption is inadequate. The resulting calcium deficiency prompts an increase in production and secretion of parathyroid hormone (PTH). PTH acts at the level of the kidney by facilitating an increase in tubular calcium reabsorption and stimulating renal production of 1,25-dihydroxyvitamin D, the hormonally active form of vitamin D. With continued deficiency, unusually high levels of PTH allow osteoclast activation so that bone can serve as a calcium source. In addition, the continued presence of high levels of circulating PTH

causes phosphate to be wasted via the kidney. The calcium phosphate product in the circulation decreases and becomes inadequate to mineralize the bone properly, potentially leading to osteopenia and osteoporosis. At the same time, osteoblasts deposit a rubbery collagen matrix layer on the skeleton. This surface cannot provide sufficient structural support. The clinical effect is osteomalacia. This abnormal collagen matrix can absorb fluids and expand. With expansion, pressure builds under the richly innervated periosteal covering. This process likely, at least in part, explains the origin of the constant dull bone ache often reported in patients with osteomalacia. In these patients, minimal pressure applied with a fingertip on the sternum, anterior tibia, radius, or ulna elicits a painful response. Because vitamin D deficiency symptoms overlap considerably with those of fibromyalgia, one condition is often mistaken for the other. Vitamin D deficiency has also been long recognized as a cause of muscle weakness and muscle aches and pain in all ages. Aside from osteomalacia and localized bone pain, antigravity muscle weakness, difficulty rising from a chair or walking, and pseudofractures also are noted in the person with vitamin D deficiency. These findings resolve with appropriate treatment. Vitamin D deficiency also contributes to the development of hypocalcemia and hypophosphatemia. In this situation, unless the vitamin D deficiency is addressed, replacing calcium or phosphate alone does not restore the body to homeostasis.

The preferred test for assessment of vitamin D status is measurement of serum 25-hydroxyvitamin D (25(OH)D). The results of this test are minimally influenced by recent dietary intake or recent sun exposure, and it is considered the most accurate functional indicator of vitamin D stores. The serum level of the biologically active form of vitamin D, 1,25-dihydroxyvitamin D ($1,25(OH)_2D$), is not an accurate indicator of nutritional vitamin D status because levels of $1,25(OH)_2D$ typically are not altered until vitamin D deficiency is well advanced. The cost of testing ranges from $50 to $200.

Opinions differ on what constitutes deficiency. Physiologic deficiency is defined as a level of serum 25(OH)D that is sufficiently low to cause an increase in parathyroid hormone (PTH) levels. Production and secretion of PTH increases to correct low calcium levels via increased bone turnover and accelerated bone loss, effects that clearly occur later in the disease process. Clinical studies have revealed that increased PTH levels occur with 25(OH)D levels of 20 ng/mL (50 nmol/L). As a result, most laboratories report the normal range to be 20 to 100 ng/mL (50 to 250 nmol/L); however, the preferred minimum level is likely 35 to 40 ng/mL (87.5 to 100 nmol/L).

Vitamin D_3 is the preferred form of the micronutrient for the treatment of vitamin D deficiency and for maintenance of vitamin D levels. Because vitamin D_3 is stored in fat and has a long half-life, low-dose (400–800 IU per day) vitamin D_3 supplementation is not sufficient to correct a deficiency. Approximately 100 IU given daily for 3 months will increase the 25(OH)D level by just 1 ng/mL (2.5 nmol/L); considered in multiples of 100 IU, 400 IU taken for 3 months will increase the level by 4 ng/mL (10 nmol/L).

For treatment of vitamin D deficiency in adults, a dose of 50,000 IU of vitamin D_3 by mouth once per week for at least 8 weeks is advised, with extension of this course to 16 weeks if the initial 25(OH)D level was below 30 ng/mL. For long-term prevention, patients should be given 50,000 IU of vitamin D_3 once or twice per month plus 1000 to 2000 IU of vitamin D_3 daily. Consuming a diet rich in vitamin D-containing foods and exposing the skin to a sensible and safe level of sunlight can aid in preventing the condition. A confirmation of vitamin D correction should be obtained after the recommended length of high-dose repletion therapy.

Excessive supplementation, but not excessive sun exposure, can cause vitamin D toxicity, leading to a variety of problems, including calcium deposition into solid organs. This is rarely seen and is usually a consequence of chronic use of $\geq$10,000 IU/d vitamin D_3.

DISCUSSION SOURCES

Holick MF. Vitamin D deficiency. *N Engl J Med* 357(3):266–281, 2007.

Holick MF. Vitamin D deficiency: What a pain it is. *Mayo Clin Proc* 78:1457–1459, 2003.

Linus Pauling Institute, Micronutrient Information Center. Vitamin D. http://lpi.oregonstate.edu/infocenter/vitamins/vitaminD.

Moyad MA. Vitamin D: A rapid review. *Medscape Today News*, http://www.medscape.com/viewarticle/589256.

Plotnikoff G, Quigley J. Prevalence of severe hypovitaminosis D in patients with persistent, nonspecific musculoskeletal pain. *Mayo Clin Proc* 78:1463–1470, 2003.

Tangpricha V, Griffing GT. Vitamin D deficiency and related disorders. *Medscape Reference*, http://emedicine.medscape.com/article/128762.

Peripheral Vascular Disease

10

Raynaud Phenomenon

1. Who is most likely to have new-onset primary Raynaud phenomenon?
   A. a 68-year-old man
   B. a 65-year-old woman
   C. a 25-year-old man
   D. an 18-year-old woman

2. All of the following are associated with secondary Raynaud phenomenon except:
   A. hypertension.
   B. scleroderma.
   C. repeated use of vibrating tools.
   D. use of beta-adrenergic antagonists.

3. Lifestyle modification for patients with Raynaud phenomenon includes:
   A. discontinuing cigarette smoking.
   B. increasing fluid intake.
   C. avoiding placing hands in warm water.
   D. discontinuing aspirin use.

4. Medications that are often helpful in relieving symptoms associated with Raynaud phenomenon include:
   A. nonsteroidal anti-inflammatory drugs (NSAIDs).
   B. angiotensin-converting enzyme inhibitors.
   C. beta-adrenergic antagonists.
   D. diuretics.

5. Which of the following is the most common presentation in a patient with Raynaud phenomenon?
   A. digital ulceration
   B. worsening of symptoms in warm weather
   C. a period of intense itchiness after blanching
   D. unilateral symptoms

Answers

1. D   3. A   5. C
2. A   4. B

Raynaud phenomenon, also known as Raynaud disease, is characterized by paroxysmal digital vasoconstriction that results in bilateral symmetrical pallor or cyanosis. The hands are nearly always involved; foot involvement is rare. A period of rubor follows this initial response. Primary Raynaud phenomenon, also known as primary Raynaud disease, is idiopathic in origin in most patients and is most often found in women. The condition usually appears between the ages of 15 and 45 years. Vasoconstriction triggers include exposure to cold relieved by warmth and, less commonly, emotional upset. Symptoms tend to be progressive, with vasospasm becoming more frequent and prolonged. There are no specific studies to help diagnose primary Raynaud disease. The diagnosis is made if recurrent episodes occur for more than 3 years without notation of associated disease or secondary cause.

Secondary Raynaud phenomenon is seen in the presence of an underlying condition, such as atherosclerosis, collagen vascular disease, and select autoimmune disease such as scleroderma; in scleroderma, this concomitant condition is a nearly universal finding. In addition, the use of vibrating tools, repeated sharp digit movement such as piano playing or typing, frostbite, tobacco, ergotamine, and beta blocker use can be contributing factors. The presentation of secondary Raynaud phenomenon is the same as that of the idiopathic condition; the degree and length of vasospasm are often more severe. Rarely, distal digital ulceration is seen.

Whatever the cause, intervention in Raynaud phenomenon is aimed primarily at preventing vasospasm by avoiding cold and other known triggers. At the onset of an episode, submerging the hands in warm water can be helpful in limiting the length and severity of vasospasm; hot water should not be used because of risk of burn. Because wound healing may be delayed and infection is common, the hands should be protected from even minor injury. Keeping the skin well lubricated can help avoid small fissures. Tobacco use exacerbates vasospasm. As a result, all forms of tobacco use should be discouraged; smoking cessation is usually associated with a stabilization of or improvement in symptoms. Biofeedback can be helpful because the patient can be taught to envision warming the digits, reducing symptoms. The dihydropyridine calcium channel blockers ("-ipine" suffix, such as amlodipine or nifedipine) and angiotensin-converting enzyme inhibitors ("-pril" suffix, such as lisinopril or fosinopril) can be used for their vasodilator effect when lifestyle modification is inadequate. In patients with secondary Raynaud phenomenon, treatment of the associated condition is important and often helps minimize episodes. Surgical intervention with distal digital sympathectomy and arterial reconstruction should be considered when more conservative therapy is unsuccessful in managing the condition.

DISCUSSION SOURCE

Hansen-Dispenza, H. eMedicine. http://www.emedicine.medscape.com/article/31197-overview, Raynaud phenomenon.

Varicose Veins

6. Which of the following does not directly contribute to the development of varicose veins?
   A. leg crossing
   B. pregnancy
   C. heredity
   D. Raynaud disease

7. When advising a woman with varicose veins about the use of support stockings, you consider that the preferred type:
   A. can be purchased in the hosiery section of a department store.
   B. is a lightweight pair and available over-the-counter.
   C. is a medium-weight to heavy-weight prescription product.
   D. is used in the form of panty hose.

8. In patients with varicose veins, which vessel is most often affected?
   A. femoral vein
   B. posterior tibial vein
   C. peroneal vein
   D. saphenous vein

9. Which of the following statements is most accurate in the assessment of a patient with varicose veins?
   A. The degree of venous tortuosity is well-correlated with the amount of leg pain reported.
   B. As the number of affected veins increases, so does the degree of patient discomfort.
   C. Symptoms are sometimes reported with minimally affected vessels.
   D. Lower-extremity edema is usually seen only with severe disease.

10. Spider varicosities are:
    A. usually symptomatic.
    B. a potential site for thrombophlebitis.
    C. responsive to laser obliteration.
    D. caused by sun exposure.

Answers

| 6. D. | 8. D. | 10. C. |
| 7. C. | 9. C. | |

Varicose veins are seen in 15% of the adult population and are most often found in the lower extremities. Tortuous, dilated, superficial veins are characteristic. An inherited venous defect of either a valvular incompetence or a weakness in the walls of the vessel likely plays a significant role. In addition, situations that cause high venous pressure, such as leg crossing, wearing of constricting garments, prolonged standing, heavy lifting, and current or prior pregnancy, contribute to their development. Women are affected twice as often as men.

The vessel most often affected is the great saphenous vein and its tributaries. Often asymptomatic, varicose veins may also be associated with leg aching but usually not severe pain. The degree of discomfort is poorly correlated with the number and appearance of the affected veins. Mild edema in the ankle area, particularly at the end of the day and in warm weather, is common. When palpated, the vein compresses easily and without pain. No specific diagnostic tests are needed with typical presentation. Various diagnostic tests are available, however, including duplex ultrasound and magnetic resonance venography; these tests are usually used to rule out deep vein obstruction as a contributor of the severity of varicose veins.

With uncomplicated varicose veins, lifestyle modification usually helps minimize the symptoms and disease progress. Attaining and maintaining normal weight helps to reduce intravenous pressure and discourage the development and progression of varicose veins. Periodic leg elevation is helpful in minimizing edema and encouraging venous return. The use of medium-weight to heavy-weight elastic support hose such as Jobst™ stockings should be encouraged. Support hose purchased in a department store or drugstore do not supply enough compression. Wearing garments that are potentially constricting, such as panty girdles and garters, should be avoided.

Various minimally invasive interventions, including endovenous laser venous ablation, are also available for varicose vein treatment. Sclerotherapy is a common procedure done for vein obliteration and involves injecting a sclerosing agent into the affected vein followed by a period of compression, which results in vessel obliteration. Surgery is often needed for symptomatic varicose veins that do not respond to conservative therapy. Patients often prefer more aggressive treatment in this condition to yield the best cosmetic outcome and to experience relief of discomfort.

Possible complications of varicose veins include superficial thrombophlebitis. Over time, varicose veins tend to dilate progressively, which can lead to secondary changes in the lower extremities, including chronic edema, skin hyperpigmentation, and development of chronic venous insufficiency. Spider varicosities are visible surface vessels usually seen with varicose veins. These vessels do not usually cause symptoms and pose no thromboembolic risk. Vessel obliteration with laser or other modalities is helpful in reducing the appearance of spider varicosities and is considered a cosmetic procedure.

DISCUSSION SOURCE

Weiss, R. eMedicine. http://www.emedicine.medscape.com/article/1085530-overview, Varicose veins.

Disorders of Coagulation

11. Which of the following is not a contributing factor to development of venous thrombophlebitis?
A. venous status
B. injury to vascular intima
C. malignancy-associated hypercoagulation states
D. isometric exercise

12. Presentation of superficial venous thrombophlebitis usually includes:
A. positive Homans sign.
B. diminished dorsalis pedis pulse.
C. a dilated vessel.
D. dependent pallor.

13. Treatment of superficial venous thrombophlebitis in a low-risk, stable patient includes use of:
A. compression stockings.
B. acetaminophen.
C. warfarin.
D. heparin.

14. In providing care for a patient with superficial thrombophlebitis, the NP considers that:
A. it is a benign, self-limiting disease.
B. the linear pattern of induration can help differentiate the process from cellulitis or other inflammatory processes.
C. a chest radiograph should be obtained.
D. limited activity enhances recovery.

15. Which of the following is the most likely to be found in deep vein thrombophlebitis (DVT)?
A. unilateral leg edema
B. leg pain
C. warmth over the affected area
D. positive obturator sign

16. A positive Homans sign is present in approximately what percentage of patients with DVT?
A. 25%
B. 33%
C. 50%
D. 75%

17. The initial diagnostic evaluation of a clinically stable patient with suspected DVT most often includes obtaining a/an:
A. impedance plethysmography.
B. iodine 125 fibrinogen scan.
C. contrast venography.
D. duplex ultrasonography.

18. Which of the following is the preferred medication to reverse the anticoagulant effects of unfractionated heparin?
A. vitamin K
B. protamine sulfate
C. platelet transfusion
D. plasma components

19. Which of the following is the preferred medication to reverse the anticoagulant effects of warfarin?
A. vitamin K
B. protamine sulfate
C. platelet transfusion
D. plasma components

20. The onset of anticoagulation effect of warfarin usually occurs how soon after the initiation of therapy?
A. immediately
B. 1 to 2 days
C. 3 to 5 days
D. 5 to 7 days

21. Compared with unfractionated heparin, characteristics of low-molecular-weight heparin (LMWH) include all of the following except:
A. more antiplatelet effect.
B. decreased need for monitoring of anticoagulant effect.
C. longer half-life.
D. superior bioavailability.

22. Which of the following is least likely to be found in patients with pulmonary embolus (PE)?
A. pleuritic chest pain
B. tachypnea
C. DVT signs and symptoms
D. hemoptysis

23. The most common method of preventing venous thromboembolism in higher risk surgical patients is the use of:
A. vitamin K.
B. LMWH.
C. vena cava filter.
D. warfarin.

24. When taken with warfarin, which of the following causes a possible increased anticoagulant effect?
A. clarithromycin
B. carbamazepine
C. pravastatin
D. sucralfate

25. When taken concomitantly with warfarin, which of the following causes a possibly decreased anticoagulant effect?
A. cholestyramine
B. allopurinol
C. cefpodoxime
D. zolpidem

26. What is the international normalized ratio (INR) range recommended during warfarin therapy as part of the management of a patient with DVT?
A. 1.5 to 2.0
B. 2.0 to 3.0
C. 2.5 to 3.5
D. 3.0 to 4.0

True or False?

____ **27.** During the first 6 weeks of the postpartum period, the childbearing woman is at increased risk for venous thrombus formation.

____ **28.** In a patient with suspected superficial thrombophlebitis in the calf, the abnormalities in the lower-extremity examination are potentially enhanced by having the patient stand for approximately 2 minutes.

____ **29.** With the use of a direct thrombin inhibitor, ongoing INR monitoring is required.

____ **30.** Prescribing a direct thrombin inhibitor is an acceptable therapeutic option to reduce the risk of recurrent DVT.

____ **31.** One of the potential serious adverse effects of unfractionated heparin is thrombocytopenia.

____ **32.** An abnormally elevated D-dimer test is highly sensitive and specific for the diagnosis of thromboembolic disease.

▶ Answers

11. D.		**14.** B.		**17.** D.	
12. C.		**15.** A.		**18.** B.	
13. A.		**16.** B.		**19.** A.	

20. C.	**25.** A.	**30.** True
21. A.	**26.** B.	**31.** True
22. D.	**27.** True	**32.** False
23. B.	**28.** True	
24. A.	**29.** False	

Blood coagulation can be activated by various pathways via the tissue factor (TF) pathway (formerly known as the extrinsic pathway) and the contact activation pathway (formerly known as the intrinsic pathway). Expressed by injured endothelial cells, TF is the clinically most significant initiator of coagulation. TF binds to and activates coagulation factor VII; the TF/factor VIIa complex then activates factor X and factor IX to factors Xa and IXa. In the presence of factor XIIa, factor IXa can also convert factor X to factor Xa. The contact activation pathway is activated when factor XII comes in contact with a foreign surface. The resulting factor XIIa activates factor XI, which activates factor IX. Factor IXa activates factor X. These pathways work together to provide maximal stimulation of factor X, which, in the presence of factor V, activates prothrombin to thrombin; this is also known as the common pathway.

Equally as important as blood coagulation is the ability of blood to avoid clot formation. In the larger arteries, clot risk is usually limited because aggregating platelets are dislodged by high-velocity blood flow and thrombus formation is avoided. In smaller arteries and veins, blood flow is slower, with platelet aggregation more likely to occur and increasing clot risk. Working against thrombus formation, TF pathway inhibitor binds to and inactivates the TF/factor VIIa/factor Xa complex. Antithrombin III inactivates circulating thrombin, whereas proteins C and S are contributors to a complex process that down regulates thrombin activity by preventing the activation of factor V. If a clot does form, circulating plasminogen is incorporated into the thrombus; healthy endothelial cells adjacent to the vessel injury site release tissue plasminogen activator and activate plasminogen to plasmin, causing thrombolysis on the clot surface and minimizing thrombus size. Meanwhile, numerous factors, including plasminogen activator inhibitor, produced by the liver and endothelial cells, inhibit fibrin degradation by plasmin to limit thrombolysis.

The Virchow triad of stasis, injury to the vascular intima, and abnormal coagulation leading to clot usually contributes to the development of vessel inflammation and the resulting thrombophlebitis. The lower extremities are most often affected.

Thrombophlebitis, presence of coagulated blood or thrombus in a vein with resulting inflammation, can occur in superficial or deep veins. Risk factors for superficial thrombophlebitis include local trauma, prolonged travel or rest, presence of varicose veins, history of prior episodes, and use of estrogen-containing hormonal contraceptives or postmenopausal hormone therapy. Owing to the increased platelet stickiness noted in late pregnancy through the first 6 weeks postpartum, this time also marks a period for increased thrombotic risk.

Characteristics of superficial thrombophlebitis usually include a localized, tender, dilated, thrombosed vessel, causing a linear area of redness, often in the popliteal fossa. Homans sign is absent. Having the patient stand for 2 minutes before examination enhances the findings because less severe cases might be missed on supine examination. Superficial thrombophlebitis is often considered a benign condition; however, this condition is likely a marker of further clotting issues. Extension into a deep vein, the vessels that act as conduits to return blood to the heart, is typically present, however, in 45% of patients with the condition. In particular, superficial, noninfectious thrombophlebitis in hospitalized patients is more likely to be associated with DVT and PE. Until proven otherwise, a patient with superficial thrombophlebitis should be assumed to have deep vein involvement. Compression duplex venous ultrasonography should be performed to help rule out concurrent DVT.

Because disordered coagulation tends to occur in multiple locations simultaneously, superficial thrombophlebitis is often accompanied by DVT in a different location or extremity; the study should not be limited to the affected area. Serial studies are often needed if initial examination findings are negative but symptoms persist. Although direct venography is the most sensitive and specific test, its use has been limited because these less invasive tests have become available. Magnetic resonance direct thrombus imaging provides an accurate noninvasive modality in DVT diagnosis.

Further PE evaluation should be undertaken based on clinical findings, such as shortness of breath or friction rub. Coagulation studies should be obtained, particularly if there is a history of previous episodes without such evaluation. D-dimer, a degradation product produced by plasmin-mediated proteolysis of cross-linked fibrin, is often elevated in DVT and PE. The test has significant limitations, however, because d-dimer levels can be elevated whenever the coagulation and fibrinolytic systems are activated and are falsely elevated in the presence of high rheumatoid factor levels.

After the diagnosis of superficial thrombophlebitis is confirmed, intervention is dictated by DVT risk factors and patient history. In the absence of risk factors and history of similar episodes, warm packs, compression hose, and NSAIDs can be used to treat superficial thrombophlebitis. Ambulation should be encouraged because rest promotes stasis and enhances coagulation, although leg elevation when at rest is helpful in managing symptoms and edema. In the presence of prior episodes, a history of DVT, decreased mobility, hypercoagulability, or extensive saphenous vein involvement, subcutaneous LMWH therapy should be initiated, with consideration for long-term warfarin use. The inflammation associated with superficial thrombophlebitis usually subsides within 2 weeks, with a firm cord remaining for a much longer period. As with DVT, collateral venous flow develops over the next few months.

Acute DVT usually involves the veins of the lower extremities and pelvis. PE, a potentially fatal condition, is largely a sequela of DVT. Long-term sequelae of DVT include chronic venous insufficiency and venous ulceration.

Because the triad of venous stasis, vessel wall injury, and altered coagulation state is the primary mechanism underlying DVT (as noted with superficial thrombophlebitis), risk factors include prolonged rest, recent trauma, recent surgery (especially hip replacement and select additional orthopedic surgery), pregnancy, and the peripartum period. The hypercoagulation state associated with many malignancies also presents considerable risk. The use of hormone-containing contraceptives (combined [estrogen/progestin] oral contraceptive, topical patch, or vaginal ring) and postmenopausal hormone therapy can increase DVT risk, particularly in cigarette smokers. Disorders of coagulation, such as factor V Leiden mutation and protein C and S and antithrombin III deficiencies, are recognized as a cause of DVT in otherwise healthy adults.

Because the presentation of DVT varies, making the diagnosis from clinical presentation alone is problematic (Table 10–1). Only a few patients with suspected DVT have the diagnosis supported, unless the Virchow triad of venous stasis, vessel wall injury, and coagulation abnormalities is present. With regard to risk and clinical presentation, Table 10–2 provides a guide for estimating clinical suspicion.

To establish the diagnosis and develop an appropriate plan of intervention, a thorough diagnostic evaluation is needed in patients suspected to have DVT. Because of cost and the invasive nature of the test and the risk of allergy to the contrast medium associated with contrast venography, long considered the standard for DVT diagnosis, noninvasive tests are used more commonly. Compression duplex ultrasound is the most common first-line diagnostic technique in DVT. Magnetic resonance direct thrombus imaging is the diagnostic test of choice for suspected iliac vein or inferior vena caval thrombosis. In the second or third trimester of pregnancy, magnetic resonance imaging (MRI) is also more accurate than duplex ultrasound because the gravid uterus alters Doppler venous flow characteristics.

Levels of d-dimer are elevated in DVT with high sensitivity but low specificity; similar results are found with recent surgery, trauma, myocardial infarction, pregnancy, and metastatic cancer. When findings are positive in DVT, the degree of d-dimer elevation depends on the size of the clot. A lower risk patient with a normal d-dimer level is unlikely to have DVT. A growing body of knowledge compels the NP to consider an underlying clotting disorder in a person with DVT, and testing for protein S, protein C, antithrombin III, fibrinogen, lupus anticoagulant, factor V Leiden, prothrombin 20210A mutation, antiphospholipid antibodies, and other thrombophilia forms is appropriate, particularly with a personal history or strong family history of prior thromboembolic episodes. These tests should be obtained before initiating anticoagulation therapy.

Therapy for patients with DVT should be aimed at minimizing the risk of PE and extension of peripheral thrombus. Anticoagulation therapy with medications, usually with a heparin form first followed by warfarin (Coumadin), should be prescribed. These products are aimed at allowing natural fibrinolysis action and clot resolution to occur and minimizing

TABLE 10-1
Clinical Presentation of Deep Vein Thrombophlebitis (DVT)

Finding	Comment
Edema	Usually unilateral (best true-positive finding)
	Bilateral calf measurement with comparative readings helpful in clinical assessment
Leg pain	Usually described as a tugging pain, heaviness, ache
	Present in ~50% of patients with DVT
	Degree of pain does not correlate well with extent of thrombus
Homans sign	Pain on dorsiflexion of the foot
	Present in about one-third of patients with DVT and up to half without DVT
Pulmonary embolus (PE) signs and symptoms	Present in ~10% of patients with DVT, but likely PE concurrently present in a higher percentage
Warmth over area of thrombosis	Relatively rare
Venous distention and prominence of subcutaneous veins	Relatively uncommon
Fever	If present, typically mild
Tenderness over and adjacent to the affected area	Found in ~75% of patients with DVT
	Also can be found in many conditions other than DVT
	Degree of tenderness does not correlate well with extent of thrombus

Source: Patel, K. eMedicine. http://www.emedicine.medscape.com/article1911303-overview, Deep Vein Thrombosis.

TABLE 10-2
Wells Clinical Prediction Guide in Deep Vein Thrombophlebitis (DVT)

CLINICAL PARAMETER	SCORE
Active cancer (treatment ongoing, within 6 mo, or palliative therapy)	1
Paralysis or recent plaster or other similar limb immobilization	1
Recently bedridden for >3 days or major surgery <4 weeks earlier	1
Localized tenderness along distribution of the deep venous system	1
Entire leg swelling	1
Calf swelling >3 cm compared with asymptomatic leg	1
Pitting edema (greater in the symptomatic leg)	1
Collateral superficial veins (nonvaricose)	1
Alternative diagnosis (as likely or greater than that of DVT)	-2

TOTAL OF SCORES
High probability: Score ≥3
Moderate probability: Score 1–2
Low probability: Score 0

Wells Clinical Prediction Guide in Pulmonary Embolus (PE)

CLINICAL PARAMETER	SCORE
Clinical signs/symptoms of DVT	3
No alternative diagnosis likely or more likely than PE	3
Heart rate >100 bpm	1.5
Immobilization or surgery in the past 4 weeks	1.5
Previous history of DVT or PE	1.5
Hemoptysis	1
Cancer actively treated within past 6 months	1

SCORING
Probability of PE is high if total score >6; moderate, if 2–6; and low, if <2

Source: Adapted from Anand SS, Wells PS, Hunt D, et al. Does this patient have deep vein thrombosis? *JAMA*279:1094–1099, 1998.

risk for clot extension; heparin and warfarin do not have intrinsic thrombolytic activity.

Direct thrombin inhibitors (DTIs), including the oral product dabigatran (Pradaxa), can also be considered as an alternative to heparin and warfarin for treatment of DVT and PE, particularly in patients who have previously undergone parenteral anticoagulant treatment. The use of these agents, particularly for stroke prevention in rate-controlled atrial fibrillation, is growing due to the ease of use and predictable anticoagulant effect that eliminates the need for ongoing therapeutic monitoring. The use of these agents can also be considered to reduce the risk of recurrence of DVT and PE. DTIs have a number of limitations and should be avoided or used with caution in certain patient populations, such as elderly patients.

Because rapid-onset anticoagulation is needed in DVT therapy, heparin is usually the initial treatment (Table 10–3). A naturally occurring acidic carbohydrate, heparin potentiates antithromboplastin III (a naturally occurring antithrombotic agent) and inhibits the activity of numerous coagulating factors. Its effect on thrombus formation is immediate, in contrast to warfarin, which usually requires 3 to 5 days of use before therapeutic levels are reached and clinical effect is seen.

Heparin is available in the standard unfractionated form, with an average molecular weight of 15,000 daltons, and a low-molecular-weight heparin (LMWH), with a molecular weight of 4000 to 6500 daltons. Enoxaparin (Lovenox), dalteparin (Fragmin), and ardeparin (Normiflo) are examples of LMWH. LMWH selectively enhances factor Xa and accelerates antithrombin III activity; because of limited bleeding risk, monitoring of partial thromboplastin time is not required during its use. LMWH has additional advantages, including superior bioavailability, a longer half-life that allows for twice-a-day dosing, ease of calculating dosage, and limited antiplatelet effect. LMWH is more expensive, however, than unfractionated heparin. Patients with an isolated calf vein DVT who are clinically stable with few risks for a further embolic process and with access to careful provider follow-up should be considered for initial outpatient treatment with self-administered injections of LMWH twice a day. In the absence of this scenario, inpatient admission and heparin anticoagulation are indicated. Length of therapy is usually about 5 days, and therapy is discontinued when heparin has been given for 5 days or until international normalized ratio (INR) is greater than 2.0 as a result of the concomitant warfarin therapy. LMWH is often used for DVT prophylaxis for high-risk surgical and medical patients.

Besides the obvious increased risk for bleeding events with its use, another problematic adverse effect is heparin-induced thrombocytopenia (HIT), a serious condition with potentially life-threatening consequences. Expert consultation on the management of a person who has HIT is required, for both immediate management and advice managing future thromboembolic events.

Long-term warfarin therapy usually follows an initial heparin course in thromboembolic disease. Warfarin acts against coagulation factors II, VII, IX, and X as a result of vitamin K antagonism. Warfarin is highly (99%) protein

TABLE 10-3
Indications and Length of Warfarin Treatment

Condition	INR	Duration of Therapy
ACUTE VENOUS THROMBOSIS		
First episode	2.0–3.0	3–6 mo
High risk of recurrence	2.0–3.0	Indefinitely
With antiphospholipid syndrome or other thrombophilia or coagulopathy	3.0–4.0	Lifelong
PREVENTION OF SYSTEMIC EMBOLUS		
Tissue heart valves	2.0–3.0	3 mo
Valvular heart disease with history of thrombotic event	2.0–3.0	Indefinitely
Mechanical heart valve (if initially indicated by valve type)	2.5–3.5	Indefinitely
Acute myocardial infarction	2.0–3.0	As deemed by concomitant clinical problems
ATRIAL FIBRILLATION		
Chronic or intermittent	2.0–3.0	Lifelong for chronic or intermittent atrial fibrillation
Cardioversion	2.0–3.0	With cardioversion, for 3 weeks before and 4 weeks after conversion to sinus rhythm

INR, international normalized ratio.
Source: Family Practice Notebook. http://www.fpnotebook.com/HemeOnc/Pharm/CmdnPrtcl.htm, Coumadin protocol.

bound, primarily to albumin, and has a narrow therapeutic range. To avoid problems with warfarin therapy, patients must be well informed of the drug-to-drug and drug-to-food interactions (Table 10–4). Because cigarette smoking likely increases thrombotic risk while reducing efficacy of warfarin, developing a smoking cessation plan is important.

Prothrombin time is used as the measure of the efficacy of warfarin and is reported as an INR. INR prolongation is seen in about 48 to 72 hours after the first warfarin dose (Table 10–5). Warfarin anticoagulant therapy is usually prescribed for at least 3 to 6 months after the first DVT episode. Studies have supported long-term low-intensity (INR 1.5 to 2.0) warfarin anticoagulation to minimize thrombus risk even after a first DVT episode. With a second episode, abnormal clotting should be suspected, and anticoagulant therapy should be lifelong. In the presence of a clotting disorder, such as factor V Leiden mutations or antiphospholipid antibodies, anticoagulation should also be lifelong.

Approximately 2% to 10% of patients taking warfarin develop a problematic bleeding episode. This complication is rarely seen, however, in patients with INR of 2.0 to 3.0. In the presence of significant bleeding in patients taking warfarin, the drug should be discontinued, and vitamin K should be given promptly. Vitamin K has little effect on hemostasis, however, until 24 hours after its administration. If immediate action is needed, such as in the case of hemorrhage or bleeding into an enclosed space, fresh frozen plasma must be given. If anticoagulation therapy is continued after the bleeding crisis, response to warfarin may fluctuate, which necessitates close monitoring.

Thrombolytic therapy with streptokinase or a similar product is also a therapeutic option for DVT. This treatment is usually reserved for patients with extensive iliofemoral venous thrombus and low risk for bleeding.

With a mortality rate of 20% to 40%, PE is a feared complication of DVT. The diagnosis is often missed, however, because the presentation is nonspecific. PE presentation usually includes dyspnea, pleuritic chest pain, pleural friction rub, and accentuation of the pulmonic component of S_2 heart sound; tachypnea (respiratory rate ≥ 16/min) and tachycardia are nearly universal findings. DVT signs and symptoms are often noted, but their absence should not eliminate the consideration of PE. Hemoptysis, cyanosis, and change in level of consciousness are rarely encountered but are often considered to be an expected part of the presentation. The use of the Wells predictive scale can be

TABLE 10-4
Warfarin: Drug and Food Interactions

Note: The concomitant use of warfarin with one of the following medications is not contraindicated. The prescriber and patient need to be aware, however, of the impact of concurrent use on anticoagulation state.

Increased Anticoagulant Effect	Decreased Anticoagulant Effects	Variable Effect
Alcohol (particularly in presence of liver disease)	Barbiturates	Phenytoin—increased and decreased effects noted, and increase in phenytoin level
Amiodarone	Carbamazepine	
Cimetidine	Chlordiazepoxide	
Clofibrate	Cholestyramine	
Cotrimoxazole	Griseofulvin	
Erythromycin	Rifampin	
Clarithromycin	Sucralfate	
Fluconazole	Azathioprine	
Isoniazid	Cyclosporine	
Metronidazole	Trazodone	
Miconazole		
Omeprazole, other proton pump inhibitors		
Piroxicam		
Propafenone		
Propranolol		
Acetaminophen (inconsistent)		
Ciprofloxacin		
Disulfiram		
Itraconazole		
Quinidine		
Tamoxifen		
Tetracyclines including doxycycline, minocycline		

Source: Indiana University School of Medicine Division of Clinical Pharmacology. http://medicine.iupui.edu/clinpharm/ddis/table.asp, P450 drug interaction table.

TABLE 10-5

Warfarin: Initiation of Therapy and Long-Term Management

- Warfarin's anticoagulation effect takes at least 3 days of use to achieve. If immediate anticoagulation effect is needed, initiate heparin therapy while also starting warfarin 5–10 mg qd for 2 days, then reduce to 5 mg qd. Check INR daily; when at goal, discontinue heparin.
- If there is no need for immediate anticoagulation, warfarin should be initiated at 5 mg/d, anticipating therapeutic effect in ~4 days. In older adults, initiate warfarin at 4 mg/d, anticipating therapeutic effect in 6–7 days.
- If INR is not within goal during warfarin therapy, check for adherence to recommended therapy before adjusting dose and use of medications or foods that may interfere with warfarin effect.

INR GOAL 2.0–3.0	ACTION
At desired range	Repeat INR at interval determined by duration of therapeutic INR and underlying condition • 4–6 weeks if stable condition and typically therapeutic INR • At least weekly when underlying condition can affect coagulation state (e.g., malignancy, clotting disorder, use of medications that can influence warfarin effect)
INR <2.0	• Increase total weekly dose by 5%–20% • Repeat INR two to three times/week until within desired range
INR 3.0–3.5	• Decrease total weekly dose by 5%–15% • Repeat INR two to three times/week until within desired range
INR 3.6–4.0	• Consider withholding 1 daily dose, decrease total weekly dose by 10%–15% • Repeat INR two to three times/week until within desired range
INR >4.0 without complications and no indication for rapid reversal of anticoagulation effect	• Consider withholding 1 daily dose, decrease total weekly dose by 10%–20% • Repeat INR two to three times/week until within desired range
INR >4.0 and need for rapid reversal of anticoagulant effect	• Vitamin K 2.5–5 mg PO x 1–2 doses or 3 mg subcutaneous (SC) or slow intravenous (IV) route

INR GOAL 2.5–3.5	ACTION
At desired range	• Repeat INR at interval determined by duration of therapeutic INR and underlying condition 4–6 weeks if stable. Repeat INR at interval determined by duration of therapeutic INR and underlying condition • 4–6 weeks if stable condition and typically therapeutic INR • At least weekly when underlying condition can affect coagulation state (e.g., malignancy, clotting disorder, use of medications that can influence warfarin effect)
INR <2.0	• Increase weekly dose by 10%–20% • Repeat INR two to three times/week until within desired range
INR 2.0–2.4	• Increase weekly dose by 5%–15% • Repeat INR two to three times/week until within desired range
INR 3.5–4.6	• Decrease weekly dose by 5%–15% • Repeat INR two to three times/week until within desired range
INR 4.7–5.2	• Consider withholding 1 dose, decrease weekly dose by 10%–20% • Repeat INR two to three times/week until within desired range
INR >5.2 without complications and no indication for rapid reversal of anticoagulation effect	• Withhold 1–2 doses, decrease weekly dose by 10%–20% • Repeat INR two to three times/week until within desired range
INR >5.2 or need for rapid reversal of anticoagulant effect	• Vitamin K 2.5 mg PO x 1–2 doses or 3 mg SC or slow IV route

INR, international normalized ratio.
Source: Family Practice Notebook. http://www.fpnotebook.com/HemeOnc/Pharm/CmdnPrtcl.htm, Coumadin protocol.

helpful in forming the diagnosis (see Table 10–2). The use of d-dimer testing in PE diagnosis has the same limitations as noted in DVT diagnosis. Imaging with spiral CT pulmonary angiography is a helpful confirmatory test.

In treating patients with PE, thrombolytic therapy is often used, followed by heparin and then warfarin therapy for a minimum of 3 months. If the patient is not a candidate for long-term anticoagulation therapy, or if clotting occurs despite adequate anticoagulation therapy, a vena cava filter is usually used to minimize the risk of future PE. Follow-up is recommended as needed to monitor INR and the underlying clinical condition. Additional therapies for long-term anticoagulation include the use of oral factor Xa inhibitors such as rivaroxaban (Xarelto). Given the proliferation of warfarin alternatives, prudent practice dictates keeping abreast of current evidence-based practice in this area.

DISCUSSION SOURCES

Ferri F. Pulmonary Embolism. In: Ferri F. *Practical Guide to the Care of the Medical Patient*, 8. Philadelphia: Elsevier Mosby; 2011.

Ouellette, D.R. eMedicine. http://www.emedicine.medscape.com/article/300901-workup, Pulmonary Embolism Workup.

Patel, K. eMedicine. http://www.emedicine.medscape.com/article/1911303-overview, Deep Vein Thrombosis.

Spence, R.K. eMedicine. http://emedicine.medscape.com/article/210467-overview, Nonplatelet Hemostatic Disorders.

Peripheral Vascular Disease

33. Which of the following is the most potent risk factor for lower-extremity vascular occlusive disease?
    A. hypertension
    B. older age
    C. cigarette smoking
    D. leg injury

34. Clinical presentation of advanced lower-extremity vascular disease includes all of the following except:
    A. resting pain.
    B. absent posterior tibialis pulse.
    C. blanching of the foot with elevation.
    D. spider varicosities.

35. Drug therapy that had previously thought to worsen symptoms in lower-extremity arterial vascular disease includes the use of:
    A. beta2-agonists.
    B. calcium channel antagonists.
    C. direct thrombin inhibitors.
    D. beta-adrenergic antagonists

36. Typically, the earliest sign of lower-extremity venous insufficiency is:
    A. edema.
    B. altered pigmentation.
    C. skin atrophy.
    D. shiny skin.

37. Comprehensive treatment for a person with peripheral occlusive arterial disease and diabetes mellitus includes all of the following except:
    A. daily aspirin use.
    B. lipid lowering with an HMG-CoA reductase inhibitor (statin).
    C. application of a topical antimicrobial to the affected area.
    D. maintenance of glycemic control.

38. Treatment options for venous stasis ulcers in the lower extremities include:
    A. cleansing with hydrogen peroxide.
    B. applying Burow solution.
    C. prescribing a systemic corticosteroid.
    D. applying a moisture-retaining dressing.

39. Cilostazol (Pletal) should be used with great caution in the presence of which of the following diagnoses?
    A. diabetes mellitus
    B. heart failure
    C. hypertension
    D. dyslipidemia

40. Clinical presentation of acute lower-extremity atherosclerotic arterial disease most likely includes:
    A. pain and paresthesia.
    B. pallor and pulselessness.
    C. poikilothermy.
    D. paralysis or loss of limb strength.

41. More common etiologies of acute lower-extremity atherosclerotic arterial disease include:
    A. arterial embolism with underlying atrial fibrillation.
    B. chronic venous insufficiency.
    C. extension of venous thrombosis.
    D. vessel trauma.

42. In ordering imaging studies in a patient with peripheral vascular disease, the use of radiocontrast medium can potentially result in:
    A. hepatic failure.
    B. renal failure.
    C. bone marrow suppression.
    D. thrombocytopenia.

43. The anticipated result of débridement as part of the treatment of venous stasis ulcers includes all of the following except:
    A. enhanced tissue granulation.
    B. encouragement of reepithelialization.
    C. reduction of bacterial burden.
    D. prevention of peripheral arterial disease.

True or False

_____ 44. In the treatment of a venous stasis ulcer that is not responding to standard therapy, additional therapeutic options include hyperbaric oxygen therapy (HBOT).

_____ **45.** A few as 3 days of malnutrition in the form of inadequate protein-calorie intake can impair normal wound-healing mechanisms.

Answers

33. C.	38. D.	43. D.
34. D.	39. B.	44. True
35. D.	40. A.	45. True
36. A.	41. A.	
37. C.	42. B.	

Peripheral vascular disease (PVD) refers to a group of conditions in which there is a reduction of blood flow to the extremities. With PVD peripheral vascular disease, the venous, arterial, or lymphatic system is often affected. Risk factors for arterial occlusive disease, caused by extensive atherosclerosis, include diabetes mellitus, hypertension, and hyperlipidemia; tobacco use is the most potent risk factor, in particular in progressive disease. In the absence of these risk factors, peripheral arterial occlusive disease is rare except in advanced age; the condition is found in 10% of older adults. Clinical presentation usually includes a patient complaint of claudication, which is a reproducible ischemic muscle pain where pain is worse with exertion and usually responds promptly to cessation of the trigger activity. Claudication is caused by the inability of the diseased vessel to vasodilate and allow for increased blood flow to handle the metabolic demands associated with physical activity.

Disease caused by atherosclerosis in the distal aorta or iliac, femoral, or popliteal arteries results in the most common clinical form and is typically called lower-extremity occlusive disease. Presentation varies according to the area of vessel disease and dysfunction (Table 10–6). Atherosclerotic and calcific lesions usually cause occlusive disease of the aorta and its branches. Disease is often asymmetrical because the distribution of obstructive lesions usually occurs in segments, rather than continuously.

The diagnosis of lower-extremity occlusive disease is made from clinical presentation and select diagnostic studies. Doppler ultrasonography is often used first line to confirm the diagnosis and monitor disease progress. Magnetic resonance angiography has largely replaced standard angiography as the "gold standard" of PVD imaging. High-definition computerized tomography (CT) with contrast is also an option. In studies that require the use of contrast, assessment of renal function preprocedure is critical because the risk of contrast-induced renal impairment is greatest in the presence of diffuse arterial disease. Angiography, although an invasive

TABLE 10-6
Clinical Presentation of Lower-Extremity Vascular Occlusive Disease

Patient Presentation	Clinical Significance
Burning sensation or ache with walking	Usually indicates femoropopliteal arterial disease
Pain in calf, hip, or buttock with activity, relieved by rest	Classic report in intermittent claudication
Foot pain at rest	Blood flow to extremity ≤10% of normal; indicates profound disease and gangrene risk
Numbness, coldness, pain in extremity	More common than claudication report in the older adult
Absent posterior tibialis pulse	This pulse is always present in a healthy adult
	Dorsalis pedis pulse absent in ~5% of healthy adults
Nail thickening	Because numbness is often also a problem, meticulous nail hygiene while minimizing injury is needed
	Onychomycosis is often seen in PVD
Absent dorsalis pedis and tibial pulses	Proximal pulses may remain palpable even in presence of significant occlusive disease
	≤10% of normal blood flow to extremity
Blanching of foot with elevation, poor capillary return, dependent rubor	Most common with long-standing poorly controlled diabetes mellitus
Ache in anterior tibial muscles, foot, and metatarsal arch with activity	Can be confused with peripheral neuropathy
Sexual dysfunction	Most common in presence of smoking, hyperlipidemia, diabetes mellitus
	PVD contributes to its development but is likely one of many influencing factors

PVD, peripheral vascular disease.
Source: Rowe, V.L. eMedicine. http://emedicine.medscape.com/article/460178-clinical#a0217, Peripheral arterial occlusive disease.

procedure, gives the best measure of the extent of the disease; the information gained from angiography is sometimes needed before clinicians proceed with percutaneous treatment or surgery.

Because patients with lower-extremity arterial occlusive disease usually have other health problems, prevention and intervention measures, such as aggressive risk factor reduction—including cessation of tobacco use and blood pressure, glucose, and lipid control—help improve overall well-being. In addition, the presence of concomitant disease, such as cardiovascular or cerebrovascular disease, often limits the patient's ability to be physically active. Exercise such as walking helps to minimize symptoms and should be encouraged; although exercise was previously thought to enhance collateral blood flow, the benefit is now recognized as being a result of improving oxygen extraction for the skeletal muscles. Meticulous skin care is needed to avoid breakdown, and periodic podiatric care is recommended. In the presence of PVD, skin and nail disruptions are particularly difficult to heal.

Pharmacotherapy for individuals with lower-extremity arterial occlusive disease often yields variable results. The use of pentoxifylline (Trental), a medication thought to reduce blood viscosity and improve blood flow by altering the ability of red blood cells to pass through diseased vessels, can be helpful in increasing exercise tolerance. Outcomes with pentoxifylline use are variable; patients without diabetes mellitus and milder symptoms seem to gain the most benefit. Cilostazol (Pletal), a medication that impairs platelet aggregation and increases vasodilation, is often helpful but has limitations. Its use is contraindicated in heart failure and carries an approximately 20% rate of adverse effects, including headache, dizziness, and diarrhea. The use of these medications does not alter the course of the disease, but rather reduces symptoms. Daily aspirin and statin therapy is usually indicated as part of a comprehensive plan to reduce cardiovascular risk; concomitant control of diabetes mellitus, which is often present, is critical. The use of beta blockers (beta adrenergic antagonists) has been historically noted to worsen claudication symptoms; the use of the drug class in patients with PVD was at one time discouraged. However, the use beta blockers of often is recommended to treat the concomitant conditions including cardiovascular disease found in the person with PVD.

Clopidogrel (Plavix) has been used in therapy for lower-extremity arterial occlusive disease, particularly in patients who are allergic to aspirin or do not tolerate aspirin or have an underlying hypercoagulable state; its use prevents fibrinogen binding and may reduce the risk of thrombus formation. Warfarin therapy with a goal INR of 2.0 to 3.0 is occasionally used for certain patients with high thrombus risk, particularly patients who have undergone a vascular procedure. The use of vasodilators and anticoagulants does not appear to alter the natural history of the disease. Surgical evaluation for percutaneous or open procedures should be part of the care of patients with lower-extremity occlusive disease; medical management of concomitant problems, such as cardiovascular

disease and diabetes mellitus, needs to be optimized preoperatively, and surgical intervention for other forms of vascular disease also needs to be considered. Angioplasty, grafting procedures, and/or vascular stenting can help improve blood flow and minimize symptoms and complications. Owing to the complexity of care, intervention for peripheral arterial ulcers usually requires specialty consultation.

Although lower-extremity arterial occlusive disease is characterized by a predictable, slower, progressive process, acute occlusion can occur. Caused by embolic, thrombotic, or traumatic events, acute limb ischemia usually manifests with the so-called six Ps: pain, paresthesia (the two most common manifestations), pallor, pulselessness, poikilothermy (variation in limb temperature), and paralysis. When acute limb ischemia is caused by arterial embolism, the origin of the clot is usually the heart, with underlying atrial fibrillation. When caused by arterial thrombosis, chronic arteriosclerotic occlusive disease is usually at the core of the problem. Prompt assessment is needed to support the diagnosis. In the presence of acute arterial occlusion, anticoagulation therapy with heparin is standard along with consideration of procedural intervention to relieve the obstruction.

Chronic venous insufficiency is a common sequela of DVT and leg trauma, although the absence of this history is noted in about 25% of patients. There is decreased venous return because of vessel damage, and lower-extremity edema is usually the earliest sign. Symptoms usually include leg aching and itchiness. Over time, the edema progressively worsens; this results in the development of thin, shiny, atrophic skin, often with brown pigmentation. Subcutaneous tissue thickens and becomes fibrous.

The stage is set for stasis ulceration. Inflamed pruritic patches usually precede the formation of an irregular ulceration with a clean base. Yellow eschar is occasionally found. Therapies enhancing venous flow (i.e., limb elevation, exercise, and compression therapy) improve oxygen transport to the skin and subcutaneous tissues, decrease edema, and reduce inflammation and can be utilized for any patient with symptoms and signs of chronic venous disease. Compression therapy has long been considered an important part of venous ulcer therapy; high compression bandages, exerting 30 to 30 mm Hg at the ankle, are most effective. The use of a flexible compression bandage is preferred over a rigid compression dressing such as an Unna boot. If compression therapy is not successful when used alone, high-dose pentoxifylline therapy can be added to compression therapy. Pentoxifylline used as an adjunct to compression is more effective than medication without compression. When used without compression, it is more effective than placebo or no treatment at a dose of 800 mg three times a day.

Although no particular wound care regimen has been associated with more rapid ulcer healing, ulcer débridement, various topical products, and hyperbaric oxygen are formidable options to consider when deciding on a wound care treatment plan. Wound débridement is an essential component in the management of venous ulcers. The presence of devitalized tissue increases the potential for local bacterial infection and sepsis. Removal of necrotic tissue and fibrinous debris in venous ulcers aids in the formation of healthy granulation tissue and enhances reepithelialization. Surgical débridement is occasionally needed, especially if an advanced therapy such as a bioengineered skin graft is being considered. Slow-release antiseptic bandages are helpful in reducing bacterial burden. Moisture-retaining dressings improve pain and have utility in autolytic débridement.

Wounds that fail to heal are typically hypoxic. Multiple components of the wound healing process are affected by oxygen concentration or gradients, which explains why hyperbaric oxygen therapy (HBOT) can be an effective therapy to treat chronic wounds. HBOT significantly increases the oxygen saturation of plasma, raising the partial pressure available to tissues. HBOT should be used in conjunction with a complete wound healing care plan. As with all chronic wounds, other underlying host factors (large vessel disease, glycemic control, nutrition, infection, presence of necrotic tissue, fluid off-loading) must be simultaneously addressed in order to have the highest chance of successful healing and functional capacity.

Nonhealing wounds not only lack oxygen, but also are deficient in viable nutrients. Adequate nutrition is an often-overlooked requirement for normal wound healing. Address protein-calorie malnutrition and deficiencies of vitamins and minerals. Inadequate protein-calorie nutrition, even after just a few days of starvation, can impair normal wound-healing mechanisms. For healthy adults, daily nutritional requirements are approximately 1.25 to 1.5 g of protein per kilogram of body weight and 30 to 35 calories/kg; these requirements are increased in the presence of sizable wounds.

The prognosis for healing of chronic wounds varies with the etiology of the wound and the general health status of the patient. If wound healing continues to be unsuccessful, a biopsy specimen of the lesion should be obtained to rule out malignancy. Given the complexity of care in patients with venous ulcers or chronic wounds, a referral to specialty wound care is usually indicated. Indications for a specialty wound care referral include arterial insufficiency, nonhealing ulcers, ulcer recurrence, persistent stasis dermatitis, and suspected contact dermatitis.

DISCUSSION SOURCES

Alguire, P.C. UpToDate. http://www.uptodate.com/contents/medical-management-of-lower-extremity-chronic-venous-disease?source=search_result&search=medical+management+of+lower+extremity&selectedTitle=1~150, Medical management of lower extremity chronic venous disease, accessed 2/12/13.

Chahin, C. eMedicine. http://www.emedicine.medscape.com/article/423649-overview, Imaging in Lower-Extremity Atherosclerotic Arterial Disease.

Latham, E. eMedicine. http://www.emedicine.medscape.com/article/1464149-overview#aw2aab6b7, Hyperbaric oxygen therapy.

Stillman, R. eMedicine. http://www.emedicine.medscape.com/article/194018-treatment#a25, Wound care treatment & management.

Torre, J. eMedicine. http://www.emedicine.medscape.com/article/1298452-overview, Chronic Wounds.

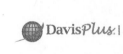 **See full color images of this topic on DavisPlus at http://davisplus.fadavis.com | Keyword: Fitzgerald**

Endocrine Disorders

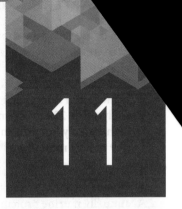

11

Diabetes Mellitus

1. Which of the following characteristics applies to type 1 diabetes mellitus (DM)?
   A. Significant hyperglycemia and ketoacidosis result from lack of insulin.
   B. This condition is commonly diagnosed on routine examination or work-up for other health problems.
   C. Initial response to oral sulfonylureas is usually favorable.
   D. Insulin resistance (IR) is a significant part of the disease.

2. Which of the following characteristics applies to type 2 DM?
   A. Major risk factors are heredity and obesity.
   B. Pear-shaped body type is commonly found.
   C. Exogenous insulin is needed for control of disease.
   D. Physical activity enhances IR.

3. You consider prescribing insulin glargine (Lantus®) because of its:
   A. extended duration of action.
   B. rapid onset of action.
   C. ability to prevent diabetic end-organ damage.
   D. ability to preserve pancreatic function.

4. After use, the onset of action of lispro (Humalog®) occurs in:
   A. less than 30 minutes.
   B. approximately 1 hour.
   C. 1 to 2 hours.
   D. 3 to 4 hours.

5 Which of the following medications should be used with caution in a person with suspected or known sulfa allergy?
   A. metformin
   B. glyburide
   C. rosiglitazone
   D. NPH insulin

6. The mechanism of action of metformin (Glucophage®) is as:
   A. an insulin-production enhancer.
   B. a product virtually identical in action to sulfonylureas.
   C. a drug that increases insulin action in the peripheral tissues and reduces hepatic glucose production.
   D. a facilitator of renal glucose excretion.

7. Generally, testing for type 2 DM in asymptomatic, undiagnosed individuals older than 45 years should be conducted every _____.
   A. year.
   B. 3 years
   C. 5 years
   D. 10 years

8. You are seeing 17-year-old Cynthia. As part of the visit, you consider her risk factors for type 2 DM would likely include all of the following except:
   A. obesity.
   B. Native American ancestry.
   C. family history of type 1 DM.
   D. personal history of polycystic ovary syndrome.

9. Criteria for the diagnosis of type 2 DM include:
   A. classic symptoms regardless of fasting plasma glucose measurement.
   B. plasma glucose level of 126 mg/dL (7 mmol/L) as a random measurement.
   C. a 2-hour glucose measurement of 156 mg/dL (8.6 mmol/L) after a 75 g anhydrous glucose load.
   D. a plasma glucose level of 126 mg/dL (7 mmol/L) or greater after an 8 hour or greater fast on more than one occasion.

10. The mechanism of action of pioglitazone is as: *Acto)*
   A. an insulin-production enhancer.
   B. a reducer of pancreatic glucose output.
   C. an insulin sensitizer.
   D. a facilitator of renal glucose excretion.

...g should be the goal measure-
...on with DM and hypertension?
...an 140 mm Hg systolic and less
...lic
...to or greater than 7%
...g/dL (11.1 to 16.6 mmol/L)
...(HDL) 35 to 40 mg/dL

...for a patient with DM, microalbuminuria
...measurement should be obtained:
   A. annually if urine protein is present.
   B. periodically in relationship to glycemia control.
   C. yearly.
   D. with each office visit related to DM.

13. The mechanism of action of sulfonylureas is as:
   A. an antagonist of insulin receptor site activity.
   B. a product that enhances insulin release.
   C. a facilitator of renal glucose excretion.
   D. an agent that can reduce hepatic glucose production.

14. When caring for a patient with DM, hypertension and
    persistent proteinuria, the NP prioritizes the choice of
    antihypertension and prescribes:
   A. furosemide.
   B. methyldopa.
   C. fosinopril.
   D. nifedipine.

15. Clinical presentation of type 1 DM usually includes all
    of the following except:
   A. report of recent unintended weight gain.
   B. ketosis.
   C. thirst.
   D. polyphagia.

16. Which of the following should be periodically moni-
    tored with the use of a biguanide?   metformin
   A. creatine kinase (CK)
   B. alkaline phosphatase (ALP)
   C. alanine aminotransferase (ALT)
   D. creatinine (Cr)

17. Which of the following should be periodically moni-
    tored with the use of a thiazolidinedione?   TZD
   A. CK
   B. ALP
   C. ALT → liver
   D. Cr

18. All of the following are risks for lactic acidosis in
    individuals taking metformin except:
   A. presence of chronic renal insufficiency.
   B. acute dehydration.
   C. radiographic contrast dye use.
   D. history of allergic reaction to sulfonamides.

19. Secondary causes of hyperglycemia potentially
    include the use of all of the following medications
    except:
   A. high dose niacin.
   B. systemic corticosteroids.
   C. high dose thiazide diuretics.
   D. low dose angiotensin receptor blockers.

20. Hemoglobin A1c best provides information on glucose
    control over the past:
   A. 1 to 29 days
   B. 21 to 47 days.
   C. 48 to 63 days.
   D. 64 to 90 days.

21. Which of the following statements is not true concern-
    ing the effects of exercise and IR?
   A. Approximately 80% of the body's insulin-
      mediated glucose uptake occurs in skeletal
      muscle.
   B. With regular aerobic exercise, IR is reduced by
      approximately 40%.
   C. The IR-reducing effects of exercise persist for
      48 hours after the activity.
   D. Hyperglycemia can occur as a result of aerobic
      exercise.

22 to 25. With an 8 a.m. dose of the following insulin forms,
followed by and inadequate dietary intake and/or excessive
energy use, at approximately what time would hypoglycemia
be most likely to occur?

22. Lispro _____ 830-930

23. Regular insulin _____ b/u 10-11am

24. NPH insulin _____ 6142 +10m

25. Insulin glargine (Lantus) _____ unlikely no peak

26. The meglitinide analogues are particularly
    helpful adjuncts in type 2 DM care to minimize
    risk of:
   A. fasting hypoglycemia.
   B. nocturnal hyperglycemia.
   C. postprandial hyperglycemia.
   D. postprandial hypoglycemia.

27. What is the most common adverse effect noted with
    alpha-glucosidase inhibitor use?
   A. gastrointestinal upset
   B. hepatotoxicity
   C. renal impairment
   D. symptomatic hypoglycemia

28. Which of the following statements best describes the Somogyi effect?
    A. Insulin-induced hypoglycemia triggers excess secretion of glucagon and cortisol, leading to hyperglycemia.
    B. Early morning elevated blood glucose levels result in part from growth hormone and cortisol-triggering hepatic glucose release.
    C. Late evening hyperglycemia is induced by inadequate insulin dose.
    D. Episodes of postprandial hypoglycemia occur as a result of inadequate food intake.

29. Intervention in microalbuminuria for a person with DM includes: (More than one can apply.)
    A. improved glycemic control.
    B. strict dyslipidemia control.
    C. use of an optimized dose of an angiotensin-converting enzyme inhibitor (ACEI) or angiotensin receptor blocker (ARB).
    D. The use of an ACEI with an ARB.

30. Hemoglobin A1c should be tested:
    A. at least annually for all patients.
    B. at least two times a year in patients who are meeting treatment goals and who have stable glycemic control.
    C. monthly in patients whose therapy has changed or who are not meeting glycemic goals.
    D. only via standardized laboratory testing because of inaccuracies associated with point-of-service testing.

31. The mechanism of action of the DPP-4 inhibitors is as:
    A. a drug that increases levels of incretin, increasing synthesis and release of insulin from pancreatic beta cells.
    B. a product virtually identical in action to sulfonylureas.
    C. a drug that increases insulin action in the peripheral tissues and reduces hepatic glucose production.
    D. a facilitator of renal glucose excretion.

32. The mechanism of action of exenatide (Byetta®) is as:
    A. a drug that stimulates insulin production in response to increase in plasma glucose.
    B. a product virtually identical in action to sulfonylureas.
    C. a drug that increases insulin action in the peripheral tissues and reduces hepatic glucose production.
    D. a facilitator of renal glucose excretion.

33. You see an obese 25-year-old man with acanthosis nigricans and consider ordering:
    A. FBS.
    B. LFT.
    C. RPR.
    D. ESR.

34. The use of a thiazolidinedione is not recommended in all of the following clinical scenarios except:
    A. a 57-year-old man who is taking a nitrate.
    B. a 62-year-old woman with heart failure.
    C. a 45-year-old man who is using insulin.
    D. a 35-year-old patient with newly diagnosed type 2 DM.

35. In an older adult with type 2 DM with gastroparesis, the use of which of the following medications should be avoided?
    A. insulin glargine (Lantus)
    B. insulin aspart (NovoLog®)
    C. glimepiride (Amaryl®)
    D. exenatide (Byetta)

36. Metformin should be discontinued for the day of and up to 48 hours after surgery because of increased risk of:
    A. hypoglycemia.
    B. hepatic impairment.
    C. lactic acidosis.
    D. interaction with most anesthetic agents.

37. All the following medications are recommended for treatment of concomitant hypertension when seen with type 2 DM except:
    A. beta blockers.
    B. calcium channel blockers
    C. alpha adrenergic receptor antagonist.
    D. angiotensin receptor blockers.

38. Which of the following best describes the physical activity recommendations such as brisk walking for a 55-year-old woman with newly diagnosed type 2 diabetes mellitus? (More than one can apply.)
    A. The goal should be for a total increased physical activity of 150 min per week or more.
    B. Increased physical activity is recommended for at least 30 minutes per day, at least three times per week with no more than 48 hours without exercise.
    C. Some form of resistance exercise such as lifting dumbbells or using an exercise band should be included at least three times per week.
    D. Vigorous aerobic or resistance activity is potentially contraindicated in the presence of proliferative or severe nonproliferative retinopathy due to the possible risk of vitreous hemorrhage or retinal detachment.

39. In teaching a patient with type 2 diabetes mellitus about using rapid-acting insulin to help with the management of post-prandial hyperglycemia, the NP advises that the usual dose is ___ unit per 15 grams of carbohydrate.
    A. 1
    B. 2
    C. 3
    D. 4

40. Which of the following patients has impaired glucose tolerance?
    A. a 70-year-old man with a fasting glucose of 109 mg/dl (6.05 mmol/L)
    B. an 84-year-old woman with a 1 hour post-prandial glucose of 98 mg/dl (5.44 mmol/L)
    C. a 33-year-old man with a hemoglobin A1c of 5.4%
    D. a 58-year-old woman with a 2 hour post-prandial glucose of 152 mg/dl (8.44 mmol/L)

41. Mr. Samuels is a 58-year-old man with type 2 DM who is using a single 10 unit daily dose of the long-acting insulin glargine. His fasting blood glucose has been between 141 to 180 mg/dL (7.8 to 10 mmol/L). Which of the following best describes the next step in his therapy?
    A. Continue on the current glargine dose.
    B. Increase his glargine dose by 4 units per day.
    C. Increase his glargine dose by 1 unit per day.
    D. Increase his glargine dose by 6 units per day.

42. Which of the following classes of medications is commonly recommended as part of first line therapy in the newly diagnosed person with type 2 diabetes?
    A. Alpha-glucosidase inhibitor
    B. Meglitinide
    C. Thiazolidinedione
    D. Biguanide

43. Pertaining to the use of sliding scale insulin in response to elevated blood glucose, which of the following best describes current best practice?
    A. The use of this type of sliding-scale insulin therapy is discouraged as this method treats hyperglycemia after it has already occurred.
    B. Sliding scale insulin in response to elevated glucose is a safe and helpful method of treating hyperglycemia.
    C. Delivering insulin in this manner is acceptable within the acute care hospital setting only.
    D. The use of the sliding insulin scale is appropriate in the treatment of type 1 DM only.

44. In a healthy person, what percentage of the body's total daily physiological insulin secretion is released as basally?
    A. 10%
    B. 25%
    C. 50%
    D. 75%

45. Five years or more after type 2 diabetes mellitus diagnosis, which of the following medications is less likely to be effective in controlling plasma glucose?
    A. Metformin
    B. Pioglitazone
    C. Glipizide
    D. Insulin

46. The use of which of the following medications has the potential for causing the greatest reduction in HbA1c?
    A. A biguanide
    B. A thiazolidinedione
    C. A sulfonylurea
    D. An insulin form

47. Which of the following best describes ethnicity and insulin sensitivity?
    A. Little variation exists in insulin sensitivity among different ethnic groups.
    B. African Americans are typically less sensitive to the effects of insulin when compared to people of European ancestry.
    C. Mexican Americans are likely the most insulin sensitive ethnic group residing in North America.
    D. The degree of insulin sensitivity has little influence on insulin production.

48. Recommended A1c goal in a 79-year-old woman with a 20-year history of type 2 diabetes mellitus who has difficulty ambulating, uses a walker, and has a cardiac ejection fraction of 35% and a history of heart failure should be equal to or less than:
    A. 7%
    B. 7.5%
    C. 8%
    D. 8.5%

49. Consideration should be given to setting A1c goal in a 22-year-old man with a 8-year history of type 1 diabetes mellitus who has not comorbid conditions equal to or at less than:
    A. 5.5%
    B. 6%
    C. 6.5%
    D. 7%

50. The use of exenatide has been associated with the development of: (Byetta)
    A. leukopenia.
    B. pancreatitis.
    C. lymphoma.
    D. vitiligo

51. The International Diabetes Federation's diagnostic criteria for metabolic syndrome include:
    A. an obligatory finding of persistent hyperglycemia.
    B. notation of ethnic-specific waist circumference measurements.
    C. documentation of microalbuminuria.
    D. a family history of type 2 DM.

52. Metformin has all of the following effects except:
    A. improved insulin-mediated glucose uptake.
    B. modest weight loss with initial use.
    C. enhanced fibrinolysis.
    D. increased LDL cholesterol production.

53. Cardiovascular effects of hyperinsulinemia include:
    A. decreased renal sodium reabsorption.
    B. constricted circulating volume.
    C. greater responsiveness to angiotensin II.
    D. diminished sympathetic activation.

54. Which of the following is an unlikely consequence of untreated metabolic syndrome and IR in a woman of reproductive age?
    A. hyperovulation
    B. irregular menses
    C. acne
    D. hirsutism

55. Acanthosis nigricans is commonly noted in all of the following areas except:
    A. groin folds.
    B. axilla.
    C. nape of the neck.
    D. face. Except

Answers

1. A.	26. C.
2. A.	27. A.
3. A.	28. A.
4. A.	29. A, B, C
5. B.	30. B.
6. C.	31. A.
7. B.	32. A.
8. C.	33. A.
9. D.	34. D.
10. C.	35. D.
11. A.	36. C.
12. C.	37. C.
13. B.	38. A, B, C, D
14. C.	39. B.
15. A.	40. D.
16. D.	41. B.
17. C.	42. D.
18. D.	43. A.
19. D.	44. C.
20. D.	45. C.
21. D.	46. D.

22. Approximately 8:30 to 9:30 a.m. (with peak of insulin dose)

23. Approximately 10 to 11 a.m. (with peak of insulin dose)

24. Approximately 2 to 10 p.m. (with peak of insulin dose)

25. Because insulin glargine (Lantus) has no peak, an episode of hypoglycemia is unlikely. If hypoglycemia were to occur, the episode could be protracted if left untreated because of the protracted duration of activity of the medication.

47. B.
48. C.
49. B.
50. B.
51. B.
52. D.
53. C.
54. A.
55. D.

Type 1 diabetes mellitus (DM) is polygenetic disease that results from autoimmune induced pancreatic beta cell destruction with resulting insulin deficiency. This disease usually occurs in persons younger than 30 years, with symptomatic presentation often comprising involuntary weight loss and the classic "polys": polydipsia, polyphagia, and polyuria. If type 1 DM is associated with ketoacidosis, DM presentation can be dramatic, with severe dehydration, abdominal pain, vomiting, and decreased level of consciousness. In any event, prompt intervention with appropriate insulin therapy is indicated. Lifelong insulin therapy is required, most often through the use of basal insulin with boluses of short-acting insulin to provide coverage for carbohydrate intake with meals and snacks. This can be done with multiple insulin injections or through the use of an insulin pump (Table 11–1).

Insulin resistance (IR) is a genetically predetermined and environmentally modified condition that is central to the pathogenesis of type 2 DM. In IR, there is a reduced sensitivity in the tissues to insulin's action at a given concentration, which causes a subnormal effect on glucose metabolism. Hyperglycemia results, which stimulates pancreatic insulin production in an effort to reduce the blood glucose level. Euglycemia occurs, albeit in the presence of hyperinsulinemia. Elevated fasting insulin levels are noted to be an independent predictor for ischemic heart disease. When coupled with acquired or lifestyle characteristics that contribute to IR, such as obesity, physical inactivity, and high carbohydrate (more than 60% of total calories) diet, the body has greater difficulty maintaining a normal blood glucose level. Over time, generally after many years of IR, pancreatic beta cell deficiency usually occurs, resulting in impaired glucose tolerance, hyperglycemia, and the diagnosis of type 2 DM.

Numerous conditions are seen in conjunction with IR. Increased IR is inversely related to decreased urinary uric acid clearance; this leads to a dramatic increase in the rate of gout. Most women with polycystic ovary syndrome have IR. Acanthosis nigricans, hyperpigmentation of the skin often in the neck and axilla, is also correlated with IR. This finding is most common in post puberty and young adults with IR and DM risk. A personal history of birth weight that was low for gestational age is also correlated with increased risk of IR. Polycystic ovary syndrome (PCOS) is largely an IR consequence. As anovulation is a consequence of PCOS, this condition is the leading cause of endocrine-based female infertility. When IR is reduced, ovulation often resumes with resulting enhanced fertility. In addition, when IR is reduced, acne and hirsutism, usually a consequence of hyperandrogenism associated with PCOS, are usually improved.

IR is recognized as contributing to a prothrombotic and proatherogenic state. Plasminogen activator inhibitor, produced by the liver and endothelial cells, inhibits fibrin degradation by plasmin and enhances clot formation; increased levels are found in atherosclerotic lesions. High levels of triglyceride, very low density lipoprotein (VLDL), and oxidized low density lipoprotein (LDL) stimulate the production of plasminogen activator inhibitor. Plasminogen activator inhibitor levels are significantly correlated with increased body

TABLE 11-1
Insulin: Type, Onset, Peak, and Duration of Action

Insulin Type	Onset of Action	Peak	Duration of Action
Short-acting, rapid onset of action (Lispro insulin solution [Humalog])	15–30 min, give within 15 min or right after meals	30 min–2.5 hr	3–6.5 hr
Short-acting, rapid onset of action (Aspart insulin solution [NovoLog])	10–20 min, give 5–10 min before meals	1–3 hr	3–5 hr
Short-acting, rapid onset of action (Insulin glulisine [Apidra®])	10–15 min, give within 15 min or right after meals	1–1.5 hr	3–5 hr
Short-acting (Regular [Humulin R®, Novolin R®])	30 min–1 hr	2–3 hr	4–6 hr
Intermediate-acting (NPH [Novolin N®, Humulin N®])	1–2 hr	6–14 hr	16–24 hr
Long-acting (Insulin glargine solution [Lantus])	Clinical effect about 1 hr after injection	None	≥24 hr
Long-acting (Insulin detemir solution [Levemir®])	Unknown, not stated in product information but appears to be about 1–2 hr from PK graphics	6–8 hr (minimal peak)	Dose dependent; 12 hr for 0.2 units/kg, 20 hr for 0.4 units/kg. Albumin bound

Source: Comparisons of insulins based on U.S. product information (2006). Prescribers Letter Detail-Document #220309. Available at: Prescribersletter.com

mass and high plasma insulin levels, whereas levels are reduced when endogenous insulin levels are reduced by exercise, weight loss, or insulin-sensitizing medications, such as metformin and thiazolidinediones.

Although the correlation of obesity with IR and type 2 DM is well established, not all body fat types and distribution are equally problematic. Some persons with IR and type 2 DM are of normal weight, whereas others with IR never develop hyperglycemia. Obesity dramatically increases the risk of diabetes in a person with IR, however. "Apple-shaped" or central abdominal obesity comprises metabolically active fat and is associated with high insulin levels, IR, and high mobilization rate of free fatty acids; high insulin levels are often associated with increased appetite. This genetic makeup helped increase the likelihood of survival in times of famine. In these times of plentiful food, however, IR helps promote fat storage.

Patients with type 2 DM are most often asymptomatic at onset. As a result, the American Diabetes Association (ADA) recommends periodic fasting plasma glucose screening every 3 years in all adults, regardless of appearance of risk; the rationale for this testing interval is that type 2 DM is unlikely to develop in a 3-year interval if initial glucose was normal. Testing should be considered at a younger age or be done more frequently in individuals with or with acquisition of type 2 DM risk factors (Table 11–2).

When a fasting plasma glucose threshold level of 126 mg/dL or greater (7.0 mmol/L or greater) after an 8-hour fast is used, this testing is 98% specific and 40% to 88% sensitive for type 2 DM. Typically, wide-scale screening done according to these guidelines yields a 6% true-positive rate. Additional ADA diagnostic criteria for type 2 DM include a casual (random)

plasma glucose level of 200 mg/dL or greater (11.1 mmol/L or greater) with classic diabetic symptoms, or those with an oral glucose tolerance result of 200 mg/dL or greater (11.1 mmol/L or greater) at 2 hours. Glycosylated (or glycated) hemoglobin, also known as hemoglobin A1c (or simply A1c), increases in proportion to the amount of circulating glucose. The most abundant glycohemoglobin subtype of hemoglobin A_1 is A1c, which constitutes about 4% to 6% of the body's total hemoglobin. Glycohemoglobin circulates as part of the red blood cell for about 90 to 120 days, the length of the red blood cell's life span. As a result, measurement of hemoglobin A1c provides a method for evaluating glucose control over time; the measurement best reflects blood glucose trends over the preceding 90 days but best measures glucose control in the past 28 to 42 days. Correlation with average plasma glucose and hemoglobin A1c is an important clinical tool and can be used for reinforcement in patient counseling. The ADA advises that hemoglobin A1c can be used as a tool for diagnosing DM, with a measure equal to or greater than 6.5% consistent with the diagnosis. The test should be repeated in an asymptomatic adult with glucose less than 200 mg/dL (less than 11.1 mmol/L). A repeat test is not needed in the presence of DM symptoms or glucose levels of 200 mg/dL or greater (11.1 mmol/L or greater) (Table 11–3).

Sadly, patients with increased risk for type 2 DM are missed due to lack of testing. Patients with impaired glucose tolerance (IGT), impaired fasting glucose (IFG), or an A1c of 5.7% to 6.4% should be identified and treated with lifestyle modification including a target weight loss of 7% of body weight and referred increasing physical activity to at least 150 min per week; adding metformin therapy is also a consideration. These

TABLE 11-2
Diabetes Mellitus Testing Recommendations

Criteria for Diabetes Testing in Asymptomatic Adults

Testing should be considered in all adults who are overweight (BMI ≥25 kg/m2*) and have additional risk factors:
- Physical inactivity
- First degree relative with type 2 diabetes
- Members of a high risk ethnic population (e.g., African American, Latino, Native American, Asian American, Pacific Islander)
- Women who delivered a baby weighing >9 lb (4.08 kg) or were diagnosed with gestational DM (GDM) (screen women with recent dx GDM at 6–12 weeks postpartum)
- Hypertension (≥140/90 mmHg or on therapy for hypertension)
- HDL cholesterol level <35 mg/dL (0.90 mmol/L) and/or a triglyceride level >250 mg/dL (2.82 mmol/L)
- Women with polycystic ovary syndrome
- A1c ≥5.7% (.057 proportion), impaired glucose tolerance (IGT), or impaired fasting glucose (IFG) on previous testing
- Other clinical conditions associated with insulin resistance (e.g., severe obesity, acanthosis nigricans)
- History of cardiovascular disease (CVD)

In the absence of the above criteria, testing diabetes should begin at age 45 years.

If results are normal, testing should be repeated at least at 3 year intervals, with consideration of more frequent testing depending on initial results and risk status.

*At risk BMI may be lower in some ethnic groups.
Source: American Diabetes Association Clinical Practice Recommendations, *Diabetes Care* January 2014; 37: Supplement 1 S1; doi:10.2337/dc14-S001.

TABLE 11-3
Diagnosis of Diabetes Mellitus, Categories of Increased Risk for Diabetes

	Plasma Glucose	Oral Glucose Tolerance Test (OGTT)	A1c
Diabetes mellitus	Fasting (no caloric intake for ≥8 h) ≥126 mg/dL (≥7.0 mmol/L) Random ≥200 mg/dL (≥11.1 mmol/L) with symptoms including polyphagia, polyuria, polydipsia, and unexplained weight loss or hyperglycemic crisis	2-hr plasma glucose ≥200 mg/dL (≥11.1 mmol/L) after a 75 G glucose load	A1c ≥6.5% No special patient preparation, can be done nonfasting, no protracted time needed to test like OGTT, improved standardization of A1c measurement. A1c repeat recommended in asymptomatic adult with glucose <200 mg/dL (<11.1 mmol/L) Repeat not needed in presence of DM symptoms and/or glucose levels ≥200 mg/dL (≥11.1 mmol/L)
Categories of increased risk for diabetes (impaired fasting glucose {IFG}, impaired glucose tolerance {IGT}, prediabetes)	IFG=100 mg/dL (5.6 mmol/L) to 125 mg/dL (6.9 mmol/L)	IGT=140 to 199 mg/dL (7.8–11.0 mmol/L) on the 75 G OGTT	A1c=5.7%–6.4%

Source: American Diabetes Association Clinical Practice Recommendations, Diabetes Care January 2014 37:Supplement 1 S1; doi:10.2337/dc14-S001.

International Expert Report on the Role of the A1c Assay in the Diagnosis of Diabetes. Available at: care.diabetesjournals.org/site/misc/DC09-9033.pdf, accessed 8/21/13.

treatment options are demonstrated to minimize the risk of progression to type 2 diabetes.

Therapeutic lifestyle changes are critically important for a person with DM. Tobacco use in any form should be discouraged due to its obvious cardiovascular risk. Because approximately 80% of the body's insulin-mediated glucose uptake occurs in muscle and is enhanced by physical activity, a regular program of aerobic exercise such as brisk walking should be prescribed. Exercise reduces IR by approximately 40%, with the effects persisting for up to 48 hours after the activity, and aids in weight maintenance. People with diabetes should be advised to perform at least 150 minutes per week of moderate-intensity aerobic physical activity at 50% to 70% of maximum heart rate. Exercise should be spread over at least 5 days per week with no more than 2 consecutive days without exercise; the insulin sensitizing effects of physical activity wane after 48 hours. In the absence of contraindications, people with type 2 diabetes should be encouraged to perform resistance training at least twice per week. Cardiac stress testing should be considered for the previously sedentary individual at moderate to high risk for cardiovascular disease or other patients who are clinically indicated who want to undertake vigorous aerobic exercise that exceeds the demands of everyday living.

For a person with type 1 or type 2 DM, current ADA recommendations advise a diet of 300 mg or less of cholesterol per day, 8% to 9% or less of total dietary calories per day from saturated fat with similar proportions of polyunsaturated and monounsaturated fats, and 25 to 30 g of dietary fiber per day. Calories from protein should be no more than 10% to 20% of the daily total.

Weight loss improves insulin sensitivity and reduces blood pressure; improvement is not related to the degree of weight loss. Eating frequent, small, high-fiber meals and foods with a low glycemic index and smaller serving sizes should be encouraged. Dietary fat should be limited, but not eliminated, with emphasis on decreasing saturated fats, while using monounsaturated fat. A pound of fat contains approximately 3500 stored calories. A deficit of 500 to 1000 calories per day would lead to a 1 to 2 lb (0.45 to 0.9 kg) weight loss per week. (Table 11–4). In addition to the appropriate A1c for the patient, an additional important marker is the achievement of at least 50% or greater of fasting, postprandial, and bedtime glycemic goals through a combination of therapeutic lifestyle

TABLE 11-4
DM Type 2: Additional Care Considerations

A	Aspirin 75–162 mg/d (use clopidogrel (Plavix®) 75 mg/d in aspirin allergy), ACEI or ARB Counsel about moderation or abstinence in alcohol and/or recreational drug intake
B	Beta blocker or alpha-beta blocker therapy as indicated by cardiovascular risk and complications
C	Cholesterol—Controlling therapy to reach the following goals: • LDL ↓100 mg/dL (2.6 mmol/L), perhaps ↓70 mg/dL (1.8 mmol/L), HDL ↑45 mg/dL (1.2 mmol/L) men, ↑55 mg/dL (1.4 mmol/L) women • Alternative, moderate-intensity stain therapy to reduce LDL 30–50% or high intensity statin therapy to lower LDL by greater than 50% as determined by patient's estimated 10-year ASCVD risk Check fasting lipid profile annually, consider less often if evidence of stability. Creatinine (renal function)—Check serum creatinine, calculated glomerular filtration rate (GFR), and urine microalbumin annually
D	Diet—Limit *trans* and saturated fats, healthiest foods in appropriate amounts every meal. Medical nutritional therapy (MNT) with a registered dietician advisable. Dental care—Reinforce ongoing dental care and treatment of dental disease
E	Exercise/increase physical activity, if not contraindicated, to at least 150 min per week of moderate activity such as walking, best in the form of ≥30 mins, ≥5 times per week at 50%–70% of maximum heart rate with no more than 2 consecutive days without exercise. In addition, resistance training ≥2 times per week. Vigorous aerobic or resistance activity is potentially contraindicated in the presence of proliferative or severe nonproliferative retinopathy due to the possible risk of vitreous hemorrhage or retinal detachment. Eye exam (dilated) annually, increase frequency as dictated by developing retinopathy or other eye problems.
F	Foot examination (visual) with every visit, teach protective foot behavior, comprehensive lower extremity sensory exam annually using 10-g monofilament with ≥1 of the following; vibration using a 128 Hz tuning fork, pinprick sensation, ankle reflexes or vibration threshold.
G	Goals—Periodically review overall goals of care with patient

Source: American Diabetes Association Clinical Practice Recommendations, Diabetes Care January 2014 37: Supplement 1 S1; doi:10.2337/dc14-S001.
Massachusetts Guidelines for Adult Diabetic Care. Available at: http://files.hria.org/files/DB723.pdf

changes and medications. Drug choices in type 2 DM are quite varied. Cost and efficacy are considerable factors in choosing the most appropriate drug(s). If initial A1c is equal to or greater than 2% above goal, at least two drugs will likely be needed. An inexpensive, well-tolerated, efficacious initial drug combination is metformin and a sulfonylurea; this is the most commonly used drug combination for the treatment of type 2 DM. Critical to safe practice is the recognition of a given medications mechanism of action, adverse effect profile, and cost (Table 11–5 and Fig. 11–1).

Metformin, a biguanide, improves insulin-mediated glucose uptake and metabolic parameters such as fibrinolysis. The anticipated A1c reduction with intensified or maximum safe and tolerated dose, with metformin use is about 1% to 2%; an A1c of 9% prior to metformin initiation can be reduced to 7% or 8% with its use. One of the most commonly reported adverse effects with metformin use is gastrointestinal upset including diarrhea. This can be minimized by titrating the dose upward over a 2 to 3 week time period, using the extended release rather than intermediate release form of the medication and by taking the metformin dose with a meal. An increased body of knowledge demonstrates that metformin use in early metabolic syndrome can help in delaying the onset of type 2 DM.

One area of concern with metformin use has been the rare development of lactic acidosis, a potentially fatal illness, during its use. In a patient with normal renal function, lactic acid produced in the body, likely slightly enhanced with metformin use, is excreted via the kidneys without causing harm. In a person with renal impairment, metformin and lactic acid are cleared less effectively. Any condition that potentially reduces renal perfusion, including hypovolemia, heart failure, or advanced age, increases the metformin-associated lactic acidosis risk. The time period around the use of radiocontrast and surgery is considered a risk due to alterations in hydration. With consideration of all of these factors, the risk of lactic acidosis with metformin use is likely overstated; best estimates are a rate of greater than 3 in 100,000 per patient treated. At the same time, in order to minimize the risk of lactic acidosis, warnings associated with metformin use include avoiding use in the presence of renal impairment, heart failure, and age greater than 80 years. In addition, regardless of patient age, metformin use should be discontinued for the day of surgery, radiocontrast use, or other condition potentially impacting hydration status and only reintroduced when hydration status and renal function is back to baseline.

The sulfonylureas (SU) are a drug class that includes medication such as glipizide (Glucotrol®), glyburide (DiaBeta®), glimepiride (Amaryl). These drugs act as insulin secretagogue resulting in the release of insulin for pancreatic beta cells. Anticipated A1c reduction with intensified use is approximately 1% to 2%. Since the medication is renally eliminated, the sulfonylurea dose should be adjusted in the presence of renal impairment. The SUs require functioning pancreatic beta cells to be clinically effective. Due to declining beta cell function, these medications are typically less effective after 5 or more years post type 2 DM diagnosis and in older adults. In addition, the presence of severe hyperglycemia inhibits

TABLE 11-5
Medications Used in the Treatment of Type 2 Diabetes Mellitus

Medication	Mechanism of Action A1c Reduction	Comment
Sulfonylurea (SU) Examples: Glipizide (Glucotrol®), glyburide (DiaBeta®), glimepiride (Amaryl®)	Insulin secretagogue Anticipated A1C reduction with intensified use=1%–2%	Adjust dose in renal impairment Use with caution with sulfonamide allergy, though cross-allergy risk is low. Potentially photosensitizing Typically less effective after ≥5 years T2DM dx, older adults, in the presence of severe hyperglycemia
Biguanide Example: Metformin (Glucophage®)	Reduces hepatic glucose production and intestinal glucose absorption, insulin sensitizer via increased peripheral glucose uptake and utilization Anticipated A1C reduction with intensified use=1%–2%	Monitor creatinine (Cr), do not initiate or continue with impaired renal function. Avoid use in presence of heart failure. Rare risk of lactic acidosis, most often with impaired renal function, hypovolemia, low perfusion state, and/or advanced age (>80 years) With radiocontrast use, surgery, or other condition that can potentially

Continued

TABLE 11-5

Medications Used in the Treatment of Type 2 Diabetes Mellitus—cont'd

Medication	Mechanism of Action A1c Reduction	Comment
Biguanide (Metforming)—cont'd		alter hydration status, omit day of and ≥48 h post-study, -procedure, -condition, and reinitiate once baseline renal function has been reestablished. Little hypoglycemia risk when used as a solo product. Metformin use increases risk of vitamin B_{12} deficiency due to B_{12} malabsorption, risk appears dose- and length of therapy–dependent. Metformin therapy for prevention of type 2 diabetes can be considered in those at highest risk for diabetes, such as those with multiple risk factors, especially if demonstrated progression of hyperglycemia (i.e., A1C ≥6% [0.06 proportion]) despite lifestyle interventions, those with BMI >35 kg/m², age <60 years, and women with prior GDM.
Thiazolidinedione (TZD, glitazones) Examples: Pioglitazone (Actos®), rosiglitazone (Avandia®)*	Insulin sensitizer via action at PPAR-γ receptors found in muscle, adipose, and other tissue Anticipated A1C reduction with intensified use=1%–2%	Rare risk (<0.5%) of hepatic toxicity with use. Monitor ALT periodically. Edema risk, particularly when used with insulin or SU. TZD use can cause or exacerbate heart failure. Do not initiate use in presence of heart failure, monitor at-risk patients carefully. In consideration of cardiovascular risk, use with insulin or nitrates not recommended. Pioglitazone use in excess of 1 year may be associated with an increased risk of bladder cancer. For additional information, see www.fda.gov/Drugs/DrugSafety/ucm259150.htm
Glucagon-like peptide (GLP)-1 agonist (incretin mimetics) Examples: Exenatide (Byetta®, Bydureon®), liraglutide (Victoza®) Injection only	Stimulates insulin production in response to increase in plasma glucose, inhibits postprandial glucagon release Slows gastric emptying, often leading to appetite suppression and weight loss Anticipated A1C reduction with intensified use=1%–2%	Major adverse effect=N/V, usually better with dose adjustment, continued use; contraindicated in gastroparesis Adjunct to improve glycemic control in T2DM when not adequately controlled with biguanide and/or sulfonylurea. Per FDA advisory, clinicians are advised to promptly discontinue exenatide use and to advise patients using product to seek care if acute pancreatitis symptoms (persistent abdominal pain, usually with vomiting)

TABLE 11-5

Medications Used in the Treatment of Type 2 Diabetes Mellitus—cont'd

Medication	Mechanism of Action A1c Reduction	Comment
		occur with drug's use. Exenatide use not recommended with pancreatitis history. Use with caution in patient with mild-moderate renal impairment (creatinine clearance [Cr Cl]=30 to 50 mL/min [0.50–0.835 mL/s]). Do not use with Cr Cl<30 mL/min (<0.50 mL/s). Exenatide approved as add-on therapy with insulin glargine, with or without metformin in T2DM with inadequate glycemic control on insulin glargine alone.
Dipeptidyl peptidase-4 (DPP-4) inhibitor Examples: Sitagliptin (Januvia®), saxagliptin (Onglyza®), linagliptin (Tradjenta®), alogliptin (Nesina®)	Increases levels of incretin, increasing synthesis and release of insulin from pancreatic beta cells and decreasing release of glucagon from pancreatic alpha cells Anticipated A1C reduction with intensified used=0.6%–1.4%	Dose adjustment required in renal impairment. Well-tolerated, little hypoglycemia risk, weight-neutral Indicated to improve glycemic control, in combination with metformin or TZD Per FDA advisory, monitor patients carefully for the development of pancreatitis after initiation or dose increases of sitagliptin or sitagliptin/metformin. DPP-4 inhibitor use has not been studied in patients with a history of pancreatitis.
Sodium-glucose cotransporter 2 (SGLT2) inhibitor Canagliflozin (Invokana), dapagliflozin (Farxiga)	Lowers renal glucose threshold, increased urinary glucose excretion Anticipated A1C reduction with intensified use= 0.7%–1%	Increased risk of genital candidiasis with use. Less clinical effect with renal impairment.
Alpha-glucosidase inhibitors Examples: Acarbose (Precose®), miglitol (Glyset®)	Delays intestinal carbohydrate absorption by reducing postprandial digestion of starches and disaccharides via enzyme action inhibition Anticipated A1C reduction with intensified use=0.3%–0.9%	Taken with first bite of a meal Helpful in management of postprandial hyperglycemia Does not enhance insulin secretion or sensitivity. GI adverse effects an issue Avoid use in inflammatory bowel disease, impaired renal function.

insulin releases. Thus, a SU will appear to be less clinically effective during a hyperglycemic episode, such as during an acute illness, and its original effectiveness will resume once the blood sugar control improves.

Various additional oral and noninsulin injectable therapies are available for the treatment of type 2 DM. To prescribe these medications appropriately and effectively, the prescriber must know the mechanism of action, indications, anticipated adverse effects, contraindications, and anticipated benefit with the available medications (Table 11-5).

Insulin therapy is indicated for all patients with type 1 DM and patients with type 2 DM with insulinopenia; short-term insulin therapy is indicated when type 2 DM is initially diagnosed, particularly with glucose values greater than 250 to 300 mg/dL (greater than 13.9 to 16.7 mmol/L). Insulins come in many forms, from short-acting to long-acting forms with different onsets, peaks, and durations of action (Tables 11–5 and 11–6). The clinician needs to be aware of the characteristics of each insulin form and how these different products contribute to glycemic control. Keep in mind that the A1c

Algorithm for Drug Therapy in Type 2 Diabetes Mellitus

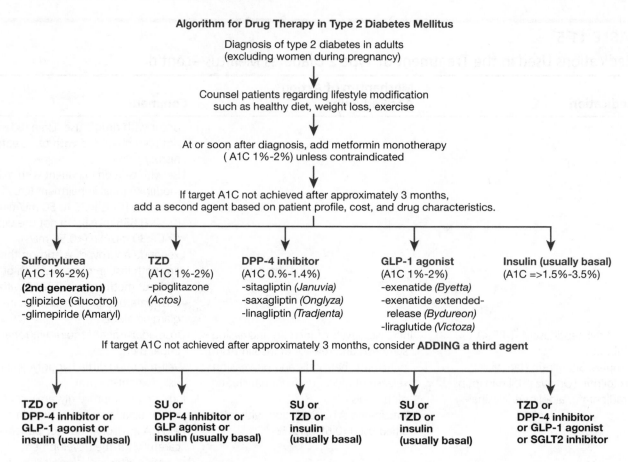

Diagnosis of type 2 diabetes in adults
(excluding women during pregnancy)

↓

Counsel patients regarding lifestyle modification
such as healthy diet, weight loss, exercise

↓

At or soon after diagnosis, add metformin monotherapy
(A1C 1%-2%) unless contraindicated

↓

If target A1C not achieved after approximately 3 months,
add a second agent based on patient profile, cost, and drug characteristics.

Sulfonylurea	TZD	DPP-4 inhibitor	GLP-1 agonist	Insulin (usually basal)
(A1C 1%-2%)	(A1C 1%-2%)	(A1C 0.%-1.4%)	(A1C 1%-2%)	(A1C =>1.5%-3.5%)
(2nd generation)	-pioglitazone	-sitagliptin *(Januvia)*	-exenatide *(Byetta)*	
-glipizide (Glucotrol)	*(Actos)*	-saxagliptin *(Onglyza)*	-exenatide extended-	
-glimepiride (Amaryl)		-linagliptin *(Tradjenta)*	release *(Bydureon)*	
			-liraglutide *(Victoza)*	

If target A1C not achieved after approximately 3 months, consider **ADDING** a third agent

TZD or	SU or	SU or	SU or	TZD or
DPP-4 inhibitor or	**DPP-4 inhibitor or**	**TZD or**	**TZD or**	**DPP-4 inhibitor**
GLP-1 agonist or	**GLP agonist or**	**insulin**	**insulin**	**or GLP-1 agonist**
insulin (usually basal)	**insulin (usually basal)**	**(usually basal)**	**(usually basal)**	**or SGLT2 inhibitor**

Note: Safe practice dictates that the prescriber be well informed as to the risks and benefits of all medications prescribed and be aware of the clinical indications for emerging therapies. See Table 11-5 for background information on these medications and prescribing information on each product for full details. Metformin with sulfonylurea therapy is usually the first line 2-drug therapy due to reasonable cost and clinical efficacy.

Figure 11-1 Algorithm for drug therapy in type 2 diabetes mellitus. Note: TZD should not be used with insulin.

lowering potential is nearly limitless, as the dose can be adjusted easily in response to persistent hyperglycemia. All currently available insulin forms are true bioidentical hormones—that is, replacing what the body would release naturally in the absence of insulinopenia. With insulin use, two conditions that can result in early morning hyperglycemia can occur. The Somogyi effect occurs when an insulin-induced hypoglycemia triggers excess secretion of glucagon and cortisol; this leads to hyperglycemia. Intervention is aimed at lowering the inappropriately high insulin dose, usually the dinnertime dose of intermediate-acting insulin. The dawn phenomenon is a result of reduced insulin sensitivity developing between 5 and 8 a.m., caused by earlier spikes in growth hormone. The net result is cortisol release, which triggers hepatic glucose secretion and early morning hyperglycemia. Intervention for the dawn phenomenon includes splitting the evening intermediate insulin dose between dinner and bedtime. Alternative interventions include switching to a bedtime dose of insulin glargine or an insulin pump.

DM is the leading cause of chronic renal failure. After the diagnosis of DM is made, periodic screening of renal function should be done (Table 11–7). Often serum creatinine measurement is used for this purpose. An increase in creatinine is

not seen, however, until at least 50% of the nephrons are not functioning. An elevated creatinine level is a late rather than early indicator of renal damage. A far more sensitive indicator of diabetic nephropathy is the presence of proteinuria, a harbinger of progressive renal failure. Urine protein consists of many forms, including the most abundant, albumin, and immunoglobulin, haptoglobin, and light chains. The standard dipstick test is sensitive to 100 to 150 mg/L of urine albumin, an earlier marker of progressive renal failure than serum creatinine, but still a later disease marker. The persistent presence of a small amount of albumin (microalbumin) is considered a predictor of glomerular dysfunction associated with diabetic nephropathy.

Microalbuminuria can precede development of DM by 10 years. With type 2 DM, the patient should be screened for microalbuminuria at onset of disease, with an annual recheck if results are normal. Collection of a first morning specimen is important because normal daily activity may cause a low level of protein spillage into the urine, creating a false-positive result. The diagnosis of microalbuminuria should be confirmed by obtaining at least two positive results from three collections in a 3 to 6 month period; results should be correlated with serum creatinine level. Intervention includes

TABLE 11-6
When to Use Insulin in DM Treatment

TYPE 1 DM	TYPE 2 DM
• All patients • Basal insulin (50% of total daily insulin requirements) with adjustments for meals and snacks (50% of total daily insulin requirements) via multiple injections or pump	• At time of diagnosis to help achieve initial glycemic control, particularly when glucose values >250–300 mg/dL (13.9–16.7 mmol/L) • When acutely ill • In critically ill surgical and nonsurgical patients with type 1 or type 2 DM, blood glucose levels should be kept generally 140 mg/dL–180 mg/dL (7.8–10 mmol/L). Overtreatment and undertreatment of hyperglycemia represent major safety concerns. • When ≥2 oral agents at optimized use are inadequate to maintain glycemic control

Source: American Diabetes Association Clinical Practice Recommendations, Diabetes Care January 2014; 37:Supplement 1 S1; doi:10.2337/dc14-S001.

tightening of glycemic control to appropriate goal for overall patient condition, controlling elevated blood pressure, treatment of dyslipidemia, and addition of a medication recommended for use in individuals with concomitant type 2 DM and hypertension according to the ADA recommendations, including angiotensin-converting enzyme inhibitors (drugs whose names have the "-pril" suffix—lisinopril, enalapril, others), angiotensin receptor blockers (drugs whose names have the "-sartan" suffix), beta blockers (drugs whose names have the "-lol" suffix—metoprolol, atenolol), alpha-beta blockers (also "-lol" suffix—carvedilol, others), and calcium channel blockers (amlodipine [Norvasc®], diltiazem [Cardizem®, others], verapamil [Calan®, Verelan®, others]). Although use of beta blockers and alpha-beta blockers in patients with DM was discouraged or contraindicated in the past, current practice supports the use of this drug class

TABLE 11-7
Guidelines for Adult Diabetes Mellitus Care

		Frequency	Description/Comments
HEALTH HISTORY AND PHYSICAL EXAMINATION	Blood pressure (BP), height and weight	Every 3–6 mo	Goal BP <140/<90, initiate measures to lower at this level with lifestyle modification and medication.
	Dilated eye examination	Annual, more often with progressive retinopathy	Refer to eye care specialist
	Foot examination	Initial/annual	Visual examination without shoes and socks every routine diabetes visit
	Comprehensive lower extremity sensory examination	Initial/annual	Teach protective foot behavior if sensation diminished. Refer to podiatrist if indicated
	Dental examination	Every 6 mo	Refer to a dentist, reinforce ongoing dental care
	Smoking, tobacco use status	Ongoing	Check every visit. Encourage smoking cessation
LABORATORY TESTS	A1c	Every 3–6 mo	Goal A1c according to individual benefit/ risks
	Fasting/postprandial blood glucose	As indicated	Compare laboratory results with glucose self-monitoring

Continued

TABLE 11-7

Guidelines for Adult Diabetes Mellitus Care—cont'd

		Frequency	**Description/Comments**
	Fasting lipid profile	Annual, consider less often with stable levels	As part of comprehensive plan to reduce cardiovascular disease risk
	Urine microalbumin/ creatinine	Initial/annual	If abnormal, recheck (2 in a 3-mo period, then treat if 2 out of 3 collections show elevated levels
	Serum creatinine	Annual	Measure annually for estimation of glomerular filtration rate
	EKG	Initial	If patient ≥40 y.o. or DM ≥10 yr
	Thyroid assessment	Initial/as indicated	Thyroid palpitation, thyroid function test(s) if indicated
RECOMMENDED IMMUNIZATIONS	Influenza	Annually in anticipation of seasonal influenza	Influenza vaccine form should be guided by standard vaccine practice.
	Antipneumococcal vaccine	Recommended	See latest recommendations on use of PCV23 and PCV13 vaccines.
	Hepatitis B vaccine	If < 60 y.o. at time as DM diagnosis, immunize as soon as possible after diagnosis	If ≥60 y.o., at the discretion of the treating clinician based on increased need for assisted blood glucose monitoring in long-term care facilities, likelihood of acquiring hepatitis B infection, its complications or chronic sequelae, and likelihood of immune response to vaccination
SELF-MANAGEMENT SKILLS AND PATIENT COUNSELING	Review self-management skills	Initial/ongoing	Reinforce healthy habits, monitoring, sick day care
	Review treatment plan	Initial/ongoing	Check self-monitoring log book, diet, physical activity, and medications
	Review education plan	Initial/ongoing	Refer for diabetes self-management education as indicated
	Review nutrition plan	Initial/ongoing	Refer for medical nutrition therapy as indicated
	Review physical activity plan	Initial/ongoing	Assess/prescribe based on patient's health status
	Tobacco use	Annual/ongoing	Assess readiness, counsel about cessation. Refer to smoking cessation program.
	Psychosocial adjustment	Initial/ongoing	Suggest diabetes support group. Counsel and refer as indicated

TABLE 11-7

Guidelines for Adult Diabetes Mellitus Care—cont'd

	Frequency	Description/Comments
Sexuality/erectile dysfunction	Annual/ongoing	Discuss diagnostic evaluation and therapeutic options
Preconception/pregnancy	Initial/ongoing	Need for tight glucose control 3–6 mo preconception. Consider early referral to high risk prenatal care

Source: American Diabetes Association Clinical Practice Recommendations, Diabetes Care January 2014 37: Supplement 1 S1; doi:10.2337/dc14-S001.

because of its ability to reduce the target population's considerable cardiovascular risk. In the presence of type 2 diabetes mellitus, dyslipidemia and hypertension must be aggressively treated to minimize risk of cardiovascular disease. Daily aspirin use is recommended to counteract the proinflammatory and prothrombotic effects of IR.

Known by numerous names, such as syndrome X, Reaven's syndrome, the "deadly quartet," metabolic cardiovascular syndrome, and cardiovascular dysmetabolic syndrome, the term metabolic syndrome is now most commonly used to describe a complex health problem that usually includes three or more of the following: obesity, blood pressure problems, dyslipidemia, and glucose intolerance (Table 11–8). Various definitions for

metabolic syndrome have been offered by well-regarded groups, including the World Health Organization (WHO). Although the definitions offered by these groups are similar, the nuanced differences in them have led to confusion, particularly when attempting to compare data from studies using different definitions. Also uncertain was which, if any, of the definitions best detected persons at risk of cardiovascular disease (CVD) and DM.

To facilitate the use of a single definition, the International Diabetes Federation (IDF) has issued a global consensus statement, proposing a consensus definition of metabolic syndrome that reflects input from experts on six continents in the fields of diabetes, cardiology, endocrinology, genetics,

TABLE 11-8

Diagnostic Criteria for Metabolic Syndrome

World Health Organization	Adult Treatment Panel (ATP) III	International Diabetes Federation
Insulin resistance (type 2 diabetes mellitus or impaired fasting glucose) plus ≥2 of the following • Abdominal/central obesity defined as a waist-to-hip ratio >0.90 (men), >0.85 (women), or BMI ≥30 kg/m² • Hypertriglyceridemia ≥150 mg/dL (≥1.7 mmol/L) • Low HDL cholesterol <35 mg/dL (<0.9 mmol/L) for men, or <39 mg/dL (<1 mmol/L) for women • High BP ≥140/90 mm Hg or documented use of antihypertensive therapy	≥3 of the following • Waist circumference: >102 cm (>40 in) in men, >88 cm (>35 in) in women • Hypertriglyceridemia ≥150 mg/dL (≥1.7 mmol/L) • Low HDL cholesterol <40 mg/dL (<1.036 mmol/L) for men, <50 mg/dL (<1.295 mmol/L) for women • BP ≥130/ ≥85 mm Hg or documented use of antihypertensive therapy • Fasting glucose ≥100 mg/dL (≥5.6 mmol/L)	Central obesity, defined as ethnic-specific waist circumference European, sub-Saharan African, Eastern Mediterranean, Middle Eastern (Arabic) ancestry • Men ≥94 cm (≥37 in) • Women ≥80 cm (≥31.5 in) South Asian, Chinese, ethnic South and Central American ancestry • Men ≥90 cm (≥35.5 in) • Women ≥80 cm (≥31.5 in) Japanese ancestry • Men ≥90 cm (≥35.5 in) • Women ≥80 cm (≥31.5 in) with ≥2 of the following • Abnormal triglycerides ≥150 mg/dL (≥1.7 mmol/L)

Continued

TABLE 11-8

Diagnostic Criteria for Metabolic Syndrome—cont'd

World Health Organization	Adult Treatment Panel (ATP) III	International Diabetes Federation
• Microalbuminuria with urinary albumin-to-creatinine ratio 30 mg/g, or albumin excretion rate 20 mcg/min		• HDL-cholesterol <40 mg/dL (<1.03 mmol/L) in men, <50 mg/dL (<1.29 mmol/L) in women • BP ≥130 mm Hg systolic or ≥85 mm Hg diastolic or treatment of previously diagnosed hypertension • Fasting glucose ≥100 mg/dL (≥5.6 mmol/L) or previous diagnosis of type 2 diabetes or impaired glucose tolerance

BMI—body mass index; BP—blood pressure; HDL—high density lipoprotein.

and nutrition. The IDF diagnostic criteria for metabolic syndrome closely resemble the current ATP III definition but with stricter criteria for glucose intolerance and ethnic differences when defining central obesity; this definition does not include any measure of IR, and hyperglycemia is not an obligatory component, which sets it apart from the definitions offered by WHO and EGIR. The majority of individuals with type 2 DM have metabolic syndrome. Treatment should follow accordingly.

DISCUSSION SOURCES

American Association of Clinical Endocrinologists' Comprehensive Diabetes Management Consensus Statement, *Endocr Pract* 2013;19 (Suppl 1):1-48

American Diabetes Association Clinical Practice Recommendations, Diabetes Care January 2014 37:Supplement 1 S1; doi:10.2337/dc14-S001.

Massachusetts Guidelines for Adult Diabetic Care. www.mass.gov/.../diabetes/diabetes-guidelines-exec-summary.doc.

International Diabetes Federation. A new worldwide definition of the metabolic syndrome. www.idf.org/webdata/docs/IDF_Meta_def_final.pdf.

Riethof M, Flavin PL, Lindvall B, Michels R, O'Connor P, Redmon B, Retzer K, Roberts J, Smith S, Sperl Hillen J. Institute for Clinical Systems Improvement. Diagnosis and Management of Type 2 Diabetes Mellitus in Adults. http://bit.ly/Diabetes0412. https://www.aace.com/files/algorithm-07-11-2013.pdf

See full color images of this topic on DavisPlus at **http://davisplus.fadavis.com** | **Keyword: Fitzgerald**

Heatstroke

56. Risk factors for heatstroke include all of the following except:
    A. obesity.
    B. use of beta-adrenergic antagonists.
    C. excessive activity.
    D. use of a vasodilator.

57. Possible adverse outcomes from heatstroke include:
    A. rhabdomyolysis.
    B. anemia.
    C. hypernatremia.
    D. leukopenia.

58. Laboratory findings in heatstroke usually include:
    A. elevated total creatine kinase.
    B. anemia.
    C. metabolic alkalosis.
    D. hypokalemia.

59. Intervention for patients with heatstroke includes:
    A. total body ice packing.
    B. rehydration.
    C. fluid restriction.
    D. potassium supplementation.

Answers

56.	D.	58.	A.
57.	A.	59.	B.

Heatstroke is a life-threatening emergency caused by a failure of the body's thermoregulatory system, usually in response to extreme environmental and personal factors. In exertional heatstroke, the illness has been triggered by exercise in a warm environment that adds to the thermal load produced by the muscular contraction. In addition, a protracted period of exercise, such as running a marathon or participating in a long football practice, usually poses greatest risk. Nonexertional heatstroke is noted in the presence of extreme environmental heat, usually defined as more than 10°F (12.2° C) greater than is typical for the given geographic area for more than 3 days, and poses a particular risk to segments of the population who have the most difficulty with body temperature self-regulation including the very young (infants) and the elderly.

Risk factors for heatstroke include the use of medications that alter adrenergic activity and possibly decrease cardiac output (negative inotrope), such as tricyclic antidepressants (drugs whose names have the "-triptyline" suffix), beta-adrenergic antagonists, or beta blockers (drugs whose names have the "-lol" suffix), and vasoconstrictors, such as oral decongestants. The use of these products negates the body's normal attempts to decrease core temperature, such as increasing cardiac output and cutaneous vasodilation. Obesity limits the ability of the body to dissipate heat and is considered a heatstroke risk factor. In addition, as mentioned previously, extremes of age, very young or very old, with the associated difficulties in maintaining body temperature, increases heatstroke risk. Alcohol use also increases risk. Adequate hydration with nonalcoholic fluids, particularly water, coupled with dressing lightly helps to minimize heatstroke risk.

Individuals who participate in strenuous activity during hot weather should be warned about early heatstroke symptoms, such as extreme increase in heart rate, headache usually described as pounding, and difficulty breathing. If any of these symptoms occur, the physical activity should be discontinued immediately, and the person should move to a shady location and drink cool water. If symptoms do not dissipate rapidly, help should be sought.

Assessment of a patient with heatstroke includes a complete evaluation of electrolytes, hematologic parameters, and liver enzymes. Total creatine kinase (CK) level is typically elevated, owing to skeletal muscle injured by muscle cramping and convulsion releasing this enzyme. Because of the release of this intracellular electrolyte with tissue damage, hyperkalemia is common; potentially life-threatening levels can be reached. Heatstroke can lead to a transient polycythemia caused by volume constriction, hyponatremia with Na^+ level of less than 120 mEq/L (less than 120 mmol/L), and stress-induced leukocytosis.

Intervention for a patient with heatstroke includes controlled cooling by the use of tepid sprays and fanning or by the application of cold packs to select areas such as the axillae, neck, and groin. Rapid cooling by total body ice packing is discouraged because this can stimulate cutaneous vasoconstriction, inhibiting heat loss. Rehydration should be aggressive, but with careful monitoring because of the risk of pulmonary edema from reduced cardiac output.

Optimally, a patient with heatstroke should be admitted to the hospital for at least 24 hours after stabilization because of the risk of late complications, including one of the most feared complications: rhabdomyolysis, a condition of rapid muscle tissue destruction. As the muscle breaks down, large amounts of myoglobin and other cellular products are released into circulation to be excreted by the kidney. Renal hypoperfusion from low blood pressure is common. As a result, about 50% of patients with rhabdomyolysis develop acute renal failure. In heatstroke, the presence of myoglobinuria is an early indicator of rhabdomyolysis. Typically, the patient also complains of muscle pain and weakness. Treatment of rhabdomyolysis is aimed at treating the potentially life-threatening consequences, such as renal failure and profound hyperkalemia.

DISCUSSION SOURCES

Centers for Disease Control and Prevention. Extreme heat: a prevention guide to promote your personal health and safety. www.bt.cdc.gov/disasters/extremeheat/heat_guide.asp.

Helman, R, Habal, R, http://emedicine.medscape.com/article/166320, heatstroke.

Obesity

60. Obesity is defined as having a body mass index (BMI) equal to or greater than _____ kg/m².
    A. 25
    B. 30
    C. 35
    D. 40

61. An example of an appropriate question to pose to a person with obesity who is in the precontemplation change stage is:
    A. "How do you feel about your weight?"
    B. "What are barriers you see to losing weight?"
    C. "What is your personal goal for weight loss?"
    D. "How do you envision my helping you meet your weight loss goal?"

62. An example of an appropriate question to pose to a person with obesity who is in the contemplation change stage is:
    A. "How do you feel about your weight?"
    B. "What are barriers you see to losing weight?"
    C. "What is your personal goal for weight loss?"
    D. "How do you envision my helping you meet your weight loss goal?"

63. When advising a person who will be using orlistat (Xenical®, Alli®) as part of a weight loss program, the NP provides the following information about when to take the medication:
    A. within an hour of each meal that contains fat.
    B. before any food with high carbohydrate content.
    C. only in the morning, to avoid sleep disturbance.
    D. up to 3 hours after any meal, regardless of types of food eaten.

64. The action of which of the following is believed to be most responsible for the sensation of satiety?
    A. norepinephrine
    B. epinephrine
    C. dopamine
    D. serotonin

65. A pound of fat contains approximately _____ stored calories.
    A. 2500
    B. 3000
    C. 3500
    D. 4000

66. The commonly recommended physical activity level of 10,000 steps per day is roughly the equivalent of walking _____ miles.
    A. 1 to 2
    B. 2 to 3
    C. 3 to 4
    D. 4 to 5

67. With the use of weight loss medications, if the patient has not achieved a 5% weight loss by week ___ of treatment, the therapy should be discontinued.
    A. 6
    B. 12
    C. 18
    D. 24

68. In a person with obesity, weight loss of _____% or more yields an immediate reduction in death rates from cardiovascular and cerebrovascular disease.
    A. 5
    B. 10
    C. 15
    D. 20

69. When counseling about malabsorptive bariatric surgery, the NP provides the following information:
    A. Most people achieve ideal BMI postoperatively.
    B. The most dramatic weight losses are seen in the first few postoperative months.
    C. The death rate directly attributable to surgery is about 10%.
    D. Weight loss will continue for years postoperatively in most patients.

70. The use of which of the following medications is often associated with weight gain?
    A. risperidone (Risperdal®)
    B. topiramate (Topamax®)
    C. metformin (Glucophage)
    D. sitagliptin (Januvia®)

71. You are counseling a patient who is considering gastric bypass surgery for weight loss. You advise the following. (More than one can apply.)
    A. Calcium absorption will be reduced.
    B. Rapid weight loss after obesity surgery can contribute to the development of gallstones.
    C. Chronic constipation is a common postoperative adverse effect.
    D. Lifelong vitamin B12 supplementation is recommended.

72 to 75. Weight loss medications: True or false?

____ 72. Lorcaserin (Belviq®) should not be used with medications that have serotonergic effect.

____ 73. Phentermine/ topiramate (Qsymia®) carries a warning about potential teratogenic effects.

____ 74. Phentermine's mechanism of action in weight loss is as a product that reduces GI motility.

____ 75. In general, weight lost post gastric bypass is significantly more when compared with the postoperative course of a restrictive procedure such as adjustable gastric band.

76. Which of the following are possible consequences of obesity? (More than one can apply.)
    A. Obstructive apnea
    B. Steatohepatitis
    C. Female infertility
    D. Endometrial cancer

◗ Answers

60. B.	66. D.	72. True
61. A.	67. B.	73. True
62. B.	68. B.	74. False
63. A.	69. B.	75. True
64. D.	70. A.	76. A, B, C, D
65. C.	71. A, B, D	

Rates of obesity, usually defined as a body mass index (BMI) of 30 kg/m² or greater (Table 11–9), in North America are currently at record levels and are projected to double over the next 30 years; this mirrors the overall increase in overweight and obesity rates worldwide. Although no specific endocrine disorder, including thyroid dysfunction, is usually found in obese individuals, the cause of the overweight and obese condition is likely a combination of environmental, genetic, and behavioral influences. Consequences of overweight and obesity include increased risk of all-cause morbidity and mortality, greater healthcare cost, lower workforce productivity, and increased workplace absentee rates and employer costs. Direct healthcare cost increases related to obesity are attributable largely to well-known obesity-related disease, including gallbladder disease, coronary heart disease, DM, osteoarthritis, and dyslipidemia. Less commonly known consequences

TABLE 11-9
Classification of Overweight and Obesity

Body Mass Index (kg/m²)	WHO Classification	CDC Description
<18.5	Underweight	Underweight
18.5–24.9	Grade 1 overweight	Healthy weight
25–29.9	Grade 2 overweight	Overweight
30–39.9	Grade 3 overweight	Obesity
≥40		Extremely obese

of obesity include an increase in sleep apnea risk, a reduction in female fertility, and nonalcoholic fatty liver including steatohepatitis. Obesity is also associated with increased risks of cancers of the esophagus, postmenopausal breast, endometrium, colon and rectum, kidney, pancreas, thyroid, gallbladder, and possibly other cancer types; the correlation between these cancers and obesity is likely, in part, due to the chronic inflammatory state caused by increased adiposity. Less tangible are issues of social and workplace discrimination.

Often, persons who are overweight or obese assume that only dramatic weight loss can produce healthy results. In reality, a 10% body weight loss yields a nearly immediate improvement of death rates from heart disease and stroke. Clinical improvement in osteoarthritis and asthma symptoms and a reduction in sleep apnea symptoms are usually noted.

The NP is well situated to help a person with obesity. For a person who desires weight loss, a first step is the discussion of achievable, reasonable goals. A first step can be simply to help the person halt weight gain or to lose 5% to 10% of total body weight. Slow, steady weight loss usually leads to long-term health benefit and risk reduction. A pound of fat contains approximately 3500 stored calories. A deficit of 500 to 1000 calories per day would lead to a 1 to 2 lb (0.45 to 0.9 kg) weight loss per week. Physical activity is often the most difficult part of a comprehensive weight reduction program. The idea of a protracted walking or other exercise regimen is quite daunting for a person who is obese. Although 30 minutes or more of aerobic activity on 5 days or more per week is typically recommended, an exercise prescription of 3 to 5 minutes of increased physical activity five to six times per day would likely yield the same results and be much better tolerated. A pedometer can also be used to measure objectively the number of steps taken; the goal should be 10,000 per day, or the equivalent of walking 4 to 5 miles. A pedometer is one method of quantifying how physically active in day-to-day behavior and deliberate exercise the person is. In addition, increased physical activity improves overall cardiac health and improves insulin sensitivity.

A comprehensive approach to obesity treatment that includes behavior modification and pharmacotherapy that result in decreased food intake and increased energy expenditure can lead to long-term success. Asking about readiness for change at every clinical visit can help facilitate success (Table 11–10).

TABLE 11-10
Facilitating Change in the Care of a Person Who Is Overweight or Obese

Stage	Questions to Ask	As the Provider, You Can:
PRECONTEMPLATION (NOT INTERESTED IN CHANGE)	• How do you feel about your weight? • How does your weight affect you? • Are you considering/planning weight loss now? • On a scale of 0–10, how ready are you to start a weight loss program?	Validate and acknowledge • This will take working together but can be done. Restate position, leave the door open • It's up to you to make the decision to lose weight. I cannot do this for you, but I am here to help you.
CONTEMPLATION (THINKING ABOUT CHANGE)	• What are the pros and cons of weight loss? • Where are you on the scale of 0–10 as far as ready? • What are barriers/supports you envision? • How do you view me as helping?	Praise and validate • I am happy that you want to deal with this issue and feel ready to do so. Try to shift decisional balance • I am here to help you and point you in the direction of other sources of support. Arrange follow-up

Continued

TABLE 11-10

Facilitating Change in the Care of a Person Who Is Overweight or Obese—cont'd

Stage	Questions to Ask	As the Provider, You Can:
PREPARATION FOR CHANGE	• What is your usual food and activity pattern? • What is your personal goal for weight loss? • Health goal? • Cosmetic goal?	Help set small behavioral goals related to diet, physical activity Assist in compiling food and activity diaries Begin to negotiate goal weight Identify support system Help set a date to start
MAKING CHANGE *MAINTAINING CHANGE* *DEALING WITH RELAPSE*	• How can I help? • What is getting in your way? • What is making this work?	Teach nutritional tactics to help control obesity • Learn energy values of different foods Monitor food consumption by keeping a food diary; reduce portion size Read and understand nutrition labels on foods • Learn new habits of food purchasing • Eliminate high-calorie foods from grocery list Limit fats and oils in cooking, recipes; high-calorie or "calorie-dense" foods Increase physical activity

Source: Center for Disease Control and Prevention, Obesity, available at http://www.cdc.gov/obesity/.

Pharmacotherapy is an important tool in weight management. Many antiobesity drugs are available. Orlistat (Xenical, Alli) is taken with meals and contributes to weight loss by reducing dietary fat absorption by approximately 30%. The fat passes undigested, and weight loss is facilitated. The medication is taken three times daily with or within 1 hour of a meal that contains fat. The most common adverse effect is gastrointestinal disturbance, including loose stools and oily anal seepage. Older medications, sympathomimetics such as dexamphetamine and phentermine (Fastin®, others), work with norepinephrine and dopamine, reducing the appetite, with resulting reduction in food intake. Sleep disturbances and nervousness rank among the most adverse effects associated with the use of these medications.

Qsymia is a fixed dose combination of phentermine and topiramate that is FDA approved for weight management in adults with an initial BMI of 30 kg/m2 or greater or 27 kg/m2 or greater when accompanied by weight-related comorbidities such as hypertension, type 2 DM, or dyslipidemia. The effect of phentermine is likely mediated by release of catecholamines, including norepinephrine in the hypothalamus, resulting in reduced appetite and decreased food consumption. The precise mechanism of action of topiramate on weight management is not known; the use of this medication has been associated with appetite suppression and satiety. Due to the topiramate portion of Qsymia, women of reproductive potential should have a negative pregnancy test before starting Qsymia and monthly thereafter during Qsymia

therapy and use a highly effective form of contraception while taking the medication.

Lorcaserin (Belviq) is believed to decrease food consumption and promote satiety by selectively activating 5-HT2C receptors on anorexigenic neurons located in the hypothalamus. Given this medication's mechanism of action, it is used with other medications with serotonergic properties such as the triptans, monoamine oxidase inhibitors (MAOIs), selective serotonin reuptake inhibitors (SSRIs), selective serotonin norepinephrine reuptake inhibitors (SNRIs), dextromethorphan, tricyclic antidepressants (TCAs), bupropion, lithium, tramadol, tryptophan, and St. John's wort. With weight loss drugs, the medication should be discontinued if the patient has not achieved a 5% weight loss by week 12 of treatment; in this circumstance, the weight loss medication is unlikely to be helpful in weight reduction.

As with many other weight loss approaches, weight loss plateaus and then may slowly increase, particularly if lifestyle modification does not include increased activity and decreased caloric intake.

The use of certain medications can result in weight gain. These medications include atypical or second generation antipsychotics (risperidone [Risperdal], olanzapine [Zyprexa®], others), select antiepileptics (valproate [Depakote®], carbamazepine [Tegretol®], others), and corticosteroids (prednisone, methylprednisolone, others). The use of these medications is occasionally necessary in a person with obesity. The patient should be advised about the risk, and weight-controlling efforts would need to be intensified.

Numerous surgical options are available for obesity intervention. The most common options include gastric bypass and adjustable laparoscopic band. The ideal candidate for a bariatric surgical procedure is a person with BMI equal to or greater than 40 kg/m² or BMI equal to or greater than 35 kg/m² who also has DM, hypertension, dyslipidemia obstructive sleep apnea, cardiovascular disease, gastroesophageal reflux, degenerative joint disease, fatty liver (steatohepatitis), or other obesity-related conditions in whom behavioral and pharmacological therapy has failed. Contraindications to bariatric surgery include untreated or unstable mental health conditions, active drug or alcohol abuse, poor adherence to advised health regimens, and concomitant health conditions that would pose significant operative risk. The Roux-en-Y gastroplasty, or gastric bypass, is one of the more common restrictive/malabsorptive bariatric surgeries. With gastric bypass, not only is the stomach size dramatically reduced, thus limiting intake, the food that is eaten no longer passes over the duodenum, the part of the gastrointestinal tract where calories are normally absorbed. The adjustable laparoscopic band procedure, in which the stomach volume is restricted, is an intervention that does not lead to malabsorption because food still passes through the duodenum, but rather restricts the amount of calories that can be ingested. High-calorie soft or liquid foods, such as milkshakes and ice cream, can pass through the band, however, and the calories in these foods are absorbed.

A person considering bariatric surgery must have a realistic idea regarding the anticipated outcome. In a well-selected patient population, the average weight loss with the gastric band procedure is approximately 40% to 60% of excess body weight. With gastric bypass, the expected weight loss is approximately 70% to 80% of excess body weight. With either procedure, most of that weight is lost within the first 3 years after surgery, and the most dramatic weight losses are seen in the first months postoperatively. With either procedure, future weight regain can occur if recommended dietary and physical activity guidelines are not followed. About 85% of patients lose a great deal of weight without major complications and maintain this loss long-term. About 10% have a significant short-term problem after the surgery (e.g., reoperation, long hospital stay, insufficient weight loss, persistent gastrointestinal upset), but most do well in the long-term. Less than 5% have major unresolved problems over time, including, for some and rarely, death as a direct result of the surgery. With all bariatric surgery, but in particular the malabsorptive procedures, expert consultation on continued micronutrient supplementation should be sought to avoid anemia and other health problems. Micronutrient supplementation is needed post procedure; this supplementation usually includes vitamin B12, iron, zinc, calcium, protein, and most fat soluble vitamins. Given the alteration in the GI tract post gastric bypass, absorption of certain medications is altered. In particular, the use of combined oral contraceptives (estrogen/progestin-containing) is not recommended post gastric bypass due to risk of contraceptive failure related to lower drug absorption. Study on other medications is ongoing.

DISCUSSION SOURCES

Center for Chronic Disease Prevention and Health Promotion. Overweight and obesity. www.cdc.gov/nccdphp/dnpa/obesity.
Hamdy O, Griffing G. Obesity Treatment and Management. http://emedicine.medscape.com/article/123702-treatment.

Thyroid Disorders

77. Increased risk of thyroid disorder is found in individuals who are:
    A. obese.
    B. hypertensive.
    C. treated with systemic corticosteroids.
    D. elderly.

78. A 48-year-old woman with newly diagnosed hypothyroidism asks about a "natural thyroid" medication she read about online and provides the drug's name, desiccated thyroid. As you counsel her about this medication, you consider all of the following except:
    A. This product is contains a fixed dose of T3 and T4.
    B. The medication is a planted-based product.
    C. Its pharmacokinetics differ significantly when compared to levothyroxine.
    D. The majority of the study on treatment for hypothyroidism has been done using levothyroxine.

79. Hypothyroidism most often develops as a result of:
    A. primary pituitary failure.
    B. thyroid neoplasia.
    C. autoimmune thyroiditis.
    D. radioactive iodine exposure.

80. Which is following is the least helpful test for the assessment of thyroid disease?
    A. Total T4
    B. TSH
    C. Free T4
    D. Antithyroid antibodies

81. Physical examination findings in patients with Graves' disease include:
    A. muscle tenderness.
    B. coarse, dry skin.
    C. eyelid retraction.
    D. delayed relaxation phase of the patellar reflex.

82. The mechanism of action of radioactive iodine in the treatment of Graves' disease is to:
    A. destroy the overactive thyroid tissue.
    B. reduce production of TSH.
    C. alter thyroid metabolic rate.
    D. relieve distress caused by increased thyroid size.

83. Which of the following medications is a helpful treatment option for relief of tremor and tachycardia seen with untreated hyperthyroidism?
    A. propranolol
    B. diazepam
    C. carbamazepine
    D. verapamil

84. In prescribing levothyroxine therapy for an elderly patient, which of the following statements is true?
    A. Elderly persons require a rapid initiation of levothyroxine therapy.
    B. TSH should be checked about 2 days after dosage adjustment.
    C. The levothyroxine dose needed by elderly persons is 75% or less of that needed by younger adults.
    D. TSH should be suppressed to a nondetectable level.

85. Thyroid stimulating hormone (TSH) is released by the:
    A. thyroid follicles.
    B. adrenal cortex.
    C. hypothalamus
    D. anterior lobe of the pituitary.

86. In the report of a thyroid scan done on a 48-year-old woman with a thyroid mass, a "cold spot" is reported. This finding is most consistent with:
    A. autonomously functioning adenoma.
    B. Graves' disease.
    C. Hashimoto's disease.
    D. thyroid cyst.

87. You advise a 58-year-old woman with hypothyroidism about the correct use of levothyroxine. She also takes a calcium supplement. All of the following information should be shared with the patient except:
    A. Take the medication on an empty stomach.
    B. To help with adherence, take your calcium supplement at the same time as your thyroid medication.
    C. You should to take the medication at approximately the same time every day.
    D. Do not take your medication with soy milk.

88. The findings of a painless thyroid mass and TSH level of less than 0.1 IU/mL in a 35-year-old woman is most consistent with:
    A. autonomously functioning adenoma.
    B. Graves' disease.
    C. Hashimoto's disease.
    D. thyroid malignancy.

89. A fixed, painless thyroid mass accompanied by hoarseness and dysphagia should raise the suspicion of:
    A. adenomatous lesion.
    B. Graves' disease.
    C. Hashimoto's disease.
    D. thyroid malignancy.

90. Which of the following is the most cost-effective method of distinguishing a malignant from a benign thyroid nodule?
    A. ultrasound
    B. magnetic resonance imaging
    C. fine-needle aspiration biopsy
    D. radioactive iodine scan

91. Possible consequences of excessive levothyroxine use include:
    A. bone thinning.
    B. fatigue.
    C. renal impairment.
    D. constipation.

92. Optimally, at what interval should TSH be reassessed after a levothyroxine dosage is adjusted?
    A. 1 to 2 weeks
    B. 2 to 4 weeks
    C. 4 to 6 weeks
    D. 6 to 8 weeks

93. As part of an evaluation of a 3-cm, round, mobile thyroid mass, you obtain a thyroid ultrasound scan revealing a fluid-filled structure. The most likely diagnosis is:
    A. adenoma.
    B. thyroid cyst.
    C. multinodular goiter.
    D. vascular lesion.

94. Periodic routine screening for hypothyroidism is indicated in the presence of which of the following clinical conditions?
    A. digoxin use
    B. male gender
    C. Down syndrome
    D. alcoholism

95 to 111. Identify each of the following findings as associated with hyperthyroidism, hypothyroidism, or both.

____ **95.** heat intolerance

____ **96.** smooth, silky skin

____ **97.** goiter

____ **98.** frequent, low-volume, loose stools

____ **99.** secondary hypertriglyceridemia

____ **100.** amenorrhea or oligomenorrhea

____ **101.** coarse, dry skin

____ **102.** menorrhagia

____ **103.** hyperreflexia with a characteristic "quick out–quick back" action at the patellar reflex

____ **104.** proximal muscle weakness

____ **105.** tachycardia with hypertension

_____ **106.** hyporeflexia with a characteristic slow relaxation phase, the "hung-up" reflex

_____ **107.** coarse hair with tendency to break easily

_____ **108.** thick, dry nails

_____ **109.** constipation

_____ **110.** atypical presentation in an elderly person

_____ **111.** change in mental status

112. The use of which of the following medications can induce thyroid dysfunction?
A. Sertraline
B. Venlafaxine
C. Bupropion
D. Lithium

113 to 115. Match the condition with the laboratory results: hypothyroidism, hyperthyroidism, or subclinical hypothyroidism

_____ **113.** TSH=8.9 mIU/L (0.4 to 4.0 mIU/L); free T4= 15 pmol/L (10 to 27 pmol/L)

_____ **114.** TSH less than 0.15 mIU/L (0.4 to 4.0 mIU/L); free T4=79 pmol/L (10 to 27 pmol/L)

_____ **115.** TSH= 24 mIU/L (0.4 to 4.0 mIU/L); free T4= 3 pmol/L (10 to 27 pmol/L)

Answers

77.	D.	**97.**	Both
78.	B.	**98.**	Hyperthyroidism
79.	C.	**99.**	Hypothyroidism
80.	A.	**100.**	Hyperthyroidism
81.	C.	**101.**	Hypothyroidism
82.	A.	**102.**	Hypothyroidism
83.	A.	**103.**	Hyperthyroidism
84.	C.	**104.**	Hyperthyroidism
85.	D.	**105.**	Hyperthyroidism
86.	D.	**106.**	Hypothyroidism
87.	B.	**107.**	Hypothyroidism
88.	A.	**108.**	Hypothyroidism
89.	D.	**109.**	Hypothyroidism
90.	C.	**110.**	Both
91.	A.	**111.**	Both
92.	D.	**112.**	D.
93.	B.	**113.**	Subclinical hypothyroidism
94.	C.		
95.	Hyperthyroidism	**114.**	Hyperthyroidism
96.	Hyperthyroidism	**115.**	Hypothyroidism

Thyroid hormone acts as a cellular energy release catalyst and is essential to normal body function. When assessing a patient with thyroid dysfunction, the NP should look for signs of excessive energy release in hyperthyroidism or decreased energy release in hypothyroidism. Hyperthyroidism or hypothyroidism signs and symptoms often are present in the history and physical examination (Table 11–11).

TABLE 11-11
Comparison of Hyperthyroidism With Hypothyroidism

	Hyperthyroidism	Hypothyroidism
CHARACTERISTICS	Excessive energy release, rapid cell turnover	Reduced energy release, slow cell turnover
CAUSES	Graves' disease, thyroiditis, metabolically active thyroid nodule	Post autoimmune thyroiditis (>95% in North America), primary pituitary failure (rare world-wide). Dietary iodine deficiency most common reason for hypothyroidism worldwide but relatively uncommon in North America.
NEUROLOGICAL	Nervousness, irritability, memory problems	Lethargy, disinterest, memory problems
WEIGHT	Weight loss (usually modest, present in ~50%, approximately 5–10 lb [2.3–4.5 kg])	Weight gain (usually 5–10 lb [2.3–4.5 kg] largely fluid, little fat))
ENVIRONMENTAL RESPONSE	Heat intolerance	Chilling easily, cold intolerance
SKIN	Smooth, silky skin	Coarse, dry skin
HAIR	Fine hair with frequent loss	Thick, coarse hair with tendency to break easily
NAILS	Thin nails that break with ease	Thick, dry nails
GASTROINTESTINAL	Frequent, low volume, loose stools, hyperdefecation	Constipation

Continued

TABLE 11-11

Comparison of Hyperthyroidism With Hypothyroidism—cont'd

	Hyperthyroidism	Hypothyroidism
MENSTRUAL	Amenorrhea or low volume menstrual flow	Menorrhagia
REFLEXES	Hyperreflexia with a characteristic "quick out–quick back" action	Overall hyporeflexia with characteristic slow relaxation phase, the "hung-up" patellar deep tendon reflex
MUSCLE STRENGTH	Proximal muscle weakness	Usually no change
	Tachycardia	Bradycardia in severe cases

Although thyroid disease likely exists in less than 7% of the population, a high index of suspicion should be maintained for individuals at particular risk. Risk factors and associated conditions include the following:

- Down syndrome: Hypothyroidism
- Elderly age: Hypothyroidism or hyperthyroidism with a high propensity for atypical presentation in either situation
- Use of certain medications causing an alteration in thyroid function, including iodide (hypothyroidism), amiodarone, lithium (capable of inducing both hyperthyroidism and hypothyroidism), interferon-alpha, interluken-2, lithium (capable of inducing thyroiditis)
- Female gender: Hyperthyroidism or hypothyroidism; because most thyroid dysfunction is autoimmune in nature, these diseases are more common in women than in men, as are most autoimmune diseases
- Postpartum period: A transient hypothyroidism is common, as is a transient thyroiditis
- Personal and/or family history of autoimmune disease, such as pernicious anemia, vitiligo, and type 1 DM: Hyperthyroidism and hypothyroidism
- History of head and neck irradiation or surgery: Hypothyroidism

Using the currently available highly sensitive and specific test form, the measurement of TSH, also known as thyrotropin) is the most helpful thyroid test, particularly when diagnosing the condition in the outpatient setting. TSH is produced and released by the anterior lobe of the pituitary with secretion stimulated by thyrotropin-releasing hormone through a negative feedback loop in response to amount of circulating thyroid hormone (T4). Because only a small fraction of T4 circulates free, with 99.7% bound to T4-binding globulin or other plasma proteins, the unbound portion of T4, or free T4, is metabolically active. The measurement of free T4 is the most helpful test to confirm an abnormal TSH level. Approximately 40% of T4 is converted in periphery to triiodothyronine (T3). Compared with T4, T3 is likely four times more metabolically active; T_4 is often referred to as a prodrug for T3.

Serum total T4 is a commonly performed but less than helpful test to assess thyroid function. Numerous factors can cause an increase or decrease in total T4; however, that is not indicative of a change in metabolic status. These factors include a change in thyroxine-binding globulin (TBG) levels, the principal carrier protein of T3 and T4. The use of certain medications, including exogenous estrogen (oral contraceptives, postmenopausal hormone therapy), opioids, and selective estrogen receptor modifiers (tamoxifen, raloxifene) can cause an alteration in TBG levels, resulting in an increase or decrease in total T4 (the total of protein-bound and free T4), but no change in the metabolically active free T4; these results are metabolically insignificant. As a result, the clinical usefulness of total T4 measurement is limited with results that can lead to errors in clinical judgment.

The likelihood of normal free T4 if TSH level is normal is greater than 98%. In the small remainder, pituitary disorder is the likely cause. If the clinician suspects thyroid disorder, and TSH level is normal, it should be assumed that the hypothalamic-pituitary-thyroid axis is intact, with no further testing required. TSH level is increased in hypothyroidism; a 50% decrease in T4 concentration can yield a 90-fold increase in TSH. Conversely, TSH level is decreased in hyperthyroidism. If TSH level is elevated, hypothyroidism should be confirmed by obtaining free T4 level. If TSH is low or undetectable, hyperthyroidism should be confirmed with a measurement of free T4.

Because thyroid disease can produce low-level symptoms attributed to other conditions, especially stress, fatigue, and a variety of self-limiting illnesses, the issue of routine testing for thyroid disorder with TSH has been long debated. Clinical Preventive Services Guidelines and other authorities advise that there is insufficient evidence to recommend for or against routine screening for all asymptomatic lower risk adults, for thyroid disease.

Chronic lymphocytic thyroiditis, also known as Hashimoto's thyroiditis, is the most common inflammatory disease of the thyroid and the leading cause of hypothyroidism in parts of the world where iodine deficiency is uncommon, such as North America. This condition likely has a genetic predisposition as an inherited dominant trait and is often linked with other autoimmune disorders, such as systemic lupus erythematosus, pernicious anemia, rheumatoid arthritis, DM, and Sjögren's syndrome. The condition is most often seen in women 30 to 50 years old; clinical presentation often includes a diffusely enlarged, firm thyroid with fine nodules, neck pain, and tightness. This Hashimoto goiter may regress over time; many individuals first present with the condition in the hypothyroid state, which necessitates the use of T4 replacement in the form of levothyroxine (Levothroid®, Levoxyl®, Synthroid®, Unithroid®, generic). Antimicrosomal thyroid antibodies, also known as antithyroid antibodies, likely reflecting cell-mediated immunity, are found in nearly all patients with Hashimoto's thyroiditis. Environmental iodine deficiency is the most common cause of hypothyroidism on a worldwide basis.

With an 8:1 female-to-male ratio, Graves' disease is the most common form of thyrotoxicosis, or hyperthyroidism. The age at onset is usually 20 to 40 years, and there is a significant correlation with autoimmune diseases such as pernicious anemia, myasthenia gravis, and type 1 DM. Clinical presentation of Graves' disease includes diffuse thyroid enlargement, exophthalmos, nervousness, tachycardia, and heat intolerance. Thyroid scan reveals a large "hot" (metabolically active) gland with heterogeneous uptake. Treatment of Graves' disease includes the use of antithyroid preparations such as methimazole or propylthiouracil; the use of both drugs carries a hepatotoxicity warning. Once euthyroid status is achieved, radioactive iodine for thyroid ablation is usually the next step in therapy. Subsequent hypothyroidism is the norm, necessitating the use of levothyroxine. Expert consultation is advised in caring for the person with hyperthyroidism.

Subclinical hypothyroidism is diagnosed based on the presence of an elevated TSH level and a normal free T4 level in the absence of or with minimal symptoms. Given that fatigue, often reported by a person with untreated or undertreated hypothyroidism, is so common in this condition, mild hypothyroidism is likely a more appropriate term for this condition. Goiter, or chronic thyroid enlargement, usually caused by hypertrophic or degenerative changes, is a common finding but is also found in many individuals with normal thyroid function or other forms of thyroid disease.

The prevalence of subclinical hypothyroidism varies by age and gender, and ranges from estimations of 1% to 10% of the overall population to 20% in women 60 years and older. In men 74 years and older, the prevalence has been reported as more than 15%. Most of these patients have TSH values of 5 to 10 mIU/L; 50% to 80% have evidence of antithyroid or antithyroperoxidase antibodies. The estimated prevalence of this disorder is about 7% in women and 3% in men among community-dwelling individuals 60 to 89 years old. There is a 2% to 5% likelihood of development of overt hypothyroidism per year if clinical findings are consistent with subclinical hypothyroidism.

The treatment of subclinical hypothyroidism is a matter of differing approaches; some authorities recommend levothyroxine therapy in the presence of antithyroid antibodies versus a watch-and-wait approach, with periodic TSH and free T4 testing every 6 months. When TSH level increases to more than 10 mIU/L, even in the presence of a normal free T4 level, a significant increase in LDL, increasing cardiovascular disease risk, is often noted, and levothyroxine therapy should be initiated. The American Association of Clinical Endocrinologists guidelines recommend treatment of patients with TSH greater than 5 mIU/L if the patient has a goiter, or if thyroid antibodies are present. The presence of symptoms compatible with hypothyroidism, infertility, pregnancy, or plans to become pregnant in the near future also favors treatment.

In the treatment of subclinical hypothyroidism, T4 replacement is prescribed in the form of levothyroxine (Levothroid, Levoxyl, Synthroid, Unithroid, generic). The anticipated dosage of thyroid replacement with levothyroxine for an adult with clinically detected hypothyroidism is 1.6 mcg/kg/d, based on ideal body weight; actual body weight should be used for the person who is underweight. A lower dose is recommended for older adults. In the presence of subclinical hypothyroidism, a relatively low levothyroxine dose is often sufficient because some thyroid function remains. Over time, thyroid failure progresses, and the patient's levothyroxine requirement typically increases.

In the treatment of hypothyroidism, T_4 replacement is needed in the form of levothyroxine (Levothroid, Levoxyl, Synthroid, Unithroid, generic). The anticipated dosage of thyroid replacement for an adult is 75 to 125 mcg of levothyroxine, or about 1.6 mcg/kg/d; ideal body weight should be used for this calculation as this lean body mass, even in the presence of obesity, best reflects levothyroxine needs; for the person who is underweight, actual body weight should be used. For an elderly person, the anticipated dosage is 75% or less of the adult dosage. Because this drug has a long half-life, the effects of a dosage adjustment would not cause a change in TSH for approximately five to six drug half-lives. Hence, the recommended testing interval post adjustment of a levothyroxine form is 6 to 8 weeks. The levothyroxine dose should be titrated so that TSH is within normal limits. All levothyroxine forms are acceptable, but due to its narrow therapeutic index, the same brand or generic should be taken. If the brand or generic form changes, the TSH should be checked 6 to 8 weeks after the adjustment.

Animal-derived desiccated thyroid such as Armour® thyroid contains T4 and T3; drug levels vary substantially throughout the day in those taking desiccated thyroid. The majority of study on thyroid treatment has been done with levothyroxine, a bioidentical hormone. There are no controlled trials supporting the preferred use of desiccated thyroid hormone over levothyroxine in the treatment of hypothyroidism or any other thyroid disease. Desiccated thyroid is animal-sourced, either bovine (cow) or porcine (pig) in nature; the use of the medication would likely pose difficulties for certain ethnic and religious groups as well as vegans and vegetarians.

In established hypothyroidism, thyroid hormone requirements tend to remain stable over time. Once an adequate replacement dose has been determined, periodic TSH measurements should be done after 6 months and then at 12-month intervals, or more frequently if the clinical situation dictates otherwise. Certain factors can influence thyroid hormone requirements, however. When levothyroxine is taken at the same time as iron, calcium, aluminum-containing antacids, sucralfate, cow or soy milk, and virtually any dairy product, its absorption can be impaired; ingestion of these medications should be separated by several hours. When levothyroxine is taken with rifampin, phenytoin, carbamazepine, and phenobarbital, its metabolism can be increased with resulting reduction of free T4. Levothyroxine should be taken at the same time every day on an empty stomach with water only. If the dose is taken upon arising, no food should be taken for ideally 1 hour post levothyroxine dose. If this is impractical, taking the medication 4 hours after eating with a 1 hour wait post dose is acceptable.

A thyroid nodule is a mass within the gland; the term nodule is not specific to any particular thyroid condition. The evaluation of a palpable thyroid nodule presents a challenge. In the absence of hyperthyroidism symptoms, the presentations of benign and malignant thyroid lesions are typically the same; the risk that any thyroid nodule is malignant is about 5%. A history of head or neck irradiation, localized pain, dysphonia, hemoptysis, regional lymphadenopathy, or a hard fixed mass should raise suspicion. Initial testing for a person with a thyroid nodule should include obtaining a TSH measurement. A metabolically active or "hot" nodule has a low risk of malignancy and can cause a reduction in TSH production from the pituitary. A thyroid scan can identify areas of increased uptake. Fine needle aspiration biopsy is advised, regardless of TSH results, and is more helpful and cost effective in arriving at a definitive diagnosis than ultrasound or thyroid scan. A properly performed fine needle aspiration biopsy has a false-negative rate of less than 5% and a false-positive rate of about 1%.

DISCUSSION SOURCES

ATA/AACE Guidelines for Hypothyroidism in Adults. https://www.aace.com/files/hypothyroidism_guidelines.pdf

American Association of Clinical Endocrinologists. AACE/AAES Medical/Surgical Guidelines for Clinical Practice: Management for Thyroid Cancer. www.aace.com/files/thyroid-carcinoma.pdf,

Fatourechi V, Subclinical Hypothyroidism: An Update for Primary Care Physicians. *Mayo Clin Proc* 2009;84(1):65-71.

Mayo Clin Proc 84(1): 65–71, 2009. Hyperthyroidism and Other Causes of Thyroidtoxicosis: Management Guidelines of the American Thyroid Association and American Association of Clinical Endocrinologists, available at https://www.aace.com/files/hyperguidelinesapril2013.pdf

▪ Hyperlipidemia

116. A 78-year-old woman has hypertension, a 100 pack per year history of cigarette smoking, peripheral vascular disease, and reduced renal function (GFR equal to 47 mL/min/1.73 m²). Triglyceride level is 280 mg/dL (3.164 mmol/L); high-density lipoprotein (HDL) level is 48 mg/dL (1 mmol/L); and low-density lipoprotein (LDL) level is 135 mg/dL (3.5 mmol/L). Which of the following represents the most appropriate pharmacological intervention for this patient's lipid disorders?
    A. Due to her age and comorbidity, no further intervention is required.
    B. Moderate intensity statin therapy is the preferred treatment option.
    C. A resin should be prescribed.
    D. The use of ezetimibe (Zetia®) will likely be sufficient to achieve dyslipidemia control.

117. You examine a 46-year-old male who is a one-half pack per day cigarette smoker with hypertension. He has no evidence of clinical atherosclerotic cardiovascular disease (ASCVD), and his estimated 10-year ASCVD risk is 10%. His lipid profile is as follows: HDL level is 48 mg/dL (1.24 mmol/L); LDL level is 192 mg/dL (4.9 mmol/L); and triglyceride level is 110 mg/dL (1.3 mmol/L). He had been on a low-cholesterol diet for 6 months when these tests were taken. Which of the following represents the best next step?
    A. No further intervention is required.
    B. A fibrate should be prescribed.
    C. A low-intensity 3-hydroxy-3-methylglutaryl–coenzyme A (HMG-CoA) reductase inhibitor should be prescribed.
    D. A high-intensity 3-hydroxy-3-methylglutaryl–coenzyme A (HMG-CoA) reductase inhibitor regimen should be initiated.

118. You examine a 64-year-old man with hypertension and type 2 DM. Lipid profile results are as follows: HDL level is 38 mg/dL (1 mmol/), LDL level is 135 mg/dL (3.5 mmol/L), and triglyceride level is 180 mg/dL (1.9 mmol/L). His estimated 10-year ASCVD risk is 5%. His current medications include a sulfonylurea, a biguanide, an angiotensin-converting enzyme inhibitor, and a thiazide diuretic, and he has acceptable glycemic and blood pressure control. He states, "I really watch the fats and sugars in my diet." Which of the following is the most appropriate advice?
    A. No further intervention is needed.
    B. His lipid profile should be repeated in 6 months.
    C. Lipid-lowering drug therapy with a moderate intensity statin should be initiated.
    D. The patient's dietary intervention appears adequate.

119. When providing care for a patient taking an HMG-CoA reductase inhibitor, initial evaluation when starting medication includes checking which of the following serological parameters?
    A. potassium
    B. alanine aminotransferase
    C. bilirubin
    D. alkaline phosphatase

120. When prescribing a fibrate, the NP expects to see which of the following changes in lipid profile?
    A. marked decrease in LDL level
    B. increase in HDL level
    C. no effect on triglyceride level
    D. increase in very low density lipoprotein (VLDL) level

121. When prescribing niacin, the NP expects to see which of the following changes in lipid profile?
    A. marked decrease in LDL level
    B. increase in HDL level
    C. no effect on triglyceride level
    D. increase in VLDL level

122. In prescribing niacin therapy for a patient with hyperlipidemia, the NP considers that:
    A. postdose flushing is often reported.
    B. hepatic monitoring is not warranted.
    C. low-dose therapy is usually effective in increasing LDL level.
    D. drug-induced thrombocytopenia is a common problem.

123. With the use of ezetimibe (Zetia), the NP expects to see:
    A. a marked increase in HDL cholesterol.
    B. a reduction in LDL cholesterol.
    C. a significant reduction in triglyceride levels.
    D. increased rhabdomyolysis when the drug is used in conjunction with HMG-CoA reductase inhibitor.

124. With ezetimibe (Zetia), which of the following should be periodically monitored?
    A. ALP
    B. lactate dehydrogenase (LDH)
    C. CPK
    D. No special laboratory monitoring is recommended.

125. With the use of a lipid-lowering resin, which of the following enzymes should be periodically monitored?
    A. ALP
    B. LDH
    C. AST
    D. No particular monitoring is recommended.

126. All of the following are risks for statin-induced myositis except:
    A. advanced age.
    B. use of a low-intensity statin therapy with a resin.
    C. low body weight.
    D. high-intensity statin therapy.

127. What is the average LDL reduction achieved with a change in diet as a single lifestyle modification?
    A. less than 5%
    B. 5% to 10%
    C. 11% to 15%
    D. 16% to 20% or more

128. You are seeing a patient who is taking warfarin and cholestyramine and provide the following advice:
    A. "Take both medications together."
    B. "You need to have additional hepatic monitoring tests while on this combination."
    C. "Separate the cholestyramine from other medications by at least 2 hours."
    D. "Make sure you take these medications on an empty stomach."

129. Which of the following medications is representative of high-intensity statin therapy?
    A. pravastatin 40 mg
    B. rosuvastatin 20 mg
    C. simvastatin 40 mg
    D. lovastatin 20 mg

130. Which of the following daily doses has the lowest lipid-lowering effect?
    A. simvastatin 10 mg
    B. rosuvastatin 5 mg
    C. atorvastatin 10 mg
    D. pravastatin 40 mg

131. Untreated hypothyroidism can result in which of the following changes in the lipid profile?
    A. increased HDL and decreased triglycerides
    B. increased LDL and total cholesterol
    C. increased LDL, total cholesterol, and triglycerides
    D. decreased LDL and HDL

132. A program of regular aerobic physical activity can yield which of the following changes in the lipid profile?
    A. increases HDL, lowers VLDL and triglycerides
    B. lowers VLDL and LDL
    C. increases HDL, lowers LDL
    D. lowers HDL, VLDL, and triglycerides

133. The anticipated effect on the lipid profile with high-dose omega-3 fatty acid use includes:
    A. increase in HDL.
    B. decrease in LDL.
    C. decrease in total cholesterol.
    D. decrease in triglycerides.

134. The anticipated effect on the lipid profile with plant stanol and sterol use includes:
    A. increase in HDL.
    B. decrease in LDL.
    C. decrease in select lipoprotein subfractions.
    D. decrease in triglycerides.

135. For patients with documented coronary heart disease, the American Heart Association advises intake of approximately ____ of eicosapentaenoic acid (EPA) and docosahexaenoic acid (DHA) per day, preferably from oily fish.
    A. 500 mg
    B. 1 g
    C. 2 g
    D. 4 g

136. Which of the following is an example of moderate-intensity statin therapy?
    A. fluvastatin 10 mg
    B. atorvastatin 10 mg
    C. simvastatin 10 mg
    D. pravastatin 20 mg

Answers

116. B.	122. A.	128. C.	134. B.
117. D.	123. B.	129. B.	135. B.
118. C.	124. D.	130. A.	136. B.
119. B.	125. D.	131. C.	
120. B.	126. B.	132. A.	
121. B.	127. B.	133. D.	

Treatment of hyperlipidemia is an important part of cardiovascular and cerebrovascular risk reduction. Intensive therapeutic lifestyle changes should be the first line of therapy. Dietary advice includes reducing saturated fat and cholesterol intake and adding dietary options to enhance LDL lowering, such as adding plant stanols and sterols and increasing intake of viscous or soluble fiber. Most adults achieve only a 5% to 10% reduction in LDL cholesterol with dietary advice as a single intervention. Weight management and a program of regular aerobic exercise should be prescribed for overall health. Dietary lipid improvement is often enhanced if coupled with exercise; since physical activity reduces insulin resistance, the anticipated improvement in the lipid profile includes an increase in HDL and reduction of triglycerides.

Pharmacological intervention in hyperlipidemia is likely to be needed in patients with considerable cardiovascular and cerebrovascular risk, including patients with DM, hypertension, and existing vascular disease. The choice of a lipid-lowering agent should be guided by the effect of the agent on the lipid profile.

Recommendations from the American College of Cardiology (ACC) and American Heart Association (AHA) no longer advise on the use of multiple medications to attain LDL-C levels below certain targets. Instead, the guidelines recommend statin treatment for four major groups in which therapy for atherosclerotic cardiovascular disease (ASCVD) risk reduction outweighs the risk of drug-induced adverse events. These groups include those: 1) with clinical ASCVD; 2) with primary elevations of LDL-C 190 mg/dL or higher; 3) with diabetes aged 40 to 75 years, with LDL-C 70 to 189 mg/dL, and without ASCVD; or 4) without clinical ASCVD or diabetes with LDL-C 70 to 189 mg/dL and estimated 10-year ASCVD risk of 7.5% or higher. Patient risk factors and 10-year risk of a cardiovascular event (based on the Pooled Risk Equation) help determine the intensity of statin therapy. High intensity statin therapy will lower LDL-C by 50% or more (e.g., atorvastatin 40 to 80 mg, rosuvastatin 20 to 40 mg), while moderate-intensity statin therapy will lower LDL-C by 30% to less than 50% (e.g., simvastatin 20 to 40 mg; atorvastatin 10 to 20 mg; pravastatin 40 to 80 mg; or rosuvastatin 5 to 10 mg). The ACC/AHA guidelines recommend the following statin intensity for each risk group:

- Clinical ASCVD: high-intensity statin for age 75 years or younger, or moderate-intensity statin for age over 75 years or if not a candidate for high-intensity statin
- LDL-C of 190 mg/dL or less: high-intensity statin (or moderate-intensity statin if not a candidate for high-intensity statin)
- Diabetes (type 1 or 2) and age 40 to 75 years: moderate intensity statin (high-intensity statin if 10-year ASCVD risk of 7.5% or less)
- 10-year ASCVD risk of 7.5% or less and age 40 to 75 years: moderate-to-high intensity statin

ACC/AHA guidelines note that the benefit of statin therapy in prevention of cardiovascular events is less clear in other patient groups. Causes of secondary dyslipidemia should be considered and eliminated or minimized, usually through lifestyle intervention or treatment of the underlying cause, or both.

DISCUSSION SOURCES

American Heart Association. Fish oil and omega-3 fatty acids. www.heart.org/HEARTORG/GettingHealthy/NutritionCenter/HealthyDietGoals/Fish-and-Omega-3-Fatty-Acids_UCM_303248_Article.jsp

American Heart Association. Managing abnormal blood lipids: A collaborative approach. http://circ.ahajournals.org/cgi/content/full/112/20/3184,

National Heart, Lung, and Blood Institute. Adult Treatment Panel III (ATP III) Guidelines: National Cholesterol Education Program Adult Treatment Panel III guidelines for lipid goals. www.nhlbi.nih.gov/guidelines/cholesterol/index.htm, a

Stone NJ, Robinson J, Lichtenstein AH, et al. ACC/AHA guideline on the treatment of blood cholesterol to reduce atherosclerotic cardiovascular risk in adults: A report of the American College of Cardiology/American Heart Association Task Force on Practice Guidelines. *Circulation* 2014;129(25 Suppl 2):S1-45.

Addison's Disease

137. A 34-year-old woman complains of progressive weakness, fatigue, poor appetite, and weight loss. She has also noticed the development of hyperpigmentation, mainly on the knuckles, elbows, and knees. All of the following blood tests can be used to help confirm a diagnosis of Addison's disease except:
    A. sodium.
    B. potassium.
    C. cortisol.
    D. folate.

138. The hormone cortisol plays a role in all of the following processes except:
    A. maintaining glucose control.
    B. maintenance of thyroid function.
    C. suppressing the immune response.
    D. helping the body respond to stress.

139. Which of the following is a mineralocorticoid?
    A. cortisol
    B. aldosterone
    C. insulin
    D. hydrocortisone

140. Secondary adrenal insufficiency can occur with the presence of a diseased or malfunctioning:
    A. pituitary gland.
    B. thyroid.
    C. pancreatic beta cells.
    D. hypothalamus.

141. A 43-year-old man is experiencing an acute adrenal crisis and presents with prominent nausea, vomiting, and low blood pressure. He appears cyanotic and confused. The most appropriate treatment is an injection of:
    A. epinephrine.
    B. insulin.
    C. adrenaline.
    D. hydrocortisone.

142. A 24-year-old female runner is diagnosed with Addison's disease. In counseling her about exercise, you recommend:
    A. tapering her running to only 10 minutes per day for 2 to 3 days per week.
    B. ceasing any prolonged strenuous exercise.
    C. ensuring an ample amount of sodium is ingested.
    D. switching to a nonimpact exercise.

Answers

137. D.	139. B.	141. D.	142. C.
138. B.	140. A.		

Addison's disease is a disorder that occurs when there is an inadequate amount of hormones produced by the adrenal glands. The condition occurs in all age groups and has a similar prevalence in male and female genders. The adrenal glands, located on top of each kidney, are responsible for producing a variety of hormones. Glucocorticoid hormones, such as cortisol, play a role in maintaining glucose control, suppressing the immune response, and helping the body respond to stress. Mineralocorticoid hormones, such as aldosterone, regulate sodium and potassium balance. Sex hormones in males (androgens) and females (estrogens) are involved in sexual development and sex drive. Patients with Addison's disease (also called adrenal insufficiency or hypocortisolism) do not produce enough cortisol and, in some cases, aldosterone.

Primary adrenal insufficiency refers to when the adrenal gland is damaged and hinders production of hormones. This can be the result of a number of reasons including an autoimmune response that attacks the glands, infections (such as tuberculosis, HIV, or fungal infections), hemorrhage or blood loss, tumors, or the use of anticoagulants. A key risk factor for the autoimmune-type of Addison's disease is the presence of other autoimmune conditions. These include chronic thyroiditis, dermatitis herpetiformis, Graves' disease, hypoparathyroidism, hypopituitarism, myasthenia gravis, type 1 diabetes, and vitiligo. Genetic defects are likely responsible for causing this condition.

Secondary adrenal insufficiency can occur if the pituitary gland is diseased. The pituitary gland produces adrenocorticotropic hormone (ACTH), which stimulates the adrenal cortex to produce its hormones. Inadequate production of ACTH can lead to insufficient production of hormones from the adrenal gland. Secondary adrenal insufficiency can also occur in those who have been taking systemic corticosteroids for a chronic condition (such as asthma or arthritis) for a protracted time period (usually longer than two weeks and typically at higher dose) and then abruptly stop taking the corticosteroids.

Symptoms of Addison's disease can be wide and varied and usually develop slowly, often over several months. Gastrointestinal impacts may include chronic diarrhea, nausea and vomiting, or loss of appetite resulting in weight loss. Dermatological changes include paleness or darkening of the skin in some places that causes the skin to have a patchy appearance. Other signs include muscle weakness, fatigue, slow or sluggish movement, hypoglycemia, low blood pressure, fainting, and salt craving.

During an Addisonian crisis, or acute adrenal failure, the signs and symptoms appear suddenly. These can include pain in the lower back, abdomen, or legs, severe vomiting and diarrhea leading to dehydration, low blood pressure, loss of consciousness, and hyperkalemia.

Laboratory evaluation for Addison's disease includes checking blood levels of potassium, sodium, cortisol, and ACTH. An ACTH stimulation test can be used to confirm the diagnosis. This test involves injecting synthetic ACTH and comparing the level of cortisol before and after injection.

Damage to the adrenal gland will show limited or no response to synthetic ACTH. Patients typically present with low blood pressure. An abdominal CT scan can be used to evaluate the size of the adrenal glands and identify any abnormalities. Additionally, an MRI scan of the pituitary gland can be used to identify secondary adrenal insufficiency.

Symptoms of the disease are usually controlled with corticosteroid replacement therapy, which can include a combination of glucocorticoids (cortisone, prednisone, or hydrocortisone) and mineralocorticoids (fludrocortisone). Oral treatments are preferred, though injections may be needed if the patient is vomiting and cannot retain oral medications. An ample amount of sodium is also recommended, especially during heavy exercise, in hot climates, and during gastrointestinal upsets, such as diarrhea. During an Addisonian crisis, an immediate injection of hydrocortisone is needed along with supportive treatment for low blood pressure. With proper hormone replacement therapy, most people with Addison's disease can lead normal lives. Expert consultation is required to provide appropriate care for the person with Addison's disease.

DISCUSSION SOURCE

Betterle C, Morlin L. Autoimmune Addison's disease. *Endocr Dev* 20:161–172, 2011.

Cushing's Syndrome and Cushing's Disease

143. A 46-year-old woman complains of fatigue, weakness, lethargy, decreased concentration and memory, and increased facial hair over the past 12 months. She also reports gaining over 30 pounds (13.6 kg) in the past 2 months. She has a history of asthma with repeated flares during the past 6 months requiring multiple courses of prednisone therapy. A likely diagnosis for this patient is:
    A. type 2 diabetes.
    B. Cushing's syndrome.
    C. Cushing's disease.
    D. central obesity.

144. Cushing's syndrome results from an excess of:
    A. luteinizing hormone.
    B. follicle stimulating hormone.
    C. cortisol.
    D. aldosterone.

145. A first-line approach to treat Cushing's syndrome in a 56-year-old woman who has been taking oral corticosteroids to treat rheumatoid arthritis for the past 2 years is:
    A. gradually tapering corticosteroid use.
    B. referral for surgery.
    C. consider radiation therapy.
    D. prescribe mifepristone.

146. Untreated Cushing's syndrome can lead to all of the following except:
    A. rheumatoid arthritis.
    B. hypertension.
    C. type 2 diabetes.
    D. osteoporosis.

147. Cushing's disease is the specific type of Cushing's syndrome that is caused by:
    A. long-term exposure to corticosteroids.
    B. a benign tumor of the adrenal gland.
    C. a benign pituitary tumor.
    D. an ectopic tumor that produces ACTH.

148. The most commonly recommended treatment of Cushing's disease is:
    A. tapering or ceasing corticosteroid use.
    B. eliminating trigger medications.
    C. antineoplastic therapy.
    D. surgical intervention.

Answers

143. B.	145. A.	147. C.	148. D.
144. C.	146. A.		

Cushing's syndrome occurs when the body is exposed to elevated levels of cortisol for an extended period of time. The most common cause of Cushing's syndrome is the result of long-term use of high-dose corticosteroids, though the body can also produce an excessive amount of cortisol from the adrenal gland. Cortisol plays various roles in the body, including regulation of blood pressure, helping the body cope with stress, and regulating the metabolism of proteins, carbohydrates, and fats.

The hallmark signs of Cushing's syndrome include progressive weight gain and fatty tissue deposits, particularly around the midsection and upper back, in the face (moon face), and between the shoulders (buffalo hump). Other signs include pink or purple stretch marks (striae) on the abdomen, thighs, breasts, and arms; thinning, fragile skin that bruises easily; slow healing of cuts, insect bites, and infections; and acne. Those with Cushing's syndrome often experience fatigue, muscle weakness or myopathy, depression, anxiety, and irritability, new or worsened high blood pressure, glucose intolerance that can lead to diabetes, headache, and bone loss. Women with this condition report thicker and more visible body and facial hair (hirsutism), as well as irregular or absent menstrual periods.

An exogenous cause of Cushing's syndrome is the long-term use of high doses of corticosteroids, such as prednisone, for the treatment of inflammatory conditions (e.g., rheumatoid arthritis, lupus, and asthma). Corticosteroid exposure can result from the use of oral medications, inhalers, nasal sprays, and skin creams. Repeated injections of corticosteroid for joint or back pain can also lead to development of this condition. The most common reason for Cushing's syndrome is protracted (greater than 2 weeks) use of higher dose system corticosteroids. These drugs have the same effect as cortisol and are often prescribed at doses that attain supraphysiological levels in the body.

Endogenous causes of Cushing's syndrome can also occur. Overproduction of cortisol can occur from one or both adrenal glands, or can be due to overproduction of adrenocorticotropic hormone (ACTH), which is produced by the pituitary gland and regulates cortisol production. Overproduction of ACTH can occur due to a pituitary gland tumor (pituitary adenoma) or an ectopic ACTH-secreting tumor (such as in the lung). Cushing's disease is a specific form of Cushing's syndrome caused by a benign tumor on the pituitary gland that overproduces ACTH. Overproduction of cortisol can also occur from a benign tumor of the adrenal cortex (adrenal adenoma) or, more rarely, an adrenocortical carcinoma.

Diagnosis of Cushing's syndrome can be difficult, particularly when endogenous in origin. For patients with long-term use of high-dose corticosteroids, Cushing's syndrome is usually suspected as a result of this exposure. For patients without a history of long-term corticosteroid use, urine, blood, and saliva tests can evaluate cortisol levels. MRI or CT scans can be used to detect abnormalities of the pituitary or adrenal glands. These tests can also help rule out other medical conditions with similar signs and symptoms, such as polycystic ovary syndrome, depression, eating disorders, and alcoholism. Expert consultation is advised.

Without intervention, Cushing's syndrome is associated with increased rates of cardiovascular events (heart failure or myocardial infarction) and infection. In addition, this condition can lead to osteoporosis, hypertension, type 2 diabetes, frequent and unusual infections, and loss of muscle mass. Treatment is designed to reduce the level of cortisol in the body. For patients taking long-term treatment of corticosteroids, tapering the dose as soon as possible is recommended. Abrupt discontinuation of long-term corticosteroid therapy can lead to adrenal crisis; therefore reducing its use to a low or maintenance dose is the safest initial intervention. For endogenous Cushing's syndrome, surgical resection is the primary treatment of choice to remove a tumor of the adrenal gland overproducing cortisol, or to remove a tumor of the pituitary gland or other sites that are overproducing ACTH. For those with Cushing's disease, first-line treatment is transsphenoidal surgery, which results in an approximately 80% cure rate. Often surgery is curative, though radiation therapy may be needed in conjunction with surgery. Radiation therapy is an option for those who are not suitable candidates for surgery. Cortisol replacement therapy is often used following surgery to provide a normal physiological level of cortisol. In most cases, this treatment can be tapered over time as the body returns to normal adrenal hormone production.

Certain medications can be used to control cortisol production. These include mitotane (Lysodren®), and metyrapone (Metopirone®). Mifepristone (Korlym®) has been approved for use in patients with endogenous Cushing's syndrome and type 2 diabetes or glucose intolerance and have failed surgery or cannot have surgery. This agent does not impact the production of cortisol but blocks the effects of cortisol on tissues.

DISCUSSION SOURCES

Prague JK, May S, Whitelaw BC. Cushing's syndrome. *BMJ* 346:f945, 2013. Available at: www.bmj.com/content/346/bmj .f945

Castinetti F, Morange I, Conte-Devolx B, Brue T. Cushing's disease. *Orphanet J Rare Dis* 7:41, 2012. Available at: www.ncbi.nlm.nih .gov/pmc/articles/PMC3458990/pdf/1750-1172-7-41.pdf

Renal Disorders

12

Renal Failure

1. All of the following electrolyte disorders are commonly found in a person with chronic renal failure except:
A. hypernatremia.
B. hypercalcemia.
C. hyperkalemia.
D. hypophosphatemia.

2. All of the following are common precipitating factors in acute renal failure except:
A. anaphylaxis.
B. infection.
C. myocardial infarction.
D. type 1 diabetes.

3. Common causes of chronic renal failure include all of the following except:
A. type 2 diabetes.
B. recurrent pyelonephritis.
C. hypotension.
D. polycystic kidney disease.

4. The use of which of the following medications can precipitate acute renal failure in a patient with bilateral renal artery stenosis?
A. corticosteroids
B. angiotensin II receptor antagonists
C. beta-adrenergic antagonists
D. cephalosporins

5. A 78-year-old man presents with fatigue and difficulty with bladder emptying. Examination reveals a distended bladder but is otherwise unremarkable. The blood urea nitrogen (BUN) is 88 mg/dL (31.4 mmol/L); the creatinine is 2.8 mg/dL (247.5 µmol/L). This clinical assessment is most consistent with:
A. prerenal azotemia.
B. acute glomerulonephritis.
C. acute tubular necrosis.
D. postrenal azotemia.

6. A 68-year-old woman with heart failure presents with tachycardia, S_3 heart sound, and basilar crackles bilaterally. Blood pressure is 90/68 mm Hg; BUN is 58 mg/dL (20.7 mmol/L); creatinine is 2.4 mg/dL (212.1 µmol/L). This clinical presentation is most consistent with:
A. prerenal azotemia.
B. acute glomerulonephritis.
C. tubular necrosis.
D. postrenal azotemia.

7. Which of the following is found early in the development of chronic renal failure?
A. persistent proteinuria
B. elevated creatinine level
C. acute uremia
D. hyperkalemia

8. You see a 63-year-old man with a suspected upper gastrointestinal bleed. Expected laboratory findings would include:
A. elevated BUN; elevated serum creatinine.
B. normal BUN; elevated serum creatinine.
C. elevated BUN; normal serum creatinine.
D. lowered BUN; elevated serum creatinine.

9. Angiotensin-converting enzyme inhibitors can limit the progression of some forms of renal disease by:
A. increasing intraglomerular pressure.
B. reducing efferent arteriolar resistance.
C. enhancing afferent arteriolar tone.
D. increasing urinary protein excretion.

10. Objective findings in patients with glomerulonephritis include all of the following except:
A. edema.
B. urinary red blood cell (RBC) casts.
C. proteinuria.
D. hypotension.

11. An increase in creatinine from 1 to 2 mg/dL is typically seen with a _____ loss in renal function.
A. 25%
B. 50%
C. 75%
D. 100%

12. Creatinine clearance usually:
A. approximates glomerular filtration rate (GFR).
B. does not change as part of normative aging.
C. is greater in women compared with men.
D. increases with hypotension.

13. Creatinine is best described as:
A. a substance produced by the kidney.
B. a product related to skeletal muscle metabolism.
C. produced by the liver and filtered by the kidney.
D. a by-product of protein metabolism.

14. Guidelines recommend considering initiating treatment with an erythropoiesis-stimulating agent (ESA) for patients with chronic renal failure and a hemoglobin (Hg) level:
A. less than 8.5 mg/dL.
B. less than 9.0 mg/dL.
C. less than 10 mg/dL.
D. less than 11.5 mg/dL.

15. Which of the following hemograms would be expected for a 75-year-old woman with anemia and chronic renal failure?
A. Hg=9.7 g/dL (12 to 14 g/dL); MCV=69 fL (80 to 96 fL); reticulocytes=0.8% (1% to 2%).
B. Hg=10.2 g/dL (12 to 14 g/dL); MCV=104 fL (80 to 96 fL); reticulocytes=1.2% (1% to 2%).
C. Hg=9.4 g/dL (12 to 14 g/dL); MCV=83 fL (80 to 96 fL); reticulocytes=0.7% (1% to 2%).
D. Hg=10.4 g/dL (12 to 14 g/dL); MCV=94 fL (80 to 96 fL); reticulocytes=2.6% (1% to 2%).

16. Which of the following is the most likely candidate to initiate dialysis due to chronic kidney disease (CKD)?
A. A 46-year-old man with hypertension and GFR=42 mL/min
B. A 64-year-old woman with type 2 diabetes and GFR=28 mL/min
C. A 76-year-old man with anemia and GFR=55 mL/min
D. A 58-year-old woman with heart disease and GFR=46 mL/min

Answers

1. D.	7. A.	13. B.
2. D.	8. C.	14. C.
3. C.	9. B.	15. C.
4. B.	10. D.	16. B.
5. D.	11. B.	
6. A.	12. A.	

Renal failure can be either acute or chronic. In acute renal failure, a precipitating event or cause is often easily identifiable. Acute renal failure can occur due to various conditions that result in: 1) decreased blood flow to the kidneys (e.g., due to blood or fluid loss, blood pressure medications, heart disease, infection, or severe allergic reaction); 2) damage to the kidneys (e.g., glomerulonephritis, hemolytic uremic syndrome, infection, lupus, or nephrotoxic medications); or 3) urine blockage in the kidneys (e.g., various cancers, enlarged prostate, or kidney stones). Causes of chronic renal failure include type 1 or type 2 diabetes mellitus, high blood pressure, glomerulonephritis, polycystic kidney disease, and recurrent pyelonephritis.

With prerenal azotemia, the most common cause of acute renal failure, the kidneys are hypoperfused, which often leads to acute tubular necrosis. Reasons for this hypoperfusion include: decreased circulating volume, as seen in patients with dehydration and acute blood loss; decreased cardiac output, as seen in patients with heart failure; or excessive sequestering of fluid, as seen in patients with burns. Postrenal azotemia is caused by obstruction to urine flow and is an uncommon cause of renal failure. In intrinsic renal failure, there is disease within the kidney at the levels of the renal tubules, glomeruli, interstitium, or vessels. Etiologies include glomerulonephritis and acute interstitial nephritis. Laboratory findings in these more common forms of acute renal failure vary (Table 12–1).

Typical findings in renal failure include increased serum creatinine and blood urea nitrogen (BUN) levels. Creatinine is the end product of creatine metabolism, which arises from skeletal muscle. Because creatinine excretion by a healthy kidney is very efficient, measurement of creatinine is used as a surrogate marker of kidney function; creatinine production equals creatinine excretion. As the kidney fails, the creatinine level increases. BUN is derived from the breakdown of protein from dietary or other sources. BUN level typically increases (uremia) more rapidly than creatinine level in response to decreased renal perfusion and can increase from prerenal, renal, and postrenal causes of kidney failure. In particular, elevated BUN level with a normal creatinine level is occasionally found in patients with healthy kidneys but with severe dehydration. In addition, upper GI bleeding usually causes a marked increase in BUN level without corresponding increase in creatinine as the gut digests and absorbs proteins found in the blood. Electrolyte disorders commonly associated with renal failure include hyperkalemia, hypercalcemia, and hypernatremia.

Anemia is typically seen in patients with chronic renal failure. Erythropoietin, a glycoprotein growth factor produced primarily by the kidneys, is normally released in the bloodstream and binds with receptors in the bone marrow to stimulate the production of erythrocytes (red blood cells [RBCs]). With end-stage renal disease, erythropoietin response is reduced because of limited supply; that is, as the kidney fails, erythropoietin production declines. In addition, as is common in chronic illness, RBC life span is shortened.

TABLE 12-1

Etiology of and Findings in Acute Renal Failure

Disease Causing Acute Renal Failure	Typical Etiology	Laboratory Findings
Acute glomerulonephritis	Poststreptococcal infection, autoimmune diseases	BUN:Cr ratio >20:1 Urinalysis: renal casts, RBCs
Acute interstitial nephritis	Allergic reaction, drug reaction	BUN:Cr ratio <20:1 Urinalysis: WBC casts, eosinophils
Acute tubular necrosis	Hypotension, nephrotoxins	BUN:Cr ratio <20:1 Urinalysis: granular casts, renal tubular cells

BUN— blood urea nitrogen; Cr—creatinine; RBCs—red blood cells; WBC—white blood cell.

These factors result in a normocytic, normochromic anemia in the presence of a low reticulocyte count, the characteristics of anemia of chronic disease. This problem is treated with recombinant erythropoietin, transfusion, and correction of additional anemia risk factors. Guidelines recommend considering treatment with an erythropoiesis-stimulating agent (ESA) for dialysis and nondialysis adult patients when hemoglobin levels are less than 10 g/dL (less than 100 g/L). In general, treatment should target a hemoglobin level not exceeding 11.5 g/dL.

Chronic kidney disease can be classified into five stages based on glomerular filtration rate (GFR). Dialysis and kidney transplantation should be considered for those approaching Stage 4 (GFR=15 to 29 mL/min) who have advanced kidney damage. Those at Stage 4 are likely to develop serious complications of CKD, including hypertension, anemia, and cardiovascular disease. For those at Stage 5 (GFR less than 15 mL/min) or end-stage renal disease, the kidneys have lost nearly all of their ability to perform and the person will require dialysis or transplantation for survival.

DISCUSSION SOURCES

National Kidney Foundation Kidney Disease Outcomes Quality Initiative. www.kidney.org/professionals/kdoqi/index.cfm.

Kliger AS, Foley RN, Goldfarb DS, et al. KDOQI US commentary on the 2012 KDIGO clinical practice guideline for anemia in CKD. *Am J Kidney Dis* 2013. www.kidney.org/Professionals/kdoqi/pdf/KDOQI_Commentary_on_KDIGO_Anemia.pdf.

Glomerulonephritis

17. Risk factors for acute glomerulonephritis include all of the following except:
    A. bacterial endocarditis.
    B. Goodpasture's syndrome.
    C. Crohn's disease.
    D. polyarteritis.

18. Poststreptococcal glomerulonephritis typically occurs how long following a bacterial pharyngitis infection?
    A. 4 to 6 days
    B. 1 to 2 weeks
    C. 3 to 4 weeks
    D. 2 months

19. Diagnostic confirmation of glomerulonephritis typically requires:
    A. urinalysis plus a CBC with differential.
    B. abdominal CT scan.
    C. kidney ultrasound.
    D. kidney biopsy.

20. A 35-year-old man presents with edema of the face, hands, and ankles along with hypertension (175/115 mm Hg). He reports urine that is darkly colored and foamy. You suspect acute glomerulonephritis and would expect urinalysis results to include all of the following findings except:
    A. elevated level of protein.
    B. presence of red blood cells.
    C. presence of renal casts.
    D. abnormally high glucose levels.

21. A 47-year-old woman with lupus erythematosus is diagnosed with acute glomerulonephritis. Treatment options include all of the following except:
    A. systemic corticosteroids.
    B. systemic antimicrobials.
    C. immune suppressors.
    D. plasmapheresis.

22. A complication of glomerulonephritis is:
    A. type 2 diabetes.
    B. nephrotic syndrome.
    C. pyelonephritis.
    D. bladder cancer.

Answers

17. C.	19. D.	21. B.
18. B.	20. D.	22. B.

Glomerulonephritis is a condition caused by inflammation of the glomeruli in the kidneys. Glomeruli are responsible for removing waste and excess electrolytes and fluid from the bloodstream. Glomerulonephritis can be acute or chronic, with signs and symptoms including pink or cola-colored urine due to hematuria, foamy urine due to proteinuria, hypertension, edema of the face, hands, feet and abdomen, and possibly anemia. The acute condition can develop as a result of infection, immune diseases (e.g., lupus, Goodpasture's syndrome, or IgA nephropathy), or vasculitis (e.g., polyarteritis or Wegener's granulomatosis). Poststreptococcal glomerulonephritis can develop 1 to 2 weeks following pharyngitis caused by group A beta-hemolytic streptoccocal t infection ("strep throat") when an overproduction of antibodies produced from the infection settle in the glomeruli and cause inflammation. Those with bacterial endocarditis are also at high risk of developing glomerulonephritis, while some viral infections have also been implicated (e.g., HIV, hepatitis B or C). If left untreated, glomerulonephritis can lead to kidney failure, high blood pressure, blood electrolyte disorders, and nephrotic syndrome. Though the cause of chronic glomerulonephritis is unclear, genetics and changes to the immune system can play a role. The chronic condition is more often found in young men who also experience hearing and vision loss.

Diagnosis involves a urinalysis and blood analysis. Urine will typically contain red blood cells and red blood cell casts, as well as the presence of white blood cells and elevated levels of protein. Elevated serum creatinine and BUN would typically be found and indicate impaired renal function (Table 12–1). Imaging studies, such as a CT scan or kidney ultrasound, can be used to evaluation the status of renal damage. A kidney biopsy is needed to confirm the diagnosis of glomerulonephritis.

Acute glomerulonephritis is often self-limiting. The goal of treatment is to manage the underlying cause of glomerulonephritis and protect the kidneys from any further damage. Antihypertensive medications can be used to lower blood pressure. Antimicrobials are used if an infection is suspected, while systemic corticosteroids and immune-suppressing drugs can reduce inflammation. For worsening cases due to an immune disorder, plasmapheresis should be considered to remove antibodies and other toxic proteins from the blood that are causing inflammation in the kidney. In cases with associated acute kidney failure, dialysis may be required to remove excess fluid and control high blood pressure.

DISCUSSION SOURCES

Radhakrishnan J, Cattran DC. The KDIGO practice guideline on glomerulonephritis: Reading between the (guide)lines—Application to the individual patient. *Kidney Int* 82:840–856, 2012.

Parmar MS. Acute glomerulonephritis. http://emedicine.medscape.com/article/239278-overview.

Urinary Tract Infection

23. Which of the following is most likely to be part of the clinical presentation of an otherwise healthy 27-year-old woman with uncomplicated lower urinary tract infection (UTI)?
    A. urinary frequency
    B. fever
    C. suprapubic tenderness
    D. lower gastrointestinal (GI) upset

24. Compared to younger women, uncomplicated UTI in an elderly woman is more likely to be associated with each of the following signs and symptoms except:
    A. new onset urinary incontinence.
    B. delirium.
    C. weakness.
    D. hematuria.

25. A 36-year-old afebrile woman with no health problems presents with dysuria and frequency of urination. Her urinalysis findings include results positive for nitrites and leukocyte esterase. You evaluate these results and consider that she likely has:
    A. purulent vulvovaginitis.
    B. a gram-negative UTI.
    C. cystitis caused by *Staphylococcus saprophyticus*.
    D. urethral syndrome.

26. The most likely causative organism in community-acquired UTI in women during the reproductive years is:
    A. *Klebsiella* species.
    B. *Proteus mirabilis*.
    C. *Escherichia coli*.
    D. *Staphylococcus saprophyticus*.

27. Which urine culture result is needed to confirm a UTI in an asymptomatic woman who has not had recent use of a urinary catheter?
    A. 10^2 cfu/mL or more
    B. 10^3 cfu/mL or more
    C. 10^4 cfu/mL or more
    D. 10^5 cfu/mL or more

28. You see a 34-year-old woman with an uncomplicated UTI. She is otherwise healthy but reports having a sulfa allergy. Appropriate therapy would include:
    A. TMP-SMX.
    B. amoxicillin.
    C. azithromycin.
    D. ciprofloxacin.

29. The notation of alkaline urine in a patient with a UTI may point to infection caused by:
    A. *Klebsiella* species.
    B. *P. mirabilis*.
    C. *E. coli*.
    D. *S. saprophyticus*.

30. Which of the following is the most accurate information in caring for a 40-year-old man with cystitis?
    A. This is a common condition in men of this age.
    B. A gram-positive organism is the likely causative pathogen.
    C. A urological evaluation should be considered.
    D. Pyuria is rarely found.

31. Evidence-based factors that prevent or minimize the risk of UTIs include all of the following except:
    A. male gender.
    B. longer urethra-to-anus length in women.
    C. timed voiding schedule.
    D. zinc-rich prostatic secretions.

32. Hemorrhagic cystitis is characterized by:
    A. irritative voiding symptoms.
    B. persistent microscopic hematuria.
    C. the presence of hypertension.
    D. elevated creatinine and BUN levels.

33. A 44-year-old woman presents with pyelonephritis. The report of her urinalysis is least likely to include:
    A. WBC casts.
    B. positive nitrites.
    C. 3+ protein.
    D. rare RBCs.

34. An example of a first-line therapeutic agent for the treatment of pyelonephritis is:
    A. amoxicillin with clavulanate.
    B. trimethoprim-sulfamethoxazole.
    C. ciprofloxacin.
    D. nitrofurantoin.

35. With fluoroquinolone use, length of antimicrobial therapy during uncomplicated pyelonephritis is typically:
    A. 5 days.
    B. 1 week.
    C. 2 weeks.
    D. 3 weeks.

36. Risk factors for UTI in women include:
    A. postvoid wiping back to front.
    B. low perivaginal lactobacilli colonization.
    C. hot tub use.
    D. wearing snug-fitting pantyhose.

37. All of the following can negatively impact perivaginal lactobacilli colonization except:
    A. recent antimicrobial use.
    B. exposure to the spermicide nonoxynol-9.
    C. estrogen deficiency.
    D. postcoital voiding.

38. In children and the elderly, which of the following conditions can contribute to bladder instability and increase the risk of a UTI?
    A. constipation
    B. upper respiratory tract infection
    C. chronic diarrhea
    D. efficient bladder emptying

39. Which of the following is not a gram-negative organism?
    A. *E. coli*
    B. *K. pneumoniae*
    C. *P. mirabilis*
    D. *S. saprophyticus*

40. You see a 70-year-old woman in a walk-in center with a chief complaint of increased urinary frequency and dysuria. Urinalysis reveals pyuria and positive nitrites. She mentions she has a "bit of kidney trouble, not too bad." Recent evaluation of renal status is unavailable. In considering antimicrobial therapy for this patient, you prescribe:
    A. nitrofurantoin.
    B. fosfomycin.
    C. ciprofloxacin.
    D. doxycycline.

Answers

23. A.	29. B.	35. B.
24. D.	30. C.	36. B.
25. B.	31. C.	37. D.
26. C.	32. A.	38. A.
27. D.	33. C.	39. D.
28. D.	34. C.	40. C.

The urinary tract, adjacent to the bacteria-rich lower GI tract, produces and stores urine. The periurethral area is typically colonized with gut and other flora, some capable of causing urinary tract infection (UTI). Although the process of urination usually flushes bacteria from the urethral orifice, periurethral pathogens occasionally enter the urethra and ascend, reaching the bladder and resulting in UTI; this is the most common route for UTI acquisition. Rarely, hematogenous UTI occurs when a pathogen is delivered to the urinary tract via the bloodstream from a distant source of infection, such as the lungs in a patient with pneumonia and bacteremia.

UTIs can involve mucosal tissue (cystitis) or soft tissue (pyelonephritis, prostatitis). Anatomically, the infection can be limited to the lower urinary tract (cystitis involving the bladder and urethra) or the upper tract (pyelonephritis). Complicated UTI can occur in either the upper or the lower urinary tract, but is accompanied by an underlying condition that increases the risk for failing therapy, such as obstruction, urological dysfunction, or resistant pathogens. Most UTIs occur via an ascending route.

UTI is typically diagnosed by clinical presentation and a few physical examination and laboratory findings. In an otherwise healthy woman, history of the present illness usually reveals a complaint of dysuria, often reported as an internal discomfort, with urinary frequency and urgency, but without fever or constitutional symptoms. Although suprapubic tenderness and pain are often considered part of the clinical presentation, this is found in only about 20% of women with an uncomplicated UTI. Back pain, fever, nausea, and vomiting are more often associated with pyelonephritis, an upper urinary tract infection, and, in rare cases, with cystitis, a lower urinary tract infection; many patients with pyelonephritis also report lower UTI symptoms. Although vaginal infection and irritation can cause dysuria, most women who have dysuria without vaginal discharge have a UTI, not vaginitis.

UTIs are one of the most common types of infection in the elderly, occurring in both the community and long-term care settings. Symptomatic UTI can include the classic symptoms of dysuria but can also include new onset incontinence, confusion or dementia, and muscle weakness. Factors that predispose older patients to UTIs include the use of urinary catheters and external urine collection devices, and age-related neurological conditions that impair bladder emptying.

Hemorrhagic cystitis is characterized by large quantities of visible blood in the urine. Its etiology can be bacterial infection or infection with adenovirus types 7, 11, 21, and 35 and influenza A, or it can be a result of radiation, cancer chemotherapy, or certain immunosuppressive medications. The clinical presentation usually depends on its origin; with all causes, irritative voiding symptoms are typically reported. When the disease is infectious in origin, signs and symptoms of infection may also be encountered. Adenovirus is a common cause and is self-limiting in nature. Hemorrhagic cystitis is often confused with glomerulonephritis, but hypertension and abnormal renal function are absent in the former.

Acute pyelonephritis is an infection of the renal parenchyma and renal pelvis, caused by ascending cystitis; most episodes are uncomplicated and not accompanied by risk of treatment failure such as obstruction, urological dysfunction, or a multidrug-resistant uropathogen. Irritative voiding symptoms similar to symptoms of cystitis, fever, flank pain, an acutely ill appearance, costovertebral tenderness, and pyuria are usually reported; GI upset including vomiting is often noted. WBC with differential usually reveals leukocytosis, neutrophilia, and bandemia.

Urine dipstick testing is commonly done in the outpatient setting when UTI is suspected because it is simple and convenient and yields immediate results. Leukocyte esterase, nitrites, protein, and blood are the important features in evaluating for UTI. The presence of leukocyte esterase on a urine dipstick is equivalent to 4 WBCs or more per high-power field (HPF). Nearly all (96% or more) patients with UTI have pyuria equivalent to more than 10 WBCs/HPF. Some uropathogens are capable of reducing dietary nitrates in the urine to nitrite; this is an indirect test for bacteriuria. When this finding is coupled with a leukocyte esterase response, the likely offending organism is a gram-negative pathogen (*E. coli*, *Proteus* species, *Klebsiella pneumoniae*). The nitrite test result is occasionally falsely negative in UTI with a low colony count or with recently voided or dilute urine. In addition, this test does not detect organisms unable to reduce nitrate to nitrite, such as enterococci, staphylococci, or adenovirus. Small amounts of protein and RBCs may also be positive on dipstick testing in cases of UTI (Table 12–2).

Urine culture is important when diagnosis is unclear, or UTI is recurrent. The presence of more than one organism often indicates a contaminated urine specimen, and collection and testing should be repeated. The presence of 10^5 or more colony-forming units (CFUs) per milliliter of bacteria is the traditional diagnostic indicator for UTI. In the presence of dysuria and other symptoms for UTI, more than 10^2 CFU/mL confirms the diagnosis.

Certain factors protect against or increase the risk for UTI. Male sex is recognized as a potent protective factor, in part because of the longer urethral length than in women; women with a shorter urethra-to-anus length appear to be at increased UTI risk. In contrast to the periurethral area in women, the male periurethral area does not support bacterial growth. Zinc-rich prostatic secretions are antibacterial, further discouraging pathogen growth.

In either sex, efficient emptying helps prevent urine stagnation and minimizes UTI risk. Factors that alter efficient bladder emptying, such as cystocele, rectocele, and benign prostatic hyperplasia, increase UTI risk. In addition, robust fucosyltransferase activity, an enzyme found in the periurethral and perivaginal area, discourages bacterial adherence; the presence of relatively few bacterial adhesion receptor sites in the bladder and urethra has a similar effect. Women with these receptors who do not have mucosal secretion of the fucosyltransferase enzyme to help block bacterial adherence are more likely to have colonization with *E. coli* and other coliforms from the rectum and less likely to have lactobacilli in the periurethral area; this situation results in frequent episodes of cystitis. The urothelial receptors can also be found in the upper urinary tract, increasing the risk of pyelonephritis. Women who are nonsecretors of ABO blood group antigens show enhanced adherence of pathogenic *E. coli* to urothelial cells compared with women who are secretors of these antigens; this becomes a major UTI risk factor when coupled with spermicide use or frequent vaginal sexual intercourse.

A woman who is exposed to the spermicide nonoxynol-9, either through vaginal use or with a male partner who uses condoms with this spermicide, is at increased risk of UTI. The proposed mechanism of this risk is the antibacterial effect of the spermicide—reducing lactobacilli, a normal component of the periurethral flora. Lactobacilli produce hydrogen peroxide and lactic acid, providing the periurethral area and vagina with a pH that inhibits bacterial growth, blocks potential sites of attachment, and is toxic to uropathogens. In postmenopausal women, estrogen deficiency leads to a marked reduction in lactobacilli colonization in the vaginal-perineal areas; topical estrogen use results in re-establishment of the normal protective flora and a reduction of UTI risk. Recent antimicrobial use potentially increases UTI risk by the same mechanism.

Voiding at regular intervals with efficient bladder emptying, wiping patterns, and postcoital voiding have not been shown to provide UTI protection. In addition, use of hot tubs, wearing pantyhose, douching, and obesity have not been shown to increase UTI risk. In children and elderly adults, constipation has been noted to contribute to bladder instability and helps encourage UTI development.

TABLE 12-2

Common Urinalysis Dipstick Findings in Urinary Tract Infection

Finding	Significance	Comment
Color	Typically pale yellow to colorless	Change in urine color is not synonymous with UTI or disease
Clarity	Typically clear	Pyuria causes urinary turbidity
Odor	Mild characteristic odor	Rancid or ammonia odor in urea-splitting organism (e.g., *P. mirabilis*)
Specific gravity (SG)	Dilute urine: SG ≤1.008 Concentrated urine: SG >1.020	Dilute or concentrated urine can influence results of urine chemical test strip testing
Leukocyte esterase	Test for enzyme present in WBCs	Positive results indicate presence of neutrophils >5 WBCs/HPF, an indicator of UTI, reported sensitivity of 75%–90%; results not valid in neutropenic patients; decreased sensitivity with increased urinary glucose concentration, high urinary SG, and presence of antimicrobial in urine
Nitrites	Surrogate marker for bacteriuria; presence indicates bacterial reduction of dietary nitrates to nitrites by select gram-negative uropathogens including *E. coli, Proteus* spp Normally absent in sterile urine and infection caused by enterococci, staphylococci	Best done on well-concentrated urine such as first AM void; for nitrites to be present, urine should be held in bladder for ≤1 hr for nitrate-to-nitrite conversion to occur; dietary nitrate intake must be adequate; false-negative result possible with low colony count UTI
Protein	Dipstick testing most sensitive for albumin	Common in febrile response or represents presence of protein-containing substance such as WBCs, bacteria, mucus; in UTI, usually trace to 30 mg/dL (1$^+$), seldom ≥100 mg/dL
pH	Average pH 5–6 Acid pH 4.5–5.5 Alkaline pH 6.5–8	If alkaline urine is found in presence of UTI symptoms and positive leukocyte esterase, likely that a urea splitting organism such as *Proteus* is allowing urea to be split into CO_2 and ammonia, causing increase in urine's normally acid pH
Red blood cells (RBCs)	Low number of RBCs noted Gross hematuria rare in uncomplicated UTI, but may be present in infection complicated by nephrolithiasis	Microscopic hematuria common with UTI, but not in urethritis or vaginitis

UTI—urinary tract infection; WBCs—white blood cells.

Most episodes of community-acquired cystitis in women, the most commonly encountered UTI, are caused by enteric gram-negative rods from the Enterobacteriaceae group, such as *E. coli, P. mirabilis,* and less commonly encountered *K. pneumoniae. Staphylococcus saprophyticus,* a gram-positive organism, and *E. coli* accounted for more than 90% of the uropathogens in one study of more than 4000 urine isolates obtained from women of reproductive age with cystitis during a 5-year period. These organisms are usually susceptible to fluoroquinolones such as ciprofloxacin and levofloxacin, though increasing resistance rates by community uropathogens are mitigating their effectiveness. Growing rates of resistance to trimethoprim-sulfamethoxazole (TMP-SMX, Bactrim®) have been exhibited by the organisms that most often cause UTI, potentially reducing the usefulness of this inexpensive medication. Nitrofurantoin and fosfomycin are effective alternatives in treating cystitis, especially in areas with high TMP-SMX resistance and/or for those with a sulfa allergy. Long-standing resistance to the beta-lactams, including ampicillin, compounds the problem.

Factors influencing the development of multidrug-resistant *E. coli* strains in part include liberal use of antimicrobials, particularly TMP-SMX, to treat UTI and other infections in adults and to provide prophylaxis against select opportunistic infections in patients with HIV. In children, attendance at day care, age younger than 3 years, and repeated antimicrobial use, particularly TMP-SMX and beta-lactams for respiratory infections, are risk factors for infection with a resistant uropathogen; child-to-child and child-to-parent transmission of the organism often occurs. Also, the more liberal use of ciprofloxacin in recent years, triggered in part by the decrease in cost when this medication became available in a generic form, is a great cause for alarm as *E. coli* resistance to the fluoroquinolone antimicrobial class has gradually increased.

Current treatment recommendations for UTI therapy in younger women without comorbid conditions include the use of a short course (3 to 7 days) of an antimicrobial with significant activity against gram-negative (*E. coli*) and select gram-positive (*S. saprophyticus*) organisms. Treatment for pyelonephritis is also focused on coverage of gram-negative pathogens, usually for 5 to 7 days with a fluoroquinolone or 2 weeks with certain other antimicrobials (Table 12–3).

Although *E. coli* is the most common uropathogen in the community and in elderly persons living in long-term care,

P. mirabilis and *K. pneumoniae* account for approximately one-third of all infections in this age group. Length of antimicrobial treatment in elderly persons with uncomplicated UTI should be 7 to 10 days for women and 10 to 14 days for men; short-course therapy is not recommended. First-line therapy includes TMP-SMX or fluoroquinolones; nitrofurantoin should not be used in elderly patients because safe and effective use of the product requires a minimal creatinine clearance of 60 mL/min. In an elderly patient with impaired renal function, the fluoroquinolone dosage potentially needs adjustment, but is considered to be a safe, effective, first-line intervention.

UTI prophylaxis should be considered for women of reproductive age who experience two or more symptomatic UTIs within 6 months or three or more UTIs over 12 months and for women with fewer infections but with severe discomfort. Continuous prophylaxis with daily TMP-SMX has been shown to be effective in the management of recurrent

TABLE 12-3
Urinary Tract Infection Therapies

Type of Infection	Usual Pathogens	Regimens
Acute, uncomplicated UTI (cystitis, urethritis) in nonpregnant women	*E. coli* (gram-negative, most common pathogen), *S. saprophyticus* (gram-positive), enterococci (gram-positive)	PRIMARY If local *E. coli* resistance to TMP-SMX <20% and no allergy, then TMP-SMX-DS bid × 3 days; if sulfa allergy, nitrofurantoin × 5 days or fosfomycin × one dose. All plus pyridium. If local *E. coli* resistance to TMP-SMX >20% or sulfa allergy, ciprofloxacin, levofloxacin, or moxifloxacin 3 days, nitrofurantoin × 5 days or fosfomycin ×1 dose. All plus pyridium. Moxifloxacin and gemifloxacin not labeled for use in UTI.
Recurrent UTI (≥3/yr)	*E. coli, S. saprophyticus,* enterococci, other pathogens possible	PRIMARY Eradicate organisms, then TMP-SMX 1 SS tablet qd long-term. ALTERNATIVE TMP-SMX 1 DS tablet postcoitus or 2 DS tablets at first sign of UTI. For recurrent UTI in postmenopausal women, consider use of estrogen cream, also consider urological factor, such as cystocele, residual urine volume, incontinence.
Acute uncomplicated pyelonephritis suitable for outpatient therapy (Note: Obtain urine and blood cultures before initiating antimicrobial therapy.)	*E. coli,* enterococci	PRIMARY Ciprofloxacin 500 mg bid, ciprofloxacin ER 1000 mg qd, levofloxacin 750 mg qd, ofloxacin 400 mg bid, or moxifloxacin 400 mg qd, all for 7 days (levofloxacin 750 mg approved for 5 days). Moxifloxacin and gemifloxacin not labeled for use in UTI. ALTERNATIVE Amoxicillin with clavulanate, cephalosporin, or TMP-SMX-DS, all for 14 days. Beta-lactams are not as effective as fluoroquinolones.

TMP-SMX—trimethoprim-sulfamethoxazole; UTI—urinary tract infection.
Source: Gilbert DN, Moellering RC, Eliopoulos GM, Chambers HF, Saag MS. *The Sanford Guide to Antimicrobial Therapy*, ed. 44. Sperryville, VA: Antimicrobial Therapy, Inc., 2014, p. 36.

uncomplicated cystitis. Alternatives to continuous prophylaxis include self-administered single-dose therapy at symptom onset, or a single-dose treatment postcoitus. Before UTI prophylaxis is initiated, resolution of the previous UTI should be confirmed by a negative urine culture 1 to 2 weeks after treatment. The method prescribed depends on the frequency and pattern of recurrences and on patient preference.

Choice of an antimicrobial agent for recurrent UTI should be based on susceptibility patterns of the strains causing the patient's previous UTIs and on patient history of drug allergies or intolerance. Long-term TMP-SMX or nitrofurantoin therapy has been used successfully for many years. Compared with TMP-SMX, nitrofurantoin has the advantage of lower rates of resistance by the more common UTI pathogens. At the same time, long-term prophylaxis with nitrofurantoin should be used with caution due to a risk of pulmonary fibrosis. It is important to note that antimicrobial prophylaxis does not appear to change the natural history of recurrences as most women reestablish their pattern and frequency of UTIs within 6 months of discontinuing prophylaxis. The use of a fluoroquinolone for UTI prophylaxis has gained some popularity; concern about emerging resistance is an issue. UTI prophylaxis in a postmenopausal woman should also include a topical or vaginal estrogen to encourage lactobacilli recolonization. Postmenopausal women with recurrent infections should be evaluated for potentially correctable urologic factors, including cystocele, incontinence, and an elevated residual urine volume.

Cranberry and blueberry juice intake has been touted as a helpful measure to reduce the rate of recurrent infections. These juices were initially believed to cause high levels of benzoic acid that resulted in urinary acidification and bacteriostatic action. However, meta-analyses of clinical studies demonstrated that cranberry or blueberry juice is not as effective as initially thought and showed no significant benefit in reducing the occurrence of symptomatic UTIs when compared to placebo, water, or no treatment.

DISCUSSION SOURCES

Gilbert DN, Moellering RC, Eliopoulos GM, Chambers HF, Saag MS. *The Sanford Guide to Antimicrobial Therapy*, ed. 44. Sperryville, VA: Antimicrobial Therapy, Inc., 2014, p. 36.

Gupta K, Hooton TM, Naber KG, et al. International clinical practice guidelines for the treatment of acute uncomplicated cystitis and pyelonephritis in women: A 2010 update by the Infectious Diseases Society of America and the European Society for Microbiology and Infectious Diseases. *Clin Infect Dis* 52:e103–e120, 2011.

Bladder Cancer

41. Long-term use of which medication has been possibly associated with increased risk for bladder cancer?
    A. pioglitazone
    B. saxagliptin
    C. rosuvastatin
    D. clopidogrel

42. Which of the following is not a risk factor for bladder cancer?
    A. occupational exposure to textile dyes
    B. cigarette smoking
    C. occupational exposure to heavy metals
    D. long-term aspirin use

43. A 68-year-old man presents with suspected bladder cancer. You consider that its most common presenting sign or symptom is:
    A. painful urination.
    B. fever and flank pain.
    C. painless gross hematuria.
    D. palpable abdominal mass.

44. In a person diagnosed with superficial bladder cancer without evidence of metastases, you realize that:
    A. the prognosis for 2-year survival is poor.
    B. a cystectomy is indicated.
    C. despite successful initial therapy, local recurrence is common.
    D. systemic chemotherapy is the treatment of choice.

45. Persistent microscopic hematuria would be the primary finding in about ___% of individuals with bladder cancer.
    A. 10
    B. 20
    C. 30
    D. 40

46. Preferred therapy for nonmuscle-invasive bladder cancer without evidence of metastases is:
    A. cystectomy.
    B. intravesical chemotherapy only.
    C. transurethral resection with intravesical chemotherapy.
    D. systemic chemotherapy.

Answers

41. A.	43. C.	45. B.
42. D.	44. C.	46. C.

Bladder cancer is the sixth most common type of cancer in the United States, and the second most common urologic malignancy after prostate cancer. It is usually a disease that occurs later in life—the mean age at diagnosis is 65 years—and it is more common in men. Risk factors include cigarette smoking, which accounts for most cases, family history of bladder cancer, arsenic exposure (mainly occurring outside the United States), and exposure to industrial chemicals, including paints, dyes, and solvents. Certain medications, such as the anticancer treatment cyclophosphamide and the diabetes medication pioglitazone, can also increase the risk for bladder cancer. Primary prevention of bladder cancer through risk reduction is critical.

Gross painless hematuria is the most common presenting sign of bladder cancer; persistent microscopic hematuria is the only finding in about 20% of individuals presenting with the disease. Irritative voiding symptoms and urinary frequency without fever are reported occasionally. Abdominal mass is palpable only with advanced disease.

Patients suspected of bladder cancer are referred to an urologist to perform a cystoscopy. A biopsy sample is taken via transurethral resection during the cystoscopy for analysis. Cytology can also be used to detect the presence of cancer cells in the urine.

Most patients with newly diagnosed bladder cancer have superficial disease (nonmuscle-invasive bladder cancer). Transurethral resection is used to remove bladder cancers that are confined to the inner lining of the bladder, or a partial cystectomy may be needed to remove the tumor and a small portion of the bladder. Treatment also includes a single immediate instillation of intravesical chemotherapy (e.g., mitomycin C). Subsequent therapy is based on patient risk factors. Meticulous follow-up is critical because recurrence is often seen, necessitating repeat procedures. Long-term survival is the norm with this noninvasive form of the disease. With invasive disease, treatment is dictated by type of tumor, degree of invasion, and presence of metastatic disease; long-term survival is based on numerous factors.

DISCUSSION SOURCES

Diagnosis, Evaluation and Follow-Up of Asymptomatic Microhematuria (AMH) In Adults: AUA Guideline, www.auanet.org/education/guidelines/asymptomatic-microhematuria.cfm.

Rodriguez Faba O, Gaya JM, Lopez JM, et al. Current management of non-muscle-invasive bladder cancer. *Minerva Med* 104: 273–286, 2013.

Urinary Incontinence

47. Patients with urge incontinence often report urine loss:
A. with exercise.
B. at night.
C. associated with a strong sensation of needing to void.
D. as dribbling after voiding.

48. Patients with urethral stricture often report urine loss:
A. with exercise.
B. during the day.
C. associated with urgency.
D. as dribbling after voiding.

49. Patients with stress incontinence often report urine loss:
A. with lifting.
B. at night.
C. associated with a strong sensation of needing to void.
D. as dribbling after voiding.

50. Factors that contribute to stress incontinence include:
A. detrusor overactivity.
B. pelvic floor weakness.
C. urethral stricture.
D. urinary tract infection (UTI).

51. Factors that contribute to urge incontinence include:
A. detrusor overactivity.
B. pelvic floor weakness.
C. urethral stricture.
D. UTI.

52. Pharmacological intervention for patients with urge incontinence includes:
A. doxazosin (Cardura®).
B. tolterodine (Detrol®).
C. finasteride (Proscar®).
D. pseudoephedrine.

53 to 55. Match the most appropriate behavioral intervention with each form of urinary incontinence.

53. urge incontinence

54. stress incontinence

55. functional incontinence
A. having an assistant who is aware of voiding cues and helps with toileting activities
B. establishing a voiding schedule and gentle bladder stretching
C. Kegel exercises and pelvic floor rehabilitation with biofeedback

56. Which form of urinary incontinence is most common in elderly persons?
A. stress
B. urge
C. iatrogenic
D. overflow

57. Common adverse effects of musculotropic relaxants used in the treatment of urinary incontinence include:
A. dry mouth and constipation.
B. nausea.
C. headaches.
D. syncope.

58. You see an 82-year-old woman with early onset dementia and urge incontinence. Which of the following medications is least likely to contribute to worsening mental status?
A. oxybutynin (Ditropan®)
B. tolterodine (Detrol)
C. darifenacin (Enablex®)
D. solifenacin (VESIcare®)

59. A 64-year-old woman presents with urge incontinence and has not been able to tolerate treatment with anticholinergic agents. You recommend the use of which of the following? More than one can apply
A. botulinum toxin injections.
B. fesoterodine fumarate (Toviaz®).
C. mirabegron (Myrbetriq®).
D. finasteride (Proscar)

Answers

47. C.	52. B.	57. A.
48. D.	53. B.	58. C.
49. A.	54. C.	59. A, C
50. B.	55. A.	
51. A.	56. B.	

Urinary incontinence (UI) is the involuntary loss of urine in sufficient amounts to be a problem. This condition is often thought by many women to be a normal part of aging. In reality, numerous treatment options are available after the cause of urinary incontinence is established (Table 12–4). In all cases, urinalysis and urine culture and sensitivity should be obtained. Further diagnostic testing should be directed by

TABLE 12-4
Types of Urinary Incontinence

Type of Urinary Incontinence	Etiology and Population Most Often Affected	Clinical Presentation	Treatment Options
Urge incontinence	Detrusor overactivity causing uninhibited bladder contractions. Most common form of incontinence in elders.	Strong sensation of needing to empty the bladder that cannot be suppressed, often coupled with involuntary loss of urine.	Avoiding stimulants, gentle bladder stretching by increasing voiding interval by 15–30 min after establishing a half-hour voiding schedule, cautious fluid ingestion (sips of fluid rather than large amounts ingested rapidly). Add agent to reduce bladder contraction such as an anticholinergic; options include tolterodine (Detrol), oxybutynin (Ditropan), solifenacin succinate (VESIcare), darifenacin (Enablex), fesoterodine fumarate (Toviaz). Alternatives to anticholinergics include mirabegron (Myrbetriq) and botulinum toxin injections.
Stress incontinence	Weakness of pelvic floor and urethral muscles. Most common form of incontinence in women; rare in men, occasionally noted post prostate/bladder surgery.	Loss of urine with activity that causes increase in intra-abdominal pressure such as coughing, sneezing, exercise.	Support to the area through the use of a vaginal tampon, urethral stents, periurethral bulking agent injections, and pessary use. Kegel and other similar exercises most helpful in younger patients. Pelvic floor rehabilitation with biofeedback, electrical stimulation and bladder training. Surgical intervention can be helpful in well-chosen patients. Topical and systemic estrogen therapy formerly recommended for this condition, now recognized as not helpful and perhaps contributing to stress incontinence symptoms. When both urge and stress incontinence is present, the term mixed urinary incontinence is often used.

Continued

TABLE 12-4

Types of Urinary Incontinence—cont'd

Type of Urinary Incontinence	Etiology and Population Most Often Affected	Clinical Presentation	Treatment Options
Urethral obstruction	Obstruction of bladder outflow through urethral obstruction (prostatic, stricture, tumor) resulting in urinary retention with overflow and detrusor instability. Most commonly found in older men.	Dribbling postvoid coupled with urge incontinence on presentation.	Treatment of urethral obstruction.
Functional incontinence	Associated with inability to get to the toilet or lack of awareness of need to void.	Usually in person with mobility issues or altered cognition. Worsened by no availability of a helper to assist in toileting activities.	Ameliorated by having assistant who is aware of voiding cue and is available to help with toileting activities.
Transient incontinence	Associated with acute event such as delirium, UTI, medication use, restricted activity.	Presentation consistent with underlying process.	Treatment of underlying process, discontinuation of offending medication.

patient presentation. If UTI is present, treatment with the appropriate antimicrobial is indicated.

Urge incontinence (also called overactive bladder) is the most common form of urinary incontinence in elderly persons. Behavioral therapy, including a voiding schedule and gentle bladder stretching, are helpful. Pharmacological intervention is indicated in conjunction with behavioral therapy (Table 12–4). Tolterodine (Detrol) and solifenacin succinate (VESIcare) are examples of selective muscarinic receptor antagonists that block bladder receptors and limit bladder contraction. Helpful in the treatment of urge incontinence, the use of these products is associated with a decrease in the numbers of micturitions and of incontinent episodes, along with an increase in voiding volume. Oxybutynin (Ditropan) is a nonselective muscarinic receptor antagonist that blocks receptors in the bladder and oral cavity, with activity similar to that of tolterodine; adverse effects include dry mouth and constipation. Darifenacin (Enablex) and fesoterodine fumarate (Toviaz) are newer anticholinergic agents approved for urge incontinence. Compared to older agents, darifenacin is associated with fewer adverse effects, such as confusion, and is likely more helpful in older patients with underlying dementia. Mirabegron (Myrbetriq), a beta-3 adrenoceptor agonist, has been shown to be effective in treatment-naïve patients as well as those who fail therapy with anticholinergic agents. Botulinum toxin injections in the bladder have also been approved and can be effective for those who fail or are intolerant of pharmacologic treatment.

Other forms of incontinence can be treated by behavioral therapy, treating the underlying cause of incontinence, and/or surgery (e.g., urethral obstruction or stress incontinence) (Table 12–4).

DISCUSSION SOURCES

Vasavada SP, Carmel ME, Rackley R. Urinary incontinence. Available at http://emedicine.medscape.com/article/452289.

Gormley EA, Lightner DJ, Burgio KL, et al. Diagnosis and treatment of overactive bladder (non-neurogenic) in adults: AUA/SUFU guideline, 2012. www.auanet.org/common/pdf/education/clinical-guidance/Overactive-Bladder.pdf.

◗ Renal Stones

60. Risk factors for renal stones include all of the following except:
    A. male gender.
    B. vegetarian diet.
    C. family history of renal stones.
    D. obesity.

61. Medications known to increase the risk of renal stones include all of the following except:
    A. hydrochlorothiazide.
    B. moxifloxacin.
    C. topiramate.
    D. indinavir.

62. The most common renal stones are composed of:
A. calcium.
B. uric acid.
C. sodium.
D. iron.

63. Struvite stones are typically found in people:
A. with type 2 diabetes.
B. who live in colder climates.
C. who abuse alcohol.
D. with a history of kidney infections.

64. Common symptoms of renal stones include all of the following except:
A. pink, red, or brown urine.
B. sharp pain in the back or lower abdomen.
C. marked febrile response.
D. pain while urinating.

65. The preferred method to identify the location of small renal stones is:
A. x-ray.
B. abdominal ultrasound.
C. CT scan.
D. radionuclide scan.

66. You see a 58-year-old man diagnosed with a kidney stone who reports pain primarily during urination. You consider all of the following except:
A. improved hydration.
B. alpha blocker use.
C. prescribing a diuretic
D. analgesia use.

67. A 63-year-old man presents with abdominal pain, pain during urination, and red urine. Imaging reveals a renal stone in the ureter. An appropriate treatment option would be:
A. percutaneous nephrolithotomy.
B. shock wave lithotripsy.
C. insertion of a nephrostomy tube.
D. insertion of a catheter.

68. The most effective strategy for preventing renal stones is:
A. daily exercise.
B. adequate hydration.
C. limiting coffee consumption.
D. smoking cessation.

69. You see a 58-year-old woman who is being treated for a renal stone. Analysis of a stone passed in the urine reveals that it is composed of calcium oxalate. In counseling the patient about preventing future stones, you consider all of the following except:
A. reducing sodium in her diet.
B. limiting consumption of beets, rhubarb, nuts, and chocolate.
C. encouraging getting her daily calcium requirements from food.
D. if calcium supplements are needed, this medication should be taken on an empty stomach.

Answers

60. B.	64. C.	68. B.
61. B.	65. C.	69. D.
62. A.	66. C.	
63. D.	67. B.	

Renal stones (also known as kidney stones or renal lithiasis) are one of the most common urinary tract disorders, accounting for more 1 million annual visits to healthcare providers and more than 300,000 visits to emergency departments in the United States. Kidney stones form when the urine becomes highly concentrated with mineral and acid salts, such as calcium, oxalate, and phosphorus, which eventually crystallize. Men are more likely to have renal stones than women. Other risk factors include family history of kidney stones, chronically poor fluid intake, dehydration, certain diets (i.e., high in protein, sodium, and sugar), and being overweight or obese. Health conditions associated with a higher risk of renal stones include hypercalciuria, cystic kidney disease, hyperparathyroidism, renal tubular acidosis, cystinuria, and gout. Certain medications can also increase the risk of renal stones, including diuretics, calcium-based antacids, indinavir (for HIV infection), and topiramate.

Calcium stones are the most common and can occur in two forms: calcium oxalate (caused by high calcium and oxalate excretion) or calcium phosphate (caused by high urine calcium and alkaline urine). Oxalate is a substance that occurs naturally in some fruits and vegetables as well as nuts and chocolate. Uric acid stones form when urine is persistently acidic. These stones form in people who do not drink enough fluids or who lose too much fluid, eat a high protein diet, or who have gout. Purines derived from animal protein in the diet can cause elevated levels of uric acid in the urine. Other types of stones include struvite stones (resulting from kidney infections) and cystine stones (cause by a genetic disorder that causes cystine to pass through the kidneys and into the urine).

Symptoms can depend on the size of the stone. People who have small stones that pass easily through the urinary tract often have no have any symptoms. Others can experience pain while urinating; have pink, red or brown urine; or feel a sharp pain in the back or lower abdomen. Pain can come in waves and fluctuate in intensity. Some will experience nausea and vomiting associated with the pain, which can last a short or long time. Some patients will have a persistent urge to urinate and/or are urinating more often than usual.

Diagnosis involves a urinalysis to check for the presence of substances that form stones and rule out other conditions that can cause the symptoms, such as infection. Imaging with either an x-ray or CT scan can confirm the diagnosis and show stone locations. X-rays can miss small kidney stones whereas a CT scan will reveal even tiny stones. Stones that pass through the urine can be analyzed to reveal the makeup of the stone. This information can be used to determine a plan for preventing further kidney stones.

Treatment will depend on the size of the stone as well as whether the stones are causing pain or blocking the urinary tract. Small stones typically pass through the urinary tract without treatment, though analgesics can be prescribed to alleviate the pain. An alpha blocker can be used to relax the muscles in the ureter in order to pass the stone more quickly and with less pain. Intravenous hydration is needed if the patient experiences nausea and vomiting and is unable to maintain hydration with oral intake. Several options are available if more urgent measures are needed. Shock wave lithotripsy (SWL) generates shock waves that travel through the body to break up the stones into smaller pieces that more readily pass through the urinary tract. For stones located in the ureter, ureteroscopy can be used to retrieve the stone or break a stone into smaller pieces with a laser. For larger stones located in the kidney, percutaneous nephrolithotomy can be used to break up the stone with shock waves followed by the use of a nephrostomy tube to drain urine and stone fragments directly from the kidneys.

Proper hydration is the optimal method to prevent renal stones, with a recommendation of drinking 2 to 3 liters (67 to 100 oz.) of fluid per day. Water and citrus drinks are preferred for prevention. For those with calcium oxalate or calcium phosphate stones, prevention can also include reducing sodium and animal protein while getting enough calcium from food sources. If calcium supplements are used, these should be taken with meals. Calcium oxalate stones can be prevented by reducing intake of oxalate-rich foods, such as rhubarb, beets, okra, spinach, Swiss chard, sweet potatoes, nuts, tea, chocolate, and soy products. For those with uric acid stones, limiting animal protein will help prevent further stone formation.

DISCUSSION SOURCES

National Kidney and Urologic Diseases Information Clearinghouse (NKUDIC). Kidney stones in adults. http://kidney.niddk.nih.gov/kudiseases/pubs/stonesadults.

Wolf JS Jr. Nephrolithiasis. http://emedicine.medscape.com/article/437096.

Hematological and Select Immunological Disorders

13

Anemia

1. Worldwide, which of the following is the most common type of anemia?
   A. pernicious anemia
   B. folate-deficiency anemia
   C. anemia of chronic disease
   D. iron-deficiency anemia

2. Most of the body's iron is obtained from:
   A. animal-based food sources.
   B. recycled iron content from aged red blood cells (RBCs).
   C. endoplasmic reticulum production.
   D. vegetable-based food sources.

3. Which of the following is most consistent with iron-deficiency anemia?
   A. low mean corpuscular volume (MCV), normal mean corpuscular hemoglobin (MCH)
   B. low MCV, low MCH
   C. low MCV, elevated MCH
   D. normal MCV, normal MCH

4. One of the earliest laboratory markers in evolving macrocytic or microcytic anemia is:
   A. an increase in RBC distribution width (RDW).
   B. a reduction in measurable hemoglobin.
   C. a low MCH level.
   D. an increased platelet count.

5. A 48-year-old woman developed iron-deficiency anemia after excessive perimenopausal bleeding, successfully treated by endometrial ablation. Her hematocrit (Hct) level is 25%, and she is taking iron therapy. At 5 days into therapy, one possible observed change in laboratory parameters would include:
   A. a correction of mean cell volume.
   B. an 8% increase in Hct level.
   C. reticulocytosis.
   D. a correction in ferritin level.

6. A healthy 34-year-old man asks whether he should take an iron supplement. You respond that:
   A. this is a prudent measure to ensure health.
   B. iron-deficiency anemia is a common problem in men of his age.
   C. use of an iron supplement in the absence of a documented deficiency can lead to iatrogenic iron overload.
   D. excess iron is easily excreted.

7. Which of the following is the best advice on taking ferrous sulfate to enhance iron absorption?
   A. "Take with other medications."
   B. "Take on a full stomach."
   C. "Take on an empty stomach."
   D. "Do not take with vitamin C."

8. A 40-year-old woman with pyelonephritis is taking two mediations: ciprofloxacin and ferrous sulfate (for iron-deficiency anemia). She asks about taking both medications. You advise that:
   A. she should take the medications with a large glass of water.
   B. an inactive drug compound is potentially formed if the two medications are taken together.
   C. she can take the medications together to enhance adherence to therapy.
   D. the ferrous sulfate potentially slows gastrointestinal motility and results in enhanced ciprofloxacin absorption.

9. One month into therapy for pernicious anemia, you wish to check the efficacy of the intervention. The best laboratory test to order at this point is a:
   A. Schilling test.
   B. hemoglobin measurement.
   C. reticulocyte count.
   D. serum cobalamin.

10. A woman who is planning a pregnancy should increase her intake of which of the following to minimize the risk of neural tube defect in the fetus?
    A. iron
    B. niacin
    C. folic acid
    D. vitamin C

11. Risk factors for folate-deficiency anemia include:
    A. menorrhagia.
    B. chronic ingestion of overcooked foods.
    C. use of nonsteroidal antiinflammatory drugs.
    D. gastric atrophy.

12. Folate-deficiency anemia causes which of the following changes in the RBC indices?
    A. microcytic, normochromic
    B. normocytic, normochromic
    C. microcytic, hypochromic
    D. macrocytic, normochromic

13. Pernicious anemia is usually caused by:
    A. dietary deficiency of vitamin B_{12}.
    B. lack of production of intrinsic factor by the gastric mucosa.
    C. RBC enzyme deficiency.
    D. a combination of micronutrient deficiencies caused by malabsorption.

14. Pernicious anemia causes which of the following changes in the RBC indices?
    A. microcytic, normochromic
    B. normocytic, normochromic
    C. microcytic, hypochromic
    D. macrocytic, normochromic

15. Common physical examination findings in patients with pernicious anemia include:
    A. hypoactive bowel sounds.
    B. stocking-glove neuropathy.
    C. thin, spoon-shaped nails.
    D. retinal hemorrhages.

16. You examine a 47-year-old man who presents with difficulty initiating and maintaining sleep and chronic pharyngeal erythema with the following results on hemogram:
    Hemoglobin (Hgb) = 15 g
    Hct = 45%
    RBC = 4.2 million mm³
    MCV = 108 fL
    MCHC = 33.2 g/dL

    These values are most consistent with:
    A. pernicious anemia.
    B. alcohol abuse.
    C. thalassemia minor.
    D. Fanconi disease.

17. You examine a 22-year-old woman of Asian ancestry. She has no presenting complaint. Hemogram results are as follows:
    Hgb = 9.1 g (normal 12 to 14 g)
    Hct = 28% (normal 36% to 42%)
    RBC = 5 million mm³ (normal 3.2 to 4.3 million mm³)
    MCV = 68 fL (normal 80 to 96 fL)
    MCHC = 33.2 g/dL (normal 32 to 36 g/dL)
    RBC distribution width (RDW) = 13% (normal ≤15%).
    Reticulocytes = 1.5%

    This is most consistent with the laboratory assessment of:
    A. iron-deficiency anemia.
    B. Cooley anemia.
    C. alpha-thalassemia minor.
    D. hemoglobin Barts.

18. A 68-year-old man who is usually healthy presents with new onset of "huffing and puffing" with exercise for the past 3 weeks. Physical examination reveals conjunctiva pallor and a hemic murmur. Hemogram results are as follows:
    Hgb = 7.6 g
    Hct = 20.5%
    RBC = 2.1 million mm³
    MCV = 76 fL
    MCHC = 28 g/dL
    RDW = 18.4%
    Reticulocytes = 1.8%

    The most likely cause of these finding is:
    A. poor nutrition.
    B. occult blood loss.
    C. malabsorption.
    D. chronic inflammation.

19. You examine a 57-year-old woman with rheumatoid arthritis who is on disease-modifying antirheumatic disease but continues to have poor disease control and find the following results on hemogram:
    Hgb = 10.5 g
    Hct = 33%
    RBC = 3.1 million mm³
    MCV = 88 fL
    MCHC = 32.8 g/dL
    RDW = 12.2%
    Reticulocytes = 0.8%

The laboratory findings are most consistent with:
    A. pernicious anemia.
    B. anemia of chronic disease.
    C. beta-thalassemia minor.
    D. folate-deficiency anemia.

20. You examine a 27-year-old woman with menorrhagia who is otherwise well and note the following results on hemogram:

Hgb = 10.1 g
Hct = 32%
RBC = 2.9 million mm ^{3}
MCV = 72 fL
MCHC = 28.2 g/dL
RDW = 18.9%

Physical examination is likely to include:
A. conjunctiva pallor.
B. hemic murmur.
C. tachycardia.
D. no specific anemia-related findings.

21. Results of hemogram in a person with anemia of chronic disease include:
A. microcytosis.
B. anisocytosis.
C. reticulocytopenia.
D. macrocytosis.

22. When prescribing erythropoietin supplementation, the NP considers that:
A. the adrenal glands are its endogenous source.
B. the addition of micronutrient supplementation needed for erythropoiesis is advisable.
C. its use is as an adjunct in treating thrombocytopenia.
D. with its use, the RBC life span is prolonged.

23. In the first weeks of anemia therapy with parenteral vitamin B_{12} in a 68-year-old woman with hypertension who is taking a thiazide diuretic, the patient should be carefully monitored for:
A. hypernatremia.
B. dehydration.
C. hypokalemia.
D. acidemia.

24. Which of the following conditions is unlikely to result in anemia of chronic disease?
A. rheumatoid arthritis
B. peripheral vascular disease
C. chronic renal insufficiency
D. osteomyelitis

25. In health, the ratio of hemoglobin to hematocrit is usually:
A. 1:1.
B. 1:2.
C. 1:3.
D. 1:4.

26. An increase in the normal variation of RBC size is known as:
A. poikilocytosis.
B. granulation.
C. anisocytosis.
D. basophilic stippling.

27. Erythropoietin is a glycoprotein that influences a stem cell to become a:
A. lymphocyte.
B. platelet.
C. neutrophil.
D. red blood cell.

28. Intervention in anemia of chronic disease most often includes:
A. oral vitamin B_{12}.
B. treatment of the underlying cause.
C. transfusion.
D. parenteral iron.

29. Poikilocytosis refers to alterations in a red blood cells:
A. thickness.
B. color.
C. shape.
D. size.

30. Which of the following is not consistent with anemia of chronic disease (ACD)?
A. NL RDW
B. NL MCHC
C. Hct less than 24%
D. NL to slightly elevated serum ferritin

31. In children younger than age 6 years, accidental overdose of iron-containing products is:
A. easily treated.
B. a source of significant GI upset.
C. worrisome but rarely causes significant harm.
D. a leading cause of fatal poisoning in the age group.

32. When counseling a patient about the neurological alterations often associated with vitamin B_{12} deficiency, the NP advises that:
A. these usually resolve within days with appropriate therapy.
B. if present for longer than 6 months, these changes are occasionally permanent.
C. the use of parenteral vitamin B_{12} therapy is needed to ensure symptom resolution.
D. cognitive changes associated with vitamin B_{12} deficiency are seldom reversible even with appropriate therapy.

33. When the cause of a macrocytic anemia is uncertain, the most commonly recommended additional testing includes which of the following?
A. haptoglobin and reticulocyte count.
B. Schilling test and gastric biopsy.
C. methylmalonic acid and homocysteine.
D. transferrin and prealbumin.

Anemia: True or False?

34. Anemia in children is potentially associated with poorer school performance.

35. During pregnancy, folic-acid requirements increase twofold to fourfold.

36. The red blood cell content is approximately 90% hemoglobin.

37. Approximately 90% of the body's erythropoietin is produced by the kidney.

38. The body's normative response to anemia is reticulocytopenia.

▌Answers

1. D.	14. D.	27. D.
2. B.	15. B.	28. B.
3. B.	16. B.	29. C.
4. A.	17. C.	30. C.
5. C.	18. B.	31. D.
6. C.	19. B.	32. B.
7. C.	20. D.	33. C.
8. B.	21. C.	34. True
9. B.	22. B.	35. True
10. C.	23. C.	36. True
11. B.	24. B.	37. True
12. D.	25. C.	38. False
13. B.	26. C.	

Anemia is defined as a decrease in the oxygen-carrying capability of the blood. This condition is not a disease, but rather a sign of an underlying process. Anemia occurs only in the presence of a clinical insult severe enough to disturb the normal hematological homeostatic mechanisms and exceed the body's ample hematological reserves.

The clinical presentation of anemia is highly variable, and compensation is common because most anemias are usually gradual in onset. In addition, the oxyhemoglobin-dissociation curve is moved to the right as the hemoglobin level decreases, with the oxygen molecule given up more freely by the RBC. As a result, symptoms of anemia seldom occur, unless the hemoglobin level decreases to less than 10 g/dL.

The health history usually reveals clues about the cause of the anemia (i.e., excessive menstrual flow, acute blood loss). Patients frequently report deep, sighing respiration with activity, often associated with a sensation of rapid, forceful heart rate; this is likely a reflection of the decreased oxygen-carrying capability of the blood and a corresponding compensatory mechanism. Fatigue, headache, and decreased exercise tolerance are often present. Poor school performance and learning difficulties have been reported in children with anemia. In patients at risk for or who have coronary artery disease, anginal symptoms are commonly reported.

The physical examination usually contributes little to the diagnosis, unless the anemia is severe. Pallor of the skin and mucous membranes is an unreliable indicator and is usually seen only when the hemoglobin is less than 8 g/dL. In elderly persons and in individuals with coronary artery disease, signs of heart failure (i.e., distended neck veins, rales, tachycardia, right upper quadrant abdominal tenderness, hepatomegaly) are often seen with severe anemia. An early systolic murmur, also known as a hemic murmur, is often heard, owing in part to the increase in blood flow over the heart valves. Neurological findings, such as paresthesia; stocking-glove neuropathy; difficulty with balance; and, in extreme cases, confusion, can be found in patients with vitamin B_{12} deficiency. Less commonly, mental status changes are noted in folate-deficiency anemia.

In evaluating the hemograms of patients with anemia, the following questions should be answered to ascertain the origin of the anemia (Table 13–1).

- What are hemoglobin (hgb), hematocrit (hct), and red blood cell (RBC) values? These values should be proportionately decreased. Normally, the hemoglobin-to-hematocrit ratio is 1:3, so that in health, 1 g of hemoglobin is equivalent to 3% points of hematocrit. Hemoglobin is an iron-containing protein responsible for the transportation of oxygen and other gases. The hematocrit value reflects the percentage of RBCs in a given volume of blood; the value is influenced by the body's hydration status. This ratio is usually violated only in severe dehydration, where the hematocrit is artificially elevated (e.g., hgb 12 g, hct 39%), or overhydration, where the hematocrit is artificially decreased (e.g., hgb 12 g, hct 32%).

- What is the RBC size? This is reflected by the mean corpuscle volume (MCV); the method of categorizing anemia is known as Wintrobe's classification. Using this classification, anemias are categorized as being microcytic (abnormally low MCV), normocytic (MCV within normal parameters), or macrocytic (abnormally high MCV). The RBC maintains its size and color throughout its 90- to 120-day lifespan.

- Is the RBC abnormally small (microcytic or low MCV)? Ninety percent of the RBC volume is composed of hemoglobin. As a result, hemoglobin is the major contributor to cell size; microcytosis is seen in patients with anemia in whom hemoglobin synthesis is impaired, such as in presence of iron-deficiency anemia and the thalassemias. In addition, because hemoglobin gives RBCs their characteristic red color, small (microcytic) and pale (hypochromic) go together. A microcytic cell will also have a low mean hemoglobin concentration (MCH).

- Is the RBC abnormally large (macrocytic)? Impaired RNA and DNA synthesis in young erythrocytes most commonly cause macrocytosis. Folic acid and vitamin B_{12} contribute significantly to RNA and DNA synthesis in the developing RBC. A lack of either or both of these micronutrients can result in macrocytic anemia. Because hemoglobin synthesis is not the issue, macrocytic cells

TABLE 13-1
Hemogram Evaluation in Anemia

Laboratory Parameter	Comment
What are hgb and hct, RBC values?	Values should be proportionately decreased. Normally, hgb:hct ratio is 1:3. • 10 g = 30% • 12 g = 36% • 15 g = 45%
What is the RBC size?	Wintrobe's classification of anemia by evaluation of mean corpuscle volume (MCV) • Microcytic: Small cell with MCV <80 fL • Normocytic: Normal size cell with MCV 80–96 fL • Macrocytic: Abnormally large cell with MCV >96 fL
What is the RBC's hemoglobin content?	Reflected by mean cell hemoglobin (MCH), mean cell hemoglobin concentration (MCHC) • Hemoglobin is the source of the cell's color ("-chromic") • Normochromic: Normal color—MCHC 31–37 g/dL • Hypochromic: Pale—MCHC <31 g/dL
What is the RDW?	Index of variation in RBC size (normal 11.5%–15%) Abnormal value: >15%, indicating that new cells differ in size (smaller or larger) compared with older cells. This is one of the earliest laboratory indicators of an evolving microcytic or macrocytic anemia.
What is the reticulocyte percentage or count?	The body's normal response to anemia is to attempt correction via increasing the number of new cells (reticulocytes). Normal response to anemia is reticulocytosis. Because the reticulocyte MCV >96 fL, marked reticulocytosis can cause RDW to increase transiently.

are usually of normal color (normochromic or MCH within normal limits).

• Is the RBC of normal size (normocytic)? In these anemias, the cells are made under ordinary conditions with sufficient hemoglobin; there is no problem with RNA, DNA, or hemoglobin synthesis. Acute blood loss and anemia of chronic disease result in a normocytic, normochromic anemia.

• What is the RDW (RBC distribution width)? RDW reflects the degree of variation in RBC size; this is often reported as anisocytosis on RBC morphologic study. RDW measurement is elevated when RBCs are of varying sizes, which implies that cells were synthesized under varying conditions. In iron-deficiency anemia, normal-sized cells produced before iron depletion continue to circulate until their 90- to 120-day life span ends. Meanwhile, new, microcytic, iron-deficient cells containing less hemoglobin are produced. There is wide variation in cell size (newer cells are smaller, and older cells are larger) and an increase in RDW. Because minor variation in cell size is normal, RDW is considered increased only when it is greater than 15%. An elevated RDW is often the first abnormal finding in the hemogram of a person with an evolving microcytic or macrocytic anemia. Poikilocytosis refers to a variation in RBC shape and is not specific to any anemia type but usually occurs with more severe anemia.

• What is the hemoglobin content (color) of the cell? The hemoglobin content of the cell is reflected in the MCH, reported as a percentage of the cell's volume. Because hemoglobin gives RBCs their characteristic red color, the suffix "-chromic" is used to describe the MCH. When a cell has a normal MCH, it is of normal color, or normochromic. When there is an impairment of hemoglobin synthesis, such as in iron-deficiency anemia or thalassemia, the cells are pale or hypochromic and the MCH is low. RBCs seldom are hyperchromic, or containing excessive amounts of hemoglobin.

• What is the percentage of reticulocytes? The body's normal response to anemia is to attempt correction via increasing the number of new cells (reticulocytes). The body's normal response to anemia is reticulocytosis, or an increase in the percentage of circulating reticulocytes to greater than the 1% to 2% noted in health. The notation of reticulocytopenia, or an abnormally low reticulocyte percentage, is evidence of inadequate hemopoiesis.

Because the reticulocyte MCV >96 fL, marked reticulocytosis can cause RDW to increase transiently.

Worldwide, iron deficiency is the most common reason for anemia (Table 13–2). Because an estimated 8 years of poor iron intake is needed in adults before iron-deficiency anemia occurs, diet is rarely the etiology in developed countries. Chronic blood loss causing a wasting of the RBCs' recyclable iron, the body's most important iron source, is the most common cause. Occult gastrointestinal blood loss, such as from an oozing gastritis or gastrointestinal malignancy, is a common cause, as is excessive menstrual flow. Lower and upper GI tract evaluation is recommended to diagnose the cause of IDA in men ≥50 and in postmenopausal women. Men and postmenopausal women require 1 mg of iron each day. During reproductive years, women require 1.5 to 3 mg/d of iron, in part because of the monthly loss of RBCs with the menses.

TABLE 13-2
Identifying Common Anemias

Anemia Type	Description	Example
Normocytic (MCV 80–96 fL), normochromic anemia with normal RDW Most common etiology: Acute blood loss or anemia of chronic disease (ACD)	Cells made under ordinary conditions with sufficient hemoglobin. This yields cells that are normal size (normocytic), normal color (normochromic), and about the same size (normal RDW)	72 y.o. man with an acute gastrointestinal bleed (acute blood loss) 32 y.o. woman with newly diagnosed lupus erythematosus (ACD) Hgb 10.1 g (12–14 g) Hct 32% (36%–43%) RBC 3.2 million mm3 (4.2–5.4 million) MCV 82 fL (81–96 fL) MCHC 34.8 g/dL (31–37 g/dL) RDW 12.1% (11.5%–15%)
Microcytic (MCV <80 fL) hypochromic anemia with elevated RDW Most common etiology: Iron-deficiency anemia	Small cell (microcytic) owing to insufficient hemoglobin (hypochromic) with new cells smaller than old cells (elevated RDW)	68 y.o. man with erosive gastritis Hgb 10.1 g (12–14 g) Hct 32% (36%–43%) RBC 3.2 million mm3 (4.2–5.4 million) MCV 72 fL (81–96 fL) MCHC 26.8 g/dL (31–37 g/dL) RDW 18.1% (11.5%–15%)
Microcytic (MCV <80 fL) hypochromic anemia with normal RDW Most common etiology: Alpha or beta thalassemia minor At-risk ethnic groups for alpha thalassemia minor: Asian, African ancestry At-risk ethnic groups for beta thalassemia minor: African, Middle Eastern, Mediterranean ancestry	Through genetic variation, small (microcytic), pale (hypochromic) cells that are all around the same size (normal RDW)	27 y.o. man of African ancestry Hgb 11.6 g (14–16 g) Hct 36.7% (42%–48%) RBC 6.38 million mm3 (4.7–6.10 million) MCV 69.5 fL (81–99 fL) MCH 22 pg (27–33 pg) RDW 13.8% (11.5%–15%)
Macrocytic (MCV >96 fL) normochromic anemia with elevated RDW Most common etiology: Vitamin B$_{12}$ deficiency, pernicious anemia, folate-deficiency anemia	Abnormally large (macrocytic) cell owing to altered RNA: DNA ratio, hemoglobin content normal (normochromic), new cells larger than old cells (elevated RDW)	52 y.o. woman with untreated pernicious anemia Hgb 10.2 g (12–14 g) Hct 32% (36%–43%) RBC 3.2 million mm3 (4.2–5.4 million) MCV 125.5 fL (81–99 fL) MCH 31 pg (27–33 pg) RDW 18.8% (11.5%–15%)
Drug-induced macrocytosis usually without anemia Etiology: Use of select medications such as carbamazepine (Tegretol), zidovudine (AZT), valproic acid (Depakote), phenytoin (Dilantin), alcohol, others. Reversible when use of offending medication is discontinued	Abnormally large (macrocytic) cell owing to altered RNA: DNA ratio, hemoglobin content normal (normochromic), new cells usually same size as old cells (normal RDW)	32 y.o. woman who is taking phenytoin Hgb 12 g (12–14 g) Hct 37% (36%–43%) RBC 4.2 million mm3 (4.2–5.4 million) MCV 105.5 fL (81–99 fL) MCH 31 pg (27–33 pg) RDW 12.8% (11.5%–15%)

In all these circumstances, these iron requirements are achievable with a well-balanced diet. Because 1 mL of packed RBCs contains 1 mg of iron, losses of 2 to 3 mL of blood per day through chronic, low-volume gastrointestinal bleeding, repeated phlebotomy, or persistent excessive menstrual flow can lead to iron deficiency.

The laboratory diagnosis of iron-deficiency anemia is supported by the following findings (Table 13–3):

- Early in the disease process: Low to normal hgb, low hct, and low to normal total RBC count; normocytic, possible hypochromic; RDW greater than 15%, a new iron-deficient cells are produced.
- Low serum iron level: Reflecting iron concentration in circulation. Serum iron is reflective of iron intake during the past 24 to 48 hours and can be falsely elevated because of recent high levels of dietary iron ingestion or self-prescribed oral iron supplementation.
- Elevated total iron-binding capacity (TIBC): A measure of transferrin, a plasma protein that easily combines with iron. When more of transferrin is available for binding, the TIBC level increases, reflecting iron deficiency.
- Iron saturation less than 15%: Calculated by dividing the serum iron level by the TIBC.
- Low serum ferritin level: This is the body's major iron storage protein. Ferritin depletion is one of the first laboratory markers of iron deficiency as stores are depleted prior to abnormal cells being formed.
- Absence of iron from bone marrow, if aspiration is done.

- Later disease: Microcytic, hypochromic anemia with low RBC count and elevated RDW greater than 15%. A decrease in hemoglobin or RBC indices is a late rather than an early marker of disease.

Therapy for patients with iron-deficiency anemia involves not only iron replacement, but also treatment of the underlying cause. Drug interactions are common (Table 13–4).

Iron use without a distinct clinical indication, including the use of iron-fortified multiple vitamins, is not recommended because this can lead to an iatrogenic iron overload. Iron overload has been hypothesized to be a cardiovascular risk factor. A lower rate of cardiovascular disease has been noted in frequent blood donors with relatively low levels of stored iron compared with age-matched controls. In addition, cardiovascular disease rates in women equal rates in men 5 to 10 years after menopause, a time when ferritin levels in women and men are equal.

Reticulocytosis begins quickly after initiation of iron therapy, with the reticulocyte count peaking 7 to 10 days into therapy. Hemoglobin increases at a rate of 2 g/dL every 3 weeks in response to iron therapy and is likely to take 2 months to correct if the underlying cause of the anemia has been successfully treated. As a result, the following laboratory tests may be used to evaluate the resolution of iron-deficiency anemia: reticulocytes at 1 to 2 weeks to ensure marrow response to iron therapy, hemoglobin at 6 weeks to 2 months to ensure anemia recovery, and ferritin at 2 months after measure of normal hemoglobin (or 4 months after initiation

TABLE 13-3
Drug Interactions With Oral Iron Therapy

Drug	Effect	Comment
Antacids	Decreased iron absorption	Separate use by ≥2 hr
Caffeine	Decreased iron absorption	Separate use by ≥2 hr
Fluoroquinolones (ciprofloxacin, moxifloxacin, levofloxacin, others)	Decreased fluoroquinolone effect	Avoid concurrent use or separate doses by ≥6 hr
Levodopa	Decreased levodopa and iron effect	Separate medications by as much time as possible; increase levodopa dose as needed
Select antihypertensives (ACE inhibitors, methyldopa)	Decreased antihypertensive effect	Separate medications by ≥2 hr, monitor BP. Additional effect with IV iron: when ACE inhibitors are given concurrently, increased risk of systemic reaction to iron (fever, arthralgia, hypotension); concurrent use should be avoided
Tetracyclines including doxycycline	Decreased tetracycline and iron effect	Do not use concurrently, or separate by ≥3–4 hr
Levothyroxine (Synthroid, Unithroid, Levoxyl, generic) o	Decreased levothyroxine effect	Take levothyroxine ≥2 hr before or 4 hr after iron dose
Histamine-2 receptor antagonists	Decreased dietary iron absorption	Less significant when compared to proton pump inhibitor use
Proton pump inhibitor	Decrease dietary iron absorption	Potentially significant contributor to iron and other micronutrient deficiencies, particularly with protracted use

Source: PL Detail-Document, Treatment of Vitamin B12 Deficiency. Pharmacist's Letter/Prescriber's Letter. August 2011.

TABLE 13-4
Oral Vitamin B$_{12}$ Drug Interactions

Drug	Effect
Aminoglycosides	With concomitant use, decreased vitamin B$_{12}$ absorption
Colchicine	With concomitant use, decreased vitamin B$_{12}$ absorption
Potassium supplements	With concomitant use, decreased vitamin B$_{12}$ absorption
Ascorbic acid	Potential to destroy vitamin B$_{12}$ if taken within 1 hr of oral vitamin B$_{12}$ ingestion
Proton pump inhibitor	With concomitant use, decreased vitamin B$_{12}$ absorption, particularly with protracted use

Source: Vitamin B12 (cyanocobalamin) Drug Interactions, available at http://www.drugs.com/drug-interactions/cyanocobalamin,vitamin-b12.html.

of iron therapy) to ensure documentation of replenished iron stores.

A number of oral iron (Fe) forms are available, including ferrous gluconate and ferrous sulfate. Either is acceptable as a supplement. Enteric-coated iron should be avoided. Although this Fe form is often reported as causing less gastrointestinal upset, iron is best absorbed in the duodenum. The use of enteric-coated iron results in relatively little of the dose being properly absorbed. In addition, the duodenum is relatively refractory to iron absorption for about 6 hours post exposure to a high iron dose. As a result, oral iron should be dosed no sooner than every 6 hours; twice-daily supplementation is usually adequate to correct iron deficiency. Oral iron overdose is the most common cause of fatal childhood overdose. The source of this iron is usually from an adult's prescription, most often the child's mother. The use of carbonyl iron has been advocated due to its slow rate of GI absorption, yielding less toxicity in overdose. A typical adult iron dose for anemia correction is 50 to 60 mg of elemental iron taken orally twice a day for 3 to 6 months. Ascorbic acid is an enhancer of iron absorption and can reverse the inhibiting effects of substances such as tea and calcium. Ascorbic acid (vitamin C) taken at the same time as ferrous sulfate can help with iron absorption. To minimize adverse GI effects, iron supplements are often taken often taken with food; this can result in as much as a two-thirds reduction in iron absorption. Taking iron on an empty stomach allows for maximum absorption. Due to safety concerns and high cost, parenteral iron use should be limited to individuals who are unable to ingest, tolerate, or properly absorb oral iron.

The thalassemias are a genetically based blood disorder where the body makes an abnormal hemoglobin form. Hemoglobin is made of two proteins: alpha globin and beta globin. In alpha thalassemia, the alteration is in the genes or genes related to alpha globin, and in beta form, it is an alteration on the beta globin. Alpha thalassemias occur most commonly in persons from Southeast Asia, the Middle East, China, and Africa. Beta thalassemias occur in persons of Mediterranean origin and, to a lesser extent, in Chinese people, other Asians, and African Americans. The thalassemia majors are life-threatening conditions that are identified in early life; two altered genes are inherited, one from each parent. The thalassemia minors (thal minor or thal trait), where one defective gene has been inherited, result in a mild microcytic hypochromic anemia. Because there is no micronutrient deficiency, the RDW and platelets are within normal limits. Given the risk of passing the altered genes to offspring if both members of a couple are affected with thal minor, prior genetic counseling is recommended. Otherwise, people with a thal minor have no particular health risks.

The most common causes of macrocytic anemia are folic-acid (folate) deficiency and vitamin B$_{12}$ deficiency. When macrocytosis with anemia is detected on hemogram, the usual next step is to obtain a serum vitamin B$_{12}$. Often labs bundle this test with a serum folate, although folic acid deficiency is much less common. When the diagnosis of macrocytic anemia is uncertain, additional testing is recommended; elevated serum methylmalonic acid (MMA) and homocysteine levels are found with pernicious anemia, whereas elevated homocysteine levels with normal MMA levels are found in folic-acid deficiency.

Folic acid (pteroylglutamic acid) is a water-soluble B complex vitamin found in abundance in peanuts, fruits, and vegetables. Through a complex reaction, folic acid is reduced to folate. Folate donates 1 carbon unit to oxidation at various levels, reactions vital to proper DNA synthesis. During times of accelerated tissue growth and repair, such as in childhood, pregnancy, recovery from serious illness, and recovery from hemolytic anemia, folic-acid requirements increase from the baseline of twofold to fourfold. Folate deficiency causes a macrocytic, normochromic anemia.

The most common causes of folic acid–deficiency anemia are inadequate dietary intake, seen in elderly, alcohol abusers, and impoverished persons and in persons with decreased ability to absorb folic acid, which occurs with malabsorption syndromes such as sprue and celiac disease. Folic-acid deficiency can be avoided with a healthy diet featuring folate-rich fruits and vegetables. In addition, many foods, including most flours, are folic-acid supplemented, further reducing risk.

Folic acid transfers readily through the placenta to the fetus, with fetal levels usually higher than maternal levels; there is evidence that pregnancy is a maternal folate–depleting event. Repeated or multiple pregnancies, in particular, cause depletion of maternal folate stores. Folate deficiency during pregnancy can be largely avoided through the consistent use of prescriptive prenatal vitamins, each tablet usually containing 0.8 to 1 mg of folic acid. Over-the-counter prenatal vitamins contain significantly less of this micronutrient, usually about 0.4 mg per tablet. Supplementation should continue through lactation because approximately 0.5 mg/d of folic acid is transferred to breast milk. Accumulation of the vitamin in human milk takes precedence over maintaining maternal folate levels.

Maternal folic-acid deficiency is a teratogenic state, particularly during neural tube formation. To reduce the rate of neural tube defects in the fetus, a woman planning a pregnancy should be advised to take additional amounts of folic acid, 0.4 mg/d, for 3 months before conception. This recommendation should be extended to all women capable of conception. Over-the-counter multivitamin or diet supplementation with vitamin-fortified foods can easily supply the recommended folate dose. If a woman has a history of giving birth to an infant with a neural tube defect, the folic-acid dose should be increased to 4 mg/d for 3 months before conception and continued at least through the first 12 weeks of pregnancy. If the pregnancy is unplanned or preconception counseling was not sought, initiating folic-acid supplementation during the first 7 weeks of pregnancy seems to offer some neural tube protection. Folic-acid supplementation can be supplied by a prescription prenatal vitamin supplement. If a pregnant woman cannot tolerate the prenatal vitamin supplement because of nausea, a common condition, she likely would be able to take folic acid alone without difficulty. A growing body of knowledge points to genetic factors in metabolizing and using folic acid as a possible contributor to the risk of neural tube defect.

Recommendations for folic-acid replacement for adults range from 0.5 to 1 to 5 mg/d, the usual dose being 1 mg/d. The underlying cause of the folate deficiency must also be treated.

Reticulocytosis occurs rapidly, with a peak at 7 to 10 days into folic-acid therapy. The hematocrit level increases by 4% to 5% per week and generally returns to normal within 1 month. Leukopenia and thrombocytopenia resolve within 2 to 3 days of therapy. A repeat hemogram in 1 to 2 months assists in monitoring of therapeutic effect. Resolution of the related signs and symptoms generally follows the time frame needed for the resolution of the anemia.

Vitamin B_{12}, a member of the cobalamin family, is found in abundance in foods of animal origin and is essential to the development of the RBC. When vitamin B_{12} is ingested orally, it binds with intrinsic factor, a glycoprotein produced by the gastric parietal cells, and is transported systematically. Within the portal blood flow, the vitamin is attached to transcobalamin II, a polypeptide synthesized in the liver and ileum. Intrinsic factor is not absorbed, and the new compound is transported to the bone marrow and other sites, where it is available for use in RBC formation. Two additional glycoproteins, transcobalamin I and III, combine with vitamin B_{12} and are used in the formation of granulocytes. In synergy with folic acid, vitamin B_{12} plays an essential role in RBC DNA synthesis. When deficiencies of either of these micronutrients exist, DNA synthesis in the RBC is impaired, which leads to the distinct changes in the RBC, macrocytosis, and bone marrow.

Vitamin B_{12} therapy should be initiated when the diagnosis is made. Usually there is a brisk hematological response, and the anemia is resolved within 2 months. Reversal of neurological abnormalities is generally slower, but improvement is seen quickly. If neurological abnormalities associated with pernicious anemia have been present for more than 6 months, the changes are occasionally permanent even with appropriate vitamin B_{12} repletion therapy.

Vitamin B_{12} is available generically and in oral and injectable forms. The parenteral form is preferred because of its excellent absorption. In oral form, vitamin B_{12} is erratically absorbed in the distal portion of the small intestine, which can potentially lead to treatment failure. The usual initial vitamin B_{12} dosage is 100 mcg/d intramuscularly for the first week, then weekly for the first month, and then 100 mcg monthly for the rest of the patient's life. Traditionally, doses of 1000 mcg per injection have been used. A cyanocobalamin dose of more than 100 mcg in a single injection exceeds the binding capacity of transcobalamin II; however, the excess is excreted via the kidney and wasted. Concomitant administration of folic acid, iron, vitamin C, and other micronutrients is often needed to help with hematological recovery. When vitamin B_{12} deficiency is to be treated orally, a higher dose, 1000 mcg/d, is needed. Vitamin B_{12} is also available in a nasal gel, usually used weekly at a dose of 500 mcg. When the cause of macrocytic anemia has not yet been established, a prudent course of action is to give parenteral vitamin B_{12} initially while giving folic acid, 1 to 2 mg/d. With this plan, no intervention time is lost. After the appropriate diagnosis is established, the correct vitamin supplement is continued; drug interactions should be noted (Table 13–4).

The hematological response is generally rapid after therapy is begun. Reticulocytosis is brisk and peaks at 5 to 7 days. Hypokalemia, caused by serum-to-intracellular potassium shifts, is common if the anemia was particularly severe and is most likely seen with the peak of reticulocytosis. Monitoring serum potassium daily during the first week of therapy is important, especially in patients receiving diuretic therapy, at other risk of hypokalemia, or taking digoxin. If hypokalemia occurs, oral potassium replacement at 40 mEq/d is usually sufficient. Concomitant oral iron therapy is indicated if there is an iron deficiency or low iron stores. Full hematological recovery usually takes about 2 months.

Reversal of the signs and symptoms of vitamin B_{12} deficiency is generally rapid. A sense of improved well-being is usually reported within 24 hours of the onset of treatment. Neurological changes, if present for less than 6 months, reverse quickly. Neurological reversal is likely impossible, however, if these changes have been present for a protracted period.

Anemia is often noted in persons with select chronic health problems, such as acute and chronic inflammatory conditions (infection, arthritis), renal insufficiency, and hypothyroidism. In part, this condition, known as anemia of chronic disease (ACD), is caused by reduced erythropoietin response in the marrow, resulting in RBC hypoproliferation. In ACD, micronutrient deficiency is not an issue; this yields a normocytic, normochromic anemia. Seldom does ACD result in a severe anemia; usually hct is ≥24%.

Worldwide, anemia of chronic disease is second only to iron deficiency in occurrence. Bone marrow can be suppressed as a result of the use of certain drugs, including cancer chemotherapy agents. Because normal RBC death occurs without the production of new RBC forms, anemia can occur. When glomerular filtration rate declines to less than 30 to 40 mL/min, renal erythropoietin synthesis is reduced; a hypoproliferative normochromic, normocytic anemia develops, usually with a hemoglobin level of 8 g/dL or greater. That is, as the kidney fails, erythropoietin production declines, and anemia of chronic disease develops.

Recombinant human erythropoietin (epoetin alfa) is used in the treatment of anemias associated with end-stage renal disease, HIV, and cancer chemotherapy and other forms of anemia of chronic disease. The drug can be administered parenterally (subcutaneously or intravenously) three times per week with an expected increase in hematocrit of approximately 4% over 2 weeks. Iron therapy is also needed, unless iron overload is present. Patient symptoms, such as altered exercise capacity and sexual function, which are often attributed to renal disease, are often attenuated if hemoglobin level is appropriately corrected to 11 to 12 g/dL with the use of recombinant human erythropoietin (epoetin alfa); correction beyond this hemoglobin level has been associated with increased thrombotic risk without additional health benefit.

DISCUSSION SOURCES

Desai, S. *Clinician's Guide to Laboratory Medicine: Pocket.* Houston, TX: MD2B, 2009.

Gentili, A., Besa, E. http://emedicine.medscape.com/article/200184-overview, Folic Acid Deficiency.

Harper, J., Besa, E. http://emedicine.medscape.com/article/202333, Iron deficiency anemia.

A Physician's Guide to Oral Iron Supplements, http://www.anemia.org/professionals/feature articles/content.php?contentid=306&sectionid=15.

Schick, P., Besa, E. http://emedicine.medscape.com/article/204930, Pernicious Anemia.

◗ Anaphylaxis

39. Tom is a 19-year-old man who presents with sudden onset of edema of the lips and face and a sensation of "throat tightness and shortness of breath" after a bee sting. Physical examination reveals inspiratory and expiratory wheezing. Blood pressure is 78/44 mm Hg, heart rate is 102 bpm, and respiratory rate is 24/min. His clinical presentation is most consistent with the diagnosis of:
    A. urticaria.
    B. angioedema.
    C. anaphylaxis.
    D. reactive airway disease.

40. Your priority in caring for Tom, the aforementioned patient, is to:
    A. administer a rapidly acting oral antihistamine.
    B. administer parenteral epinephrine.
    C. initiate vasopressor therapy.
    D. administer a parenteral systemic corticosteroid.

41. Which of the following food-based allergies is likely to be found in adults and children?
    A. milk
    B. egg
    C. soy
    D. peanut

42. A person with latex allergy also often has a cross-allergy to all of the following except:
    A. banana.
    B. avocado.
    C. kiwi.
    D. romaine lettuce.

43. The most common clinical manifestation of systemic anaphylaxis typically is:
    A. dizziness.
    B. airway obstruction.
    C. urticaria.
    D. gastrointestinal upset.

44. Second-line drug intervention in the presence of anaphylaxis should be:
    A. oral diphenhydramine.
    B. nebulized albuterol.
    C. nebulized epinephrine.
    D. oral prednisone.

45. Which of the following is the best answer regarding anaphylaxis?
    A. Adults usually do not develop new anaphylaxis triggers such as food allergies.
    B. Peanuts are the primary food that can cause a severe allergic reaction.
    C. Future anaphylactic reactions will become increasingly more severe.
    D. Trace amounts of an allergen in a food can cause a severe anaphylactic reaction.

46. Increased risks for fatal reactions from anaphylaxis include all of the following except:
    A. personal history of asthma.
    B. delay in administering epinephrine
    C. age in the teen years.
    D. delay in administering antihistamines.

47. Which of the following plays an essential role in type 1 hypersensitivity?
    A. immunoglobulin E
    B. immunoglobulin A
    C. immunoglobulin G
    D. immunoglobulin F

48. Of the following medications, which is least likely to be implicated as a trigger for anaphylaxis?
    A. ibuprofen
    B. amoxicillin
    C. acetaminophen
    D. aspirin

49. The time to highest blood concentration (Cmax) of epinephrine is shorter when the medication is given:
    A. intramuscularly in the vastus lateralis.
    B. subcutaneously in the abdominal wall.
    C. intramuscularly in the deltoid.
    D. intramuscularly into the gluteus.

50. The use of a systemic corticosteroid in the treatment of anaphylaxis is primarily helpful for:
    A. treatment of the most acute symptoms.
    B. minimization of a protracted allergic response.
    C. prevention of future episodes.
    D. reducing the risk of fatality associated with the event.

Answers

39. C.	43. C.	47. A.
40. B.	44. A.	48. C.
41. D.	45. D.	49. A.
42. D.	46. D.	50. B.

Anaphylaxis is an acute, life-threatening systemic reaction with varied mechanisms, clinical presentations, and severity; this is a manifestation of a type I hypersensitivity. Anaphylaxis usually results from an immunoglobulin E (IgE)-immune—mediated reaction; however, nonimmunologic events often cause sudden release of mediators from mast cells and basophils. Vasodilation, increased capillary permeability, and smooth muscle contraction occurs; new inflammatory cells are attracted to the area, which then perpetuates the systemic reaction. The more rapidly anaphylaxis develops, the more likely the reaction is to be severe and potentially life threatening. Clinical presentations are unpredictable, and initial mild symptoms can rapidly progress to a life-threatening situation. Increased risks for fatal reactions include being a teen or young adult, having asthma, and failing to administer epinephrine promptly. Quick recognition of the signs and symptoms of anaphylaxis and immediate implementation of a prioritized action plan are essential.

Urticaria and angioedema are most commonly reported findings in anaphylaxis (Table 13–5); however, respiratory compromise and cardiovascular collapse are of greatest concern because they are the most frequent cause of death from anaphylaxis. Hemodynamic collapse can occur rapidly with little or no cutaneous or respiratory manifestation. Although the diagnosis of anaphylaxis usually involves two or more organ systems (i.e., skin plus respiratory), anaphylaxis may

TABLE 13-5
Frequency of Occurrence of Signs & Symptoms of Anaphylaxis

Signs & Symptoms	Percent
CUTANEOUS	
Urticaria and angioedema	85–90
Flushing	45–55
Pruritus without rash	2–5
RESPIRATORY	
Dyspnea, wheeze	45–50
Upper airway angioedema	50–60
Rhinitis	15–20
Dizziness, syncope, hypotension	30–35
ABDOMEN	
Nausea, vomiting, diarrhea, cramping pain	25–30
MISCELLANEOUS	
Headache	5–8
Substernal pain	4–6
Seizure	1–2

Source: http://www.aaaai.org/Aaaai/media/MediaLibrary/PDF%20Documents/Practice%20and%20Parameters/Anaphylaxis-2010.pdf, accessed 2/25/13.

present with single-organ involvement, such as a respiratory event or hypotension alone.

Anaphylaxis includes one of three clinical scenarios:
1. The acute onset of a reaction (minutes to hours) with involvement of the skin, mucosal tissue, or both *and at least one of the following*: (a) respiratory compromise, or (b) reduced blood pressure or symptoms of end-organ dysfunction *or*
2. Two of more of the following that occur rapidly after exposure to a *likely* allergen for that patient: involvement of the skin/mucosal tissue, respiratory compromise, reduced blood pressure or associated symptoms, and/or persistent GI symptoms *or*
3. Reduced blood pressure after exposure to a *known* allergen

Foods are the most common cause of IgE-mediated anaphylaxis. Eight foods account for 90% of all food-allergic reactions in the United States: peanuts, tree nuts, fish, shellfish, milk, eggs, wheat, and soy. Food allergy is more common in children than adults. Food allergy in adults can reflect persistence of childhood allergies or may be a new sensitization. Milk, egg, wheat, and soy allergies often resolve in children; peanut, tree nut, fish, and shellfish can resolve but more likely persist. Fatal food allergic reactions are usually caused by peanuts, tree nuts, fish, and shellfish but have also occurred from milk, egg, seeds, and other foods.

Medications are another potential source for IgE and non-IgE—mediated anaphylaxis. Antibiotics (particularly penicillin), aspirin, and nonsteroidal anti-inflammatories (NSAIDs)

TABLE 13-6
Assessment and Management of Anaphylaxis

Assess	Airway, breathing, circulation (ABC), vital signs (VS), and mental status
	Upper and lower airways, CV, skin, and GI
Administer epinephrine	No contraindications to epinephrine in anaphylaxis
	Failure to or delay in use associated with fatalities
	Aqueous 1:1000 concentration (1 mg/mL), IM preferred
	Adult dose 0.2–0.5 mL (mg); autoinjector 0.3 mg, ≥25–30 kg
	Child dose 0.01 mL (mg)/kg; autoinjector 0.15 mg, app 15–30 kg
	May repeat every 5–10 minutes if needed
Activate EMS	Notify others; usually need to call 911
Airway maintenance	Ensure airway patent; use oxygen as indicated
Circulatory maintenance	Epinephrine first line, IV fluids, vasopressors
H_1 antihistamine (AH)	Second line only; first- or second-generation AH may be used
H_2 antihistamine	Added to H_1 antihistamine may be helpful
Inhaled B-adrenergic agonist	Relieves bronchospasm and upper airway obstruction
Systemic corticosteroid	Possibly prevents recurrent or protracted anaphylaxis
Observation	Individualized; often several hours
Follow-up care	Education: diagnosis, cause, how to avoid trigger(s), recognition of S&S, action plan
	Give epinephrine autoinjector with instructions for and indications on use
	Consider referral to allergist
	Wear/carry identification indicating anaphylaxis

Source: http://www.aaaai.org/Aaaai/media/MediaLibrary/PDF%20Documents/Practice%20and%20Parameters/Anaphylaxis-2010.pdf

are the more common medications identified. Insect venoms and latex are other causes for anaphylaxis. Healthcare workers, children with spina bifida and genitourinary abnormalities, and workers with occupational exposure to latex are at increased risk for natural rubber latex-induced anaphylaxis. Cross-sensitivity may occur between natural rubber latex protein and certain fruit proteins, potentially causing a reaction if the patient eats bananas, avocados, kiwi, melons, or chestnuts.

The initial drug of choice for the management of anaphylaxis is parenteral epinephrine (Table 13–6). It reverses the effects of anaphylaxis and inhibits further mediator release and should be administered as soon as the diagnosis is suspected. The time to highest blood concentration (Cmax) when studied in asymptomatic subjects is shorter when given IM in the vastus lateralis muscle (lateral thigh) than when administered either subcutaneously or IM in the deltoid muscle. Unusually severe or refractory anaphylaxis in patients taking beta-adrenergic blockers has been reported. This might be due to a blunted response to epinephrine, an increased propensity for bronchospasm, and reduced cardiac contractility with perpetuation of hypotension. H1 antihistamines are second-line agents and do not replace epinephrine. Parenteral or oral diphenhydramine is a common option for an H1 antihistamine. However, other oral first- or second-generation H1 antihistamines can also be used. There is no direct outcome data regarding the effectiveness of any antihistamine in anaphylaxis. H2 antagonists, such as ranitidine, added to H1 antihistamines can be helpful and often are used. An inhaled beta-adrenergic agent (i.e., albuterol) is indicated for bronchospasms and/or upper airway obstruction. Systemic corticosteroids have

not been shown to be effective in altering the course of acute anaphylaxis but can prevent recurrent or protracted anaphylaxis. Length of time for observation is individualized; often it is several hours. The discharge plan should include the diagnosis, including the suspected cause for the anaphylaxis, avoidance measures, recognition of signs and symptoms, and a treatment plan. Recurrence later in the day of similar symptoms (a biphasic reaction) occurs in 1% to 23% of episodes and may occur hours (most within 10 hours) after anaphylactic resolution. A prescription for an epinephrine autoinjector with instructions should be provided, and the patient should be well-informed on its use. A bracelet or similar identification, indicating anaphylaxis history, should be worn. Consider referring to an allergist to confirm cause and to reduce risk factors for future reactions. Venom immunotherapy should be recommended for patients with systemic sensitivity to stinging insects; this is a highly (90%–98%) effective treatment option.

DISCUSSION SOURCES

The diagnosis and management of anaphylaxis practice parameter, http://www.aaaai.org/Aaaai/media/MediaLibrary/PDF%20Documents/Practice%20and%20Parameters/Anaphylaxis-2010.pdf.

Guidelines for the Diagnosis and Management of Food Allergy in the US, http://www.aaaai.org/Aaaai/media/MediaLibrary/PDF%20Documents/Practice%20Resources/Food-Allergy-Guidelines-Summary.pdf.

Food Allergy: A Practice Parameter, http://www.aaaai.org/Aaaai/media/MediaLibrary/PDF%20Documents/Practice%20and%20Parameters/food-allergy-2006.pdf.

The Food Allergy and Anaphylaxis Network, www.foodallergy.org.

Psychosocial Disorders

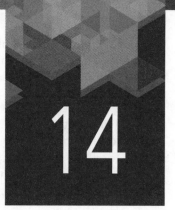

14

Alcohol Abuse

1. A 44-year-old man who admits to drinking "a few beers now and then" presents for examination. After obtaining a health history and performing a physical examination, you suspect he is a heavy alcohol user. Your next best action is to:
   A. obtain liver enzymes.
   B. administer the CAGE questionnaire.
   C. confront the patient with your observations.
   D. advise him about the hazards of excessive alcohol use.

2. Which of the following is not a component of the CAGE questionnaire?
   A. Have you ever felt you should cut down on your drinking?
   B. Have you been annoyed by people criticizing your drinking?
   C. Have you ever felt guilty about your drinking?
   D. Have you ever engaged in a violent act while drinking?

3. Which of the following contains the greatest amount of alcohol?
   A. 12 oz (360 mL) beer (9 proof)
   B. 4 oz (120 mL) wine (22 proof)
   C. 3.5 oz (105 mL) mixed drink (30 proof)
   D. 3 oz (90 mL) liquor (80 proof)

4. DSM-5 criteria for a substance use disorder include all of the following except:
   A. substance use in larger amounts or over longer period than intended.
   B. substance overuse resulting in hospitalization.
   C. craving or strong desire to use.
   D. substance use in potentially hazardous positions.

5. The *Diagnostic and Statistical Manual of Mental Disorders, 5th edition* (DSM-5) criteria for substance use tolerance includes:
   A. diminished effect with the same amount of substance used.
   B. desiring to get an amplified effect with higher doses.
   C. ability to decrease the frequency of substance use.
   D. absence of withdrawal symptoms when substance is not used for a prolonged period.

6. During an office visit, a 38-year-old woman states, "I drink way too much but do not know what to do to stop." According to Prochaska's change framework, her statement is most consistent with a person at the stage of:
   A. precontemplation
   B. contemplation
   C. preparation
   D. action

7. The NP can consider presenting treatment options and support for change after the patient has moved into which of Prochaska's stages?
   A. precontemplation
   B. contemplation
   C. preparation
   D. action

8. Lorazepam or oxazepam is the preferred benzodiazepine for treating alcohol withdrawal symptoms when there is a concomitant history of:
   A. seizure disorder.
   B. folate deficiency anemia.
   C. multiple substance abuse.
   D. hepatic dysfunction.

9. Peak symptoms of alcohol withdrawal are usually observed how long after alcohol intake is discontinued?
A. less than 12 hours
B. 12 to 24 hours
C. 24 to 36 hours
D. more than 36 hours

10. Which of the following is the most helpful approach in the care of a patient with alcoholism?
A. Advise the patient to stop drinking in a straightforward manner.
B. Counsel the patient that alcohol abuse is a treatable disease.
C. Inform the patient of the long-term health consequences of alcohol abuse.
D. Refer the patient to Alcoholics Anonymous.

11. A 42-year-old man who has a long-standing history of alcohol abuse presents for primary care. He admits to drinking 12 to 16 beers daily for 10 years. He states, "I really do not feel like the booze is a problem. I get to work every day." Your most appropriate response is:
A. "Work is usually the last thing to go in alcohol abuse."
B. "Your family has suffered by your drinking."
C. "I am concerned about your health and safety."
D. "Participating in a support group can help you understand why you drink."

12. Which of the following agents offers an intervention for the control of tremor and tachycardia associated with alcohol withdrawal?
A. phenobarbital
B. clonidine
C. verapamil
D. naltrexone

13. Which of the following is most likely to be noted in a 45-year-old woman with laboratory evidence of chronic excessive alcohol ingestion?
A. alanine aminotransferase (ALT) 202 U/L (0 to 31 U/L), mean corpuscular volume (MCV) 70 fL (80 to 96 fL)
B. aspartate transaminase (AST) 149 U/L (0 to 31 U/L), MCV 81 fL (80 to 96 fL)
C. ALT 88 U/L (0 to 31 U/L), MCV 140 fL (80 to 96 fL)
D. AST 80 U/L (0 to 31 U/L), MCV 103 fL (80 to 96 fL)

14. Which of the following is the anticipated clinical effect of acamprosate (Campral®) in the treatment of alcohol dependence?
A. modifies intoxicating effects of alcohol
B. causes unpleasant adverse effects of alcohol
C. helps to reduce the urge to drink
D. minimizes alcohol withdrawal symptoms

Answers

1. B.	6. B.	11. C.
2. D.	7. B.	12. B.
3. D.	8. D.	13. D.
4. B.	9. C.	14. C.
5. A.	10. B.	

In the US, about 18 million people have an alcohol use disorder, classified as either alcohol dependence or alcohol abuse. Additionally, a growing number of young adults (12 to 20 years of age) participate in underage drinking and are more likely to participate in binge drinking (5 drinks to less for men or 4 drinks or less for women on a single occasion). By the age of 18 years, 80% have consumed alcohol and 60% have been intoxicated.

Providing primary care for patients abusing alcohol presents many challenges; this is a complex disorder affecting an individual's family and social function, health, and employment. Often a person who is abusing alcohol minimizes its effect by pointing out that employment has not been affected. In reality, alcoholism is a progressive disease that usually affects family and personal relationships first, then health and, much later, employment. The use of an effective screening tool for alcohol abuse such as the CAGE questionnaire (Box 14–1) is critical for disease detection. An alcoholic drink is defined as 12 oz (360 mL) beer, 4 oz (120 mL) nonfortified wine, or 1 to 1.5 oz (30 to 45 mL) liquor (80 proof).

DSM-5 criteria for substance use disorder require two or more of the following within the past 12 months:
- Substance use in larger amounts or over longer period than intended
- Desire to cut down and/or has tried unsuccessfully in the past
- Excessive time spent obtaining substance, using substance, or recovering from its effects
- Craving or a strong desire to use
- Inability to maintain major role obligations
- Continued substance use despite recurrent social or interpersonal problems related to substance use

BOX 14-1
CAGE Questionnaire

Have you ever felt you ought to *Cut* down on drinking?
Have people *Annoyed* you by criticizing your drinking?
Have you ever felt bad or *Guilty* about your drinking?
Have you ever had a drink first thing in the morning to steady your nerves or get rid of a hangover? (*Eye-opener*)
■ This questionnaire can be modified for use with other forms of substance abuse by substituting *N (Normal)* for *E (Eye-opener)*; i.e., Do you ever use heroin to keep from getting sick or withdrawing?

Source: Ewing JA. Detecting alcoholism: The CAGE questionnaire. *JAMA* 252:1905–1907, 1984.

- Substance use in potentially hazardous positions
- Important social, occupational or recreational activities are given up or reduced due to substance use
- Tolerance
  - Needing more to get same effect
  - Diminished effect with the same amount
- Withdrawal
  - Set of characteristic withdrawal symptoms
  - Same or other substances taken to avoid withdrawal

Counseling the patient and family about alcoholism as a lifelong but treatable disease is a helpful clinical approach. In addition, asking about current drinking habits and associated consequences to health with each visit is important. Consistently offering assistance in accessing treatment conveys the seriousness of this life-threatening condition. As with other health problems with a behavioral component, using statements beginning with "I" is important—"I continue to be very concerned about your health and safety when I hear that you are drinking every day."

In providing primary care, the NP must maintain an attitude that, as with any substance abuse, the patient is capable of changing and achieving sobriety. Change occurs dynamically and often unpredictably. A commonly used change framework is based on the work of James Prochaska, who notes five stages of preparation for change:

- Precontemplation: The patient is not interested in change and might be unaware that the problem exists or minimizes the problem's impact.
- Contemplation: The patient is considering change and looking at its positive and negative aspects. The person often reports feeling "stuck" with the problem.
- Preparation: The patient exhibits some change behaviors or thoughts and often reports feeling that he or she does not have the tools to proceed.
- Action: The patient is ready to go forth with change, often takes concrete steps to change, but is inconsistent with carrying through.
- Maintenance/relapse: The patient learns to continue the change and has adopted and embraced the healthy habit. Relapse can occur, however, and the person learns to deal with backsliding.

As health counselor, the NP provides a valuable role in continually "tapping" the patient with a message of concern about health and safety, possibly moving the person in the precontemplation stage to the contemplation stage. After the patient is at this stage, presenting treatment options and support for change is a critical part of the NP's role.

In a person who drinks more than 1 pint of hard liquor or six beers per day, alcohol withdrawal symptoms typically begin about 12 hours after the last drink. Peak symptoms are seen at 24 to 48 hours with abatement over the next few days. The most common symptoms include anxiety or nervousness, depression, fatigue, irritability, jumpiness or shakiness, mood swings, and nightmares. Other symptoms can include clammy skin, dilated pupils, headache, insomnia, loss of appetite, nausea and vomiting, pallor, rapid heartbeat, sweating, and tremors. Abrupt withdrawal of alcohol use in an addicted person can lead to potentially life-threatening problems with autonomic hyperactivity (i.e., agitation, hallucinations, disorientation) and seizures. The most serious presentation of alcohol withdrawal is known as delirium tremens, which has significant mortality in untreated patients. Use of a benzodiazepine is helpful in managing distressing symptoms and preventing seizures. Treatment of concurrent problems, such as dehydration, malnutrition, and infection, is also warranted.

A highly motivated person with adequate social support systems and a relatively low level of alcohol addiction is likely a suitable candidate for outpatient detoxification. In this type of detoxification, the patient and support person contract with the healthcare provider about a safe plan of detoxification. This plan includes daily office visits or contact; ongoing involvement in Alcoholics Anonymous (AA), Employee Assistance Program (EPA) or similar program; counseling services; and use of a limited supply of medications for managing withdrawal symptoms.

Benzodiazepines have long been used to treat alcohol withdrawal symptoms. Chlordiazepoxide (Librium®) or diazepam (Valium®), therapeutic agents with a long half-life, are reasonable treatment options for a patient with adequate hepatic function, but agents with shorter half-lives (e.g., lorazepam) or agents that have an absence of active metabolites (e.g., oxazepam), should be used in patients with hepatic dysfunction to prevent prolonged effects. Providing a higher dose long-acting benzodiazepine, such as diazepam 20 mg on day one, followed by a dosing schedule reduced by 5 mg daily (increased if symptoms are particularly severe), is often effective and is currently favored over a fixed-dosed dose schedule. If benzodiazepine allergy or intolerance is an issue, carbamazepine offers a therapeutic alternative; atypical or standard antipsychotics play no role in managing alcohol withdrawal symptoms. Alpha-adrenergic agonists (e.g., clonidine) or beta-adrenergic antagonists (i.e., propranolol) are helpful in managing the distressing physical manifestations of alcohol withdrawal such as tachycardia and tremor. Adjunctive therapy with an anticonvulsant can be used to treat or prevent withdrawal seizures. The use of these medications does not prevent the progression of alcohol withdrawal, and these should not be used as monotherapy but only with appropriate use of a benzodiazepine. Attention must be focused on treating alcohol-induced nutritional deficiencies, in particular with high-dose vitamin B supplementation, including thiamine, pyridoxine, and folic acid, and vitamin C. Magnesium deficiency is a common correctable problem in alcohol abuse. The recommended dietary allowance for magnesium in men is 400 to 420 mg/day, while for nonpregnant and nonlactating women, it is 310 to 320 mg/day. Supportive care, including sufficient fluid intake and frequent clinical reassessment, including vital signs, is important.

Although it is tempting to rely on laboratory markers in assessing a person with alcohol abuse, typically few laboratory markers are abnormal (Table 14–1). Evaluation of hepatic

TABLE 14-1

Hepatic Enzyme Elevations and Their Significance

Enzyme Elevation	Comment, Associated Conditions	Example
Alanine aminotransferase (ALT, formerly known as SGPT)	Measure of hepatic cellular enzymes found in circulation, elevated when hepatocellular damage is present. Highly liver specific. This enzyme has circulatory half-life of 37–57 hr; levels increase relatively slowly in response to hepatic damage and clear gradually after damage ceases. See AST for contrast in this rise and fall pattern. In hepatitis A, B, C, D, or E, and drug- or industrial chemical–associated hepatitis, ALT usually increases higher than AST, with enzyme increases ≥10 times ULN. In nonalcoholic fatty liver steatohepatitis (NASH, also known as nonalcoholic fatty liver disease [NAFLD]), ALT usually increases higher than AST, with enzyme increases usually within 3 times ULN.	A 22 y.o. woman with acute hepatitis A AST 678 U/L (normal 0–31 U/L) ALT 828 U/L (normal 0–31 U/L) AST:ALT ratio <1 A 66 y.o. woman with obesity, type 2 diabetes mellitus, and nonalcoholic fatty liver disease AST 44 U/L ALT 78 U/L ALT:AST ratio >1
Aspartate aminotransferase (AST, formerly known as SGOT)	Measure of hepatic cellular enzymes found in circulation, elevated when hepatocellular damage is present. Enzyme also present in lesser amounts in skeletal muscle and myocardium. AST has circulatory half-life of ~12–24 hr; levels increase in response to hepatic damage and clear quickly after damage ceases. In alcohol-related hepatic injury AST usually increases higher than ALT. In acetaminophen overdose, massive increases in AST and ALT are often noted, >20 times ULN.	A 38 y.o. man with a 10-yr history of increasingly heavy alcohol use AST 83 U/L (normal 0–31 U/L) ALT 50 U/L (normal 0–31 U/L) AST:ALT ratio 1 A 26 y.o. man with intentional acetaminophen overdose AST 15,083 U/L (normal 0–31 U/L) ALT 10,347 U/L (normal 0–31 U/L)
Alkaline phosphatase (ALP)	Enzyme found in rapidly dividing or metabolically active tissue, such as liver, bone, intestine, placenta. Elevated levels can reflect damage or accelerated cellular division in any of these areas. Most in circulation is of hepatic origin. Levels increase in response to biliary obstruction and are a sensitive indicator of intrahepatic or extrahepatic cholestasis.	A 40 y.o. woman with acute cholecystitis AST 45 U/L (0–31) ALT 55 U/L (0–31) ALP 225 U/L (0–125)
Gamma glutamyl transferase (GGT)	Enzyme involved in the transfer of amino acids across cell membranes. Found primarily in the liver and kidney. In liver disease, usually parallels changes in alkaline phosphatase. Marked elevation often noted in obstructive jaundice, hepatic metastasis, intrahepatic cholestasis.	A 40 y.o. woman with acute cholecystitis AST 45 U/L (0–31) ALT 55 U/L (0–31) ALP 225 U/L (0–125) GGT 245 U/L (0–45)

Source: Ferri F. *Ferri's Best Test: A Practical Guide to Clinical Laboratory Medicine and Diagnostic Imaging*, ed. 3. Philadelphia, PA: Mosby; 2014.

function is often ordered by providers, who then have the dilemma of presenting an alcohol-abusing patient with a set of relatively normal test results. This situation can help reinforce further the patient's denial or minimization of the effect excessive alcohol use has on health. As previously mentioned, physical health is negatively affected by alcohol abuse later in the course of the abuse. All currently available hepatic tests indirectly measure liver function or capacity. The most commonly performed tests are measurement of hepatic enzymes, protein molecules acting as catalysts and regulating metabolism within liver cells.

Aspartate aminotransferase (AST, formerly known as SGOT) is found in large quantities in hepatocytes. Small amounts are typically found in circulation as a result of hepatic growth and repair. AST level increases in response to hepatocyte injury, as can occur in heavy alcohol use and acetaminophen misuse or overdose. This enzyme is also found in myocardium, brain, kidney, and skeletal tissue in smaller amounts; damage to these areas can result in a modest increase in AST. With a circulatory half-life ($T^1/_2$) of approximately 12 to 24 hours, AST levels increase rapidly in response to hepatic damage and clear quickly after damage ceases. AST elevation is generally found in only about 10% of problem drinkers. If AST is elevated, however, particularly coupled with normal or minimally-elevated alanine aminotransferase (ALT) and mild macrocytosis (MCV >100 fL), long-standing alcohol abuse is the likely cause. This finding is noted in about 30% to 60% of men who drink five or more drinks per day and in women at a threshold of three or more drinks per day.

Alanine aminotransferase (ALT, formerly known as SGPT) is more specific to the liver, having limited concentration in other organs. This enzyme has a longer $T^1/_2$ than AST at 37 to 57 hours. As a result, ALT levels increase slowly after the onset of hepatic injury, and elevation persists longer after hepatic damage has ceased. The greatest elevation of this enzyme is likely seen in liver injury caused by hepatitis induced by acute infection or drug reaction. This enzyme is unlikely to increase significantly if the only hepatic problem is related to alcohol abuse.

When evaluating a patient with suspected substance abuse causing hepatic dysfunction, the NP should note the degree of AST and ALT elevation. The AST-to-ALT ratio can also offer insight into the cause of hepatic enzyme elevations (Table 14–1). The hepatic enzymes generally return to baseline after 2 to 3 months of sobriety. This is an important patient teaching point because a patient who has abused alcohol for many years often believes that little health benefit is gained from sobriety. The mild macrocytosis seen in alcohol abuse also resolves after about 2 to 3 months of alcohol abstinence.

In addition to psychosocial support and counseling, many medications are available to assist in preventing relapse in an alcohol-dependent person. These products can be divided into categories by anticipated clinical effect and include medications that modify the intoxicating effects of alcohol, such as naltrexone (Revia®, Vivitrol®); medications that help to reduce alcohol craving, such as acamprosate (Campral); and medications that induce unpleasant adverse effects if alcohol is ingested, such as disulfiram (Antabuse®). Although these medications can be helpful, the therapeutic effect is generally seen only when these products are used in a motivated patient who has adequate psychosocial support and is involved in counseling. Because of its significant adverse-effect profile, disulfiram use has largely fallen out of favor. Other agents are being studied to assist alcohol-dependent persons, such as baclofen, nalmefene, and ondansetron. Treatment of underlying mental health problems such as depression with a selective serotonin reuptake inhibitor can also be helpful in maintaining sobriety.

DISCUSSION SOURCES

Ferri F. *Ferri's Best Test: A Practical Guide to Clinical Laboratory Medicine and Diagnostic Imaging*, ed. 3. Philadelphia, PA: Elsevier Mosby, 2014.

Ferri F. Management of alcohol withdrawal. In: Ferri F. *Practical Guide to the Care of the Medical Patient*, ed. 8. Philadelphia, PA: Elsevier Mosby; 2010.

Prochaska JO, Redding CA, Evers KE. The transtheoretical model and stages of change. In: Glanz K, Lewis FM, Rimer BK (eds). *Health Behavior and Health Education: Theory, Research, and Practice*, ed. 2. San Francisco, CA: Jossey-Bass; 1997.

Mayo-Smith MF, Beecher LH, Fischer TL, Gorelick DA, Guillaume JL, Hill A, Jara G, Kasser C, Melbourne J. Management of alcohol withdrawal delirium: An evidence-based practice guideline. *Arch Intern Med* 164:1405–1412, 2004.

Pratt DS, Kaplan MM. Evaluation of abnormal liver-enzyme results in asymptomatic patients. *N Engl J Med* 342:1267, 2000.

Hoffman RS, Weinhouse GL. Management of moderate and severe alcohol withdrawal syndromes, 2013. www.uptodate.com/contents/management-of-moderate-and-severe-alcohol-withdrawal-syndromes.

Substance Abuse

15. When providing primary care for a middle-aged woman with a history of prescription benzodiazepine dependence, you consider that:
    A. she is unlikely to have a problem with misuse of other drugs or alcohol.
    B. rapid detoxification is the preferred method of treatment for this problem.
    C. she likely has an underlying untreated or under-treated mood disorder.
    D. she is at significant risk for drug-induced hepatitis.

16. DSM-5 criteria for a substance abuse include all of the following except:
    A. desire to cut down and/or has tried unsuccessfully in the past.
    B. inability to maintain major role obligations.
    C. excessive time spent obtaining substance, using substance, or recovering from its effects.
    D. involved in at least one incarceration related to substance use in the past 6 months.

17. Demographic data indicate which of the following persons is most likely to misuse prescription medications?
  A. a 14-year-old male
  B. a 24-year-old female
  C. a 33-year-old male
  D. a 38-year-old male

18. Risk of benzodiazepine misuse can be minimized by use of:
  A. agents with a shorter half-life.
  B. the drug as an "as-needed" rescue medication for acute anxiety.
  C. more lipophilic products.
  D. products with longer duration of action.

19. When discontinuing benzodiazepine treatment after prolonged use, you recommend:
  A. terminating treatment immediately.
  B. decreasing the dose 20% per day.
  C. decreasing the dose 25% per week.
  D. decreasing the dose 50% per week.

20. Benzodiazepines taken concomitantly with which of the following can lead to enhanced sedation and increased risk of death?
  A. alcohol
  B. acetaminophen
  C. ibuprofen
  D. statins

21. While counseling an adolescent about the risks of marijuana use, the NP considers that:
  A. symptoms of physical and psychological dependency are rarely reported by regular users.
  B. the development of chronic obstructive airway disease is often associated with regular use.
  C. use on a daily basis among teens is significantly less common than that of alcohol.
  D. driving ability is minimally impaired with its use.

22. When assessing a person with acute opioid withdrawal, you expect to find:
  A. constipation.
  B. hypertension.
  C. hypothermia.
  D. somnolence.

23. An alternative to methadone that can be used to curb opioid withdrawal symptoms is the use of:
  A. gabapentin.
  B. buprenorphine plus naloxone.
  C. methylnaltrexone.
  D. topiramate.

24. When providing care for a middle-aged man with acute cocaine intoxication, you inquire about:
  A. feelings of anxiety.
  B. difficulty maintaining sleep.
  C. chest pain.
  D. abdominal pain.

25. Hyperthermia and a racing heart rate is a potentially life-threatening presentation for a person using:
  A. cannabis.
  B. MDMA (e.g., Molly).
  C. LSD.
  D. barbiturates.

26. Use of flunitrazepam (Rohypnol®) has been associated with:
  A. agitation.
  B. amnesia.
  C. increased appetite.
  D. hallucination.

Answers

15. C.	**19.** C.	**23.** B.
16. D.	**20.** A.	**24.** C.
17. B.	**21.** B.	**25.** B.
18. D.	**22.** B.	**26.** B.

The misuse and overuse of various mood-altering products such as alcohol, opioids, cocaine, amphetamines, and other similar products is often referred to as substance abuse. Substance abuse is a common problem, affecting 10% to 14% of primary care patients, with less than 10% being detected and appropriately treated.

The *Diagnostic and Statistical Manual of Mental Disorders*, 5th edition, defines substance abuse as a problematic pattern of substance use leading to significant impairment or distress (see Alcohol Abuse section for full description of DSM-5 criteria).

When providing healthcare, the NP should remember that substance abuse and dependence commonly means misuse of multiple agents, including alcohol, prescription drugs, and illegal agents. Many substance abusers have an underlying mental health problem, such as a mood disorder. Substance abuse, including alcoholism, is often a method of self-treatment in patients with an undetected or untreated psychiatric illness.

Young adults (18- to 25-year-olds) are most likely to misuse prescription medications, with 13% using prescription drugs for nonmedical purposes, compared to 7% of 12- to 17-year-olds and 4% of those 26 years of age and older. Compared to men, women have higher rates of misuse of prescription medications, which is most likely related partly to their more frequent use of the healthcare system. In addition, women are more likely to have mood disorders, including anxiety and depression, and, consequently, are more likely to have potential drugs of abuse such as benzodiazepines prescribed by a healthcare provider. Benzodiazepine abuse is likely less common than perceived by prescribers, however, who often fear that many patients receiving these anxiolytic agents would abuse or misuse the medications (Table 14–2). Prescribers often hesitate to use these highly effective agents

TABLE 14-2

Psychotropic Medications Typically Prescribed to Treat Anxiety, as Adjunctive Therapy in Depression with Anxiety

Medications	Pharmacokinetics	Indications	Onset of Action	Comments
Buspirone (BuSpar)	Slow onset of action (>7 days), lipophilic, T$\frac{1}{2}$ of metabolite 16 hr	Generalized anxiety syndrome, social phobia. May be used as adjunct in obsessive-compulsive disorder, posttraumatic stress disorder. Less effective in panic disorder, acute anxiety. Not helpful in alcohol withdrawal.	2–4 weeks for some relief of anxiety 4–5 weeks for full therapeutic effect	5-HT1A receptor site agonist, not a benzodiazepine (BZD), not effective as a PRN or sleep aid drug. Minimal to no effect on performance, nonsedating. No tolerance, withdrawal syndrome. No potentiation with alcohol. Little abuse potential. If anxiety is disabling, consider adding short-term BZD while awaiting other agent's action.
Lorazepam (Ativan)	Plasma peak in 1–6 hr, about half as lipophilic as diazepam (Valium) No active metabolites T$\frac{1}{2}$ 10–20 hr	Generalized anxiety syndrome, social phobia, adjunct in obsessive-compulsive disorder, posttraumatic stress disorder, panic disorder. Helpful in acute anxiety, alcohol withdrawal.	Slow onset of action, sustained effect	As with all BZDs, abuse and habituation potential.
Oxazepam (Serax)	About half as lipophilic as diazepam, slower onset of action Plasma peak in 1–4 hr No active metabolites T$\frac{1}{2}$ 3–21 hr	Generalized anxiety syndrome, social phobia, adjunct in obsessive-compulsive disorder, posttraumatic stress disorder, panic disorder. Helpful in acute anxiety, alcohol withdrawal.	Slow onset of action, relatively sustained effect	As with all BZDs, abuse and habituation potential. Good choice for elderly patients with anxiety because of short elimination T$\frac{1}{2}$ and lack of active metabolites. BZDs should be used with caution in older adults because of increased risk of fall and potential for altering mental status.
Alprazolam (Xanax)	Plasma peak in 1–2 hr About half as lipophilic as diazepam Parent compound T$\frac{1}{2}$ 12–15 hr	Generalized anxiety syndrome, social phobia, adjunct in obsessive-compulsive disorder, posttraumatic stress disorder, panic disorder. Helpful in acute anxiety, alcohol withdrawal.	Slow onset of action, relatively sustained effect	As with all BZDs, abuse and habituation potential. When prescribed, sufficient daily doses should be allotted.

Continued

TABLE 14-2

Psychotropic Medications Typically Prescribed to Treat Anxiety, as Adjunctive Therapy in Depression with Anxiety—cont'd

Medications	Pharmacokinetics	Indications	Onset of Action	Comments
Clonazepam (Klonopin)	Plasma peak in 1–2 hr About one quarter as lipophilic as diazepam No active metabolites $T\frac{1}{2}$ 18–50 hr	Generalized anxiety syndrome, social phobia, adjunct in obsessive-compulsive disorder, posttraumatic stress disorder, panic disorder. Helpful in acute anxiety, alcohol withdrawal. Absence and petit mal seizures. Anxiety and panic.	Slow onset of action, highly sustained effect	As with all BZDs, abuse and habituation potential. Protracted $T\frac{1}{2}$ may pose a problem when used in elderly adults, but helpful in younger adults to provide consistent anxiety relief.
Diazepam (Valium)	Plasma peak in 0.5–2 hr Highly lipophilic Three active metabolites with various $T\frac{1}{2}$ Desmethyldiazepam $T\frac{1}{2}$ 30–200 hr Oxazepam $T\frac{1}{2}$ 3–21 hr 3-hydroxydiazepam $T\frac{1}{2}$ 5–20 hr	Generalized anxiety syndrome, social phobia, adjunct in obsessive-compulsive disorder, posttraumatic stress disorder, panic disorder. Helpful in acute anxiety, alcohol withdrawal. Anxiety Seizures Musculoskeletal pain	Rapid onset of action, relatively sustained effect	As with all BZDs, abuse and habituation potential. Protracted $T\frac{1}{2}$ may pose a problem when used in elderly patients.

Source: Goldberg R, Posner D. Anxiety disorders: Diagnosis and management. In: Goldberg R (ed). *Practical Guide to the Care of the Psychiatric Patient*, ed. 3. Philadelphia, PA: Mosby; 2007, pp. 158–177.

because of fear of providing the patient with a potentially habituating drug with the possibility of needing increasing doses. In reality, psychological dependence does occur occasionally, but careful prescribing practices can help avoid this.

Psychological dependence on benzodiazepines is usually associated with a rapid onset agent, one that possibly gives a sensation of intoxication. In addition, prescribing at dosing intervals beyond duration of action of the drug gives alternating periods of drug effect and withdrawal. The perception of difference is significant and possibly perceived as a buildup of unpleasant anxiety followed by a period of relief or rescue provided by the patient, with the cycle repeated with each drug dose. Using a benzodiazepine as an "as needed" product increases the likelihood of abuse because this heightens the patient's awareness of drug versus no-drug state. Psychological dependence on benzodiazepines can be avoided by using a slow onset product with a long half-life, such as clonazepam. If using short-acting products, an adequate number of doses per day should be given. If a benzodiazepine is being used on an as-needed basis, the practitioner should advise a maximum number of available or prescribed doses per week, such as three to four times per week, rather than once or twice a day. This approach may help avoid benzodiazepine tolerance, a situation in which the patient requires increasingly

higher doses to reach therapeutic effect. Tolerance usually precedes physical dependence.

Physical dependence on benzodiazepines is a significant problem. When working with a patient to discontinue benzodiazepine use, the practitioner should consider reducing the dose by 25% per week. Rapid withdrawal can lead to tremors, hallucinations, seizures, and a delirium tremens-like state. The onset of withdrawal symptoms occurs a few days after the last dose in a benzodiazepine with a shorter half-life (e.g., lorazepam) and up to 3 weeks in one with a longer half-life (e.g., clonazepam).

Benzodiazepines rarely cause hepatic or renal impairment. When taken alone in overdose, benzodiazepines have a favorable toxicity profile. Sedation risk is enhanced, however, when benzodiazepines are combined with alcohol and barbiturates, leading to a potentially life-threatening condition. Accidental and intentional fatalities with benzodiazepine ingestion with alcohol often occur.

Opioid withdrawal shares many common characteristics with alcohol withdrawal. Hypertension, tachycardia, diarrhea, nausea, temperature dysregulation, fever, papillary dilation, restlessness, myalgia, lacrimation, and rhinorrhea are often reported in addition to intense cravings for opioids. Although very distressing, the condition is not life-threatening and usually resolves within a few days. Clonidine, an alpha-adrenergic agonist, helps minimize opioid withdrawal symptoms. As with any chemical dependence, long-term rehabilitation therapy is usually needed, necessitating a high level of patient desire for sobriety. Methadone, a long-acting opioid, can help curb the use of illegal drugs when used in conjunction with a comprehensive counseling and monitoring program. Buprenorphine with naloxone (Suboxone®) is a fixed-dose combination of an opioid agonist (buprenorphine) and antagonist (naloxone) that offers an alternative to methadone. Compared with methadone, this drug combination has clinically desirable qualities—such as lower abuse potential—less withdrawal discomfort, and greater safety against overdose. When used to treat addiction, methadone can be dispensed only through a qualified opioid treatment program, whereas buprenorphine with naloxone (Suboxone) can be prescribed in private practices and outpatient clinics by qualified clinicians. Although a helpful option that potentially increases access to patients with opioid addiction, this medication is most helpful when used by a motivated patient who is actively involved in a comprehensive treatment program.

Marijuana has historically been considered a drug that has potential for psychological dependence but with little potential for physical addiction. For teens in many communities, daily use of marijuana is more common than daily alcohol use. Marijuana currently being used is extremely potent, however, because of its high tetrahydrocannabinol (THC) content. After a period of abstinence, physical withdrawal symptoms are often reported among daily marijuana users. Chronic marijuana use can lead to airway obstruction similar to that found in heavy tobacco users. Individuals with marijuana intoxication, when performing activities requiring concentration or physical skills, such as operating a motor vehicle, show significant impairment.

Cocaine is a potent sympathomimetic. After cocaine ingestion, the user has an increase in heart rate and myocardial contractility and generalized vasoconstriction, causing an increase in blood pressure. In addition, cocaine preferentially constricts the coronary and cerebral vessels, creating significant risk for cerebral ischemia and stroke and myocardial ischemia and infarction. Inquiring about chest pain is prudent in caring for a patient with cocaine abuse.

Amphetamine use is second only to marijuana use in illicit drug use in the United States; methamphetamine belongs to the amphetamine drug class. These stimulants are rapidly absorbed and have a rapid onset of action (less than 1 hour), causing the desired effects of CNS stimulation, euphoria, mood elevation, and appetite suppression. Withdrawal can cause depressed mood, fatigue, vivid and disturbing dreams, sleep disturbance, increased appetite, and psychomotor agitation or retardation. MDMA (3, 4-methylenedioxymethamphetamine), also known as ecstasy or Molly (a purportedly pure drug form), is a psychoactive drug that has similarities to amphetamine and the hallucinogen mescaline. Initially popular with white adolescents and young adults, use of the drug has expanded to broader demographics. The drug increases the activity of the neurotransmitters serotonin,

dopamine, and norepinephrine, and the effects can last approximately 3 to 6 hours. In high doses, MDMA can interfere with regulation of body temperature that can lead to hyperthermia, rapid heart rate, excessive sweating, shivering, and involuntary twitching. In rare cases, the effect can lead to extreme hyperthermia with resulting liver, kidney, and cardiovascular system failure and eventual death.

Flunitrazepam (Rohypnol) is a benzodiazepine, also known as "roofies" or the "date rape drug." Flunitrazepam is particularly potent with a rapid onset of action and is not available for prescription use in North America. This product is a commonly prescribed sleep aid in other countries, however. Flunitrazepam has been misused as a drug to reduce sexual inhibition, often given without the knowledge of the recipient. Because its use can result in amnesia, sexual assault can occur, possibly without the victim's recalling the event.

DISCUSSION SOURCES

Book S, Myrick H. The diagnosis and treatment of substance abuse/dependence and co-occurring social anxiety disorder. www.psychiatrictimes.com/display/article/10168/47706.

Eating Disorders

27. Which of the following statements is true concerning anorexia nervosa?
    A. The disease affects men and women equally.
    B. Onset is usually in the mid-20s for men and women.
    C. Depression is often found concomitantly.
    D. Individuals with anorexia nervosa are aware of the extreme thinness associated with the disease.

28. DSM-5 criteria for anorexia nervosa include all of the following except:
    A. refusal to maintain body weight at or above the minimum normal weight for age and height.
    B. intense fear of gaining weight or becoming fat despite being underweight.
    C. distorted experience and significance of body weight and shape.
    D. absence of at least three consecutive menstrual cycles.

29. Treatment for anorexia nervosa usually includes:
    A. referral for parenteral nutrition evaluation.
    B. antidepressant therapy.
    C. use of psychostimulants.
    D. psychoanalysis.

30. Physical examination findings in patients with bulimia nervosa often include:
    A. body mass index (BMI) less than 75% of anticipated.
    B. dental surface erosion.
    C. tachycardia.
    D. hair that is easily plucked.

31. DSM-5 criteria for bulimia nervosa include all of the following except:
    A. eating an excessively large amount of food within a discrete amount of time.
    B. a sense of lack of control during binge eating episode.
    C. binge eating and compensatory behavior occurring at least three times per week.
    D. self-worth heavily influenced by body shape and weight.

32. Use of laxatives and diuretics by persons with bulimia nervosa will most commonly result in:
    A. hypokalemia.
    B. hypercalcemia.
    C. proteinuria.
    D. hypernatremia.

33. Which of the following is most consistent with the diagnosis of bulimia nervosa?
    A. Patients with bulimia nervosa usually present asking for treatment.
    B. Periods of anorexia often occur.
    C. Hyperkalemia often results from laxative abuse.
    D. Most patients with bulimia nervosa are significantly obese.

34. All of the following pharmacological interventions are used in the treatment of patients with bulimia nervosa except:
    A. fluoxetine (Prozac®).
    B. desipramine (Norpramin®).
    C. bupropion (Wellbutrin®).
    D. paroxetine (Paxil®).

35. Characteristics of binge eating disorder include all of the following except:
    A. lack of control over the amount and type of food eaten.
    B. behavior present for at least 6 months.
    C. marked distress, self-anger, shame, and frustration as a result of binging.
    D. purging activity after an eating binge.

36 to 40. Identify if the following characteristics are noted in anorexia nervosa, bulimia nervosa, or both disorders.

_____ 36. Parotid gland enlargement

_____ 37. Hypokalemia

_____ 38. Lanugo

_____ 39. Esophageal tears

_____ 40. Dysrhythmias

▶ Answers

36. Bulimia nervosa, possible with anorexia nervosa if binge-purging type present
37. Both anorexia nervosa and bulimia nervosa
38. Anorexia nervosa
39. Bulimia nervosa, possible with anorexia nervosa if binge-purging type present
40. Both anorexia nervosa and bulimia nervosa

Anorexia nervosa (AN) is a potentially life-threatening disease. DSM-5 criteria for AN include the following:
- Inability or refusal to maintain body weight at or above the minimum normal weight for age and height
- Intense fear of gaining weight and becoming fat despite low body weight
- Disturbance in perception of body weight and shape

A denial of the seriousness of the low body weight is often found in patients with AN. Often despite extreme thinness, a patient with AN looks in the mirror and comments on the need to lose "just a few more pounds." Amenorrhea, which is common in women with AN, contributes to establishing the diagnosis. The usual onset of AN in women is during the teens to early 20s, with ages 14 and 18 years being the most common; men with the condition typically present a few years later. AN is an overwhelmingly female disease (90%), with either gender often involved in an activity that has an emphasis on weight and shape, including wrestling, modeling, dancing, gymnastics, and swimming. Some of the activities are occasionally called appearance as well as performance sports.

Patients with AN usually exhibit one of two types of behavior. With the restricting type, a patient with AN severely limits food intake, but does not use binge eating or purging. In the binge-purge type, a patient with AN has cycles of these behaviors.

In contrast to bulimia nervosa (BN), which is a secretive disease with relatively few easily noted clinical findings, AN is usually easy to identify clinically. Besides the marked reduction in weight, muscle wasting, abdominal distention with hepatomegaly, cheilosis, oral and gum disease, coarse dry skin, and hypotension with bradycardia and hypothermia are commonly noted.

AN is a potentially life-threatening disease with a mortality rate of 5% to 20%. Hospitalization to correct fluid and electrolyte disorders and to initiate refeeding is often needed. When physiological stability is reached, AN treatment usually includes cognitive-behavioral and pharmacological and ongoing nutritional therapy. In cognitive-behavioral therapy, the focus is the disturbed eating and the patterns of thinking that help perpetuated the binge-purge cycle. To be effective, accessing care with a clinician or treatment team expert in eating disorders is critical.

Pharmacological therapy usually involves the use of antidepressants, which are thought to have an effect because of the high rate of comorbid depression. The choice of a specific agent should be guided by the principles used in choosing therapy for depression. Benzodiazepines are also sometimes used to reduce anxiety associated with eating.

27.	C.	30.	B.	33.	B.
28.	D.	31.	C.	34.	C.
29.	B.	32.	A.	35.	D.

Cyroheptadine (Periactin®) can be used before meals to enhance appetite and reduce anxiety.

BN is more common in women and typically is present for many years before the patient presents for treatment or before the disorder is noted by a healthcare provider seeing the patient for another issue. Because BN tends to be a secretive disease, few with the disease present directly requesting intervention.

According to DSM-5 criteria, a person with BN has episodes of binge eating characterized by eating excessive quantities of food in a discrete period, such as 2 hours. During this period, the person feels a lack of control over the eating for the amount and the type of food ingested. In addition, there is a recurrent compensatory behavior used to prevent excessive weight gain from a binge, such as self-induced vomiting, excessive exercise, laxative or diuretic abuse, or fasting. Binge eating and compensatory behavior occurs at least once per week for 3 months. Body weight and shape excessively influence self-worth.

A patient with BN is often identified in the clinical setting by problems with erosion of the lingual surface of the upper teeth because of excessive exposure to gastric contents during induced vomiting. Hypokalemia, caused by laxative and diuretic use, is also common. Body weight provides few clues because a patient is typically of average to slightly above average weight.

Treatment of a patient with BN usually includes cognitive-behavioral and pharmacological therapy. In cognitive-behavioral therapy, the focus is the disturbed eating and the thinking patterns that help perpetuate the binge-purge cycle. To be effective, accessing care with a clinician or treatment team expert in eating disorders is critical.

Pharmacological therapy usually involves the use of antidepressants such as selective serotonin reuptake inhibitors (SSRIs). SSRIs are usually highly successful in reducing the frequency and amount of binges, partly because of their activity at the 5-HT1A-receptor site. All antidepressants can be used except for bupropion (Wellbutrin), which can induce further bingeing or seizures in patients with BN. The choice of a specific agent should be guided by the principles used in choosing therapy for depression.

Binge eating disorder is characterized as a lack of control over the amount and type of food eaten, occurring two or more times per week for at least 6 months. The bingeing is accompanied by marked distress, self-anger, shame, and frustration as a result of the bingeing. Purging activity is not present; as a result, a person with binge eating disorder is usually obese. As with all eating disorders, treatment requires an interdisciplinary approach with contributions from healthcare providers with expertise in this area.

DISCUSSION SOURCES

Academy of Eating Disorders. Treatment. www.aedweb.org/Treatment/4021.htm#.UrR2xJso7IU.

Depression

41. Which patient presentation is most consistent with the diagnosis of depression?
    A. recurrent diarrhea and cramping
    B. difficulty initiating sleep
    C. diminished cognitive ability
    D. consistent early morning wakening

42. According to DSM-5, a diagnosis of depression must include either depressed mood or which of the following?
    A. loss of interest or pleasure
    B. recurrent thoughts of death
    C. feelings of worthlessness
    D. weight change (either increase or decrease)

43 to 45. When considering depression and thoughts about death, rank the following from most common (1) to least common (3):

43. thinking it would be fine to just die

44. having suicidal thoughts

45. making a plan to commit suicide

46. Which of the following statements is false regarding patients with depression and hypochondriasis?
    A. About 30% of patients with depression also have hypochondriasis.
    B. These patients are less likely to see a healthcare provider compared to those with depression alone.
    C. These patients are unable to process objective information that they have no particular health problem.
    D. They perceive that an existing health problem is far more serious than it is in reality.

47. Of the following individuals in need of an antidepressant, who is the best candidate for fluoxetine (Prozac) therapy?
    A. an 80-year-old woman with depressed mood 1 year after the death of her husband
    B. a 45-year-old man with mild hepatic dysfunction
    C. a 28-year-old man who occasionally "skips a dose" of his prescribed medication
    D. a 44-year-old man with decreased appetite

48. In caring for elderly patients, the NP considers that all of the following is true except:
    A. many older patients with dementia have a component of depression.
    B. dementia signs and symptoms usually evolve over months, but depression usually has a more rapid onset.
    C. with dementia, a patient is aware of difficulties with cognitive ability.
    D. treating concurrent depression can help improve symptoms of dementia.

49. Dysthymia is characterized by:
    A. suicidal thoughts.
    B. multiple incidents of harming oneself.
    C. social isolation.
    D. low level depression.

50. Which of the following is most consistent with the diagnosis of dysthymia?
    A. a 23-year-old man with a 2-month episode of depressed mood after a job loss
    B. a 45-year-old woman with "jitteriness" and difficulty initiating sleep for the past 6 months
    C. a 38-year-old woman with fatigue and anhedonia for the past 2 years
    D. a 15-year-old boy with a school adjustment problem and weekend marijuana use for the past year

51. Treatment of dysthymia typically involves:
    A. psychotherapy alone.
    B. antidepressants alone.
    C. psychotherapy plus antidepressants.
    D. electroconvulsive therapy (ECT).

52. John is a 47-year-old man who reports constant sadness following the death of his wife in a motor vehicle accident 2 weeks ago. He has not been able to function at work and avoids socializing with friends and family. You recommend:
    A. giving him time and support during this period of acute grief.
    B. weekly psychotherapy sessions.
    C. prescribing an anxiolytic to help with grief symptoms.
    D. psychotherapy plus a prescription for an antidepressant.

53. Successful treatment of a patient with reactive depression associated with a loss (e.g., death of a loved one) would expect all of the following results except:
    A. elevated mood.
    B. restored function.
    C. improved decision-making ability.
    D. elimination of sadness.

54. Drug treatment options for a patient with bipolar disorder often include all of the following except:
    A. atomoxetine (Strattera®).
    B. lithium carbonate.
    C. risperidone (Risperdal®).
    D. valproic acid (Depakote®).

55. Which of the following drugs is likely to be the most dangerous when taken in overdose?
    A. a 4-week supply of fluoxetine
    B. a 2-week supply of nortriptyline
    C. a 3-week supply of venlafaxine
    D. a 3-day supply of diazepam

56. One week into sertraline (Zoloft®) therapy, a patient complains of a new onset recurrent dull frontal headache that is relieved promptly with acetaminophen. Which of the following is true in this situation?
    A. This is a common, transient side effect of selective serotonin reuptake inhibitor (SSRI) therapy.
    B. She should discontinue the medication.
    C. Fluoxetine should be substituted.
    D. Desipramine should be added.

57. A patient has been taking fluoxetine for 1 week and complains of mild nausea and diarrhea. You advise that:
    A. this is a common, long lasting side effect of SSRI therapy.
    B. he should discontinue the medication.
    C. another antidepressant should be substituted.
    D. he should be taking the medication with food.

58. Sally is a 34-year-old married woman who is diagnosed with major depressive disorder. She feels that it is likely associated with stress resulting from her troubled marriage. She is initiated on an SSRI and reports initial improvement in symptoms. However, over the following months, the medication loses its effectiveness despite her insistence that she is being adherent with the dosing regimen. This is likely a result of:
    A. an inadequate dose of the medication.
    B. development of tolerance to the SSRI.
    C. continued or escalated stress from the troubled marriage.
    D. missed doses despite her insistence on compliance.

59. Which of the following medications is most likely to cause sexual dysfunction?
    A. vilazodone (Viibryd®)
    B. fluoxetine (Prozac)
    C. nortriptyline (Pamelor®)
    D. bupropion (Wellbutrin)

60. SSRI withdrawal syndrome is best characterized as:
    A. bothersome but not life-threatening.
    B. potentially life-threatening.
    C. most often seen with discontinuation of agents with a long half-life.
    D. associated with seizure risk.

61. Which of the following SSRIs is most likely to significantly interact with warfarin?
    A. citalopram
    B. paroxetine
    C. fluoxetine
    D. sertraline

62. Which of the following SSRIs is associated with the greatest anticholinergic effect?
    A. fluvoxamine
    B. sertraline
    C. fluoxetine
    D. paroxetine

63. Which of the following statements is true regarding depression and relapse?
    A. Without maintenance therapy, the relapse rate is typically less than 50% in the first year.
    B. The risk of relapse is less for those who have experienced multiple episodes of major depressive disorder.
    C. The risk of relapse is greatest in the first 2 months after discontinuation of therapy.
    D. Relapse rarely occurs if there is an absence of symptoms after 9 months of treatment discontinuation.

64. All of the following are risk factors for relapse except:
    A. current episode lasts more than 2 years.
    B. onset of depression occurs at younger than 20 years of age.
    C. poor recovery between episodes.
    D. absence of dysthymia preceding the episode.

65. Which of the following is most consistent with the presentation of a patient with bipolar I disorder?
    A. increased need for sleep
    B. impulsive behavior
    C. fatigue
    D. anhedonia

66. In general, pharmacological intervention for patients with depression should:
    A. be given for about 4 months on average.
    B. continue for a minimum of 6 months after remission is achieved.
    C. be continued indefinitely with a first episode of depression.
    D. be titrated to a lower dose after symptom relief is achieved.

67. Depression often manifests with all of the following except:
    A. psychomotor retardation.
    B. irritability.
    C. palpitations.
    D. increased feelings of guilt.

68. A 44-year-old man has been taking an SSRI for the past 4 months and complains of new onset of sexual dysfunction and difficulty achieving orgasm. You advise him that:
    A. this is a transient side effect often seen in the first weeks of therapy.
    B. switching to another SSRI would likely be helpful.
    C. this is a common adverse effect of SSRI therapy that is unlikely to resolve without adjustment in his therapy.
    D. he should see an urologist for further evaluation.

69. The maximum recommended dose of citalopram for patients older than 60 years of age is:
    A. 10 mg/day.
    B. 20 mg/day.
    C. 30 mg/day.
    D. 40 mg/day.

70. Which of the following agents has the longest $T^{1}/_{2}$?
    A. fluoxetine
    B. paroxetine
    C. citalopram
    D. sertraline

71. Which of the following agents should be avoided in heavy alcohol users due to a potential risk for hepatotoxicity?
    A. duloxetine
    B. desvenlafaxine
    C. escitalopram
    D. bupropion

72. Treatment with venlafaxine (Effexor®) can lead to dose-dependent increases in:
    A. heart rate.
    B. serum glucose.
    C. AST/ALT.
    D. blood pressure.

73. You see a 28-year-old man who has been diagnosed with moderate depression and has not responded well to SSRI therapy over the past 3 months. He was involved in a motor vehicle accident 2 years ago that resulted in head trauma and now occasionally experiences occasional tonic clonic seizures. When considering alternative antidepressant therapy, which of the following should be avoided?
    A. bupropion
    B. trazodone
    C. citalopram
    D. duloxetine

74. QT prolongation is a concern with higher doses of:
    A. citalopram.
    B. sertraline.
    C. venlafaxine.
    D. fluoxetine.

75. Priapism is a potential adverse effect of which of the following psychotropic medications?
    A. bupropion
    B. sertraline
    C. trazodone
    D. amitriptyline

76. When using trazodone to aid sleep, the drug should be optimally taken _____ prior to sleep.
    A. immediately
    B. 15 minutes
    C. 1 hour
    D. 2 hours

77. Patient presentation possibly common to anxiety and depression includes:
    A. feeling of worthlessness.
    B. psychomotor agitation.
    C. dry mouth.
    D. appetite disturbance.

78. Which of the following describes prescriptions for antidepressant medications written by primary care providers?
A. dose too high
B. dose too low
C. excessive length of therapy
D. appropriate length of therapy

79 to 83. Match each serotonin receptor site with its associated activity when stimulated.

79. 5-HT1A
80. 5-HT1C, 5-HT2C
81. 5-HT1D
82. 5-HT2
83. 5-HT3

A. agitation, anxiety, panic
B. antimigraine effect
C. antidepressant
D. cerebral spinal fluid production
E. nausea, diarrhea

Answers

41. D.	56. A.	71. A.
42. A.	57. D.	72. D.
43. 1	58. C.	73. A.
44. 2	59. B.	74. A.
45. 3	60. A.	75. C.
46. B.	61. C.	76. C.
47. C.	62. D.	77. B.
48. C.	63. C.	78. B.
49. D.	64. D.	79. C.
50. C.	65. B.	80. D.
51. C.	66. B.	81. B.
52. A.	67. C.	82. A.
53. D.	68. C.	83. E.
54. A.	69. B.	
55. B.	70. A.	

- Fatigue—with report of lack of energy.
- Self-worth—with report of worthlessness or inappropriate guilt.
- Concentration—with report of difficulty concentrating, trouble thinking clearly, or indecisiveness.
- Thoughts of death—the patient has had repeated thoughts about death and dying (other than the fear of dying), or has had thoughts of suicide (with or without a plan).

The symptoms cause clinically important distress or impair work, social, or personal functioning and cannot be attributed to another health condition. Other symptoms of depression are often reported. Hypochondriasis is found in at least 30% of patients; such a patient is unable to process objective information that he or she has no particular health problem. Alternatively, a person with hypochondriasis perceives that an existing health problem is far more serious than it is in reality. Suicidal ideation is occasionally present, with the patient voicing thoughts (most common) or a plan (less common) of self-harm. Most patients with depression have a passive idea of death without a plan. The patient often agrees with the statement, "If I could just die in my sleep, that would be all right," but steadfastly denies a plan of self-harm. As with any person with suicidal ideation or plan, a thorough safety evaluation should be completed and appropriate referral facilitated; this can include involuntary hospitalization for a patient who is a risk of self-harm. Inquiring about thoughts or plans of harm to others is also an important part of the patient's safety plan. All patients with a disordered mood should be made aware of local resources for emergency mental healthcare.

In an older adult, depression is sometimes mistaken for new onset or worsening dementia. A patient with dementia typically has cognitive changes that are slowly progressive over months to years, however. The cognitive changes reported by patients with depression usually have evolved over a much shorter period with the patient often accurately reporting what changes have occurred.

Anxiety is often reported by a depressed person and is a common comorbid condition. In individuals with depression, the mood disturbance occurs first, followed in several weeks by the addition of anxiety-related symptoms. Depression should be considered as the diagnosis rather than anxiety if the patient reports feeling worse while taking benzodiazepines. The concept that a person has either depression or anxiety has been largely replaced with the realization that mood disorders occur on a continuum, with most individuals with mood disorders showing features of depression and anxiety.

Psychomotor agitation with fidgeting and irritability is often found in patients with depression, especially in children and adolescents. In these age groups, this presentation is more likely than psychomotor retardation. This type of increased activity is also found in type A adults with depression.

Intervention for patients with depression includes a combination of support, counseling, and medication. Interpersonal therapy, including counseling and support, alone has a 40% to 60% efficacy with a high relapse rate. As a single therapeutic modality, this is most effective for individuals with reactive depression. Combined therapy of pharmacological

Depression is a common health problem with at least a 15% lifetime occurrence rate. DSM-5 criteria for depression include the presence of particular symptoms and findings within a 2-week period. The person has had five or more of the following symptoms, which are a definite change from usual functioning. Either depressed mood or decreased interest or pleasure must be one of the five, with findings reported by the patient or noted by others, or both:

- Mood—often with a marked diurnal variation in mood, with morning mood being more depressed than later in the day. Agitated mood and irritability are commonly noted together.
- Interests—with lack of interest or pleasure in activities normally or formerly found to be pleasurable.
- Eating—with a marked increase or decrease in appetite noted with corresponding change in weight.
- Sleep—with reports of excessive or insufficient amounts. Reports of early morning wakening, such as 3 or 4 a.m., with inability to fall back to sleep, are common.
- Motor activity—with reports of activity being agitated or retarded.

intervention and interpersonal therapy allows the patient to have effective therapy for what is now recognized as a biochemical disorder, while acquiring the cognitive skills that are helpful in dealing with what is often a chronic, relapsing condition.

Dysthymia is found in approximately 3% of the general population and is characterized by low-level daily depression with at least two of the previously identified depressive symptoms for at least 2 years in adults and 1 year in children and adolescents. DSM-5 consolidates dysthymia with chronic major depression to form the "persistent depressive disorder" category. As with people who are depressed, patients with dysthymia respond well to a combination of interpersonal and pharmacological intervention. A patient who reports a life-changing feeling with antidepressant use, often described as "feeling good to be alive for the first time," is likely dysthymic. The person's underlying personality emerges after being suppressed or altered by the debilitating effects of the low-level depression that characterizes dysthymia.

Depressed mood often follows a significant life stressor, such as death of a loved one or loss of a job; normal sadness or grief is often inappropriately labeled as depression. An important difference is that the person who is sad, as might be reported in an individual who was recently laid off from work, or the person who is grieving, such as an individual whose loved one recently died, can identify the reason for the altered mood. With the passage of time and support, most people with normative sadness or grief find that the altered mood improves. An important role for the healthcare provider is to help the bereaved person to identify the difference between the normative sadness of loss and depression. Commonly, the acutely bereaved person will mistake grief for depression. At the same time, if diagnostic criteria for depression are met beyond 1 to 3 months after the precipitating event, particularly if the bereaved is having difficulty with daily basic function, the diagnosis of complicated grief with major depression should be considered. Treatment for adjustment disorder with depressed mood lasting beyond 1 to 3 months is the same as treatment for major depression, recognizing that interpersonal therapy can be highly effective in assisting patients in dealing with loss. Although treating a reactive depression is helpful in lifting mood and restoring function, such treatment would not relieve the normal sadness associated with loss.

Primary care providers write 80% of all psychotropic prescriptions, making the acquisition of skill in prescribing these helpful medications crucial to practice. All prescription antidepressants are about equally effective if taken in therapeutic doses for sufficient lengths of time. Primary care providers tend to underdose antidepressants, however, and prescribe them for an insufficient length of therapy. Current treatment guidelines offer recommendations for length of therapy (Box 14–2). Long-term antidepressant therapy should be considered when there is a high risk of depression relapse (Box 14–3).

When prescribing an antidepressant, the provider should encourage psychotherapy or counseling to work on building skills needed to help manage this usually long-term health problem. In particular, the provider should convey the message

BOX 14-2

Length of Pharmacological Intervention in Depression

Acute plus continuation phases
- In acute phase treatment, 4–8 weeks of treatment is generally needed before concluding that a patient is partially responsive or unresponsive to a specific treatment.
- Patients successfully treated during acute phase should continue the same course of treatment for 4–9 months, preferably for a minimum of 6 months.
- Relapse highest in first 2 months after discontinuation of therapy,
- With >2 major depressive disorder episodes, 80% relapse in 1 year without treatment.
- Consider maintenance therapy as with any chronic illness.

Source: American Psychiatric Association. Practice guidelines for the treatment of patients with major depressive disorder, ed. 3, 2010. http://psychiatryonline.org/content.aspx?bookid=28&sectionid=1667485

BOX 14-3

Risks in Depression Relapse

Dysthymia preceding episode
Poor recovery between episodes
Current episode >2 yr
Onset depression <20 y.o., >50 y.o.
Family history of depression
Severe symptoms such as suicide and psychosis

to the patient that the use of psychotropics can help facilitate therapy.

When choosing an antidepressant, the prescriber should ask the following questions:
- What has worked in the past? Unless now contraindicated, this medication should be the agent of choice.
- What has worked for relatives? Certain medications seem to have greater activity at given serotonin receptor sites. Besides having heard positive comments about the medication from family members, relatives often have similar serotonin receptor site activity and response to a given medication.
- What are the most bothersome signs and symptoms of the depression? An antidepressant with activity against these or at least one that will not make these worse should be chosen. If insomnia and anxiety bother a depressed person, using a highly energizing medication is a poor choice (Tables 14–3 and 14–4).
- What are the potential drug-drug interactions? As with all medication use, a careful inventory should be taken so that potential drug-drug interactions can be avoided (Box 14–4).

TABLE 14-3
Selective Serotonin Reuptake Inhibitors (SSRIs)

SSRI	Half-life	Labeled Indications	Adverse Effect Profile	Comments
Paroxetine (Paxil)	$T^{1/2}$ 21 hr, no active metabolites	Major depressive disorder Panic disorder with or without agoraphobia Obsessive-compulsive disorder Social anxiety disorder Generalized anxiety disorder Posttraumatic stress disorder Premenstrual dysphoric disorder	Sedating (HS dosing likely best) Likely most anticholinergic effect of the SSRIs. More constipation (13%) than diarrhea (11%) Antihistamine-like, anticholinergic activity can lead to increased appetite	Helpful in depression with anxiety Elimination via renal and hepatic routes Fewer problems with limited renal/hepatic function Low mania induction in bipolar; with relatively short $T^{1/2}$ and lack of active metabolites, helpful in the treatment of depression in elderly patients Because of short $T^{1/2}$, slow tapering dose when discontinuing medication is recommended to avoid significant withdrawal syndrome
Fluvoxamine (Luvox®)	$T^{1/2}$ 16 hr No active metabolites	Obsessive-compulsive disorder Social anxiety disorder	High rate of gastrointestinal upset and sleep disturbance compared with other SSRIs	Adverse-effect profile can limit utility
Sertraline (Zoloft)	$T^{1/2}$ 26 hr Metabolite $T^{1/2}$ 62–104 hr	Major depression, obsessive-compulsive disorder, panic disorder, posttraumatic stress disorder, premenstrual dysphoric disorder, social anxiety disorder	Equal numbers find medication sedating and energizing Low rate of nervousness, anorexia	Take with food to enhance absorption
Citalopram (Celexa) Escitalopram (Lexapro)	Citalopram: Racemic compound $T^{1/2}$ ~35 hr for parent compound, metabolite $T^{1/2}$ 2 days for one, 4 days for another Escitalopram: Single isomer of citalopram with shorter $T^{1/2}$ 27–32 hr	Major depression, generalized anxiety disorders	Equal numbers reporting somnolence and insomnia. Favorable gastrointestinal profile Low rates of agitation and anorexia Due to risk of QT prolongation with citalopram, for patients >60 years of age, the maximum recommended dose is 20 mg/day, maximum 40 mg/day in all others.	Escitalopram 10 mg is therapeutically equivalent to citalopram 20–40 mg with a possibly superior adverse-effect profile
Prozac (Fluoxetine)	$T^{1/2}$ 24–72 hr Metabolite $T^{1/2}$ 4–16 days	Major depressive disorder Bulimia nervosa Obsessive-compulsive disorder	Energizing, anorexia common	Morning dosing recommended. Protracted $T^{1/2}$ can present problem in elderly patients

TABLE 14-3
Selective Serotonin Reuptake Inhibitors (SSRIs)—cont'd

SSRI	Half-life	Labeled Indications	Adverse Effect Profile	Comments
		Premenstrual dysphoric disorder Panic disorder with or without agoraphobia		Missed doses less of a problem because of protracted $T^{1}/_{2}$ Weight loss of ~3–5 lb (1.4–2.3 kg) common in early months of use, but usually not sustained long-term

Source: Posternak M, Zimmerman M. Antidepressants. In: Goldberg R (ed). *Practical Guide to the Care of the Psychiatric Patient*, ed. 3. Philadelphia, PA: Mosby; 2007, pp. 108–136.

TABLE 14-4
Selective Serotonin Norepinephrine Reuptake Inhibitors, Tricyclic, Tetracyclic, and Other Antidepressants

Agent	Half-life	Adverse Reactions	Comments
Venlafaxine (Effexor and Effexor ER) [selective serotonin and norepinephrine reuptake inhibitor, SSNRI]	5 hr for venlafaxine and 11 hr for its active metabolite (15 hr for venlafaxine extended release capsules)	Activating in larger amounts Patients often need trazodone or other agent to help with sleep Significant nausea with rapid onset of high dose Dose-dependent increases in diastolic blood pressure Average 5 mm Hg response	SSRI-like effect only in low doses, with norepinephrine uptake blockade at medium to high doses, similar to TCA effect, but with fewer adverse effects. Withdrawal syndrome similar to SSRIs
Duloxetine (Cymbalta) [selective serotonin and norepinephrine reuptake inhibitor, SSNRI]	8–17 hr	Rare liver toxicity risk, most often noted in presence of other hepatic risk factors. Few anticholinergic adverse effects	Serotonin norepinephrine reuptake inhibitor. Indicated for treatment of mood disorders and neuropathic pain
Bupropion (Wellbutrin) [selective dopamine reuptake inhibitor]	9.8 hr (3.9–24 hr) Extended-release 29 hr (20–38 hr)	Few anticholinergic effects Energizing Possible increased libido, agitation (25%) Avoid with significant manifestation of anxiety, agitation, insomnia	Blocks reuptake of dopamine at presynaptic neuron, especially in high doses, some increase in norepinephrine transmission. Dopamine receptor sites likely stimulated in substance abuse, making bupropion a helpful antidepressant for a person with a history of substance abuse. Nonaddicting and nonintoxicating Avoid use in presence of eating disorder or if anorexia is a major component of depression. Weight loss often seen (28% >5 lb [2.3 kg]) after initiation of therapy Do not give if history of or risk for seizure, closed head injury history, history of quiescent epilepsy Seizure risk worsens if dose increased rapidly

Continued

TABLE 14-4

Selective Serotonin Norepinephrine Reuptake Inhibitors, Tricyclic, Tetracyclic, and Other Antidepressants—cont'd

Agent	Half-life	Adverse Reactions	Comments
Mirtazapine (Remeron) [Tetracyclic antidepressant]	20–40 hr	Potent H1 inhibitor Weight gain common Major side effect is sedation that is worse in lower doses. Little sexual dysfunction or gastrointestinal side effect	Effect likely due to increase in central noradrenergic and serotoninergic activity Selectively stimulates 5HT1A while blocking 5HT2 and 5HT3 Higher doses more receptor site-selective and associated with fewer side effects
Tricyclic antidepressants; includes nortriptyline [Pamelor, active metabolite of amitriptyline], desipramine [Norpramin], active metabolic of imipramine)	24–32 hr	Weight gain Anticholinergic activity (blurred vision, dry mouth, memory loss, sweating, anxiety, postural hypotension, dizziness, and tachycardia) Constipation a problem, but infrequent nausea. Little sexual dysfunction	Inexpensive, more effective than SSRI in more severe depression, likely owing to its norepinephrine and serotonin activity More bothersome side-effect profile leads to high dropout rate Primary care providers seldom prescribe sufficient doses to relieve depression Taper off over 2–4 weeks to avoid TCA withdrawal symptoms; sleep disturbance, nightmares, gastrointestinal upset, malaise, irritability
Trazodone (Desyrel®, Oleptro®) [Triazolopyridine]	5 hr (3–9 hr)	Highly sedating, dizziness, favorable gastrointestinal side-effect profile. Priapism risk found in 1 in 6000 men using drug. Patient should be informed to go to emergency department promptly for painful erection lasting >30 min	Anxiolytic and antidepressant activity 5-HT2 antagonist Clinical use limited by marked sedation Effective hypnotic with little morning drowsiness at doses 25–100 mg taken 1 hr before sleep Can use in low, frequent doses as benzodiazepine alternative for generalized anxiety
Vilazodone (Viibryd) [Novel class]	25 hr	Diarrhea, nausea, vomiting and insomnia most common; no apparent effect on weight or cardiac function (e.g., QT prolongation).	Works through enhancement of serotonergic activity in the CNS through selective inhibition of serotonin uptake as well as a partial agonist of serotonergic 5-HT1A receptors

Source: Posternak M, Zimmerman M. Antidepressants. In: Goldberg R (ed). *Practical Guide to the Care of the Psychiatric Patient*, ed. 3. Philadelphia, PA: Mosby; 2007, pp. 108–136.

When choosing an antidepressant, the side-effect profile is critical. Often a given agent has a desirable side effect, such as sedation in a patient having difficulty with sleep or anxiety. In addition, the drug's half-life influences the therapeutic choice, with products with a shorter $T^1/_2$ being desirable in elderly patients and patients with hepatic disease. A younger adult could benefit from the use of a drug with a longer $T^1/_2$ if he or she skips a dose from time to time.

Another consideration in choosing an antidepressant is its toxicity when taken in overdose. A suicidal patient clearly needs hospitalization to ensure safety and appropriate treatment. As with many conditions, however, depression is a disease with episodes of improvement and deterioration. The prescriber should consider the risk of an intentional overdose.

A 2-week supply of a tricyclic antidepressant (TCA) in full therapeutic dose would likely be lethal, with significantly smaller amounts capable of causing seizures and dysrhythmias. SSRIs and atypical antidepressants have a significantly better safety profile when taken in overdose; usually more

BOX 14-4

Cytochrome P450 Isoenzyme Inhibition by Selective Serotonin Reuptake Inhibitors

CYP ISOENZYMES

	1A2	2C9	2C19	2D6	3A4
Escitalopram	0	0	0	0	0
Citalopram	+	0	0	+	0
Fluoxetine	+	++	+ to ++	+++	++
Paroxetine	+	+	+	+++	+
Sertraline	+	+	+ to ++	+	+

0 = minimal or weak inhibition; +, ++, +++ = mild, moderate, or strong inhibition.

than a 2-month supply of a full therapeutic dose is needed to cause life-threatening effects.

Antidepressants generally work by causing an increase in availability of certain neurotransmitters, such as serotonin, norepinephrine, and dopamine. This increased availability allows for greater activity at the neurotransmitter's respective receptor sites. There is evidence that interpersonal therapy also increases serotonin availability.

SSRIs are a heterogeneous group of drugs with a common mechanism of action: blocking reuptake of serotonin in the central nervous system and increasing amounts of serotonin available to postsynaptic neurons. The end effect is that more serotonin is available for action at selected receptors. Serotonin is active at numerous receptor sites (Table 14–5).

The use of serotonin norepinephrine reuptake inhibitors (SNRIs) for the treatment of depression has been increasing.

TABLE 14-5
Serotonin Activity

Serotonin Receptor Site	Activity When Activated	Comments
5-HT1A	Antidepressant, anti–obsessive-compulsive behavior, antipanic, anti–social phobia action, antibulimia effect	Action at this site basis of most antidepressant, antipanic therapy Reason that shyness often lifts with SSRI use
5-HT1C, 5-HT2C	Influence cerebrospinal fluid production, cerebral circulation Regulation of sleep Perception of pain Cardiovascular function	Reason tachycardia, dizziness, alteration of sleep patterns and change in pain perception occur with SSRI use
5-HT1D	Antimigraine activity	Triptan preparations work by stimulating this receptor site TCAs also work at this site and are helpful in preventing migraine
5-HT2	Agitation, akathisia, anxiety, panic, insomnia, sexual dysfunction Excessively upregulated in those with depression	Receptor site highly stimulated in activating SSRI such as fluoxetine. Activity at this receptor site causes sexual dysfunction associated with SSRI use Trazodone (Desyrel) antagonizes action at this site and is helpful in treatment of anxious depression and has a more favorable sexual function profile
5-HT3	When stimulated, nausea, gastrointestinal distress, diarrhea, headache	Particularly stimulated with antidepressants with poor gastrointestinal side-effect profile Products such as ondansetron (Zofran, a 5-HT3 antagonist) block activity at this site

Source: Maxmen J, Ward N. *Psychotropic Drug Facts Fast*, ed. 3. New York, NY: Norton, 2002.

These can be considered for patients who fail to respond to SSRIs and are also used to treat other conditions, such as anxiety and chronic nerve pain. These drugs block the absorption of serotonin and norepinephrine in the brain, which changes the balance of these chemicals, thereby boosting mood. Adverse effects are generally similar to those caused by SSRIs, with the most common consisting of nausea, dry mouth, dizziness, and excessive sweating. Tiredness, difficulty urinating, anxiety, constipation, insomnia, sexual dysfunction, headache, and loss of appetite have also been reported.

With all antidepressants, a receptor site-induced effect is immediate when therapy is initiated. The length of onset of therapeutic action is usually several weeks, however. This length of onset is likely associated with time needed for change in receptor site activity.

When a patient who is depressed takes antidepressants while undergoing an ongoing significant life stressor, such as family or marital discord or abuse, depressive symptoms usually subside as the medication takes effect. If the stressor continues, however, the antidepressant may appear to lose its initial effectiveness. Ongoing interpersonal therapy can be highly effective in augmenting pharmacological treatment in such situations.

In early SSRI therapy, the patient often complains of drug-related adverse effects, including headache, nausea, and diarrhea; these resolve within 2 to 6 weeks. Advising the patient that these side effects are expected, easily treatable, and transient helps avoid the problem of the patient discontinuing this important therapeutic agent. The headache is usually frontal in location and resolves with acetaminophen. Using a nonsteroidal antiinflammatory drug will likely contribute further to the gastrointestinal upset often found in the first weeks of SSRI use. Taking the medication with food can minimize nausea and diarrhea. Because of the potential chelation effect and impact of altered stomach pH on drug absorptions, taking many medications with an antacid can potentially limit the drug's effectiveness.

The use of SSRIs and other psychotropics is often associated with sexual function problems. Decreased libido and anorgasmia in either gender are often reported; erectile dysfunction in men is also common. If this is a problem, switching the patient to an a selective dopamine reuptake inhibitor such as bupropion (Wellbutrin) or a serotonin and norepinephrine reuptake inhibitor (SNRI) such as venlafaxine (Effexor®), duloxetine (Cymbalta®), or desvenlafaxine (Pristiq®), or a TCA can be considered because the use of these products is associated less often with sexual dysfunction. Vilazodone (Viibryd) is a dual-acting serotonergic agent that combines the antidepressant effects of a SSRI with partial serotonin-receptor agonist activity and provides an additional option. Additional options for SSRI sexual dysfunction include adding bupropion to the therapeutic regimen; support for this common practice is largely based on anecdotal reports. Taking a 1-day "drug holiday" from SSRI/SNRI use, with sexual activity planned for the end of the drug-free period, offers a reasonable option for a person with relatively infrequent sexual activity. This practice can lead to SSRI/SNRI-withdrawal symptoms toward the end of the drug-free period, however, with all products except fluoxetine. Given its long $T^1/_2$, this practice is unlikely to be helpful for a person taking fluoxetine.

Trazodone is used to treat depression or anxiety but has the potential to cause priapism. Its use is for mood disorder therapy, limited due to it being highly sedating. When used in patients with a sleeping disorder, trazodone should be administered about 1 hour prior to sleep for maximum effect. A withdrawal syndrome is often seen with SSRI/SNRI use longer than 5 weeks when the product is rapidly discontinued.

In SSRI/SNRI-withdrawal syndrome, there is a sudden change in the amount of serotonin available and an alteration in receptor site action. Its onset is related to the $T^1/_2$ of the drug, with three to five drug-free half-lives needed before the medication clears fully. Symptoms occur more rapidly after SSRI/SNRI discontinuation with a drug with a short $T^1/_2$ and may not occur at all in a drug with a protracted $T^1/_2$ (e.g., fluoxetine). Symptoms of SSRI/SNRI-withdrawal syndrome include dizziness, paresthesia, anxiety, nausea, sleep disturbance, and insomnia. Although disturbing and uncomfortable, this syndrome, in contrast to benzodiazepine withdrawal, is not dangerous or life-threatening and generally resolves within days to a few weeks.

Bupropion is used to treat depression as well as seasonal affective disorder (SAD) and as an aid in smoking cessation. The agent is structurally unrelated to SSRIs or TCAs and does not inhibit the activity of monoamine oxidase or the reuptake of serotonin. Bupropion blocks the reuptake of dopamine, which makes this agent especially useful for those with a history of substance abuse since dopamine receptor sites are likely stimulated in substance abuse. The drug is nonaddicting and nontoxicating and is associated with few anticholinergic effects. The most common adverse effects include headache, dry mouth, nausea, weight loss, and insomnia.

TCAs are helpful but often misunderstood and underused medications. TCAs have a more problematic side-effect profile compared with SSRIs. In addition, they require considerable prescriber skill and patient cooperation. TCAs are seldom well tolerated in a dose that is therapeutic for depression therapy. These medications are likely superior to SSRIs when depression is moderate to severe and characterized by emotional withdrawal, guilt, anorexia, and middle to late insomnia. In addition, they are effective in depressed patients who also have chronic pain, fibromyalgia, migraine, or the need for sedative or hypnotic agents. Choosing a TCA (e.g., nortriptyline [Pamelor]) with less anticholinergic effect and slowly increasing the dose helps enhance patient adherence.

If a patient with depression also has episodes of mania, bipolar I disorder is present. Bipolar disorders occur in approximately 1% of the general population. Characteristics of mania include those listed as follows. For at least 1 week, or less if hospitalized, the person's mood is persistently high, irritable, or expansive, coupled with three or more of these symptoms:

- Grandiosity or exaggerated self-esteem
- Reduced need for sleep
- Increased talkativeness
- Flight of ideas or racing thoughts
- Easy distractibility
- Psychomotor agitation or increased goal-directed activity (social, sexual, work, or school)
- Poor judgment (as shown by spending sprees, sexual misadventures, poor investments)
- The severity of the symptoms is such that there is at least one of the following: material distress impairs work, social, or personal functioning; psychotic features; and need for hospitalization to protect the person or others.

In bipolar I disorder, the patient usually presents with cycles of elevated or irritated mood lasting longer than 1 week. Bipolar I disorder is most common in women, with an onset around puberty. If a patient with depression has episodes of mania lasting fewer than 4 days with little social incapacitation, the diagnosis of bipolar II disorder is made. In patients with bipolar II disorder, the episodes of mania are relatively mild (hypomania) and are often quite productive in contrast to the low point of depression.

Further descriptors of bipolar disease include rapid cycling and cyclothymic disorder. In rapid-cycle bipolar disorder, there are four or more hypomanic, manic, mixed, or major depressive episodes in a 1-year period. In cyclothymic disorder, the mood disorder has been present for at least 2 years with episodes of mania lasting fewer than 4 days, too brief to fit standard criteria of mania or hypomania. If a TCA is given to a person with bipolar disorder, approximately 15% develop mania. This also happens when an energizing SSRI such as fluoxetine is given. Ongoing evaluation and treatment of a person with bipolar disorder requires significant expertise; expert advice should be sought. Treatment usually includes the use of mood-stabilizing medications, such as lithium carbonate, valproic acid, carbamazepine, and second generation antipsychotics such as risperidone.

DISCUSSION SOURCES

Posternak M, Zimmerman M. Depression: Identification and diagnosis. In: Goldberg R, (ed). *Practical Guide to the Care of the Psychiatric Patient*, ed. 3 Philadelphia, PA: Elsevier Mosby; 2007, pp. 86–106.

Posternak M, Zimmerman M. Antidepressants. In: Goldberg R, ed. *Practical Guide to the Care of the Psychiatric Patient*, ed. 3. Philadelphia, PA: Elsevier Mosby; 2007, pp. 108–136.

Truman C. Antidepressants. In: Goldberg R, ed. *Practical Guide to the Care of the Psychiatric Patient*, ed. 3. Philadelphia, PA: Elsevier Mosby; 2007, pp. 137–157.

American Psychiatric Association. Diagnostic and statistical manual of mental disorders: DSM-5, ed. 5. Arlington, VA: American Psychiatric Publishing, 2013.

American Psychiatric Association. Practice guidelines for the treatment of patients with major depressive disorder, ed. 3, 2010. http://psychiatryonline.org/content.aspx?bookid=28&sectionid=1667485.

Anxiety

84. Anxiety in response to a challenging life event is a natural response by the body to:
    A. help a person focus on the issue at hand.
    B. diminish the fight-or-flight response.
    C. impair decision-making under duress.
    D. provide transient improvement in physical capabilities.

85. Which of the following is most consistent with the diagnosis of generalize anxiety disorder?
    A. gastrointestinal upset
    B. difficulty initiating sleep
    C. diminished cognitive ability
    D. consistent early morning wakening

86. Conditions that commonly mimic or can worsen anxiety include all of the following except:
    A. opioid use.
    B. thyrotoxicosis.
    C. alcohol withdrawal.
    D. overuse of caffeine.

87. When prescribing a benzodiazepine, the NP considers that:
    A. the drugs are virtually interchangeable, with similar durations of action and therapeutic effect.
    B. the onset of therapeutic effect is usually rapid.
    C. these drugs have a low abuse potential in substance abusers.
    D. elderly adults will likely require doses similar to those needed by younger adults.

88. The drug buspirone (BuSpar®) has:
    A. low abuse potential.
    B. significant antidepressant action.
    C. a withdrawal syndrome when discontinued, similar to benzodiazepines.
    D. rapid onset of action.

89. A 24-year-old woman has a new onset of panic disorder. As part of her clinical presentation, you expect to find all of following except:
    A. peak symptoms at 10 minutes into the panic attack.
    B. history of agoraphobia.
    C. report of chest pain during panic attack.
    D. history of thought disorder.

90. As you develop the initial treatment plan for a woman with panic disorder, you consider prescribing:
    A. carbamazepine (Tegretol®).
    B. risperidone (Risperdal).
    C. citalopram (Celexa®).
    D. bupropion (Wellbutrin).

91. Diagnostic criteria for generalized anxiety disorder include all of the following except:
    A. difficulty concentrating.
    B. consistent early morning wakening.
    C. apprehension.
    D. irritability.

92. Which of the following is often reported by anxious patients?
    A. constipation
    B. muscle tension
    C. hive-form skin lesions
    D. somnolence

93. Pharmacological intervention in an anxiety disorder should be:
    A. generally given for about 4 to 6 months.
    B. continued for at least 6 months after remission is achieved.
    C. continued indefinitely with a first diagnosis of the condition.
    D. titrated to a highest dose recommended after symptom relief is achieved.

94. The use of which of the following drugs often mimics generalized anxiety disorder?
    A. sympathomimetics
    B. antipsychotics
    C. anticholinergics
    D. alpha-beta antagonists

95. When prescribing a benzodiazepine, the NP should consider that:
    A. the ingestion of 3 to 4 days of therapeutic dose can be life-threatening.
    B. the medication must be taken at the same hour every day.
    C. concomitant use of alcohol should be avoided.
    D. onset of therapeutic effect takes many days.

96. A middle-aged woman who has taken therapeutic dose of lorazepam for the past 6 years wishes to stop taking the medication. You advise her that:
    A. she can discontinue the drug immediately if she believes it no longer helps with her symptoms.
    B. rapid withdrawal in this situation can lead to tremors and hallucinations.
    C. she should taper down the dose of the medication over the next week.
    D. gastrointestinal upset is typically reported during the first week of benzodiazepine withdrawal.

97. Risk of benzodiazepine misuse is minimized by use of:
    A. agents with a shorter $T^1/_2$.
    B. the drug as an as-needed rescue medication for acute anxiety.
    C. more lipophilic products.
    D. products with long duration of action.

98. Which of the following statements concerning panic disorder is false?
    A. Panic disorder rarely occurs with depression.
    B. Up to 4% of the general population suffers from panic disorder.
    C. New onset panic disorder rarely occurs after 45 years of age.
    D. Family history of panic disorder is a risk factor for the condition.

99. Which of the following is true regarding panic disorder and agoraphobia?
    A. More men than women experience panic disorder without agoraphobia.
    B. More women than men experience panic disorder without agoraphobia.
    C. More men than women experience panic disorder with agoraphobia.
    D. More women than men experience panic disorder with agoraphobia.

100. Concomitant health problems found in a patient with panic disorder often include:
    A. irritable bowel syndrome.
    B. thought disorders.
    C. hypothyroidism.
    D. inflammatory bowel disease.

101. When initiating SSRI therapy for a patient with panic disorder, the NP should consider all of the following except:
    A. start with a low dose and slowly escalate doses as necessary.
    B. preferable to use agents that are more energizing than less energizing.
    C. select agents with a low rate of insomnia and akathisia.
    D. SSRI therapy can precipitate panic attacks with early use.

102. In providing primary care for a patient with posttraumatic stress disorder (PTSD), you consider that all of the following are likely to be reported except:
    A. agoraphobia.
    B. feeling of detachment.
    C. hyperarousal.
    D. poor recall of the precipitating event.

103. Among the preferred first-line pharmacological treatment options for patients with PTSD include the use of:
    A. methylphenidate (Ritalin®).
    B. oxazepam (Serax®).
    C. lithium carbonate.
    D. sertraline.

104. Which of the following therapeutic agents is commonly used to help with sleep difficulties such as insomnia associated with PTSD?
    A. duloxetine
    B. bupropion
    C. mirtazapine
    D. zolpidem

105. Which of the following is an over-the-counter herbal preparation used to relieve symptoms of depression?
    A. valerian root
    B. melatonin
    C. kava kava
    D. St. John's wort

106. In treatment-resistant patients with panic disorder, which drug class is occasionally used?
    A. atypical antipsychotic
    B. selective dopamine reuptake inhibitor
    C. monoamine oxidase inhibitor
    D. neuroleptic

107. In treating a person with panic disorder using an SSRI, the NP should consider that there is:
    A. considerable abuse potential with these medications.
    B. no significant therapeutic advantage over TCAs.
    C. a reduction in number and severity of panic attacks.
    D. significant toxicity in overdose.

108. Concomitant use of an SSRI with which of the following herbal products can potentially lead to serotonin syndrome?
    A. St. John's wort
    B. kava kava
    C. gingko biloba
    D. valerian root

109. Use of St. John's wort is known to impact the effectiveness of all of the following medications except:
    A. oral contraceptives.
    B. fluoroquinolones.
    C. cyclosporine.
    D. select antiretrovirals.

110. High doses or prolonged use of kava kava has been associated with cases of:
    A. renal impairment.
    B. hepatotoxicity.
    C. iron-deficiency anemia.
    D. hyperthyroidism.

Answers

84. A.	93. B.	102. D.
85. B.	94. A.	103. D.
86. A.	95. C.	104. C.
87. B.	96. B.	105. D.
88. A.	97. D.	106. C.
89. D.	98. A.	107. C.
90. C.	99. D.	108. A.
91. B.	100. A.	109. B.
92. B.	101. B.	110. B.

Anxiety is a normal human emotion that is an important part of fear response and helps a person focus on the issue at hand, such as anxiety associated with taking an important examination or making a presentation. Anxiety can also be protective, heightening senses when an individual encounters a dangerous situation. This is a rational, expected emotion when present for an appropriate reason and should dissipate with the cessation of the stressor. Anxiety becomes problematic, however, when it is exaggerated, is prolonged, or interferes with daily function.

Generalized anxiety disorder (GAD) is present in approximately 2% to 4% of the population. The typical age of onset is usually in the teen to young adult years; 15% have a first-degree relative with GAD. DMS-5 criteria for GAD include at least three of the following symptoms occurring on most days for 6 or more months:
- Excessive anxiety or worry (this must be present)
- Difficulty controlling worry (this must be present)
- Difficulty concentrating or mind going blank
- Sleep disturbance
- Muscle tension
- Restlessness or feeling keyed up/on edge
- Fatigue
- Irritability

Anxiety often occurs in patients with depression, making the differentiation between these two common disorders problematic. A patient with depression that has an anxious component usually reports nervous feelings after the onset of depressed mood. Also in depression, the patient has feelings of worthlessness and the feeling that situations are hopeless; patients with anxiety often report feeling "worried sick" and helpless. As with all mood disorders, anxiety most commonly occurs on a continuum.

The cardinal presenting signs of anxiety disorder are related to the hypersympathetic state. Physical manifestations include tachycardia, hyperventilation, palpitations, tremors, and sweating. When establishing the diagnosis of GAD, it is important to rule out many clinical conditions that can mimic the disorder, including thyrotoxicosis, alcohol withdrawal, or abuse of sympathomimetic drugs such as caffeine, amphetamines, and cocaine.

Treatment recommendations for pharmacological intervention in anxiety disorders are similar to the guidelines for depression therapy. Treatment should begin with a 3-month trial period of working with the patient to find the correct medication and dose that help abate symptoms. The practitioner should encourage psychotherapy to work on building skills needed to help manage a long-term health problem. In particular, the practitioner should convey the message to the patient that the use of psychotropic agents can help facilitate therapy. This acute care phase should be followed with a 6- to 12-month maintenance period, yielding a minimal treatment period of 9 months, although longer term therapy should be considered, especially if symptoms recur with depression. Choice of a therapeutic agent is guided by numerous factors, including asking about what has worked in the past and what has worked in the treatment of relatives with similar conditions.

Neurotransmitters implicated in anxiety include γ-aminobutyric acid (GABA), the brain's major inhibitory chemical, and serotonin (5-HT). Norepinephrine, dopamine, and epinephrine likely play a role as well. Drug therapy for patients with anxiety disorders includes agents that enhance GABA function, such as benzodiazepines, and products that enhance the availability of serotonin, such as SSRIs. The first-line therapy for anxiety is a SSRI. An anxiolytic, such as a benzodiazepine, is occasionally used to help with symptom management until the SSRI exerts its therapeutic effect. The SSRI choice is based on the previously identified factors when used in the treatment of depression.

The mechanism of action of benzodiazepines is as a mediator of GABA, enhancing its activity. Benzodiazepines are highly effective in the treatment of anxiety disorders. Because numerous benzodiazepines are available, choosing the appropriate agent can seem daunting. Critical differences can be found in these agents, however. Some agents, such as diazepam (Valium), are more lipophilic, entering the brain more rapidly and igniting an effect promptly. Although this may seem to be a desired therapeutic effect for severely anxious patients, this rapid ignition can also be intoxicating. More hydrophilic benzodiazepines, such as lorazepam, give reasonable therapeutic effect while having a slower onset of action and tend to be less intoxicating. In addition, with a highly lipophilic agent, excess is stored in body fat; this leaves a large repository for the drug, resulting in a longer $T^1/_2$.

As with any drug, the $T^1/_2$ should be considered. Products such as diazepam and clonazepam (Klonopin®), with a long $T^1/_2$, give sustained effect without periods of withdrawal. With drugs with a shorter $T^1/_2$, such as oxazepam (Serax), therapeutic gaps can occur. The use of drugs with a shorter $T^1/_2$ without active metabolites should be considered, however, when treating elderly persons.

One issue that needs to be considered when prescribing benzodiazepines is their abuse and misuse. Prescribers often hesitate to use these highly effective agents because of fear of providing the patient with a potentially habituating drug with the possibility of needing increasing doses. In reality, psychological dependence does occur occasionally, but careful prescribing can help avoid this.

Psychological benzodiazepine dependence is usually associated with a rapid onset agent, possibly giving a sensation of intoxication. In addition, prescribing at dosing intervals beyond the duration of action of the drug gives alternating periods of drug effect and withdrawal. The perception of difference is significant and possibly perceived as a buildup of unpleasant anxiety followed by a period of relief or rescue provided by the drug, with the cycle repeated with each drug dose. Using a benzodiazepine as an as-needed product increases the likelihood of abuse because this heightens the patient's awareness of drug versus no-drug state. Psychological benzodiazepine dependency can be avoided by using a slow-onset product such as clonazepam that has a long $T^1/_2$. If using short-acting products, the prescriber must give an adequate number of doses per day. If using on an as-needed basis, the prescriber should advise a maximal number of available or prescribed doses per week, such as three or four times per week, rather than once or twice a day. Increasing tolerance to high therapeutic dose, usually at a level two to four times the prescribed level, creates physical dependence on benzodiazepines.

When taken alone in overdose, benzodiazepines have a favorable toxicity profile. Sedation is enhanced, however, when benzodiazepines are combined with alcohol and barbiturates, leading to a potentially life-threatening condition. As a result, accidental and intentional fatalities can occur.

Physical benzodiazepine dependence is a significant problem. When working with the patient to discontinue benzodiazepine use, reducing the dose by 25% per week should be considered. Rapid withdrawal can lead to tremors, hallucinations, seizures, and a delirium tremens-like state. Onset occurs a few days after the last dose in a benzodiazepine with a shorter $T^1/_2$ (e.g., lorazepam) to up to 3 weeks in one with a longer $T^1/_2$ (e.g., clonazepam).

Panic disorder affects 2% to 4% of the general population. Average age of onset is 27 years; new onset is rare after age 45 years. There is a strong comorbidity with depression. The female-to-male ratio for panic disorder is approximately 1:1 if seen without agoraphobia. Panic disorder with agoraphobia is more common in women, however, with a ratio of 2:1. A strong family history of agoraphobia is often also reported.

Diagnostic criteria for panic disorder include recurrent and unexpected panic attacks and one or more of the panic attacks followed by at least one of the following: worry about an additional attack, pondering implications of attacks, or significant change of behavior related to attack. Panic attacks can occur with or without agoraphobia and should not be due to a substance or medical condition or accounted for by another mental disorder.

Panic attack is central to panic disorder. This is a period of intense fear or discomfort developing abruptly and peaking within 10 minutes with at least four characteristic symptoms present. Panic attack symptoms include palpitations, tachycardia, sweating, trembling, shortness of breath, choking, chest pain, chills, nausea, dizziness, and a sensation of derealization and depersonalization. Additional symptoms include fear of losing control or dying, paresthesia, and hot flashes. In addition to the characteristics mentioned, many individuals with panic disorder have problems with alcohol abuse, depression, dizziness, and chronic fatigue. Irritable bowel syndrome is often found in patients with panic disorder.

Because of the low abuse potential and favorable side-effect profile, SSRIs have become the initial treatment of choice for persons with panic disorder. SSRI use helps decrease the number and severity of panic attacks and, to a lesser degree, phobia and anxiety related to the attacks.

When using an SSRI for treating a patient with panic disorder, "start low, go slow, but get to goal" should guide therapy. Individuals with panic disorder usually do not tolerate a rapid induction or change in any therapy because of their heightened sympathetic state. An agent with an early side-effect profile that the patient is likely to tolerate should be chosen, such as a product that is less rather than more energizing with a lower rate of insomnia, nervousness, and akathisia; such agents include paroxetine (Paxil), citalopram (Celexa) or escitalopram (Lexapro®), but a more energizing SSRI such as fluoxetine (Prozac) is unlikely to be well tolerated. Also, SSRI use can precipitate panic attacks with early use, but prevent these episodes after the full therapeutic effect is realized. TCAs are occasionally used to treat panic disorder, recognizing this drug class's limitation, including toxicity in overdose and adverse effect profile. Benzodiazepine use in panic disorder is generally discouraged due to risk of habituation and abuse.

Monoamine oxidase inhibitors are the most potent drugs available for treating patients with panic disorder. Because of side effects and the need for dietary restriction while patients take the medications, their use is generally limited to individuals with treatment-resistant panic disorder. Consultation and care by a psychopharmacology team with experience in prescribing these medications is recommended.

Posttraumatic stress disorder (PTSD) is a condition that occurs after a significant single event, such as a natural disaster, being the victim of a crime, or exposure to combat conditions. It can also be precipitated by recurrent trauma, such as serving in combat, living in a war-torn area, or domestic abuse. Trauma can involve direct personal experience of an event that involves actual or threatened death or serious injury or witnessing an event that involves death, injury, or a threat to the physical integrity of another person. Horror and helplessness are expected emotions in response to a traumatic life event for at least 1 month afterward. These emotions last significantly longer in patients with PTSD, however, and are coupled with intrusive recall of the event, numbing of emotions, detachment, hyperarousal, and impaired social and occupational function. When considering military personnel with PTSD, it should be noted that they do not always respond in the same manner as civilians, and criteria for "fear, helplessness, and horror" do not always apply.

Treatment of patients with PTSD requires an interdisciplinary approach of expert providers. First-line pharmacological intervention can include the use of an SSRI or venlafaxine to treat arousal symptoms and associated depression. Treatment can also include mirtazapine (for insomnia) as well as a second-generation antipsychotic or mood stabilizers. Benzodiazepines should be used with caution because substance abuse is a common comorbid condition in patients with PTSD. Carbamazepine (Tegretol) and valproic acid (Depakote) have been used with some success in treating irritability, aggression, and impulsiveness. Clonidine (Catapres®) and propranolol (Inderal®) can be helpful in minimizing hyperarousal. Trazodone (Desyrel®) offers a nonaddicting option to enhance sleep.

Patients often choose to treat mood disorder with herbal products, which are available over-the-counter in unlimited supply. Although encouraging and facilitating patient self-care is an important part of the role of the NP, the use of herbal products should be approached with caution. Herbal medications are considered nutritional supplements and are not subject to the regulatory process common to prescription and over-the-counter medications. As a result, quality control in their production may be lacking, leading to inconsistent amounts of herbs per dose. In addition, when a patient takes an herbal product to treat symptoms of anxiety and depression, he or she is self-medicating a potentially life-threatening disease. Using herbs with prescription medications can lead to problems with drug interactions or additive effects, such as when St. John's wort is used concurrently with an SSRI. The NP and patient need to be aware of the effects, efficacy, and side-effect profiles of these products (Table 14–6).

TABLE 14-6
Over-the-Counter Herbal Products for Mood Disorders

Agent	Mechanism of Action	Comments
St. John's wort	Like MAOI-, SSRI-, TCA-like >10 active compounds	Compared with TCA, less anticholinergic effect, weight gain, less efficacy in more severe depression. Compared with SSRI, similar potential for energizing such as fluoxetine, similar efficacy in mild to moderate depression with limited study. TID–QID dosing needed; 6–8 weeks before clinical effect. Prudent to avoid concurrent use of SSRI, TCA, MAOI due to serotonin syndrome risk. Potentially photosensitizing, peripheral neuropathy in high doses. Capable of altering activity of CYP450 enzymes extensively involved in drug metabolism, and thus may interact significantly with many drugs. Can reduce serum levels of antiretrovirals (e.g., indinavir) and cyclosporine. Use can reduce effectiveness of oral contraceptives.
Kava	Action at GABA receptors similar to benzodiazepines	Satisfactory response compared with placebo, low-dose oxazepam (Serax). Sedating, can potentiate effects of alcohol. Cross-allergenic with pepper. Hepatotoxicity risk with overdose, prolonged treatment, and/or comedication.
Valerian root	Action similar to benzodiazepines	5%–10% with paradoxical stimulating effect. Available in aromatic tea, but weaker, with shorter duration of action. Less drug hangover than with benzodiazepines.

GABA—gamma-aminobutyric acid; MAOI—monoamine oxidase inhibitor; SSRI—selective serotonin reuptake inhibitor; TCA—tricyclic antidepressant.

DISCUSSION SOURCES

Goldberg RJ. *Practical Guide to the Care of the Psychiatric Patient,* ed. 3. St. Louis: Elsevier Health Sciences, 2007.

Department of Veteran Affairs, Department of Defense. VA/DoD clinical practice guideline for the management of posttraumatic stress, 2010. www.healthquality.va.gov/ptsd/CPGSummaryFINAL MgmtofPTSDfinal021413.pdf, accessed 1/15/14.

Interpersonal Violence

111. You note that a 25-year-old woman has bruises on her right shoulder. She states: "I fell up against the wall." The bruises appear finger-shaped. She denies that another person injured her. What is your best choice of statement in response to this?
   A. "Your bruises really look as if they were caused by someone grabbing you."
   B. "Was this really an accident?"
   C. "I notice the bruises are in the shape of a hand."
   D. "How did you fall?"

112. Which of the following statements is true concerning domestic violence?
   A. It is found largely among people of lower socioeconomic status.
   B. The person in an abusive relationship usually seeks help.
   C. Routine screening is indicated during pregnancy.
   D. A predictable cycle of violent activity followed by a period of calm is the norm.

113 to 118. The following questions should be answered True or False.

___ **113.** Access to a firearm by a male perpetrator is associated with increased risk of abuse toward women only in lower socioeconomic income households.

___ **114.** The NP is in an ideal position to provide counseling to both members of a couple involved in domestic violence, particularly if both members of the couple are members of the NP's practice panel.

___ **115.** Women's violence against male partners is as likely to result in serious injury as men's violence toward women.

___ **116.** Interpersonal violence is uncommon in same-sex relationships.

___ **117.** Access to a firearm increases the risk for a completed suicide.

___ **118.** Child abuse is present in about half of all homes where partner mistreatment occurs.

119. When considering characteristics of the domestic violence perpetrator, One of the best predictors of a subsequent homicide of victims of domestic violence is which of the following?
   A. history of perpetrator striking victim on the face with an open hand
   B. history of perpetrator attempting to strangle the victim
   C. perpetrator's access to kitchen knives.
   D. alcohol abuse history in the victim

Answers

111. C.	**114.** False	**117.** True
112. C.	**115.** False	**118.** True
113. False	**116.** False	**119.** B.

Interpersonal violence among family or household members (i.e., domestic violence) is found in all socioeconomic and ethnic groups. Because providers working with lower income and certain ethnic groups are perhaps more vigilant about domestic violence, however, it often appears that this abuse is more of a problem in certain groups.

Abuse can take numerous forms: psychological, financial, emotional, and physical. Acts of violence are typically thought to be against the victim, but often include destruction of property, intimidation, and threats. A cycle of tension building, including criticism, yelling, and threats followed by violence and then a quieter period of apologies and promises to change, is often seen. This cycle usually accelerates over time, however, with the violence being less predictable. Love for the perpetrator, hope that things will change, and fear of the consequences of leaving the relationship help to keep the victim in the relationship. These items also usually prevent victims from coming forth and asking for help.

As with counseling and screening for other health problems, using objective statements beginning with "I" is helpful. When a patient denies that finger-shaped bruises are caused by intentional injury by another person, the NP can simply state what is seen. This statement reinforces the assessment of abuse and allows the patient to offer more information. In a situation in which a patient is verbally abused in the NP's presence, the NP should reinforce his or her role as patient advocate by stating that the behavior is unacceptable in the NP's presence. Some providers fear that this statement can possibly precipitate another episode of abuse; however, this is unlikely.

Applying the BATHE model is helpful in framing the problem and forming a therapeutic relationship and directing intervention. Developed by Stuart and Lieberman, this model provides a guide for gathering information while helping the patient reflect on the issues at hand. The components of the model are as follows:
- BATHE
  - *B*—Background:
    - How are things at home? At work? Has anything changed? Good or bad? Anything you wish would change?

- *A*—Affect, anxiety
  - How do you feel about home life? Work? School? Life in general?
- *T*—Trouble
  - What worries you the most? How stressed are you about this problem?
- *H*—Handling
  - How are you handling the problems in your life? How much support do you get at home or work? Who gives you support in dealing with problems?
- *E*—Empathy
  - "That sounds difficult."

You might want to add SOAP to the BATHE:

- *S*—Support
  - Normalize problems, but do not minimize.
  - "Many people struggle with the same (similar) problem."
  - "What supports or resources can you use to help deal with this?"
    - Some providers may use selected self-disclosure for this. Self-disclosure usually works best in crises that are common and not of unusually tragic proportions, such as timely death or job change.
- *O*—Objectivity
  - Watch your reactions to the story. Maintain your professional composure without acting stonelike, but be mindful of "recoiling" gestures.
  - Help client with objectivity.
    - "What is the worst thing that can happen?"
    - "How likely is that?"
    - "Then what would happen?"
- Acceptance
  - Coach the client to personal acceptance.
    - "That is an understandable way to feel."
    - "I think you have done well considering the stress."
    - "I wonder if you are not being too hard on yourself."
- *A*—Acknowledge client priorities.
  - "It sounds like family is more important to you than your work."
- Acknowledge readiness or difficulty in making a change.
  - "Change is hard and sometimes very scary."
  - "It sounds to me like you are (not) ready to make a change."
- *P*—Present focus
  - Assist client in focusing on the present, without minimizing concerns of the past and future.
    - "How could you cope better?"
    - "What could you do differently?"
- What to do after you have gathered this information
  - Negotiate a problem-focused contract for behavioral change.
    - Repeat after me, "I promise not to harm myself or anyone else in any way between now and my next visit with _____."
- Homework assignment with "I" messages.
  - "I would like more help with the children."
  - "I feel really unimportant to you when _____."
  - "I feel angry when _____."
- How do you keep this to 15 minutes?
  - Focus the client, using open and close-ended questions. Tell the client how much time you have, particularly with revisit.
    - "We have ___ (fill in the blank) minutes to chat. What would you like to focus on?"
    - If client cannot focus, ask, "If one problem in your life could just disappear, what would you choose?"

Interpersonal violence is likely as common in same-sex relationships as in opposite-sex relationships. Violent behavior by a woman against a male partner is unlikely to result in injury as serious as a man's violence toward a woman, in part because of the usual disparity in body size and lower likelihood of weapon use in women. In all socioeconomic groups, access to a firearm by a perpetrator is associated with increased risk of abuse for serious or fatal injury; this is also a risk for completed suicide. The NP is in an ideal position to direct the couple to the appropriate resources for help in domestic violence but should not attempt to provide this counseling because of the complexity of this type of care. Individual treatment is the rule as long as the violent behavior continues. Child abuse is present in about half of all households in which there is partner abuse.

A history of strangulation attempts is one of the best predictors for subsequent homicide of victims of domestic violence. The probability of becoming an attempted homicide victim increases by 700%, and the probability of becoming a homicide victim increases 800% for women who have been strangled by their partner. For healthcare professionals documenting domestic violence, it is important to use the correct terminology between "strangulation" and "choking." Strangulation refers to external neck compression whereas the term choking should be reserved for internal airway blockage. It is important to note that most strangulation cases produce minor or no visible injury. Nearly all strangulation perpetrators are men, and though most abusers do not strangle to kill, they do strangle to show that they can kill.

DISCUSSION SOURCES

Stuart M, Lieberman J. *The 15-Minute Hour: Therapeutic Talk in Primary Care*, ed. 4. Philadelphia, PA: Saunders, 2008.

U.S. Department of Agriculture, Safety, Health and Employee Welfare Division. www.da.usda.gov/shmd/aware.htm, Domestic violence awareness handbook.

Female Reproductive and Genitourinary Systems

15

Contraception

1. Which of the following is a contraindication to estrogen/progestin-containing methods (combined oral contraception [COC], patch [Ortho Evra], or ring [NuvaRing])?
   A. mother with a history of breast cancer
   B. personal history of hepatitis A at age 10 years
   C. presence of factor V Leiden mutation
   D. cigarette smoking one pack per day in a 22-year-old

2. A 22-year-old woman taking a 35-mcg ethinyl estradiol COC calls after forgetting to take her pills for 2 consecutive days. She is 2 weeks into the pack. You advise her to:
   A. take the last pill missed immediately, even if this means taking 2 pills today.
   B. discard two pills and take two pills today.
   C. discard the rest of the pack and start a new pack with the first day of her next menses.
   D. continue taking one pill daily for the rest of the cycle.

3. When counseling a woman about COC use, you advise that:
   A. long-term use of COC is discouraged because the body needs a "rest" from birth control pills from time to time.
   B. fertility is often delayed for many months after discontinuation of COC.
   C. there is an increase in the rate of breast cancer after protracted use of COC.
   D. premenstrual syndrome symptoms are often improved with use of COC.

4. Noncontraceptive benefits of COC use include a decrease in all of the following except:
   A. iron-deficiency anemia.
   B. pelvic inflammatory disease (PID).
   C. cervicitis.
   D. ovarian cancer.

5. Which of the following women is the best candidate for progestin-only pill (POP) use?
   A. an 18-year-old woman who frequently forgets to take prescribed medications
   B. a 28-year-old woman with multiple sexual partners
   C. a 32-year-old woman with adequately-controlled hypertension
   D. a 26-year-old woman who wants to use the pill to help "regulate" her menstrual cycle

6. The most common reasons for discontinuing oral contraception use is breakthrough bleeding and:
   A. nausea/vomiting.
   B. inconvenience of use.
   C. cost.
   D. high failure rate.

7. A 38-year-old nulliparous woman who smokes two and a half packs a day is in an "on-and-off" relationship. The woman presents seeking contraception. Which of the following represents the most appropriate method?
   A. contraceptive ring (NuvaRing)
   B. COC
   C. contraceptive patch (Ortho Evra)
   D. vaginal diaphragm

8. Due to an increased risk of blood clots, an alternative to the contraceptive ring (NuvaRing) or patch (Ortho Evra) is preferred in all of the following women except:
   A. a 42-year-old nulliparous woman.
   B. 31-year-old woman with history of naturally occurring multiple gestation pregnancy
   C. 28-year-old who smokes one pack per day.
   D. 33-year-old woman with a family history of venous thrombosis.

9. Which of the following statements is true concerning vaginal diaphragm use?
   A. When in place, the woman is aware that the diaphragm fits snugly against the vaginal walls.
   B. This is a suitable form of contraception for women with recurrent urinary tract infection.
   C. After insertion, the cervix should be smoothly covered.
   D. The device should be removed within 2 hours of coitus to minimize the risk of infection.

10. According to the U.S. Medical Eligibility Criteria for Contraception Use, which of the following is a clinical condition in which use of a copper-containing IUD should be approached with caution?
    A. uncomplicated valvular heart disease
    B. AIDS-defining illness
    C. hypertension
    D. dysmenorrhea

11. Which of the following is the most appropriate response to a 27-year-old woman who is taking phenytoin (Dilantin) for the treatment of a seizure disorder and is requesting hormonal contraception?
    A. "A barrier method would be the preferable choice."
    B. "COC is the best option."
    C. "Depo-Provera (medroxyprogesterone acetate in a depot injection [DMPA]) use will likely not interact with your seizure medication."
    D. "Copper-containing IUD use is contraindicated."

12. Which of the following is commonly found after 1 year of using DMPA (Depo-Provera)?
    A. weight gain
    B. hypermenorrhea
    C. acne
    D. rapid return of fertility when discontinued

13 to 21. The following questions should be answered by responding yes or no.
   According to the U.S. Medical Eligibility Criteria for Contraception Use, who is a category 1 or 2 COC candidate?

_____ 13. a 22-year-old woman who smokes one pack per day

_____ 14. a 29-year-old woman with PID

_____ 15. a 45-year-old woman with tension-type headache

_____ 16. a 32-year-old woman breastfeeding a 6-month-old infant

_____ 17. a 28-year-old woman with type 1 diabetes mellitus

18 to 21. According to the U.S. Medical Eligibility Criteria for Contraception Use, who is a candidate for a copper-containing intrauterine device (IUD)?

_____ 18. a 45-year-old woman with fibroids with uterine cavity distortion

_____ 19. a 33-year-old woman who smokes two packs per day

_____ 20. a 25-year-old woman with hypertension

_____ 21. a 33-year-old woman with low-grade squamous intraepithelial lesions noted on Pap test

22. As you prescribe COC containing the progestin drospirenone (Loryna, Ocella, Vestura, Yasmin, Yaz), you offer the following advice:
    A. "Always take this pill on a full stomach."
    B. "You should not take acetaminophen when using this birth control pill."
    C. "Avoid using potassium-containing salt substitutes."
    D. "You will likely notice that premenstrual syndrome symptoms might become worse."

23. A 26-year-old mother who breastfeeds her 10-month-old child queries about contraceptives. In counseling her on the use of the progestin-only pill (POP), you mention all of the following except:
    A. the pill is taken every day.
    B. POP is a more effective contraceptive than COC.
    C. POP does not alter the quality or quantity of breast milk.
    D. POP is associated with bleeding irregularity, ranging from prolonged flow to amenorrhea.

24. By using a diaphragm with spermicide nonoxynol-9 during sexual intercourse, a woman is likely at increased risk for:
    A. cervical stenosis.
    B. urinary tract infection.
    C. increased perivaginal lactobacilli colonization.
    D. ovarian malignancy.

25. With the use of a levonorgestrel intrauterine system (Mirena), which one of the following is normally noted?
    A. endometrial hyperplasia
    B. hypermenorrhea
    C. increase in PID rates
    D. reduction in menstrual flow

26. The reduction in free androgens noted in a woman using COC can yield an improvement in:
    A. cycle control.
    B. acne vulgaris.
    C. breast tenderness.
    D. rheumatoid arthritis.

27. With DMPA in depot injection (Depo-Provera), the recommended length of use is usually:
    A. less than 1 year.
    B. no more than 2 years.
    C. as long as the woman desires this form of contraception.
    D. as determined by her lipid response to the medication.

28. Irregular bleeding associated with DMPA (Depo-Provera) can be minimized with the use of all of the following except:
    A. acetaminophen.
    B. ibuprofen.
    C. naproxen sodium.
    D. estrogen supplements.

29. When can a woman safely conceive after discontinuing COC use?
   A. immediately
   B. after 1 to 2 months
   C. after 3 to 4 months
   D. after 5 to 6 months

30. When prescribing the contraceptive patch (Ortho Evra) or vaginal ring (NuvaRing), the NP considers that:
   A. these are progestin-only products.
   B. candidates include women who have difficulty remembering to take a daily pill.
   C. there is significant drug interactions with both products.
   D. contraceptive efficacy is less than with COC.

31 to 33. Answer the following questions true or false.

____ **31.** The use of combined oral contraception (COC) reduces menstrual volume by approximately 60%, thereby reducing the risk of iron deficiency anemia.

____ **32.** Nausea with oral contraceptive use can be minimized by taking the pill on an empty stomach.

____ **33.** Calcium and vitamin D supplementation is recommended for those taking DMPA (Depo-Provera) injections to minimize the risk of a loss in bone density.

Answers

1. C.	14. Yes	23. B.	
2. A.	15. Yes	24. B.	
3. D.	16. Yes	25. D.	
4. C.	17. Yes, in the	26. B.	
5. C.	absence of	27. B.	
6. B.	advanced	28. A.	
7. D.	vascular	29. A.	
8. B.	disease	30. B.	
9. C.	18. No	31. T	
10. B.	19. Yes	32. F	
11. C.	20. Yes	33. T	
12. A.	21. Yes		
13. Yes	22. C.		

Despite the availability of numerous methods of highly reliable contraception, nearly half of all pregnancies in the United States are unplanned. Rates of continued contraception use vary greatly according to the method. Helping a woman choose an effective and acceptable form of family planning is an important part of providing healthcare.

Available for more than 5 decades, COC has been used by millions of women. This highly reliable form of contraception usually results in 1 pregnancy per 1000 women with perfect use and 50 pregnancies per 1000 women with typical use. The patch (Ortho Evra) and ring (NuvaRing) are also highly effective forms of contraception containing estrogen and progestin with reported rates of 99% efficacy when used as directed.

Contraceptive effect is achieved through the action of the COC, patch, and ring progestin and estrogen components. Progestational effects help to inhibit ovulation by suppressing luteinizing hormone (LH), thickening endocervical mucus, and hampering implantation by endometrial atrophy. Through estrogenic effects, ovulation is inhibited by suppression of follicle-stimulating hormone (FSH) and LH and by alteration of endometrial cellular structure.

When COC, ring, or patch is discontinued, fertility usually returns promptly. Contrary to common belief, there is no need to delay conception after discontinuing these contraceptive forms; prolonged combined hormonal contraceptive use is not associated with future infertility or other health problems.

Noncontraceptive benefits of combined hormonal contraception include lower rates of benign breast tumors and dysmenorrhea. Menstrual volume is reduced by about 60%, resulting in decreased rates of iron deficiency anemia. Decreased rates of endometrial, ovarian, and colon cancers are particularly noted among long-term users (more than 5 years). In part because of the endometrial thinning, COC can be safely used for an extended time without withdrawal, which is an attractive option for a woman who does not wish to menstruate or who has a health problem that is exacerbated by menstruation. Although COC is not protective against sexually transmitted infections (STIs), COC users have decreased frequency of pelvic inflammatory disease (PID), which results from thickened endocervical mucus; this results in a lower rate of future ectopic pregnancy. Decreased rates of acne, hirsutism, and ovarian cyst, as well as reduction in premenstrual syndrome and improvement in rheumatoid arthritis symptoms are also noted among COC users. Improvement in acne is usually noted after about 3 months of use, whereas improvement in hirsutism usually takes about 6 months; these improvements persist while the woman is taking COC and are usually reversible when COC is discontinued. COC is also a highly effective family planning option for a wide variety of women with chronic health problems (Table 15–1).

The highest dropout rates with COC and progestin-only pill (POP) use are in the first 3 months of use. The most frequently mentioned reasons are breakthrough bleeding (BTB) and inconvenience of use. Although BTB is bothersome, it is not harmful and does not indicate lesser contraceptive benefit. BTB can be minimized by taking COC or POP within the same 4-hour period every day. Cigarette smoking increases the likelihood of BTB and should be discouraged. BTB rate increases dramatically when pills are missed. Advice about what to do in the event of missed pills is an important part of providing contraceptive care (Table 15–2). Compared with COC use, BTB rates with the use of the contraceptive ring and patch are usually lower after the first few weeks of

TABLE 15–1

Summary of United States Medical Eligibility Criteria (USMEC) for Contraception Use: Precautions for Use of Combined Hormonal Contraceptive

Combined hormonal contraceptives (CHCs) include low-dose (<35ug ethinyl estradiol [EE]) combined oral contraceptives (COCs), combined hormonal patch (Ortho Evra), and combined vaginal ring (NuvaRing): Summary of US Medical Eligibility Criteria for Contraceptive Use

Category 4: Use Represents Unacceptable Health Risk	Category 3: Exercise Caution: Theoretical or Proven Risks Usually Outweigh Benefit	Category 2: Advantages Outweigh Risk	Category 1: No Restriction
• Venous thromboembolism • CHD, CVA • Structural heart disease • Breast cancer • Pregnancy • Postpartum <21 days • Acute hepatitis • Hepatic adenoma • Migraine with aura (any age) • Migraine without aura and age ≥35 years (for continuation) • Major surgery with prolonged immobilization • Age ≥35 and smoking ≥15 cigarettes per day • Hypertension (≥160/≥100 mm Hg or with vascular disease) • Known thrombotic mutations (factor V Leiden, prothrombin mutations, protein S, C, or antithrombin deficiency)	21-42 days postpartum, with other risk factors for VTE (such as age ≥35 years, previous VTE, thrombophilia, immobility, transfusion at delivery, BMI ≥30 mg/kg2, postpartum hemorrhage, postcesarean delivery, preeclampsia, or smoking or with lactation) • Undiagnosed vaginal bleeding • Age ≥35 and smoking less than 15 cigarettes per day • History breast cancer but no recurrence in past 5 yr • Interacting drugs (select antiepileptics such as phenytoin, carbamazepine, valproate) • Gallbladder disease • DM type 1 or type 2 ≥20 years' duration or with vascular disease • Past history breast cancer, no current disease for 5 yr • Hypertension adequately controlled without vascular disease • Untreated systolic 140–159 mm Hg or diastolic 90–99 Hg • Bariatric surgery with malabsorptive procedures (i.e., gastric bypass) for COC only • Migraine without aura and age ≥35 years (for initiation) • Rifampin or rifabutin therapy	• Age ≥40 • 21–42 days postpartum, without risk factors for VTE • Cigarette smoking < age 35 • Severe headache with oral contraceptive use • DM type 1 or type 2 without vascular disease • Major surgery without immobilization • Sickle cell disease • Hypertension (140/100–159/109 mm Hg) • Undiagnosed breast mass • Cervical cancer • Age ≥40 • Nonadherence factors • Family history lipid disorders • Family history premature MI • BMI ≥30 kg/m2 • Lactation ≥42 days without risk for VTE • Migraine without aura and age <35 years for initiation • Asymptomatic gall bladder disease	• Age menarche up to age 40 • Postpartum ≥42 days without breastfeeding • Post therapeutic or spontaneous abortion • History gestational DM • Varicose veins • Mild headache • PID, STI history • HIV • Benign breast disease • Family history breast, cervical, ovarian cancer • Cervical ectropion • Uterine fibroids • Past history ectopic pregnancy • Thyroid disease • Depression • Minor surgery without immobilization • Menorrhagia • Irregular menses • History gestational DM • Ovarian or endometrial cancer • Bariatric surgery with restrictive procedure (i.e., laparoscopic band procedure) • Broad spectrum antimicrobial and antifungal use

BMI—body mass index; CHD—congestive heart disease; CVA—cerebrovascular disease; DM—diabetes mellitus; MI—myocardial infarction.

Source: Centers for Disease Control and Prevention. United States Medical Eligibility Criteria (USMEC) for Contraception Use. www.cdc.gov/reproductivehealth/unintendedpregnancy/usmec.htm.

TABLE 15-2
Missed Combined Oral Contraceptive Pill Advice

Missed Pill Situation	Required Action	Comment
If pill missed within 12 hours of the time that should have been taken	Take today's pills immediately.	No additional or emergency contraception needed; continue with the rest of the pack.
If 1 pill missed for more than 12 hours but only 1 pill missed in a day.	Take today's pills immediately.	No additional or emergency contraception needed; continue with the rest of the pack.
If more than 1 pill missed	Take today's pill and the last forgotten pill today (2 tablets in 1 day). If she has a least 7 active pills in the pack, she has two options: 1. Take the rest of the active pills, skip the placebo pills and start the next pack of pills without interruption, and use condoms or abstain for 7 days. Or 2. Take the pills as in the pack and use condoms or abstinence until she has taken 7 of the pills in the pack.	Encourage use of EC if she has had unprotected intercourse in the prior 7 days.

EC—emergency contraception.
Source: Nelson AL, Cwiak C. Combined oral contraceptives (COCs). In: Hatcher RA, Trussell J, Nelson AL,
Cates Jr W, Kowal D, Policar MS (eds). *Contraceptive Technology*, ed. 20. New York: Ardent Media, Inc.;
2011, pp. 310–311.

use. This difference is largely due to the fact that the patch and ring do not require a daily action on the user's part, and adherence is significantly better. Therefore, the patch and ring may be preferable for women who are not as diligent in taking a pill every day. The patch and ring also contain a lower dose of estrogen and progestin than COC, which can result in fewer systemic adverse effects (e.g., headaches, breast tenderness).

Nausea with COC, patch, ring, and hormone therapy is a commonly reported adverse effect. Nausea is usually a transient problem noted in the first months of use and can be minimized by taking the medication with food or at bedtime. If vomiting occurs within 2 hours of taking COC, the dose should be retaken.

COC hormones interact with a few drugs. Interaction is noted, however, with many antiepileptic drugs (AEDs), including phenytoin, carbamazepine, phenobarbital, and primidone, potentially causing a reduction in therapeutic levels of these important medications. The BTB rate is greater in women using COC, patch, and ring and AEDs partly because of more rapid metabolism of estrogen. A woman with a seizure disorder who wishes to use hormonal contraception is likely to have a reduction in frequency and severity of seizures while using DMPA (Depo-Provera) because progestin use has long been noted to be protective against seizures. In addition, DMPA does not appear to interact with AEDs. Levonorgestrel implants appear to have the same effect. Use

of barrier methods, IUDs, or levonorgestrel-containing intrauterine systems (Mirena) does not interfere with AEDs and has no effect on seizure threshold.

The progestins used in most COC, patch, and ring formulations are testosterone derivatives. Drospirenone, found in the COC products Yasmin and Yaz, is an analogue of an aldosterone antagonist and has potassium-sparing qualities. Drospirenone should be used with caution in hepatic or renal dysfunction or with concomitant use of angiotensin receptor blocker, angiotensin-converting enzyme inhibitor, salt substitute, or potassium-sparing diuretic. Although POP inconsistently suppresses ovulation, this form of contraception likely works through thickening of endocervical mucus and through the alteration of the endometrium. POP use offers certain advantages and disadvantages compared with COC. With failure rates of up to 13%, POP is a less effective contraceptive than COC. The nausea rate with its use is significantly lower than with COC use because of the lack of estrogen. POPs are taken daily, a schedule many women find more convenient than the typically 3-weeks-on/1-week-off schedule with COC. POP must be used daily, however, for maximal efficacy. For lactating women who wish to use an oral hormonal contraceptive, POP is highly effective and does not alter the quality or quantity of breast milk. One significant disadvantage with POP use is bleeding irregularity, ranging from prolonged flow to amenorrhea.

The contraceptive patch (Ortho Evra) and contraceptive intravaginal ring (NuvaRing) contain estrogen and progestin as a birth control method in a nonoral form. Both of these methods have the advantage of infrequent dosing, with a new patch needed once a week and a new ring needed every 3 weeks. With proper use, contraceptive efficacy is similar to that of COC. Observed contraceptive failure rates are usually lower with the patch and ring likely because of greater ease of use. Adverse effects and contraindications to patch and ring use are similar to those of COC use. Women who dislike or forget to take a daily pill often welcome the opportunity to use the patch or ring. Another potential adverse effect associated with the use of the patch and ring is an increased risk of blood clots. The FDA issued a warning regarding a higher risk of venous thromboembolisms (VTEs) with patch and ring use compared with standard oral contraceptives. Therefore, it is recommended that an alternative contraceptive be used in women at higher risk of blood clots, including those over 35 years old, obese women, smokers, or those with a personal or family history of venous thrombosis.

DMPA (Depo-Provera), given every 90 days, is a highly reliable form of contraception (99.7% efficacy). DMPA is best suited for women who do not wish a pregnancy for at least 18 months because resumption of fertility is frequently delayed 6 to 12 months. When the injection is given within the first few days of menses, the contraceptive effect is immediate. When it is started 5 days after the onset of menses, a backup method of contraception should be used for 1 week. Depo-Provera may be started immediately postpartum if the woman is not breastfeeding and initiated 3 to 6 weeks postpartum if she is breastfeeding. Earlier use can diminish quantity but not quality of breast milk. Irregular bleeding, a common problem during the first few months of DMPA injection use, can be minimized by the use of a prostaglandin inhibitor such as ibuprofen, 400 mg tid, or naproxen sodium, 375 to 540 mg bid, for 3 to 5 days. Estrogen supplements, such as a 0.1-mg estrogen patch used for 7 to 10 days, can also be helpful but are seldom needed to manage this bothersome, but not dangerous, adverse effect. After 1 year of DMPA use, 30% to 50% of women have amenorrhea. According to observations from limited study, bone density is occasionally noted to be reduced in women using DMPA. This condition is largely reversible, however, when the medication is discontinued. The U.S. Food and Drug Administration (FDA) has assigned a boxed warning to DMPA, highlighting that prolonged use can result in the loss of bone density and recommending that the medication not be used for more than 2 years unless other methods cannot be used; bone density seems to normalize quickly with discontinuation of the medication. Calcium supplementation, at 1000 to 1500 mg/d, weight-bearing exercise, and vitamin D supplementation should be recommended; this advice is helpful for general bone health.

Standard IUDs, such as the copper-containing ParaGard (Copper T 380A), are an effective form of contraception with a failure rate of 0.5% to 2.2%. The mechanism of contraceptive action is not entirely understood, but it is unlikely that these are abortifacients. There is often an increase in menstrual bleeding and upper reproductive tract infection with their use, and IUDs are not widely used, in part because of the incorrect perception of the healthcare provider that few women can safely use this highly effective contraceptive method (Table 15–3). Mirena is a levonorgestrel-containing intrauterine system of drug delivery that produces marked endometrial atrophy. As a result, about 50% of Mirena users are amenorrheic at the end of 2 years of use. Thickened endocervical mucus is also noted, which limits the ascent of infection into the upper reproductive tract and minimizes PID risk. This is a particularly helpful method of contraception for women with menorrhagia.

The diaphragm, a barrier method of contraception, is placed in the vagina before intercourse. This device, which has an effectiveness rate of 88% to 94%, should be used in conjunction with a spermicide and removed no sooner than 6 hours after coitus. When properly fitted and in the appropriate position, the device should rest snugly in the vagina but without tension against the vaginal walls. The woman and her partner should be unaware of the diaphragm's presence. If either partner can feel the diaphragm, the device is either the wrong size or not properly inserted. Because a diaphragm should always be used with a spermicide, a woman with a history of recurrent urinary tract infection (UTI) is not an ideal candidate for diaphragm use. Although the thought behind this long-held advice is that the diaphragm increases UTI risk as a result of potential pressure on the woman's lower urinary tract, the risk more likely arises from the concurrent use of a spermicide. A woman who is exposed to the spermicide nonoxynol-9, either through vaginal use or with a male partner who uses condoms with this spermicide, is likely at increased risk of UTI. The proposed mechanism of this risk is the antibacterial effect of the spermicide, which is to reduce lactobacilli, a normal component of the periurethral flora. Lactobacilli produce hydrogen peroxide and lactic acid, providing the periurethral area and vagina with a pH that inhibits bacterial growth and blocks potential sites of attachment and is toxic to uropathogens.

DISCUSSION SOURCES

Cates W, Harwood B. Vaginal barriers and spermicides. In: Hatcher RA, Trussell J, Nelson AL, Cates W, Kowal D, Policar MS (eds). *Contraceptive Technology*, ed 20. New York: Ardent Media, Inc.; 2011, pp. 391–408.

Dean G, Bimla Schwarz E. Intrauterine contraceptives (IUCs). In: Hatcher RA, Trussell J, Nelson AL, Cates W, Kowal D, Policar MS (eds). *Contraceptive Technology*, ed 20. New York: Ardent Media, Inc.; 2011, pp. 151 and 154.

Raymond EG. Progestin-only pills. In: Hatcher RA, Trussell J, Nelson AL, Cates W, Kowal D, Policar MS (eds). *Contraceptive Technology*, ed. 20. New York: Ardent Media, Inc.; 2011, p. 240.

TABLE 15–3

Summary of the United States Medical Eligibility Criteria (USMEC) for Contraception Use: Precautions for the Use of Intrauterine Devices

Summary of Classification for Use of Intrauterine Devices, Including LNG-IUS (Mirena, Skyla) and Cu-IUD (Paragard)

Category 4: Use Represents Unacceptable Health Risk	Category 3: Exercise Caution: Theoretical or Proven Risk Usually Outweigh Benefit	Category 2: Advantages Outweigh Risk	Category 1: No Restriction
• Current PID (within 3 mo) • Current purulent cervicitis or chlamydia infection or gonorrhea • Unexplained vaginal bleeding • Cervical cancer, awaiting treatment • Uterine fibroids with distortion of uterine cavity • Positive antiphospholipids (LNG-IUS)	• AIDS-defining illness • Cirrhosis with severe decompensation	• High risk for HIV • HIV infection • Age less than 20 years • Nulliparous • Complicated valvular heart disease • Severe dysmenorrhea	• Immediately post first-trimester therapeutic abortion • Parous • Hypertension • Vascular disease • Uncomplicated valvular heart disease • Cervical intraepithelial neoplasia • Uterine fibroids without distortion of uterine cavity • Postpartum > 4 weeks

Source: Centers for Disease Control and Prevention. United States Medical Eligibility Criteria (USMEC) for Contraception Use, 2010 (updated 2012). www.cdc.gov/reproductivehealth/unintendedpregnancy/usmec.htm.

Trussell J, Guthrie KA. Choosing a contraceptive: Efficacy, safety, and personal considerations. In: Hatcher RA, Trussell J, Nelson AL, Cates W, Kowal D, Policar MS (eds). *Contraceptive Technology*, ed. 20. New York: Ardent Media, Inc.; 2011, pp. 50 and 65.

Bartz D, Goldberg AB. Injectable contraceptives. In: Hatcher RA, Trussell J, Nelson AL, Cates W, Kowal D, Policar MS (eds). *Contraceptive Technology*, ed. 20. New York: Ardent Media, Inc.; 2011, pp. 213, 215, and 221.

Cates W, Harwood B. Vaginal barriers and spermicides. In: Hatcher RA, Trussell J, Nelson AL, Cates W, Kowal D, Policar MS (eds). *Contraceptive Technology*, ed. 20. New York: Ardent Media, Inc.; 2011, pp. 394 and 400.

Dean G, Bimla Schwarz E. Intrauterine contraceptives (IUCs). In: Hatcher RA, Trussell J, Nelson AL, Cates W, Kowal D, Policar MS (eds). *Contraceptive Technology*, ed. 20. New York: Ardent Media, Inc.; 2011, p. 158.

Nelson AL, Cwiak C. Combined oral contraceptives (COCs). In: Hatcher RA, Trussell J, Nelson AL, Cates Jr W, Kowal D, Policar MS (eds). *Contraceptive Technology*, ed. 20. New York: Ardent Media, Inc.; 2011, pp. 264, 267, 282, 288, 308, 309, and 332.

Trussell J, Guthrie KA. Choosing a contraceptive: efficacy, safety, and personal considerations. In: Hatcher RA, Trussell J, Nelson AL, Cates W, Kowal D, Policar MS (eds). *Contraceptive Technology*, ed. 20. New York: Ardent Media, Inc.; 2011, p. 65.

Centers for Disease Control and Prevention. United States Medical Eligibility Criteria (USMEC) for Contraception Use, 2012. www.cdc.gov/reproductivehealth/unintendedpregnancy/usmec.htm, accessed 8/1/13.

Emergency Contraception

34. An 18-year-old woman requests emergency contraception after having unprotected vaginal intercourse approximately 18 hours ago. Today is day 12 of her normally 27- to 29-day menstrual cycle and she has no contraindications to the use of any currently available forms of emergency contraception. You advise her that:
   A. emergency hormonal contraception use reduces the risk of pregnancy by approximately 33%.
   B. all forms of emergency contraception must be used within 12 hours after unprotected intercourse.
   C. the likelihood of conception is minimal.
   D. insertion of a copper-containing IUD offers a effective form of emergency and ongoing contraception.

35. Which of the following is likely not among the proposed mechanisms of action of all forms of oral emergency contraception?
A. inhibits ovulation
B. acts as an abortifacient
C. slows sperm transport
D. slows ovum transport

36. A 24-year-old woman who requests emergency contraception pills wants to know the effects if pregnancy does occur. You respond that there is the risk of increased rate of:
A. spontaneous abortion.
B. birth defects.
C. placental abruption.
D. none of the above.

37. In contrast to progestin-only emergency contraception, a possible mechanism of action of ulipristal is:
A. inhibiting embryo implantation.
B. impairing sperm transport.
C. through spontaneous abortion.
D. impairing ovum transport.

38. You see a 34-year-old woman who reports having unprotected sexual intercourse 4 days ago and requests emergency contraception. She has a recent history of gonorrhea that was treated successfully. The most acceptable and effective option in this clinical scenario is:
A. progestin-only emergency contraception.
B. ulipristal.
C. copper-containing IUD.
D. nothing, as 4 days is too long for emergency contraception to be effective.

39. Which of the following statements is false?
A. Progestin-only emergency contraception can be taken as one dose or two doses.
B. Ulipristal is available by prescription only.
C. Progestin-only emergency contraception is available OTC for women 17 years old and older.
D. Ulipristal is taken in two doses 12 hours apart.

40. A woman who has used emergency contraception pills should be advised that if she does not have a normal menstrual period within _____ weeks, a pregnancy test should be obtained.
A. 1 to 2
B. 2 to 3
C. 3 to 4
D. 4 to 5

As previously mentioned, nearly half of all pregnancies are unplanned. Emergency contraception, used after coitus to minimize the risk of unintended pregnancy when a contraceptive method fails or is not used, is an effective method of minimizing the number of unintended pregnancies (Box 15–1). An estimated 800,000 annual pregnancy terminations could be

Box 15–1
Emergency Hormonal Contraception: Indications and Mechanism of Action

Candidates for Emergency Contraception	Emergency Contraception Mechanism of Action with Levonorgestrel (Plan B, Plan B One Step, Next Choice), or Ulipristal (ella®) Use

Any time unprotected sexual intercourse occurs including potential method failure (e.g., late for or missed pills, late for DMPA, dislodged or misplaced diaphragm, condom break or slippage, expelled IUD)	Depending on time taken during menstrual cycle
	■ Inhibit or delay ovulation (most likely effect)
	■ Inhibit tubal transport of egg or sperm
	■ Interfere with fertilization
	■ Possible effect on endometrium:
	  ■ With levonorgestrel use as emergency contraception, minimal to no alteration to endometrium, therefore unlikely to inhibit implantation of a fertilized egg.
	  ■ With ulipristal use as emergency contraception, changes in the endometrium can potentially alter likelihood of fertilized egg implantation.
	Unlikely mechanism of action
	■ Emergency hormonal contraception use results in minimal to no alteration to endometrium and is unlikely to inhibit implantation of a fertilized egg

Source: Trussell J, Bimla Schwarz E. Emergency contraception. In: Hatcher RA, Trussell J, Nelson AL, Cates W, Kowal D, Policar MS (eds). *Contraceptive Technology*, ed. 20. New York: Ardent Media, Inc.; 2011, pp. 113–145.

Answers

34. D.	**37.** A.	**39.** D.
35. B.	**38.** B.	**40.** C.
36. D.		

avoided if knowledge of and access to emergency contraception were widely available.

Numerous methods are available, including the use of levonorgestrel (LNG), ulipristal acetate, and copper-containing IUDs. Emergency contraception with oral hormonal agents, such as LNG and ulipristal, is highly effective, reducing the risk of pregnancy by 75% or more, according to the following model: If 100 fertile women have unprotected heterosexual intercourse in the second to third weeks of their cycles, eight typically become pregnant. One or two typically become pregnant when using emergency contraception. The most likely mechanism of action to reduce pregnancy risk is by inhibiting or delaying ovulation or impairing ovum or sperm transport.

Emergency contraception with LNG is unlikely to prevent pregnancy by preventing implantation of a fertilized ovum because the resulting minor endometrial changes would likely be insufficient to yield this result. Progestin-only emergency contraception (e.g., Plan B, Plan B One-Step, Next Choice, Next Choice One Dose) includes levonorgestrel 1.5 mg total dose. The first dose should be taken within 72 hours of unprotected sexual intercourse but can be effective up to 120 hours post intercourse. For Plan B or Next Choice, women can take both pills in a single dose or they can separate the doses by 12 hours. Plan B One-Step and Next Choice One Dose are one-dose, single-pill options. For women 17 years of age and older, these products are available as over-the-counter medication. For those under 17 years of age, a prescription is required or, in select locations, pharmacist consultation is required.

An alternative to progestin-only emergency contraception is ulipristal acetate (ella). This product works as a progesterone agonist/antagonist and thus has a direct inhibitory effect on follicular development and ovum release. In contrast with levonorgestrel, ulipristal remains effective when administered immediately before ovulation around the time of luteinizing hormone surge. Ulipristal is approved for use up to 5 days (120 hours) post unprotected sexual intercourse. However, it should be noted that endometrial alterations associated with ulipristal use could impact embryo implantation. Ulipristal is only available through a prescription and is administered as one tablet (though a repeat dose may be needed if vomiting occurs within 3 hours of the dose).

Use of oral hormonal emergency contraception would not interrupt an established pregnancy or increase risk of early pregnancy loss. If pregnancy does occur, use of this therapeutic method does not appear to be teratogenic.

A copper-containing IUD such as the ParaGard (Copper T 380A) can be inserted within 5 days after intercourse as a form of emergency contraception. Because of the risk of upper reproductive tract infections, use of a copper-containing IUD is contraindicated in the presence of STI. In addition to providing ongoing contraception, IUD insertion provides a hormone-free emergency contraception option.

Menstrual bleeding should be expected within 3 to 4 weeks of using emergency contraception. If none occurs, a pregnancy test should be done.

DISCUSSION SOURCES

Centers for Disease Control and Prevention. United States Medical Eligibility Criteria (USMEC) for Contraception Use, 2010 (updated 2012). www.cdc.gov/reproductivehealth/unintendedpregnancy/usmec.htm.

Office of Population Research & Association of Reproductive Health Professionals at Princeton University. The Emergency Contraception Website, 2012. http://ec.princeton.edu

Trussell J, Bimla Schwarz E. Emergency contraception. In: Hatcher RA, Trussell J, Nelson AL, Cates W, Kowal D, Policar MS (eds). *Contraceptive Technology*, ed. 20. New York: Ardent Media, Inc.; 2011, pp. 121, 124, 128, and 135.

Menopause

41. The average onset of perimenopause is between the ages of:
A. 35 to 40 years.
B. 40 to 45 years.
C. 45 to 50 years.
D. 50 to 55 years.

42. Which of the following statements regarding perimenopause is false?
A. Menstruation ceases during perimenopause.
B. Hot flashes and flushes are common during the week before menses.
C. Pregnancy is still possible during perimenopause.
D. Ovulation becomes more erratic during perimenopause.

43. In advising a woman about menopause, the NP considers that:
A. the average age at last menstrual period for a North American woman is 47 to 48 years.
B. hot flashes and night sweats occur in about 60% to 90% of women.
C. women with surgical menopause usually have milder symptoms.
D. follicle-stimulating hormone (FSH) and luteinizing hormone (LH) levels are suppressed.

44. Findings in estrogen deficiency (atrophic) vaginitis include:
A. a malodorous vaginal discharge.
B. an increased number of lactobacilli.
C. a reduced number of white blood cells.
D. a pH greater than 5.0.

45. A 53-year-old woman who is taking hormone therapy (HT) with conjugated equine estrogen, 0.45 mg/d, with MPA, 1.5 mg, has bothersome atrophic vaginitis symptoms. You advise that:
A. her oral estrogen dose should be increased.
B. the addition of a topical estrogen can be helpful.
C. the MPA component should be discontinued.
D. baking soda douche should be tried.

46. For a woman with bothersome hot flashes who cannot take HT, alternative options with demonstrated efficacy and limited adverse effects include the use of all of the following except:
    A. venlafaxine.
    B. sertraline.
    C. gabapentin.
    D. clonidine.

47. Absolute contraindications to postmenopausal HT include:
    A. unexplained vaginal bleeding.
    B. seizure disorder.
    C. dyslipidemia.
    D. migraine headache.

48. In advising a perimenopausal woman about HT, you consider that it may:
    A. reduce the risk of venous thrombotic events.
    B. significantly reduce serum triglyceride levels.
    C. worsen hypertension in most women.
    D. help preserve bone density.

49. Postmenopausal HT use can result in:
    A. a reduction in the rate of cardiovascular disease.
    B. an increase in the rate of rheumatoid arthritis.
    C. a reduction in the frequency and severity of vasomotor symptoms.
    D. a disturbance in sleep patterns.

50. The progestin component of HT is given to:
    A. counteract the negative lipid effects of estrogen.
    B. minimize endometrial hyperplasia.
    C. help with vaginal atrophy symptoms.
    D. prolong ovarian activity.

51. Concerning selective estrogen receptor modulator therapy such as raloxifene (Evista), which of the following statements is correct?
    A. Concurrent progestin opposition is needed.
    B. Hot flashes are reduced in frequency and severity.
    C. Use is contraindicated when a woman has a history of breast cancer.
    D. Osteoporosis risk is reduced with use.

52. During perimenopause, which of the following is likely to be noted?
    A. Symptoms are most likely in the week before the onset of the menses.
    B. The length of the perimenopausal period is predictable.
    C. Symptoms are less severe in women who smoke.
    D. Hot flashes are uncommon.

53. A 48-year-old woman complains of increased frequency and severity of hot flashes. Her last menses occurred 6 months ago. You would expect all of the following laboratory findings except:
    A. increased levels of LH.
    B. elevated levels of testosterone.
    C. reduced levels of estradiol.
    D. reduced levels of progesterone.

54. Which of the following is likely to be noted with short-term (less than 1 to 2 years) HT use in a post-menopausal woman?
    A. reduction in dementia risk
    B. significant increase in breast cancer risk
    C. minimized hot flashes.
    D. increase in cardiovascular risk

55. Which body area has the greatest concentration of estrogen receptors?
    A. vulva
    B. vascular bed
    C. heart
    D. brain

56. When counseling a 46-year-old woman who is experiencing debilitating hot flashes, you advise all of the following regarding higher and lower dose hormone replacement therapy (HT) except:
    A. current clinical guidelines recommend using the lowest effective dose possible.
    B. higher-dose HT will relieve hot flashes faster than lower-dose regimens.
    C. lower-dose HT is better tolerated than higher-dose HT.
    D. the duration of lower-dose HT is usually shorter than that of higher-dose regimens.

57. You see a 45-year-old woman who is considering HT. She has a family history of cervical dysplasia, hyperlipidemia, and VTE. You advise her on all of the following except:
    A. the use of progestin can minimize the risk of endometrial cancer for a woman on HT and who has not had a hysterectomy.
    B. supplemental estrogen should be avoided in women who are at high risk of breast cancer or uterine cancer.
    C. supplemental estrogen should be avoided in women who are at high risk of cardiovascular disease.
    D. short-term studies demonstrate that oral HT is associated with lower thromboembolic risk than transdermal forms of HT.

58. Examples of phytoestrogens include all of the following except:
    A. red clover.
    B. ginseng.
    C. vitamin E.
    D. soy products.

59. The typical HT regimen contains _____ or less of the estrogen dose of COC.
    A. one-eighth
    B. one-fourth
    C. one-half
    D. three-fourths

60. For the woman with a history of DVT who is having significant vasomotor symptoms, which of the following can be can be used for symptom management?
    A. 17- 17β-estradiol patch
    B. drospirenone
    C. estrone.
    D. paroxetine.

61. Long term calcium supplementation is recommended in postmenopausal women as its use reduces the risk of fracture by approximately:
    A. 25%.
    B. 50%.
    C. 65%.
    D. 80%.

62. In postmenopausal women, a major benefit from the use of topical or local estrogen is:
    A. decreased rate of breast cancer.
    B. reduced risk of recurrent UTIs.
    C. reduced risk of type 2 diabetes.
    D. increased levels of androgens.

63. When reviewing the use of nutritional supplements for the management of menopausal symptoms, the NP considers that:
    A. few high-quality studies support the use of these products.
    B. the use of these products is consistently reported to be helpful.
    C. the products can be safely used as long as blood hormone levels are carefully evaluated.
    D. the use of these products is associated with a greater reduction in menopausal symptoms than with prescription HT.

64. Which of the following statements is true?
    A. Many over-the-counter progesterone creams contain sterols that the human body is unable to use.
    B. All progesterones are easily absorbed via the skin.
    C. Alfalfa is an example of a phytoprogesterone.
    D. Progesterones, whether synthetic or plant-based, should not be used by a woman who has undergone a hysterectomy.

Answers

41. B.	49. C.	57. D.
42. A.	50. B.	58. C.
43. B.	51. D.	59. B.
44. D.	52. A.	60. D.
45. B.	53. B.	61. B.
46. D.	54. C.	62. B.
47. A.	55. A.	63. A.
48. D.	56. D.	64. A.

A woman's life is characterized by a series of shifts: first, a woman transitions to the reproductive years, then to the premenopausal period, and then to the menopausal and postmenopausal years. Each transition is normal, expected, and not a disease state. Perimenopause and menopause are often symptom-producing events, however.

Perimenopause is the time surrounding menopause; its onset is marked by the beginning symptoms of menopause and ends with the cessation of menses. The average age of onset of perimenopause is 40 to 45 years; it occurs earlier in cigarette smokers. Perimenopause lasts an average of 4 years but can range from a few months to 10 years. Menopause, when the final menstrual period occurs, marks another transition in a woman's reproductive life. By definition, a woman is in menopause when she has had no naturally occurring menstrual period for 12 months. The average age for a North American woman at menopause is 51.3 years, with some women living one-third of their lives after this time.

During perimenopause, menstrual irregularity is common, with the interval between periods becoming longer or shorter and flow becoming heavier or lighter. Ovulation becomes more erratic, but pregnancy is still possible. Hot flashes and sleep problems are usually worse in the week before the menses and are reported by approximately 65% to 75% of women during perimenopause. During this stage, estrogen levels are usually normal, but FSH levels are elevated. As mentioned, the woman often notes hot flashes or flushes during the week before the onset of the menses, a time when hormonal shifts are most dramatic. Because most women associate menopause symptoms with irregular or absent menstrual bleeding, these perimenopausal symptoms can be confusing as the woman is menstruating on a regular basis. Although low estrogen levels have often been implicated as the cause of perimenopausal symptoms, the shifting levels of multiple biological substances is likely implicated.

As the menopausal period progresses, LH and FSH levels increase dramatically as the anterior lobe of the pituitary sends out an abundance of these substances in an attempt to induce ovulation; the ovaries fail to respond with ovulation, sometimes leading to heavy, anovulatory menstrual bleeding. Levels of estrogen forms (estradiol, estrogen) and androgens (testosterone, progesterone, androsterone, and dehydroepiandrosterone) are reduced. Hot flashes now usually become more frequent and severe, in part induced by the FSH surge. About 80% of woman going through menopause have hot flashes, ranging in severity from mildly bothersome to debilitating. Compared with naturally occurring menopause, women with surgical menopause usually have more severe symptoms, likely because the hormonal shifts are more rapid and dramatic.

Estrogen receptors are found in high concentrations in the vulva, vagina, urethra, and trigone of the bladder. As a result, symptoms of urogenital atrophy from estrogen shifts are a common perimenopausal and menopausal problem. These receptors are found in lower concentrations in the vascular bed, heart, brain, bone, and eye—areas of the body that also exhibit changes during perimenopause and menopause.

Vasomotor symptoms can be debilitating, causing disturbed sleep, avoidance of social situations in which hot flashes occur, and numerous other problems. Women often seek advice from their healthcare provider about minimizing these symptoms. Numerous lifestyle modifications can be quite helpful (Table 15–4). When these measures are inadequate, the addition of pharmacological intervention is often appropriate.

HT, usually in the form of an estrogen supplement prescription, is likely the most commonly used and most effective therapy that has been extensively studied for hot flash management. When given during the first years after menopause, reduction of hot flashes by 80% to 95% is expected. All types and routes of administration of estrogen are effective. Although the benefit seems to be related to the dose, even low doses of estrogen are often effective. Higher doses (equivalent of 1 mg of oral estradiol) usually provide relief in about 4 weeks, whereas lower doses usually take about 8 to 12 weeks to provide similar hot flash effect. Lower-dose HT is usually better tolerated with less breast tenderness and uterine bleeding. The FDA, American College of Obstetrics and Gynecology, and the North American Menopause Society recommend using the lowest dose of HT that is effective; the length of therapy should be dictated by clinical response and kept as short as possible (Table 15–5).

As with all medication use, HT comes with the possibility for adverse effects. Endometrial cancer risk with unopposed estrogen use is considerable, with the rate of 4 to 5 per 1000 users per year, with a 5-year use risk of 2% and a 10-year use risk of 4%. As a result, unless a woman taking HT has undergone a hysterectomy, she must also take a progestin to minimize this risk. An observed increased risk of breast cancer in women who use HT has also been noted, particularly with long-term use. Supplemental estrogen use should be avoided in women who have a history of or are at high risk for cardiovascular disease, breast cancer, uterine cancer, or venous thromboembolic events and in women with active liver disease. Compared with the oral form, transdermal estrogen use is associated with a lower thromboembolic risk in short-term studies.

Many women who use oral HT continue to have symptoms of atrophic vaginitis; the addition of topical estrogen, via an estrogen-containing vaginal cream, ring, or tablet, can be helpful.

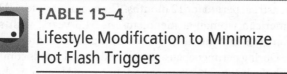

TABLE 15–4
Lifestyle Modification to Minimize Hot Flash Triggers

Hot flashes can often be reduced in number and minimized in severity with simple lifestyle changes

Hot Flash Trigger	Intervention
Spicy foods, chocolate, other foods	Keep food diary to track triggers. Avoid triggers or eat in small amounts.
Alcohol use	Note if certain amounts of types of alcohol trigger hot flashes. Restrict or avoid use.
Elevated ambient temperature and humidity	Control room temperature and humidity. Using climate control to achieve a cool room with low humidity is particularly helpful in improving sleep quality.
Tight, restrictive clothing	Dress in layers that can be removed and replaced in response to hot flashes.
Cigarette smoking	Tobacco use is associated with a marked increase in hot flashes. Smoking cessation improves overall health and reduces hot flash frequency and severity.
Hot baths or showers	Well-known hot flash trigger. Also tends to worsen dry skin, a common complaint during perimenopause and menopause. Taking a cool shower or bath minimizes hot flash risk.
Relaxation techniques, self-hypnosis	In many smaller studies, shown to be helpful in reducing hot flash severity and frequency.

Source: Nelson AL. Perimenopause, menopause and postmenopause: Health promotion strategies. In: Hatcher RA, Trussell J, Nelson AL, Cates W, Kowal D, Policar MS (eds). *Contraceptive Technology*, ed. 20. New York: Ardent Media, Inc.; 2011, pp. 737–777.

TABLE 15–5
What Estrogen Form? What Dose? How Much Relief?

The three most commonly used prescription hormone therapy agents include oral conjugated equine estrogen and oral and transdermal estradiol-17β. The amount of hot flash relief women get from each form and dose differs.

Estrogen Form	Dose (mg)	Reported Hot Flash Relief (%)
Oral conjugated estrogen	0.625	94
	0.4	78
	0.3	78
Oral 17β estradiol-	2	96
	1	89
	0.5	79
	0.25	55
Transdermal 17β estradiol	0.1	96
	0.05	96
	0.025	86

Increasing the dose of oral estrogen is seldom helpful and likely increases HT adverse effects. The use of over-the-counter vaginal lubricants and moisturizers can also afford great relief for vaginal dryness that interferes with sexual activity.

Occasionally, a woman with significant vasomotor symptoms does not or cannot use HT for relief. Low-dose antidepressant (selective serotonin reuptake inhibitors [SSRIs] and selective serotonin and norepinephrine reuptake inhibitors [SNRIs]) therapy can reduce the frequency and severity of hot flashes by 35%. Examples of options include the SNRI venlafaxine (Effexor) and the SSRIs sertraline (Zoloft) and paroxetine (Paxil). Typically, the doses given to minimize vasomotor symptoms are less than the doses used for the treatment of depression. The usual adverse effects associated with the use of these medications can be anticipated; sexual dysfunction including anorgasmia is common with SSRI and SNRI use. Gabapentin (Neurontin) has also demonstrated efficacy in reducing vasomotor symptoms. Older antihypertensives, such as methyldopa (Aldomet) and clonidine (Catapres), have been used for this purpose but demonstrate limitations of use due to undesirable side effects.

In a woman who continues to menstruate but is having significant perimenopausal symptoms, lower-dose oral contraceptives can be helpful for symptom relief and for cycle regulation. Oral contraceptives contain approximately three to four times the estrogen dose of the usual HT dose.

The prescriber and the patient need to be aware of the risks of estrogen supplementation; as with all medications, the use of HT should be approached with caution and is contraindicated in some women (Table 15–6).

Estrogen deficiency is a potent risk factor in the development of osteoporosis, which is most common in postmenopausal women. By age 80, the average woman has lost greater than 30% of her premenopausal bone density. When taken with calcium supplements, postmenopausal HT can help reduce the risk of postmenopausal fracture by 50% by minimizing further bone loss. However, because of the greater observed rate of venous thrombotic events with short-term and long-term HT use and invasive breast cancer with longer term use and because of the availability of other medications to minimize or treat bone thinning such as the bisphosphonates, HT should not be used solely for this purpose.

Because the vaginal introitus remains colonized with protective flora when HT is used, there are lower rates of urogenital atrophy and UTIs in women using this therapy. However, some women using HT continue to need topical or local estrogen in the form of a vaginal cream, tablet, or estrogen-impregnated ring (Estring) to help minimize urogenital atrophy symptoms. Topical or local estrogen use also helps reduce the risk of recurrent UTIs in postmenopausal women, likely through increasing periurethral and perivaginal colonization with lactobacilli and other protective organisms.

Women approaching and during menopause are among the greatest users of botanical and other natural-based therapies. Although a wide variety of these therapies are available for this indication, relatively few high-quality studies have

TABLE 15–6

Contraindications to and Caution With Postmenopausal Estrogen Therapy

Absolute contraindication
- Unexplained vaginal bleeding
- Acute liver disease
- Chronic impaired liver function
- Thrombotic disease
- Neuro-ophthalmological vascular disease
- Endometrial cancer (controversial—short-term use for management of severe menopausal symptoms occasionally acceptable)
- Breast cancer current, past, or suspected (controversial—short-term use for management of severe menopausal symptoms occasionally acceptable)

Use with caution, considering if benefit outweighs risk
- Seizure disorder (owing to potential drug-drug interaction)
- Dyslipidemia, particularly hypertriglyceridemia (transdermal, intravaginal hormone therapy has limited lipid impact)

Source: Goodman NF, Cobin RH, Ginzburg SB, Katz IA, Woode DE, American Association of Clinical Endocrinologists Medical Guidelines for Clinical Practice for the Diagnosis and Treatment of Menopause. *Endocr Pract* 17(suppl 6):1–25, 2011. Available at: www.aace.com/files/menopause.pdf.

been done on the safety and efficacy of these products. At the same time, many authorities, including the North American Menopause Society, view the use of botanical and other natural-based therapies as an option for assisting a woman through the menopause transition.

Phytoestrogens are chemical substances similar to estrogen, in particular estradiol, that are found in more than 300 plants, including apples, carrots, coffee, potatoes, yams, soy products, flaxseed, ginseng, bean sprouts, red clover sprouts, sunflower seeds, rye, wheat, sesame seeds, linseed, black cohosh, and bourbon. These are active substances that bind to estrogen receptor sites and have mild estrogenic effects and some antiestrogenic activity in some areas by binding and blocking to sites in the breast, colon, and rectum. Over-the-counter topical creams made of wild yam, a phytoprogesterone, are available and commonly used by women seeking relief from hot flashes. Because of poor bioavailability, however, little of the product actually reaches circulation. In limited studies of women who were breast cancer survivors, high-dose vitamin E—800 IU/d—modestly reduced the number of hot flashes. Few high-quality studies support the use of nutritional supplements for management of menopausal symptoms. Women often view these supplements as a safe alternative to drug therapy, however.

DISCUSSION SOURCES

Goodman NF. Cobin RH. Ginzburg SB. Katz IA. Woode DE. American Association of Clinical Endocrinologists Medical Guidelines for Clinical Practice for the Diagnosis and Treatment of Menopause. *Endocr Pract* 17 (suppl 6):1–25, 2011. https://www.aace.com/files/menopause.pdf.

Nelson AL. Perimenopause, menopause and postmenopause: Health promotion strategies. In: Hatcher RA, Trussell J, Nelson AL, Cates W, Kowal D, Policar MS (eds). *Contraceptive Technology*, ed. 20. New York: Ardent Media, Inc.; 2011, pp. 748, 755, 757, 758,762, 763, 765, 766, and 767.

Santen RJ. Postmenopausal hormone therapy: An endocrine society scientific statement. *J Clin Endocrinol Metabolism* 95(suppl 1): S34, 2010.

The North American Menopause Society. Position statement: The 2012 hormone therapy positions statement of the North American menopause society. *Menopause: The Journal of the North American Menopause Society* 19(3):257–271, 2012. doi:10.1097/gme.0b013e33824b970a.

Vulvovaginitis

65. Chlamydial infections occur most frequently among women in which age group?
    A. younger than 25 years
    B. 25 to 35 years
    C. 40 to 50 years
    D. over 60 years

66. Common sites of *C. trachomatis* infection in women include all of the following except:
    A. ovaries.
    B. cervix.
    C. endometrium.
    D. urethra.

67. The incubation period for *C. trachomatis* is approximately:
    A. 24 hours.
    B. 3 days.
    C. 7 to 14 days.
    D. 24 days.

68. Which of the following include characteristics of a friable cervix?
    A. presence of a dull pain, particular prior to menses
    B. a constant burning sensation
    C. presence of multiple polyps
    D. easily irritated and prone to bleeding, especially following intercourse

69. An annual screening for *C. trachomatis* infection is recommended for:
    A. all sexually active women.
    B. sexually active women 25 years of age and younger.
    C. sexually active women who have had 2 or more partners in the past 12 months.
    D. sexually active men 25 years of age and younger.

70. Which of the following is not a normal finding in a woman during the reproductive years?
    A. vaginal pH of 4.5 or less
    B. *Lactobacillus* as the predominant vaginal organism
    C. thick, white vaginal secretions during the luteal phase
    D. vaginal epithelial cells with adherent bacteria

71. Which of the following findings is most consistent with vaginal discharge during ovulation?
    A. dry and sticky
    B. milky and mucoid
    C. stringy and clear
    D. tenacious and odorless

72. What is the approximate incubation period for *Neisseria gonorrhoea*?
    A. 1 to 5 days
    B. 7 to 10 days
    C. 18 days
    D. 28 days

73. A recommended treatment for rectal gonorrhea is:
    A. oral amoxicillin.
    B. oral azithromycin.
    C. oral ciprofloxacin.
    D. ceftriaxone injection.

74. Physical examination of a 19-year-old woman with a 3-day history of vaginal itch reveals moderate perineal excoriation, vaginal erythema, and a white, clumping discharge. Expected microscopic examination findings include:
    A. a pH greater than 6.0.
    B. an increased number of lactobacilli.
    C. hyphae.
    D. an abundance of white blood cells.

75. Women with bacterial vaginosis typically present with:
    A. vulvitis.
    B. pruritus.
    C. dysuria.
    D. malodorous discharge.

76. Treatment of vulvovaginitis caused by *Candida albicans* includes:
    A. metronidazole gel.
    B. clotrimazole cream.
    C. hydrocortisone ointment.
    D. clindamycin cream.

77. A 24-year-old woman presents with a 1-week history of thin, green-yellow vaginal discharge with perivaginal irritation. Physical examination findings include vaginal erythema with petechial hemorrhages on the cervix, numerous white blood cells, and motile organisms on microscopic examination. These findings most likely represent:
    A. motile sperm with irritative vaginitis.
    B. trichomoniasis.
    C. bacterial vaginosis.
    D. condyloma acuminatum.

78. A preferred treatment option for trichomoniasis is:
A. oral metronidazole.
B. clindamycin vaginal cream.
C. topical acyclovir.
D. oral azithromycin.

79. Treatment options for bacterial vaginosis include all of the following except:
A. oral metronidazole.
B. clindamycin cream.
C. oral clindamycin.
D. oral azithromycin.

80. A 30-year-old woman presents without symptoms but states that her male partner has dysuria without penile discharge. Examination reveals a friable cervix covered with thick yellow discharge. This description is most consistent with an infection caused by:
A. *Chlamydia trachomatis.*
B. *Neisseria gonorrhoeae.*
C. human papillomavirus (HPV).
D. *Trichomonas vaginalis.*

81. Which of the following agents is active against *N. gonorrhoeae*?
A. ceftriaxone
B. metronidazole
C. ketoconazole
D. amoxicillin

82. Which of the following agents is most active against *C. trachomatis*?
A. amoxicillin
B. metronidazole
C. azithromycin
D. ceftriaxone

83. Which of the following statements is true of gonococcal infection?
A. The risk of transmission from an infected woman to a male sexual partner is about 80%.
B. Most men have asymptomatic infection.
C. The incubation period is about 2 to 3 weeks.
D. The organism rarely produces beta-lactamase.

84. Complications of gonococcal and chlamydial genitourinary infection in women include all of the following except:
A. pelvic inflammatory disease (PID).
B. tubal scarring.
C. acute pyelonephritis.
D. acute peritoneal inflammation.

85. What percentage of sexually active adults has serological evidence of human herpes virus 2 (HHV-2 or herpes simplex type 2)?
A. 5.8%
B. 14.5%
C. 18.9%
D. 35.6%

86. All of the following are likely reported in a woman with an initial episode of genital HSV-2 (HHV-2) infection except:
A. painful ulcer.
B. inguinal lymphadenopathy.
C. thin vaginal discharge.
D. pustular lesions.

87. In the person with HSV-2 infection, the virus can spread via:
A. genital secretions.
B. oral secretions.
C. normal-looking skin.
D. all of the above.

88. During asymptomatic HSV-2 infections, genital shedding of virus occurs during approximately _____ of days.
A. 10%
B. 25%
C. 50%
D. 100%

89. Diagnostic testing of a person with primary HSV-2 infection would likely show:
A. negative virological and serological test results.
B. negative virological test result and positive serological test result.
C. positive virological test result and negative serological test result.
D. positive virological and serological test results.

90. Treatment options for HSV-2 genital infection include:
A. ribavirin.
B. indinavir.
C. famciclovir.
D. cyclosporine.

91. Suppressive therapy reduces the frequency of genital herpes recurrences by:
A. 5% to 10%.
B. 20% to 25%.
C. 40% to 50%.
D. 70% to 80%.

92. Recommended comprehensive STI testing includes testing for all of the following except:
A. hepatitis B.
B. syphilis.
C. hepatitis A.
D. HIV.

Answers

65. A.	**70.** D.	**75.** D.
66. A.	**71.** C.	**76.** B.
67. C.	**72.** A.	**77.** B.
68. D.	**73.** D.	**78.** A.
69. B.	**74.** C.	**79.** D.

80. A.	85. C.	90. C.
81. A.	86. D.	91. D.
82. C.	87. D.	92. C.
83. B.	88. A.	
84. C.	89. C.	

Vulvovaginitis is one of the most common gynecological problems. Treatment is guided by presentation and causative organism (Table 15–7). Chlamydial infection is the most commonly reported STI, affecting primarily adolescents and adults younger than 25 years. The causative organism, *C. trachomatis*

TABLE 15–7
Female Genitourinary Infection

Conditions	Causative Organism	Clinical Presentation	Treatment Options
Chancroid	*H. ducreyi*	Painful genital ulcer, multiple lesions common, inguinal lymphadenitis	Primary: azithromycin 1 g orally in a single dose; or ceftriaxone 250 mg intramuscularly (IM) in a single dose. Alternative: ciprofloxacin 500 mg orally twice a day for 3 days; or erythromycin base 500 mg orally three times a day for 7 days.
Genital herpes	HSV-2, also known as herpes simplex type 2 (rarely human herpes virus 1)	Painful ulcerated lesions, lymphadenopathy, particularly with primary outbreak. Subsequent outbreaks often less severe	For primary infection (initial episode): acyclovir 400 mg PO tid for 7–10 days; or famciclovir 250 mg PO tid for 7–10 days; or valacyclovir 1 g PO bid for 7–10 days. For episodic recurrent infection: acyclovir 800 mg tid for 2 days; or 400 mg PO tid for 5 days; or famciclovir 1000 mg bid for 1 day or 125 mg PO bid for 5 days; or valacyclovir 1g PO qd for 5 days; or valacyclovir 500 mg PO bid for 5 days. For suppression of recurrent infection: acyclovir 400 mg PO bid; or famciclovir 250 mg PO bid; or valacyclovir 1 g PO qd. For patient with ≥9 recurrences per year, another treatment option is valacyclovir 500 mg qd with an increase to 1 g qd if breakthrough.
Lymphogranuloma venereum	Invasive serovar L1, L2, L3 of *C. trachomatis*	Vesicular or ulcerative lesion on external genitalia with inguinal lymphadenitis or buboes	Primary therapy: doxycycline 100 mg PO bid for 21 days. Alternative therapy: erythromycin 500 mg qid for 21 days.
Nongonococcal urethritis and cervicitis	*C. trachomatis* (50%), *Mycoplasma hominis*, *Mycoplasma genitalium* Assume concomitant infection with *N. gonorrhoeae*, unless ruled out by accurate diagnostic testing	Irritative voiding symptoms, rarely mucopurulent vaginal discharge, cervicitis, often asymptomatic	Primary therapy: azithromycin 1 g PO as a single dose; or doxycycline 100 mg PO bid for 7 days. Alternative therapy: erythromycin base 500 mg PO qid for 7 days; or ofloxacin 300 mg bid for 7 days; or levofloxacin 500 mg qd for 7 days.
Gonococcal urethritis and cervicitis	*N. gonorrhoeae* Assume concomitant infection with *C. trachomatis*	Irritative voiding symptoms, occasional purulent vaginal discharge, cervicitis	Recommended therapy: single-dose therapy for uncomplicated infection ceftriaxone 250 mg IM. Concurrently treat with azithromycin 1 g as a single dose; or doxycycline 100 mg bid for 7 days. Alternative therapy in the presence of severe beta-lactam allergy: Azithromycin 2 g as a single dose

TABLE 15–7

Female Genitourinary Infection—cont'd

Conditions	Causative Organism	Clinical Presentation	Treatment Options
Genital warts (condyloma acuminata)	Human papillomavirus	Verruca-form lesions or can be subclinical or un-recognized	Patient-applied therapy: podofilox 0.5% solution; or imiquimod 5% cream. Provider-applied therapy: liquid nitrogen or cryoprobe, trichloroacetic acid, podophyllin resin, or surgical removal.
Bacterial vaginosis	Overgrowth of anaerobes, including Gardnerella species and *Mycoplasma hominis*	Increased volume of vaginal secretions; thin, gray, homogeneous discharge; burning; pruritus On microscopic examination, vaginal pH < 4.5, clue calls, positive whiff test, few white blood cells	First-line therapies: metronidazole 500 mg bid for 7 days; or metronidazole gel 0.75%, 1 applicator (5 g) intravaginally qd for 5 days; or clindamycin cream 2%, 1 applicator (5 g) intravaginally at HS for 7 nights. Alternative regimens: metronidazole 2 g as single dose; or clindamycin 300 mg bid for 7 days; or clindamycin ovules 100 g intravaginally at bedtime for 3 days; or tinidazole 2 g PO daily for 2 days or 1 g PO daily for 5 days.
Candidiasis	*Candida albicans, Candida glabrata, Candida tropicalis*	Itching, burning, thick white-to-yellow adherent, curd-like discharge, vulvovaginal excoriation, erythema, excoriation. On microscopic examination, hyphae, pseudohyphae, pH less than 5, few white blood cells	Single-day therapy options: fluconazole (Diflucan) 150 mg PO as single dose); butoconazole 2% SR cream (Gynazole-1); tioconazole 6.5% (Vagistat-1); miconazole (Monistat) 1200 mg, as single dose vaginally. Various 3- and 7-day therapies with azole antifungal vaginal creams, suppositories, tablets (miconazole, butoconazole, terconazole [Terazol], tioconazole).
Pelvic inflammatory disease	*N. gonorrhoeae, C. trachomatis, E. coli, Mycoplasma* and *Ureaplasma* species, others	Irritative voiding symptoms, fever, abdominal pain, cervical motion tenderness, vaginal discharge	Recommended therapy for outpatient treatment: ceftriaxone 250 mg IM as a single dose plus doxycycline 100 mg bid for 14 days with or without metronidazole 500 mg bid for 14 days. Alternate oral regimens: ofloxacin 400 mg PO bid; or levofloxacin 500 mg PO qd with or without metronidazole 500 mg PO bid for 14 days. Alternate regimen should be used only with awareness of quinolone-resistant *N. gonorrhoeae*, but may be the primary treatment alternative in the presence of significant penicillin or cephalosporin allergy.
Trichomoniasis	*T. vaginalis*	Dysuria, itching, vulvovaginal irritation, dyspareunia, yellow-green vaginal discharge, cervical petechial hemorrhages ("strawberry spots") in about 30% On microscopic examination: motile organisms and white blood cells	Recommended therapy: metronidazole (Flagyl) or tinidazole (Tindamax) 2 g as a one-time dose. Alternative therapy: metronidazole, 500 mg PO bid for 7 days.

Sources: Centers for Disease Control and Prevention. Sexually Transmitted Diseases Treatment Guidelines, 2010. www.cdc.gov/std/treatment/2010/STD-Treatment-2010-RR5912.pdf.

immunotype D–K, is an obligate intracellular parasite closely related to gram-negative bacteria. This infection causes cervicitis in most infected women. About one-half have urethral infection, and one-third have endometrial involvement; despite this, many women are asymptomatic, although mucopurulent vaginal discharge, dysuria, dyspareunia, and postcoital bleeding are often reported. The organism has an incubation period of approximately 7 to 14 days.

Clinical presentation of C. trachomatis genitourinary infection in women typically includes the presence of mucopurulent discharge, often adherent to a friable cervix. Cervical motion and adnexal tenderness is usually present when there is upper reproductive tract infection such as PID. Diagnostic testing includes DNA probe endocervical testing or urinalysis for ligase chain reaction. Routine screening—that is testing that is encouraged and offered to all in a given group even in the absence of signs and symptoms—for C. trachomatis infection is recommended annually for all sexually active females age 25 years and younger. Evidence is insufficient to recommend routine screening for C. trachomatis infection in sexually active young men based on feasibility, efficacy, and cost-effectiveness. However, screening of sexually active young men should be considered in clinical settings associated with high prevalence of chlamydial infection including adolescent practices, correctional facilities, and STI clinics.

Treatment options for uncomplicated C. trachomatis infection include antimicrobials that act against intracellular organisms, such as doxycycline, erythromycin, and azithromycin. Azithromycin is preferred, given in a highly efficacious, well-tolerated, single-dose oral therapy. For uncomplicated infection, a test-of-cure following completion of the antimicrobial course is not needed unless the patient has persistent symptoms or is pregnant. In pregnancy, testing for cure should be performed 3 weeks after completion of treatment. Because reinfection is common, all women with chlamydial infection should be rescreened 3 to 4 months after completing antimicrobial treatment. If a woman presents within 12 months of the initial infection and has not been previously screened, she should be reassessed for infection regardless of whether she says the partner was treated or not.

Infections caused by the organisms Ureaplasma urealyticum and Mycoplasma genitalium present similarly as chlamydial infection. Recommended antimicrobial treatment for these infections is similar for treating C. trachomatis.

Gonorrhea, caused by the gram-negative diplococcus N. gonorrhoeae, is also a common STI. This organism has a short incubation period of 1 to 5 days and is likely to cause infection in approximately 20% of men who have sexual contact with infected women and approximately 80% of women who have sexual contact with infected men.

Most men with gonococcal infection have no symptoms. In women, presentation typically includes dysuria with a milky to purulent, occasionally blood-tinged, vaginal discharge. With anal-insertive sex, rectal infection leading to proctitis is often seen. Because the organism frequently produces beta-lactamase, the choice of a therapeutic agent should include agents with beta-lactamase stability, such as

injectable ceftriaxone (preferred) and oral cefixime. Because of increasing rates of resistance, the use of the fluoroquinolones to treat this infection is no longer recommended.

Genital herpes is a result of infection with a HHV (human herpes virus, also known as herpes simplex virus [HSV]). Most often, HSV-2 is the causative organism; HSV-1, the virus form that causes cold sores (herpes labialis), is rarely implicated. HSV-2 can infect the perioral area, however. The clinical presentation usually includes a painful ulcerated genital lesion, often accompanied by inguinal lymphadenopathy. If lesions involve the vagina or its introitus, a thin, sometimes profuse discharge accompanies the infection.

HSV-2 can be spread through contact with lesions, mucosal surfaces, genital secretions, or oral secretions. The virus can also be shed from skin that looks normal. In those with asymptomatic infections, genital shedding of the virus occurs on 10% of days, even in the absence of any signs or symptoms. Transmission most commonly occurs from an infected partner who does not have a visible sore and may not know that he or she is infected.

Diagnosis can be performed through direct (virological) or indirect (serological) testing. Viral culture is the standard for diagnosing genital herpes, which requires a collection of a sample from a sore. PCR can also be used to test for the presence of viral DNA or RNA and may allow for more rapid and accurate results. Serological approaches can detect for the presence of antibodies in the blood. In symptomatic patients, the use of direct and indirect assays can differentiate between a new infection and a newly-recognized older infection. A positive virological test with a negative serological test would suggest a new infection. Positive results for both tests would indicate a recurrent infection.

Though there is no definitive cure for herpes, antiviral therapy for recurrent outbreaks can be given as suppression therapy to reduce the frequency of recurrences, or episodically to shorten the duration of lesions. Treatment with an antiviral such as acyclovir, famciclovir, or valacyclovir for acute infection, recurrence, or suppression is highly effective. Suppressive therapy reduces the frequency of genital herpes recurrences by 70% to 80% in those who have frequent recurrences. Treatment is also effective in those who have less frequent recurrences. Suppression therapy also has the advantage of decreasing the risk for viral transmission to susceptible partners.

As with all STIs, a critical part of care is discussion of preventive strategies, including condom use and limiting the number of sexual partners. NPs should offer and encourage testing for other STIs, including HIV, hepatitis B, and syphilis. Consideration should also be given to offering testing for hepatitis C. Immunization that provides protection against hepatitis A, hepatitis B, and HPV should be offered as needed and appropriate. In patients diagnosed with chlamydia or gonorrhea, providing prescriptions or medication for the patient to take to his/her partner without clinical visit, known as Expedited Partner Therapy (EPT), should be considered.

DISCUSSION SOURCES

Centers for Disease Control and Prevention. 2010 Sexually Transmitted Diseases Surveillance (updated 2011). www.cdc.gov/std/stats10/other.htm#herpes.

Centers for Disease Control and Prevention. Genital Herpes—CDC Fact Sheet (updated 2012). www.cdc.gov/std/herpes/STDFact-Herpes.htm.

Marrazzo JM, Cates W. Reproductive tract infections, including HIV and other sexually transmitted infections. In: Hatcher RA, Trussell J, Nelson AL, Cates W, Kowal D, Policar MS (eds). *Contraceptive Technology*, ed. 20. New York: Ardent Media, Inc.; 2011, p. 602.

Centers for Disease Control and Prevention. Sexually Transmitted Diseases Treatment Guidelines, 2010. www.cdc.gov/std/treatment/2010/STD-Treatment-2010-RR5912.pdf.

Pelvic Inflammatory Disease (PID)

93. Women with PID typically present with all of the following except:
    A. dysuria.
    B. leukopenia.
    C. cervical motion tenderness.
    D. abdominal pain.

94. A 22-year-old woman complains of pelvic pain. Physical examination reveals cervical motion tenderness and uterine tenderness. Which of the following would further support a diagnosis of PID?
    A. temperature less than 100°F (37.8°C)
    B. absence of white blood cells in vaginal fluid
    C. mucopurulent vaginal discharge
    D. laboratory documentation of cervical infection with E. coli

95. The most likely causative pathogen in a 23-year-old woman with PID is:
    A. *Escherichia coli*.
    B. Enterobacteriaceae.
    C. *C. trachomatis*.
    D. *Pseudomonas*.

96. The presence of an adnexal mass in the woman with PID most likely indicates the presence of:
    A. uterine fibroids.
    B. an ectopic pregnancy.
    C. ovarian malignancy.
    D. a tubo-ovarian abscess.

97. Expected laboratory findings for the woman with PID include all of the following except:
    A. elevated ESR.
    B. elevated CRP.
    C. elevated CrCl.
    D. leukocytosis.

98. A transvaginal ultrasound in the woman with PID will likely show:
    A. tubal thickening with or without free pelvic fluid.
    B. cervical thickening.
    C. endometrial thinning.
    D. inflammation of the ovaries.

99. Which of the following is a treatment option for a 28-year-old woman with PID who has no history of medication allergy and has undergone a bilateral tubal ligation?
    A. ofloxacin with metronidazole
    B. gentamicin with cefpodoxime
    C. ceftriaxone with doxycycline
    D. clindamycin with azithromycin

100. Which of the following is a treatment option for a 30-year-old woman with PID and a history of severe hive-form reaction when taking a penicillin or cephalosporin?
    A. ofloxacin with metronidazole
    B. amoxicillin with gentamicin
    C. cefixime with vancomycin
    D. clindamycin with azithromycin

Answers

93. B.	96. D.	99. C.
94. C.	97. C.	100. A.
95. C.	98. A.	

Pelvic inflammatory disease (PID) is an infectious disease consisting of endometritis, salpingitis, and oophoritis. The condition is caused by various pathogens, including *C. trachomatis*, *N. gonorrhoeae*, *Haemophilus influenzae*, *Streptococcus* species, select anaerobes, *Mycoplasma* species, and *Ureaplasma* species; approximately 60% of infections are acquired through sexual transmission. Clinical presentation usually includes lower abdominal pain, abnormal vaginal discharge, dyspareunia, fever, gastrointestinal upset, or abnormal vaginal bleeding. An adnexal mass can be palpable when tubo-ovarian abscess is present. PID should be considered when a woman presents with new onset lower abdominal or pelvic pain coupled with at least one of the following findings on clinical examination: cervical motion tenderness, uterine tenderness, or adnexal tenderness.

Supporting laboratory findings in PID include elevated erythrocyte sedimentation rate or C-reactive protein level and leukocytosis with neutrophilia. Although diagnosis can usually be made from clinical findings, transvaginal ultrasound, if obtained, will usually demonstrate tubal thickening with or without free pelvic fluid or tubo-ovarian abscess. Ultrasound offers an acceptable imaging option and avoids the radiation burden and increased cost associated with pelvic computed tomography (CT) (Table 15–8).

TABLE 15–8
Diagnostic Criteria for PID

Empiric treatment for PID should be initiated in sexually active young women and other women at risk for STDs if they are experiencing pelvic or lower abdominal pain, if no cause for the illness other than PID can be identified, and if one or more of the following minimum criteria are present on pelvic examination: • cervical motion tenderness or • uterine tenderness or • adnexal tenderness.	One or more of the following additional criteria can be used to enhance the specificity of the minimum criteria and support a diagnosis of PID: • oral temperature >101°F (>38.3°C); • abnormal cervical or vaginal mucopurulent discharge; • presence of abundant numbers of WBC on saline microscopy of vaginal fluid; • elevated erythrocyte sedimentation rate; • elevated C-reactive protein; and • laboratory documentation of cervical infection with *N. gonorrhoeae* or *C. trachomatis*.

Treatment options differ according to patient presentation. When a woman with PID is severely ill, is pregnant, or has tubo-ovarian abscess, hospitalization for hydration and parenteral antibiotic therapy is indicated. In most situations, outpatient therapy with oral or parenteral antibiotics is sufficient. Ceftriaxone, 250 mg intramuscularly as a one-time dose, followed by doxycycline, 100 mg bid for 2 weeks with or without metronidazole 500 mg, is likely the most commonly used treatment regimen and is highly effective. The addition of metronidazole is helpful in the treatment of bacterial vaginosis that is often found in the woman with PID as well as provides activity against select anaerobes. A fluoroquinolone with or without metronidazole offers an effective oral treatment option that is a reasonable alternative in the presence of severe penicillin or cephalosporin allergy; when considering this combination, the practitioner must realize that *N. gonorrhoeae* is often quinolone-resistant.

As with all STIs, a critical part of care is discussion of preventive strategies, including condom use and limiting the number of sexual partners. NPs should offer and encourage testing for other STIs, including HIV, hepatitis B, and syphilis. Consideration should also be given to offering testing for hepatitis C. Immunization that provides protection against hepatitis A, hepatitis B, and HPV should be offered as needed and appropriate.

DISCUSSION SOURCES

Marrazzo JM, Cates W. Reproductive tract infections, including HIV and other sexually transmitted infections. In: Hatcher RA, Trussell J, Nelson AL, Cates W, Kowal D, Policar MS (eds). *Contraceptive Technology*, ed. 20. New York: Ardent Media, Inc.; 2011, p. 613.

Centers for Disease Control and Prevention. Sexually Transmitted Diseases Treatment Guidelines, 2010. www.cdc.gov/std/treatment/2010/STD-Treatment-2010-RR5912.pdf.

Condyloma Acuminatum

101. Which of the following best describes lesions associated with condyloma acuminatum?
    A. verruciform
    B. plaque-like
    C. vesicular-form
    D. bullous

102. Treatment options for patients with condyloma acuminatum include all of the following except:
    A. topical acyclovir.
    B. cryotherapy.
    C. podofilox.
    D. trichloroacetic acid.

103. Which HPV types are most likely to cause genital condyloma acuminatum?
    A. 1, 2, and 3
    B. 6 and 11
    C. 16 and 18
    D. 22 and 24

104. Which HPV types are most often associated with cervical and anogenital cancer?
    A. 1, 2, and 3
    B. 6 and 11
    C. 16 and 18
    D. 22 and 24

105. What percentage of anogenital and cervical cancers can be attributed to HPV infection?
    A. less than 30%
    B. at least 50%
    C. at least 70%
    D. 95% or greater

106. Which of the following terms describes the mechanism of action of imiquimod (Aldara)?
A. keratolytic
B. immune modulator
C. cryogenic
D. cytolytic

107. About _____ of patients with genital warts have spontaneous regression of the lesions?
A. 10%
B. 25%
C. 50%
D. 75%

Answers

101. A.	**104.** C.	**106.** B.
102. A.	**105.** C.	**107.** C.
103. B.		

Condyloma acuminatum is a verruciform lesion seen in genital warts and is an STI. The causative agent is human papillomavirus (HPV), and infection with multiple HPV types is usually seen with genital infection. Anal, penile, and cervical carcinomas can be consequences of HPV infection. Not all HPV types are correlated with malignancy, however. HPV types with high malignancy risks include types 16, 18, 31, 33, 35, 39, and 45, whereas low malignancy risks are seen with infection with types 6, 11, 40, 42, 43, 44, 54, 61, 70, 72, and 81. HPV types 6 and 11 most often cause genital warts, whereas HPV types 16 and 18 are most often associated with genital malignancies.

About 50% of patients have spontaneous regression of genital warts without intervention. The most common treatment options for genital warts include podofilox, imiquimod, trichloroacetic acid, or cryotherapy. The location of lesions can dictate therapeutic choices; imiquimod use is only indicated for external lesions. Prescribing patient-administered therapies, such as imiquimod (Aldara) or podofilox, saves the cost and inconvenience of office visits. Surgical intervention and laser ablation are typically reserved for complicated, recalcitrant lesions.

As with all STIs, a critical part of care is discussion of preventive strategies, including condom use and limiting the number of sexual partners. NPs should offer and encourage testing for other STIs, including HIV, hepatitis B, and syphilis. Consideration should also be given to offering testing for hepatitis C. Immunization that provides protection against hepatitis A, hepatitis B, and HPV should be offered as needed and appropriate.

DISCUSSION SOURCES

Centers for Disease Control and Prevention. Sexually Transmitted Diseases Treatment Guidelines, 2010. www.cdc.gov/std/treatment/2010/STD-Treatment-2010-RR5912.pdf.

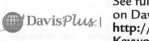
See full color images of this topic on DavisPlus at
http://davisplus.fadavis.com |
Keyword: Fitzgerald

Marrazzo JM, Cates W. Reproductive tract infections, including HIV and other sexually transmitted infections. In: Hatcher RA, Trussell J, Nelson AL, Cates W, Kowal D, Policar MS (eds). *Contraceptive Technology*, ed. 20. New York: Ardent Media, Inc.; 2011, pp. 609 and 610.

Syphilis

108. How long after contact do clinical manifestations of syphilis typically occur?
A. less than 1 week
B. 1 to 3 weeks
C. 2 to 4 weeks
D. 4 to 6 weeks

109. Which of the following is not representative of the presentation of primary syphilis?
A. painless ulcer
B. localized lymphadenopathy
C. flu-like symptoms
D. spontaneously healing lesion

110. Which of the following is not representative of the presentation of secondary syphilis?
A. generalized rash
B. chancre
C. arthralgia
D. lymphadenopathy

111. Which of the following is found in tertiary syphilis?
A. arthralgia
B. lymphadenopathy
C. macular or papular lesions involving the palms and soles
D. gumma

112. Syphilis is most contagious during which of the following?
A. before onset of signs and symptoms
B. at the primary stage
C. at the secondary stage
D. at the tertiary stage

113. First-line treatment options for primary syphilis include:
A. penicillin.
B. ciprofloxacin.
C. erythromycin.
D. ceftriaxone.

Answers

108. C.	**110.** B.	**112.** C.
109. C.	**111.** D.	**113.** A.

Caused by the spirochete *Treponema pallidum*, syphilis is a complex, multiorgan disease. Sexual contact is the usual route of transmission. The initial lesion forms about 2 to 4 weeks after contact; contagion is greatest during the secondary stage. Treatment is guided by the stage of disease and clinical manifestations (Table 15–9).

As with all STIs, a critical part of care is discussion of preventive strategies, including condom use and limiting the number of sexual partners. The NP should offer and encourage testing for other STIs, including HIV and hepatitis B. Consideration should also be given to offering testing for hepatitis C. Immunization that provides protection against hepatitis A, hepatitis B, and HPV should be offered as needed and appropriate.

DISCUSSION SOURCES

Centers for Disease Control and Prevention. Sexually Transmitted Diseases Treatment Guidelines, 2010. www.cdc.gov/std/treatment/2010/STD-Treatment-2010-RR5912.pdf.

Centers for Disease Control and Prevention. Syphilis—CDC Fact Sheet, 2012. www.cdc.gov/std/syphilis/STDFact-Syphilis.htm.

See full color images of this topic on DavisPlus at
http://davisplus.fadavis.com |
Keyword: Fitzgerald

Cervical Cancer Screening

114. You see an 18-year-old woman with a history of *C. trachomatis* infection and a total of five lifetime partners. You recommend:
    A. Pap smear only.
    B. Pap smear and HPV testing.
    C. Pap smear and STI testing.
    D. STI testing only.

115. During well-women visits for 21- to 29-year-old sexually active women who report more than 1 sex partner within the past 6 months, all of the following are appropriate screening tests except:
    A. Pap smear.
    B. HPV testing.
    C. Pelvic examination.
    D. STI screening.

TABLE 15–9

Stages of Syphilis, Clinical Manifestations, and Recommended Treatment

Stage of Syphilis	Clinical Manifestations	Treatment Options	Comment
Primary syphilis	Painless genital ulcer with clean base and indurated margins, localized lymphadenopathy	Recommended therapy: • Benzathine penicillin G 2.4 million U IM as a 1-time dose Alternative therapy in penicillin allergy: • Doxycycline 100 mg PO bid for 2 weeks; or • Ceftriaxone 1 g IM or IV q 24 h for 8–10 days	Azithromycin 2 g as a 1-time dose has been suggested, although issues of emerging resistance are concerning
Secondary syphilis	Diffuse maculopapular rash involving palms and soles, generalized lymphadenopathy, low-grade fever, malaise, arthralgias and myalgia, headache	Recommended therapy: • Benzathine penicillin G 2.4 million U IM as a 1-time dose Alternative therapy in penicillin allergy: • Doxycycline 100 mg PO bid for 2 weeks;	Also treatment for latent syphilis of greater than 1 yr duration
Late or tertiary syphilis	Gumma (granulomatous lesions involving skin, mucous membranes, bone), aortic insufficiency, aortic aneurysm, Argyll Robertson pupil, seizures	Recommended therapy: • Benzathine penicillin G 2.4 million U IM for 3 weekly doses Alternative therapy in penicillin allergy: • Doxycycline 100 mg PO bid for 4 weeks; Expert consultation advisable, especially in the face of neurosyphilis	Also treatment for latent syphilis of greater than 1 yr or unknown duration

Source: Centers for Disease Control and Prevention. Sexually Transmitted Diseases Treatment Guidelines, 2010. www.cdc.gov/std/treatment/2010/STD-Treatment-2010-RR5912.pdf.

116. A 45-year-old woman just had a normal Pap test result and has an absence of high-risk HPV. You recommend her next Pap test in:
   A. 1 year.
   B. 3 years.
   C. 5 years.
   D. 7 years.

117. Which of the following is not part of the criteria for an older woman to cease having any future Pap tests performed?
   A. over 55 years of age
   B. negative screening results on three consecutive cytology or two consecutive co-test results within 10 years
   C. the most recent cytology occurring within the past 5 years
   D. no history of cervical intraepithelial neoplasm (CIN) 2 or greater within the past 20 years

118. You see a 48-year-old woman who underwent an abdominal hysterectomy with cervical removal for uterine fibroids 6 months ago. She last had a normal Pap test 1½ years ago. You recommend her next Pap test.
   A. immediately.
   B. in 1 ½ years.
   C. in 3 ½ years.
   D. She does not need to have a pap test now or in the future.

119. You see a 24-year-old woman who received the HPV vaccine (three doses) as a teenager. She had a normal Pap test 3 years ago. You recommend:
   A. conducting a Pap test.
   B. conducting a Pap test and HPV testing.
   C. waiting 2 years for the next Pap test.
   D. ceasing future Pap tests until she turns 30 years old.

120. You see a 33-year-old woman whose Pap smear result reveals atypical cells of undetermined significance (ASC-US). She is also positive for HPV, with genotype testing revealing the presence of HPV type 16. You recommend:
   A. repeating Pap test immediately.
   B. repeating the Pap test in 3 to 4 months.
   C. referral for colposcopy.
   D. administering the HPV vaccine.

121. You see a 41-year-old woman whose Pap smear result reveals high-grade squamous intraepithelial lesion (HSIL). The HPV test is negative. You recommend:
   A. repeating the Pap test in 3 to 4 months.
   B. repeating the Pap test in 1 year.
   C. referral for colposcopy.
   D. referral for biopsy.

Answers

114. D.	117. A.	120. C.
115. B.	118. D.	121. C.
116. C.	119. A.	

Cervical cancer impacts approximately 12,000 women in the United States each year, most commonly occurring in women over the age of 30 years. The main cause of cervical cancer is the human papillomavirus (HPV), which is a common virus that is transmitted through sexual intercourse. At least half of sexually active women will have HPV at some point in their lives, though few will develop cervical cancer.

Through routine screening, follow-up, and the availability of the HPV vaccine, cervical cancer is highly preventable. There are two types of tests available for screening: cytology (Pap test or Pap smear) and HPV testing. The Pap test is used to detect precancers or cell changes on the cervix that can be identified and treated early before cancer development. The Pap test is recommended for women between 21 and 65 years of age. See Table 15–10 for recommendations on the use of cytology and HPV testing and follow-up.

DISCUSSION SOURCE

Massad LS, Einstein MH, Huh WK, et al. 2012 updated consensus guidelines for the management of abnormal cervical cancer screening tests and cancer precursors. *J Lower Genital Tract Dis* 17:S1–27, 2013. Available at: www.asccp.org/Portals/9/docs/ASCCP%20Updated%20Guidelines%20%20-%203.21.13.pdf.

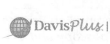

See full color images of this topic on DavisPlus at
**http://davisplus.fadavis.com |
Keyword: Fitzgerald**

TABLE 15–10
Cervical Cancer Screening Recommendations

Patient Classification	Recommendations
Ages ≤20 years: Should NOT be screened (*no Pap test should be done*)	*Regardless of age onset of sexual activity, sexual orientation, and history of sexually transmitted infection (STI), or HPV immunization status* **Pelvic examination and appropriate STI screening should be performed as indicated by clinical presentation and risk assessment.**
Ages 21–29 years: Should be screened every 3 years (*Pap test should be done*)	*Screening with cytology only* *Human papillomavirus (HPV) testing should NOT be used, either as a stand-alone test, or co-test to include reflex* **Pelvic examination and appropriate STI screening should be performed as indicated by clinical presentation and risk assessment.**
Ages 30–65 years: Should be screened at a maximum every 5 years (*Pap test should be done*)	*Screening with cytology and HPV "co-test" (preferred)* *Screening with cytology alone is acceptable every 3 years* **Pelvic examination and appropriate STI screening should be performed as indicated by clinical presentation and risk assessment.**
Age >65 years: Should NOT be screened (*no Pap test should be done*)	*If evidence of negative prior screening (3 consecutive cytology or 2 consecutive co-test results within 10 years before ceasing screening, with the most recent test occurring within the past 5 yrs) and no history of cervical intraepithelial neoplasm (CIN) 2 or greater within the past 20 years.* *Once screening is discontinued it should not be resumed* **Pelvic examination and appropriate STI screening should be performed as indicated by clinical presentation and risk assessment.**
SPECIAL CIRCUMSTANCES: Has undergone a hysterectomy with removal of cervix regardless of age: Should NOT be screened (*no Pap test should be done*)	*If no history of CIN 2 or greater, no evidence of adequate negative prior screening is needed* *Once screening is discontinued it should not be resumed* **Pelvic examination and appropriate STI screening should be performed as indicated by clinical presentation and risk assessment.**
History of CIN2, CIN3, or adenocarcinoma in situ Should be screened (*Pap test should be done*)	*Routine screening should continue for at least 20 years, even if this timeframe extends past age 65 years.*
HPV Vaccination Status (*positive or negative*) (*see recommendation*)	*Regardless of immunization status, screening should be done based on the practice recommendations*

Management of Abnormal Screening Pap Results
Follow American Society for Colposcopy and Cervical Pathology (ASCCP) Guidelines

INADEQUATE SAMPLES:
Unsatisfactory cytology
Ages 21–29 years:
(*Pap test should be repeated*)
Ages ≥30 years:
(*Pap test should be repeated*)
	• *Repeat screening after 2–4 months with cytology only*
	• *All patients with repeat screening:*
	  • *If result returns negative, screen as routine*
	  • *If result returns abnormal, manage per guideline*
	  • *If result returns unsatisfactory, refer for colposcopy*

TABLE 15–10
Cervical Cancer Screening Recommendations—cont'd

Patient Classification	Recommendations

Negative cytology with absent or insufficient endocervical/ transformation zone
Ages 21–29 years:
Ages ≥30 years:
	• *Screen as routine*
	• *If no or unknown HPV result:*
	  • *repeat screening with HPV testing (preferred); or*
	  • *if HPV not performed, repeat <u>cytology</u> in 3 years (acceptable)*
	• *If HPV result is negative, screen as routine in 1 year*
	• *If HPV result is positive, repeat <u>co-test</u> in 1 year (acceptable) or immediate genotyping*
	  • *for genotype absent HPV type 16 or 18, screen with <u>co-test</u> in 1 year*
	  • *for genotype present HPV type 16 or 18, refer for colposcopy*

ABNORMAL RESULTS: Negative cytology, Positive HPV Ages 30 to ≥65 years: *(see recommendation)*	*Option 1) repeat co-testing in 12 months;* *Option 2) immediate HPV genotype-specific testing for high risk HPV forms (HPV 16/18, others)* *Option 1 Results at 12 Months:* • *If HPV positive or low-grade squamous intraepithelial (LSIL) or greater, refer for colposcopy* • *If HPV and cytology are both negative, repeat co-testing in 3 years* • *If negative HPV and atypical squamous cells of undetermined significance (ASC-US), screen as routine in 1 year* *Option 2 Results (Immediate Genotyping):* • *If positive for HPV type 16 or type 18, refer for colposcopy* • *In absence of high-risk HPV , repeat <u>co-testing</u> in 1 year*
ASC-US cytology Ages 25 to ≥65 years: *(see recommendation)*	*HPV testing (preferred)* *or* *Repeat cytology in 1 year (acceptable)* *With results positive of high-risk HPV result, refer for colposcopy*
ASC-US or LGSIL cytology Ages 21–24 years: *(see recommendation)*	*Repeat cytology in 1 year (preferred)* *or* *Reflex HPV testing (acceptable)* *for HPV result that is positive, repeat cytology in 1 year*
ASC-US cytology, Negative HPV Ages ≥30 to ≥65 years: *(see recommendation)*	*Screen as routine per age specific recommendations*
LSIL cytology: No, Negative, or Positive HPV Ages 25 to ≥65 years: *(see recommendation)*	*If negative HPV, repeat co-test in 1 year (preferred)* *or* *If no, negative, or positive high-risk HPV result, refer for colposcopy*

TABLE 15–10
Cervical Cancer Screening Recommendations—cont'd

Patient Classification	Recommendations
Atypical squamous cells, cannot exclude high-grade squamous intraepithelial lesion (ASC-H) and high-grade squamous intraepithelial lesion (HSIL), or Atypical Glandular Cells (AGC) Ages 21 to ≥65 years: (*see recommendation*)	*Refer for colposcopy*

Older Adults

16

Demographics

1. In the elderly population, the current fastest growing group is the age range:
   A. 71 to 75 years.
   B. 76 to 80 years.
   C. 81 to 84 years.
   D. 85 years and older.

2. The age range referred to as "young old" is:
   A. 60 to 65 years.
   B. 66 to 70 years.
   C. 65 to 74 years.
   D. 70 to 80 years.

3. Which of the following is most commonly reported as the largest single source of income for elderly people?
   A. Social Security
   B. public/private pension earnings
   C. asset income
   D. family financial support

4. The poverty rate among elderly people residing in the United States can best be described as:
   A. at approximately the same level across ethnic and age groups.
   B. highest among the old old.
   C. greatest among married couples.
   D. highest among older adults depending on investment income as a substantial part of their finances.

Answers

1. D. 2. C. 3. A. 4. B.

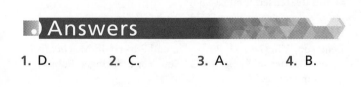

See full color images of this topic on DavisPlus at
http://davisplus.fadavis.com
Keyword: Fitzgerald DISCUSSION

The older adult population is usually classified into four groups: the young old, 65 to 74 years old; the old old, 75 to 84 years old; the oldest old, 85 to 100 years old; and the elite old, more than 100 years old. Significant increase in the population group older than 65 years is projected to occur from 2010 to 2030. This increase is largely attributable to the aging of the "Baby Boomers," the demographic born from 1946 to 1964, and to a sharp decline in mortality at older ages. Currently, the fastest growing group of older adults is those older than age 85 years.

Among elderly people residing in the United States, Social Security is mentioned as the most important source of income. Private or public pension and income from other financial investments together are mentioned as most important at less than half the frequency. In the early 1970s, the poverty rate for elderly adults was approximately 20%. Currently, the older adult demographic has an overall poverty rate of approximately 11%, which is a significant improvement. Certain groups, including the old old, women living alone, and select ethnic groups, have poverty rates double the overall rate.

DISCUSSION SOURCE

Centers for Disease Control and Prevention. National Vital Statistics Reports, United States. Available at: www.cdc.gov/nchs/nvss.htm.

Aging Theories

5. During a routine assessment of a 73-year-old man with back pain, he reveals that he has become increasingly concerned about the physical changes related to aging. He misses the ability to do physical and recreational activities that he once enjoyed. He feels that this realization has made him "cranky," which his children have mentioned to him on several occasions. You realize that this patient may be having difficulty accepting the inevitability of physical decline and death as described by:
   A. Erickson.
   B. Peck.
   C. Butler.
   D. Levinson.

6 to 10. Match the following biological theories with the key aspect.

_____ **6.** Gene theory

_____ **7.** Error theory

_____ **8.** Programmed theory

_____ **9.** Cross-link theory

_____ **10.** Somatic mutation theory

A. collagen molecules bind to each other to produce stiffness and rigidity
B. a senescence factor accumulates in the cell
C. one or more latent harmful genes become activated
D. an essential gene is destroyed and causes the cell to stop dividing
E. proteins produced in the cell accumulate more errors during aging

Answers

5. A.   7. E.   9. A.
6. C.   8. B.   10. D.

Several working theories have been developed to help explain the psychosocial and physiological changes associated with older age, as well as the developmental tasks of the elderly. Erik Erikson postulated that the major psychosocial task of late adulthood is to maintain ego integrity (holding on to one's self of wholeness) while avoiding despair. Those who succeed in accomplishing this will develop wisdom, have little regret for the life that was lived, and accept the inevitable event of death. Similarly, Robert Butler theorized that retrospection and life review in older adults can lead to serenity, candor, and wisdom. A life review can involve reminiscing, taking trips to favorite childhood places, or going through photo albums and scrapbooks. Robert Peck expanded on Erickson's theory and introduced the following three tasks faced in older age: 1) ego differentiation versus work-role preoccupation (to develop satisfaction from one's self as a person rather than through the work role); 2) body transcendence versus body preoccupation (to find psychological pleasures rather than becoming absorbed with the health problems or physical limitations imposed by aging); and 3) ego transcendence versus ego preoccupation (to feel pleasure through reflecting on one's life rather than dwelling on the limited number of years left to live). Finally, Daniel Levinson's theory of the Seasons of Life focuses on the relationship of physical changes to personality, and ultimately, individuals must come to terms with the inevitability of death.

Three theories attempt to explain the psychosocial aspects of aging. The disengagement theory views aging as a process of mutual withdrawal in which older adults voluntarily slow down their activities, such as by retiring from occupational and social endeavors. Proponents of this theory suggest that social withdrawal benefits the individual and society. In contrast, the activity theory sees a positive correlation between keeping active and aging well. Proponents of the activity theory argue that mutual social withdrawal runs counter to traditional American ideals of activity and industry. Finally, the continuity theory postulates that basic personality, attitude, and behaviors remain constant throughout the life span. Research has not been able to show if one model is superior to the other. However, a number of commonalities exist for older adults. These include adjusting to decreasing physical strength and health, adjusting to retirement and reduced income, and adjusting to the death of a partner. Furthermore, older adults must establish an affiliation with peers, adapt to social rules concerning the elderly, and establish satisfactory living arrangements.

A number of biological theories attempt to explain the process of aging. These theories can help explain the variety of factors involved in the aging process:

- Gene theory: one or multiple latent harmful genes become activated that lead to cell death.
- Error theory: as a cell ages, genes encode for proteins with an accumulation of errors and an eventual "killer" gene is produced.
- Somatic mutation theory: the destruction of a key gene causes the cell to stop dividing; longevity of the cell depends on how well the cell can repair damage to DNA.
- Programmed theory: a senescence factor accumulates in the cell and acts in a dominant fashion, leading to cell death.
- Immunological theory: an imbalance of T cells results in decreased cellular immune function; autoantibodies are produced.
- Free radical theory: unpaired electrons are produced intrinsically and extrinsically; altered biochemical reactions result in DNA damage and cell death.
- Cross-link theory: collagen molecules cross-link in tissues that produce stiffness and rigidity.
- Stress-adaptation theory: a diminished ability to cope with stress results in hypothermia, cardiac output decline, and decreased vital capacity.

DISCUSSION SOURCE

Bengtson, VL, Gans D, Putney N, and Silverstein M. _Handbook of Theories of Aging,_ ed. 2. New York: Springer Publishing Company, 2008.

Normative Age-Related Changes

11 to 15. Match the following age-related changes in the senses with the problem reported by the older adult.

____ **11.** Difficulty with appreciating the content of conversation in noisy environment

____ **12.** Decline in sense of smell

____ **13.** Painless vision change that includes central vision distortion

____ **14.** Results in near vision blurriness

____ **15.** Can result in peripheral vision loss

A. Hyposmia
B. Presbycusis
C. Presbyopia
D. Age-related maculopathy
E. Chronic glaucoma

16. A 76-year-old woman is being treated for senile cataracts. The granddaughter who is accompanying the patient expresses concern that one day she may also develop cataracts. You explain that she can reduce the risk of senile cataracts by avoiding all of the following except:
A. tobacco use.
B. alcohol abuse.
C. ocular corticosteroid therapy.
D. sunlight exposure.

17. A 81-year-old woman has early bilateral senile cataracts. Which of the following situations would likely pose the greatest difficulty for her?
A. reading the newspaper
B. distinguishing between the primary colors
C. following extraocular movements
D. reading road signs while driving

18. All of the following are consistent with normal age-related vision changes except:
A. need for increased illumination.
B. increasing sensitivity to glare.
C. washing out of colors.
D. gradual loss of peripheral vision.

19. A risk factor for primary open-angle glaucoma is:
A. postural hypotension.
B. age more than 40 years.
C. history of fungal conjunctivitis.
D. white race.

20. All of the following are risk factors for angle-closure glaucoma except:
A. Asian ethnicity.
B. female gender.
C. far-sightedness.
D. long-term use of contact lenses.

21. Besides aging, a risk factor for age-related macular degeneration is:
A. hypertension.
B. hyperlipidemia.
C. tobacco use.
D. alcohol abuse.

22. An effective method to prevent presbycusis is:
A. avoid using cotton swabs in the ear canal.
B. use of ear protection when exposed to loud noises.
C. avoid using hearing aids for a prolonged period of time.
D. regular cerumen removal.

23. A common complaint for a person with presbycusis is:
A. general diminution of hearing.
B. diminution of high-frequency hearing.
C. worsening hearing at night.
D. unable to hear low-pitched sounds.

24. A person with cerumen impaction experiences:
A. a general diminution of hearing.
B. unhampered ability in hearing low-pitched sounds.
C. pain when exposed to high-pitched sounds.
D. an ability to hear but cannot understand a conversation in a noisy environment.

Answers

11. B.	16. B.	21. C.
12. A.	17. D.	22. B.
13. D.	18. D.	23. B.
14. C.	19. B.	24. A.
15. E.	20. D.	

Normative aging results in changes in the senses. In addition, certain diseases that result in changes in the senses are more common in older adults (Table 16–1). Presbycusis is a progressive, symmetric, high-frequency, age-related sensory hearing loss that is likely caused by cochlear deterioration. Speech discrimination is usually the primary problem; an individual with presbycusis often reports the ability to hear another person talking but has limited ability to understand the content of the speech, particularly when in a noisy environment.

Distance vision poses the greatest problem for individuals with senile cataracts. As the lens becomes more opaque, near vision also deteriorates. Other visual changes of age-related cataracts include loss of ability to distinguish contrasts and progressive dimming of vision. Close vision is usually retained, and there are occasional improvements in reading ability.

Presbyopia refers to age-related vision changes caused by a progressive hardening of the lens. Patients most often complain of close vision problems, usually first manifested by difficulty with reading smaller print. Other normal age-related vision changes include a progressive yellowing of the lens and decreased flexibility of the sclera, in part leading to the perception of washing out of colors, difficulty seeing under low illumination, and increased sensitivity to glare.

TABLE 16-1

Age-Related Changes and Conditions That Result in Changes of the Senses

Condition	Etiology	Result	Comment
Presbyopia	Hardening of lens	Close vision problems	Nearly all adults ≥45 y.o. need reading glasses.
Senile cataracts	Lens clouding	Progressive vision dimming, distance vision problems, close vision usually retained and may initially improve	Risk factors: Tobacco use, poor nutrition, sun exposure, corticosteroid therapy. Potentially correctable with surgery, lens implant.
Open-angle glaucoma	Painless, gradual onset of increased intraocular pressure leading to optic atrophy	Loss of peripheral vision	≥80% of all glaucoma. Risk factors: elevated intraocular pressure, African American race, age ≥40 years. Periodic screening with tonometry, assessment of visual fields. Treatment with topical miotics, beta blockers, other drugs, or surgery effective in vision preservation.
Angle-closure glaucoma	Sudden increase in intraocular pressure	Usually unilateral, acutely red, painful eye with vision change including halos around lights; eyeball firm compared with other eyeball	Risk factors: older age, female gender, Asian ethnicity, family history, far-sightedness. Immediate referral to ophthalmology for rapid pressure reduction via medication, possible surgery.
Age-related maculopathy	Thickening, sclerotic changes in retinal basement membrane complex	Painless vision changes including distortion of central vision	Besides aging, risk factors include tobacco use, sun exposure, family history. Dry form: No treatment available except to minimize risk factors that worsen the condition. Wet form: Laser treatment and other therapies to obliterate neovascular membrane. Anti-angiogenic drugs injected in the eye to block new blood vessel development and leakage from abnormal vessels.
Hyposmia	Neural degeneration	Decline in sense of smell, usually gradual, resulting in fine taste discrimination (largely a function of smell)	Accelerated by tobacco use. Risk factors: aging, head trauma, history of chronic rhinosinusitis.
Presbycusis	Multifactorial including loss of eighth cranial nerve sensitivity	Difficult with appreciating the content of conversation in noisy environment; person can hear but cannot understand	Accelerated by excessive noise exposure. Besides aging, risk factors include family history, smoking, cardiovascular diseases, diabetes, otosclerosis, infection, and trauma. Hearing aids helpful.
Cerumen impaction	Conductive hearing loss	General diminution of hearing, easily corrected through cerumen removal	Risk factors: ear canal hairs, use of hearing aids, bony growths secondary to osteophyte or osteoma, history of impacted cerumen. Cerumen removal.

Source: Merck Manual of Geriatrics. Available at: www.merckmanuals.com/professional/geriatrics.html.

Macular degeneration is the most common cause of newly-acquired blindness and vision loss in elderly adults. Vision changes seen in macular degeneration include loss of the central vision field. This disease is seen more often in women of European descent. A history of cigarette smoking and a family history of the disease are often found as well; excessive sun exposure has also been implicated as a risk factor for macular degeneration. The ophthalmological examination reveals hard drusen or yellow deposits in the macular area. Soft drusen can also be seen. These appear larger, paler, and less distinct.

DISCUSSION SOURCE

Merck Manual of Geriatrics. www.merckmanuals.com/professional/geriatrics.htm.

See full color images of this topic on DavisPlus at
http://davisplus.fadavis.com |
Keyword: Fitzgerald

Medication Use

25. Age-related changes in an elderly adult include all of the following except:
A. total body water decreases by 10% to 15% between ages 20 and 80 years.
B. body weight as fat increases from 18% to 36% in men and from 33% to 45% in women.
C. increase in serum albumin.
D. increase in gastric pH.

26. A general principle of drug absorption in an elderly adult is best described as:
A. amount of absorption is decreased.
B. rate of absorption is changed.
C. drug absorption is altered but predictable.
D. bioavailability is altered.

27. When evaluating serum creatinine in an elderly adult, the clinician considers that:
A. this value is influenced by glomerular filtration rate.
B. age-related physiological changes do not influence this laboratory value.
C. male and female norms are equivalent.
D. an increase is an expected age-related change.

28. Anticipated age-related changes that can result in less drug effect include:
A. loss of beta-2 receptor sites.
B. lower gastrointestinal (GI) pH.
C. increased renin-angiotensin production.
D. increased GI motility.

29. When prescribing a diuretic, the NP considers that the older adult:
A. has diminished ability to conserve sodium.
B. has increased ability to excrete potassium.
C. has continued response to a thiazide despite increasing creatinine.
D. often develops allergic reaction to these products.

30. Age-related changes in the gastrointestinal system include all of the following except:
A. decreased gastric acid production.
B. decreased gastric motility.
C. increased GI surface area.
D. decreased gastric emptying.

31. Long-term proton pump inhibitor (PPI) use is associated with all of the following except:
A. increased risk of pneumonia in hospitalized patients.
B. increased risk of *C. difficile* colitis in hospitalized patients.
C. reduced absorption of calcium and magnesium.
D. increased absorption of iron and copper.

32. To avoid rebound gastric hyperacidity following discontinuation of long-term PPI use, all of the following methods can be used except:
A. gradually tapering the PPI dose.
B. switch to every-other-day dosing of PPI.
C. switch to a low-dose H_2RA therapy.
D. avoiding antacid therapy when symptoms flare.

33. Age-related renal changes in older adults potentially include all of the following except:
A. decreased glomerular filtration rate (GFR).
B. diminished renal blood flow.
C. loss of functional nephrons.
D. increased renal mass to compensate for decreased function.

34. An expected age-related change in the older adult with intact renal function is decreased muscle mass and an associated:
A. increase in serum creatinine.
B. decrease in serum creatinine.
C. minimal impact on serum creatinine.
D. increase in creatinine clearance.

35. In an older adult with advanced impaired renal function, the clinician anticipates that there is usually no need to adjust the antimicrobial dose with the use of:
A. ceftriaxone.
B. tobramycin.
C. levofloxacin.
D. vancomycin.

36. When dosing warfarin in older adults, it is important to consider:
A. a lower dose is needed due to lower serum albumin.
B. a lower dose is needed due to higher serum albumin.
C. a higher dose is needed due to lower serum albumin.
D. a higher dose is needed due to lower serum albumin.

37. Which of the following medications has little anticholinergic effect?
A. diphenhydramine
B. amitriptyline
C. chlorpheniramine
D. loratadine

38 to 41. Indicate (yes or no) which of the following adverse effects is associated with the use of anticholinergic agents in older adults.

38. Confusion

39. Hypertension

40. Urinary retention

41. Constipation

42. The process of absorption, distribution, metabolism, and elimination of a drug is known as:
   A. pharmacodynamics.
   B. drug interactions study.
   C. pharmacokinetics.
   D. therapeutic transformation.

43. The study of biochemical and physiological effects of drugs on the body or disease is called:
   A. pharmacodynamics.
   B. pharmacokinetics.
   C. biotransformation.
   D. bioavailability.

44. When considering the properties of a drug in the body, which of the following does not change as a person ages?
   A. excretion
   B. biotransformation
   C. pharmacodynamics
   D. absorption

45. When prescribing a medication, the clinician considers that half-life is the amount of time needed to decrease the serum concentration of a drug by:
   A. 25%.
   B. 50%.
   C. 75%.
   D. 100%.

46. Under ordinary circumstances, the presence of a medication in the body is needed for how many half-lives to reach steady state?
   A. 0.5 to 1
   B. 1 to 3
   C. 3 to 5
   D. 5 to 7

47. Compared with a healthy 40-year-old adult, CYP 450 isoenzyme levels can decrease by ___% in elderly adults after age 70.
   A. 10
   B. 20
   C. 30
   D. 40

48. When considering pharmacological options to treat neuropathic pain in a 72-year-old man, which of the following is the least appropriate option due to its anticholinergic effect?
   A. nortriptyline
   B. amitriptyline
   C. duloxetine
   D. venlafaxine

Answers

25. C.	33. D.	41. Y.
26. B.	34. B.	42. C.
27. A.	35. A.	43. A.
28. A.	36. A.	44. C.
29. A.	37. D.	45. B.
30. C.	38. Y.	46. C.
31. D.	39. N.	47. C.
32. D.	40. Y.	48. B.

"Start low, go slow" is geriatric prescribing advice all clinicians likely learned. Although there is wisdom in this adage, a more complete understanding of numerous age-related factors is needed for safe prescribing for elderly adults.

The Beers Criteria provide an important reference to avoid the inappropriate use of medications in the elderly population. First published in 1991 by Dr. Mark Beers and periodically updated by an interdisciplinary expert panel of the American Geriatrics Society, the criteria identify more than 50 medications or medication classes that should be avoided in older adults, a number that should be used with caution, and others that should be avoided under certain conditions. Medications deemed unconditionally inappropriate are generally to be avoided regardless of circumstances, and alternatives should be used. Medications considered for conditional use upon disease state or drug dose are likely only to be inappropriate in specific context. When prescribing medications for the elderly, checking to see if the drug is listed in the Beers Criteria is an important step in ensuring the safe use of medications.

Elderly people are a heterogeneous group who constitute a small portion of the North American population yet use approximately one-third of prescription medications and nearly three-fourths of all over-the-counter medications. Because advancing age is often accompanied by various health problems, elderly adults often have multiple healthcare providers and multiple prescribers and medications. In addition, normative age-related physiological changes can influence pharmacological responses; these changes are often accentuated by illness (Table 16–2). Financial constraints commonly cause elderly adults to use a medication less often than prescribed or to attempt to substitute. The clinician must be aware of these factors to prescribe for older adults safely and effectively.

Because the term "elder" or "elderly adult" is typically used to describe any person age 65 or older, this could imply that aging occurs only after this milestone. In reality, normal age-related changes influencing drug therapy occur gradually over decades. These changes often lead to altered pharmacokinetics; components of pharmacokinetics include drug absorption, distribution, biotransformation (metabolism), and excretion. A simple way of remembering pharmacokinetics principles is that this is what the body does to the drug. At the same time, pharmacodynamics, the study of biochemical and physiological effects of drugs or what the drug does to the body or disease, does not change over the life span. Normative age-related changes, such as the loss of the beta-2-receptor sites, result in less of a clinical effect with beta-2-agonist use, however.

TABLE 16-2
Age-Related Changes Important to Medication Use

	Age 20–30 Years	Age 60–80 Years
Percent body weight as water	60%	53%
Lean muscle mass	Baseline	≥20% reduction
Serum albumin (average)	4.7 g	3.8 g
Relative kidney weight	100%	80%
Relative hepatic blood flow	100%	55%–60%

Source: Katzung B. Special aspects in geriatric pharmacology. In: Katzung B. *Basic and Clinical Pharmacology*, ed. 12. New York: McGraw Medical; 2011 pp 1051-1060.

Although age alone likely does not alter the amount of the drug absorbed, age-related changes can significantly influence the rate of absorption. A drug's half-life ($T^1/_2$), defined as the time required for the amount of drug in the body to be reduced by one-half after a single dose of the medication is given, is often increased in older adults. As gastric acid production decreases, stomach pH increases, potentially prolonging the initial breakdown of medication made to dissolve in low pH. In addition, age-related decreases in GI blood flow, gastric motility, and gastric emptying mean that medication stays in the gut longer, whereas decreased GI surface area can lead to erratic absorption. The use of antacids in the elderly population complicates this situation by increasing stomach pH further, potentially allowing the formation of an inactive drug-antacid compound and delivering drug to absorption sites in the intestines at a variable rate; proton pump inhibitors and histamine-2 receptor antagonists also increase stomach pH.

Protracted PPI use is associated with reduced absorption of iron, vitamin B12, and other micronutrients. An increase in fracture risk of the hip, spine, wrist, and forearm has also been noted with long-term PPI use; this risk is possibly associated with the decreased absorption of calcium and magnesium during PPI use. In particular, individuals with multiple health problems when hospitalized or in long-term care who are on chronic PPI therapy have an increased risk of contracting pneumonia and of developing *C. difficile* colitis. As a result, PPI use should not extend beyond the period of time needed for the clinical condition.

Often patients report an increase in upper GI distress when discontinuing long-term PPI use. The likely cause is rebound gastric hyperacidity; this problem can be minimized by gradually tapering the PPI dose (if possible) or trying every-other-day dosing with a supplemental dose of an antacid when symptoms flare. An alternative is to try low-dose H2RA therapy with supplemental antacid use as needed. This gap therapy is usually continued for approximately 1 month.

Drug distribution can be altered by age-related changes. Serum albumin, an important plasma protein used to bind and distribute various medications, including warfarin (Coumadin) and phenytoin (Dilantin), decreases with aging. With less albumin available for drug binding, potentially more free drug is available. These changes, coupled with altered drug elimination, often lead to a decrease in the dose needed in an aging adult. The amount of the plasma protein alpha-1-acid glycoprotein, with an affinity for binding with certain medications. including propranolol, quinidine, and lidocaine, increases; as a result, less free drug is in circulation.

Age-related hepatic changes include decreased hepatic, blood flow, mass, and functioning hepatocytes and diminished activity of hepatic enzymes responsible for drug metabolism. These changes contribute to a prolonged drug $T^1/_2$ and longer duration of action than found in younger adults. In addition, ability to recover from alcohol-induced, medication-induced, or viral-induced hepatic damage is lessened.

Renal changes noted in aging are numerous. Glomerular filtration rate (GFR), the rate plasma is filtered through the glomeruli, continues at the maximal adult rate through age 50. GFR then begins a gradual decline, with approximately 80% of maximal adult rate at age 60, 70% by age 70, and 55% by age 80. GFR, coupled with reduced renal mass, loss of functional nephrons, and diminished renal blood flow, can lead to problems with drug elimination. Health problems, such as diabetes mellitus and hypertension, can compromise renal function further. As a result, having an accurate measure of renal function before prescribing is important. Formed from lean muscle, creatinine production and excretion rate are equal in health. Lean muscle mass decreases in aging; this decline parallels age-related renal function changes; this can lead to a normal serum creatinine in elderly adults when renal function is significantly impaired.

Compared with serum creatinine, creatinine clearance and GFR provide a more accurate measure of renal function, especially in an older adult. Many medications that are excreted via the renal route carry a notice of needed dose adjustment in the presence of impaired renal function, using creatinine clearance or GFR levels as the guide for appropriate dose. Creatinine clearance is most accurately measured by obtaining a 24-hour urine specimen. Given that a medication that requires dose adjustment in the presence of renal impairment often needs to be started urgently, waiting for the results of a 24-hour urine test to be collected and analyzed is often impractical. Using the Cockcroft-Gault equation provides a reasonable estimate of creatinine clearance. As creatinine clearance is reduced, dose or dosing interval adjustment of numerous medications, including angiotensin-converting enzyme inhibitors and certain antibiotics, is required. GFR can be calculated using the formula found at the National Kidney Foundation's website at www.kidney.org/professionals/kdoqi/gfr_calculator.cfm. The dosing interval of trimethoprim-sulfamethoxazole (Bactrim) needs to be adjusted in the presence of renal impairment with abnormal creatinine clearance or GFR. In contrast, ceftriaxone (Rocephin) can be used without dose or dosing interval adjustment in the presence of altered GFR or creatinine clearance.

Medications with significant systemic anticholinergic effect should be avoided in older adults because of risk of confusion, urinary retention, constipation, visual disturbance, and hypotension. If anticholinergic effect is unavoidable, a product in the class with the least amount of this effect should be chosen. A tricyclic antidepressant can be a helpful and inexpensive treatment option for the management of chronic neuropathic pain but can have significant anticholinergic effect. Compared with amitriptyline, nortriptyline has significantly less of this effect, however, and is likely a better treatment option. Serotonin-norepinephrine reuptake inhibitors (SNRIs), such as duloxetine and venlafaxine, have been found to be helpful in treating neuropathic pain. Other options for neuropathic pain include the anticonvulsants gabapentin and pregabalin, though dose adjustment based on renal function may be needed in the elderly as these drugs are renally excreted. Gabapentin is also associated with sedation and should be started at a low dose and titrated as needed. If an antihistamine is needed, loratadine offers an option with little anticholinergic effect, whereas diphenhydramine is a less attractive option, owing to its strong anticholinergic effect.

The adage, "start low, go slow" in prescribing for elderly adults has an often forgotten third part: "but get to goal." Clinicians, in their zeal to provide safe pharmacotherapeutic care for older adult patients, often prescribe enough of a medication to give anticipated adverse effects but not enough to provide the desired therapeutic effect. Knowledge of the safe and appropriate medication doses in older adults, keeping in mind the age-related effects on pharmacokinetics, is a critical part to safe prescriptive practice.

DISCUSSION SOURCES

AGS. American Geriatrics Society updated Beers Criteria for potentially inappropriate medication use in older adults. *J Am Geriatr Soc* 2012. Available at: www.americangeriatrics.org/files/documents/beers/2012BeersCriteria_JAGS.pdf.

Katzung B. Special aspects in geriatric pharmacology. In: Katzung B. *Basic and Clinical Pharmacology*, ed. 12. New York: McGraw Medical; 2011 pp 1051-1060.

Elder Maltreatment

49. When making a home visit to a bedridden 89-year-old man, you note that he is cachectic and dehydrated but cognitively intact. He states he is not receiving his medications regularly and that his granddaughter is supposed to take care of him but mentions, "She seems more interested in my Social Security check." The patient is unhappy but asks that you not "tell anybody" because he wants to remain in his home. The most appropriate action would be to:
    A. talk with the patient's granddaughter and evaluate her ability to care for the patient.
    B. visit the patient more frequently to ensure that his condition does not deteriorate.
    C. report the situation to the appropriate state agency.
    D. honor the patient's wishes because a competent patient has the right to determine care.

50. Which of the following statements is true concerning elder maltreatment?
    A. This problem is found mainly in families of lower socioeconomic status.
    B. An elderly adult who is being mistreated usually seeks help.
    C. Routine screening is indicated as part of the care of an older adult.
    D. In most instances of elder maltreatment, a predictable cycle of physical violence directed at the older adult followed by a period of remorse on the part of the perpetrator is the norm.

51. Risk factors for becoming a perpetrator of elder maltreatment include all of the following except:
    A. a high level of hostility about the caregiver role.
    B. poor coping skills.
    C. assumption of caregiving responsibilities at a later stage of life.
    D. maltreatment as a child.

52. Elder maltreatment is considered to be underreported, with an estimated ___ cases going unreported to each one case that is reported.
    A. three
    B. four
    C. five
    D. six

53. The most commonly reported form of elder maltreatment is:
    A. physical abuse.
    B. sexual exploitation.
    C. financial exploitation.
    D. neglect.

54. The daughter of a 76-year-old woman expresses concern regarding her mother's refusal for assistance in everyday living activities. The mother lives by herself and is often found with poor hygiene and reports eating one small meal a day. She also has poor adherence to her current medication regimens. This represents an example of:
    A. abandonment.
    B. self-neglect.
    C. early-onset dementia.
    D. psychological abuse.

Answers

49. C.	51. C.	53. D.
50. C.	52. C.	54. B.

The Centers for Disease Control and Prevention (CDC) defines elder maltreatment as any abuse and neglect of persons age 60 and older by a caregiver or another person in a relationship involving an expectation of trust. Elder maltreatment can take various forms (Table 16–3). Every state in the

TABLE 16-3
Forms of Elder Maltreatment

Form of Elder Maltreatment	Descriptions
Physical abuse	Elderly adult is injured by another individual, including being scratched, bitten, slapped, pushed, hit, or burned; assaulted or threatened with a weapon, including a knife, gun, or other object; or inappropriately restrained.
Sexual abuse or abusive sexual contact	Any sexual contact against elderly adult's will, including acts in which elderly adult is unable to understand the act or is unable to communicate consent. Abusive sexual contact is defined as intentional touching, either directly or through the clothing, of the genitalia, anus, groin, breast, mouth, inner thigh, or buttocks.
Psychological or emotional abuse	Any event in which elderly adult experiences trauma after exposure to threatening acts or coercive tactics. Examples include humiliation or embarrassment; controlling behavior such as prohibiting or limiting access to transportation, telephone, money, or other resources; social isolation; disregarding or trivializing needs; or damaging or destroying property.
Neglect	Failure or refusal of a caregiver or other responsible person to provide for elderly adult's basic physical, emotional, or social needs, or failure to protect elderly adult from harm. Examples include not providing adequate nutrition, hygiene, clothing, shelter, or access to necessary healthcare, or failure to prevent exposure to unsafe activities and environments.
Abandonment	Willful desertion of elderly adult by caregiver or other responsible person.
Financial abuse or exploitation	Unauthorized or improper use of resources of elderly adult for monetary or personal benefit, profit, or gain by another individual. Examples include forgery, misuse or theft of money or possessions, use of coercion or deception to surrender finances or property, or improper use of guardianship or power of attorney.
Self-neglect	This form of elder maltreatment is, as defined, instituted by the elderly adult, not another individual, and is the failure or refusal of elderly adult to address his or her own basic physical, emotional, or social needs. Examples include self-care tasks, such as nourishment, clothing, hygiene, and shelter; proper or appropriate use of medications; and managing or administering one's finances. This is also characterized by the lack of intervention to halt or modify the behavior by another individual who is often in the position to recognize the problem.

United States and many Canadian provinces have enacted legislation to protect vulnerable older adults from abuse, with a requirement for healthcare workers and others who come in contact with older adults to report this abuse to the appropriate protective authorities. Elder maltreatment is significantly underreported; for every one case reported, an estimated five other cases go unreported. Neglect is the most commonly encountered type of elder maltreatment. In times of economic difficulty, the rate of financial exploitation usually increases.

A combination of individual, relational, community, and societal factors contribute to the risk of an individual becoming a perpetrator of elder maltreatment. Understanding these factors can help identify various opportunities for prevention.

Risk factors for perpetration of elder maltreatment include a current diagnosis of mental illness or alcohol abuse, a high level of hostility about the caregiver role, poor coping skills, inadequate preparation for caregiving responsibilities, assumption of caregiving responsibilities at an early age, and maltreatment as a child. At the relationship level, additional risk factors emerge, including a high level of financial and emotional dependence on a vulnerable elder, a past experience of disruptive behavior, and lack of social support. Elder mistreatment is likely to be more prevalent in a cultural and community milieu in which tolerance of aggressive behavior and negative beliefs about aging and elderly adults exist; formal services, such as respite care for individuals providing care to elderly adults, are limited, inaccessible, or unavailable; family members are expected to care for elderly adults without seeking help from others; and individuals are encouraged to endure suffering or remain silent regarding their pain. At the institutional level, such as in a long-term care or assisted living facility, unsympathetic or negative attitudes toward residents, chronic staffing problems, lack of administrative oversight, staff burnout, and stressful working conditions are considered risk factors for elder maltreatment.

Certain factors have been identified as protection against elder mistreatment, including strong personal relationships, community support for the caregiver role, and coordinated resources to help serve elderly adults and caregivers. Factors within institutional settings that can be protective include effective monitoring systems in place; clear, understandable institutional policies and procedures regarding patient care; ongoing education on elder abuse and neglect for employees; education about and clear guidance on how durable power of attorney is to be used; and regular visits by family members, volunteers, and social workers.

DISCUSSION SOURCES

Centers for Disease Control and Prevention. Elder abuse. Available at: www.cdc.gov/violenceprevention/elderabuse/index.html.
Elder Maltreatment Alliance. Information. Available at: www.elder-maltreatment.com/information.

Orthostatic Hypotension

55. Orthostatic (postural) hypotension is defined as an excessive decrease in blood pressure (BP) with position, usually greater than _____ mm Hg systolic and _____ mm Hg diastolic.
    A. 10, 5
    B. 15, 7
    C. 20, 10
    D. 30, 15

56. Orthostatic hypotension is present in about _____% of older adults.
    A. 10
    B. 20
    C. 30
    D. 40

57. The use of which of the following medications is associated with the least risk of postural hypotension in the older adult?
    A. nifedipine
    B. furosemide
    C. clonidine
    D. lisinopril

58. Lifestyle interventions for an older adult with orthostatic hypotension should include counseling about:
    A. avoiding the use of compression stockings.
    B. minimizing salt intake.
    C. flexing the feet multiple times before changing position.
    D. restricting fluids.

59. In assessing a person with or at risk for orthostatic hypotension, the BP should be measured after 5 minutes in the supine position and then ___ and ___ minutes after standing.
    A. 1, 3
    B. 2, 4
    C. 3, 5
    D. 5, 10

Answers

55. C.	57. D.	59. A.
56. B.	58. C.	

Although not a specific disease state, orthostatic (postural) hypotension is a manifestation of abnormal blood pressure (BP) regulation. Normal BP is usually maintained by the sympathetic system causing an increase in heart rate and contractility in response to the pooling of blood in the lower extremity and trunk veins because of position change. Simultaneous parasympathetic (vagal) inhibition also increases heart rate. With continued standing, activation of the renin-angiotensin-aldosterone system and antidiuretic hormone secretion cause sodium and water retention and increase circulating blood volume. When these mechanisms do not work properly, BP control is not maintained with position change. The end result is a transient decrease in venous return, reduced cardiac output, and a decrease in BP; usually the first patient-reported effects from the decrease in BP are light-headedness, dizziness, or blurred vision that occur within seconds of changing position, most often from sitting to standing. Orthostatic hypotension is defined as an excessive decrease in BP when an upright position is assumed; the change in BP is usually greater than 20 mm Hg systolic and greater than 10 mm Hg diastolic, with resulting symptoms that occur within seconds of changing position from supine or sit to standing. This condition is present in about 20% of older adults and is a potent risk factor for falls.

Although age-related changes in the cardiovascular and cerebrovascular systems contribute to orthostatic hypotension, the use of certain medications can cause or worsen the condition. The medications most often implicated typically cause a decrease in circulating volume or peripheral vasodilation; these medications include loop diuretics, tricyclic antidepressants, calcium channel blockers, alpha-adrenergic blockers, centrally acting antihypertensives such as clonidine, and nitrates. Certain disease states that alter baseline cardiac output and vascular capacity, increasing orthostatic risk, are common in older adults; these include aortic stenosis, dehydration, peripheral vascular insufficiency, and electrolyte disturbances. Alcohol use is also a potent contributor, as is prolonged bedrest; beta blocker use is seldom implicated. Cardiac rhythm disturbances usually occur with regularity, which results in more consistent symptoms, not simply with position change, and are not a significant orthostatic hypotension contributor.

In assessing a person with or at risk for orthostatic hypotension, BP should be measured after the patient has been in a supine position for 5 minutes and then at 1 and 3 minutes after standing. Patient symptoms should be recorded. If the patient is too symptomatic or ill to stand, the maneuvers should be performed with supine to sit position change. If hypotension is accompanied by an increase of heart rate to greater than 100 bpm, altered circulating volume is the likely cause.

When orthostatic hypotension is documented, possible contributing factors, such as medications implicated in the condition, should be modified. Fluid and electrolyte imbalance, if a contributor, should be corrected. In addition, instruction about lifestyle modification to minimize risk is a critical and often overlooked intervention. This instruction includes information about moving slowly and deliberately with position change from supine to sit or supine to stand, dorsiflexing the feet multiple times before position change, and avoiding standing in one position for an excessive length of time; the use of compression stockings to enhance venous return can also be helpful. If not contraindicated by cardiac or other health issues, an increase in sodium and fluid intake usually helps increase circulating volume and minimizes orthostatic risk.

DISCUSSION SOURCES

Lanier J, Mote M, Clay E. Evaluation and management of orthostatic hypotension. *Am Fam Physician* 84(5):527–536, 2011.

Merck Manual for Health Professionals. Orthostatic Hypotension. Available at: www.merckmanuals.com/professional/cardiovascular_disorders/symptoms_of_cardiovascular_disorders/orthostatic_hypotension.html.

Falls

60. Most falls in older adults occur in:
    A. a healthcare institution.
    B. a public place.
    C. the patient's home.
    D. an outdoor setting.

61. Which of the following are identifiable risk factors for falls in the older adult? Choose all that apply.
    A. negative prior history of a fall
    B. history of a stroke
    C. current diagnosis of osteoporosis
    D. osteoarthritis of the hips

62. The NP is asked to evaluate a 77-year-old woman who recently had an unexpected fall. The patient is normally healthy and has no mobility limitations or other obvious risk factors. During the history, the NP learns that the patient did not attempt to break the fall, "I just suddenly found myself on the floor." This statement suggests:
    A. a previously undiagnosed cognitive impairment that requires further evaluation.
    B. that underlying sensory deficits (visual, hearing) are the most likely cause of the fall and require physical assessment.
    C. that a history of alcohol use or abuse should be explored.
    D. a syncopal episode requiring a cardiovascular and neurological evaluation.

63. In an older adult, the greatest risk of long-term complication is associated with fracture of the:
    A. forearm.
    B. spine.
    C. ankle.
    D. hip.

64. Fall risk in an older adult is decreased with the use of which of the following footwear?
    A. sandal
    B. jogging shoe
    C. slipper
    D. semirigid sole shoe

65. With the use of insulin, fall risk in an older adult is most likely to occur _____ of the medication.
    A. at the onset of action
    B. at the peak of action
    C. at the middle point of duration of action
    D. toward the end of anticipated duration of action

66. A 68-year-old man is taking multiple medications for various chronic conditions. Discontinuing or finding an alternative for which of the following medications will have the greatest impact in decreasing the potential for fall risk?
    A. amitriptyline
    B. sitagliptin
    C. atorvastatin
    D. aspirin

67. An older adult who has recently fallen has a(n) _____ times increased risk of falling again within the next year.
    A. 1 to 2
    B. 2 to 3
    C. 3 to 4
    D. 4 to 5

68. Which of the following is not part of the "Get Up and Go" criteria when evaluating gait and balance for a 72-year-old woman who normally uses a walker?
    A. rising from a straight-backed chair
    B. walking 10 feet without the use of a walking aid
    C. turning around after walking 10 feet
    D. returning to the chair and sitting down

69. With the use of a benzodiazepine in an older adult, the risk of fall is most likely to occur _____ of the medication.
    A. at the onset of action
    B. at the peak of action
    C. at the middle point of duration of action
    D. toward the end of anticipated duration of action

Answers

60. C.	64. D.	67. B.
61. B, C, D	65. B.	68. B.
62. D.	66. A.	69. B.
63. D.		

Falls are a significant source of morbidity and mortality in the elderly population; multiple falls are associated with increased risk of death. Approximately one-third of community-dwelling elderly adults and two-thirds of long-term care residents experience falls each year. Of elderly adults who fall, 20% to 30% sustain moderate to severe injuries that reduce mobility and independence and increase the risk of premature death. Older adults are hospitalized for fall-related injuries five times more often than they are for injuries from other causes. For adults 65 years old or older, 60% of fatal falls happen at home, 30% occur in public places, and 10% occur in healthcare institutions.

Risk factors for falls are numerous and are modifiable and nonmodifiable (Table 16–4).

Polypharmacy, in particular the use of medications associated with postural hypotension, increases fall risk. Additional risks include personal history of a stroke or fall; a person who has fallen is two to three times more likely to fall within the next year. Environmental hazards in the home, including poorly placed furnishings and inadequate lighting, often contribute to falls. Wearing thick, soft-soled shoes, such as a jogging shoe, also increases fall risk.

Comprehensive elder care should focus on minimizing modifiable fall risks. When a fall does occur, the patient should be promptly and appropriately assessed. Questions should be asked to investigate for an underlying condition that could have contributed to the fall and is amenable to intervention and often subtle age-related changes that can contribute to increased fall risk (see Table 16–4). These questions are as follows:

- What was the patient doing when he or she fell?
- Was there an aura or warning that the fall was impending?
- Was there a vision loss?

TABLE 16-4
Fall and Fracture Risk Factors in Older Adults

Postural hypotension
Sensory impairment including altered vision and hearing
Parkinsonism
Osteoporosis
Osteoarthritis
Altered gait and balance, including decreased proprioception, increased postural sway, slower righting reflexes, peripheral neuropathy, stroke
Psychotropic medication use, especially products with sedating effect
Cardiac drug use, especially products with properties that cause or contribute to postural hypotension
Environmental hazards

Source: Wachel T. Falls. In: Wachel T. *Geriatric Clinical Advisor.* Philadelphia: Mosby; 2007, pp. 77–78.

- Did the patient experience dizziness?
- Was there a loss of consciousness?
- Did the patient break the fall?
- Is this an isolated incident, or are falls occurring more frequently?
- What medications is the patient taking? In particular, notation should be made of newly added medications or increased dose of existing medications.
- Was the patient drinking alcohol or taking other potentially intoxicating medications?

The assessment of an older adult after a fall should focus on identification of possible correctable fall risk factors and fall-related injury and should include, at minimum, the following:

- Vital signs and evaluation of orthostasis.
- Cardiovascular assessment.
- Sensory assessment.
- Assessment of gait and balance, including the use of the "Get Up and Go" test, in which the elderly adult is asked to rise from a straight-backed chair, walk 10 feet using usual walking aid such as a cane if applicable, turn, and return to the chair and sit down, with the clinician observing balance with sitting and on standing, pace and stability with walking, ability to turn without staggering, and time to complete the task.
- Survey for fall-related injuries.

The most common fall-related injuries are osteoporotic fractures of the hip, spine, or forearm. Of all fall-related fractures, hip fractures are the most serious and lead to the greatest number of health problems and deaths.

Nonpharmacological interventions to prevent falls include the following:

- Review medications; assess doses, and eliminate high-risk drugs that can contribute to falls (Table 16–5).
- Evaluate for postural hypotension.
- Provide prevention and treatment interventions for osteoporosis.
- Recommend proper footwear, avoiding slippers, sandals, and soft-soled jogging shoes in favor of an enclosed toe, tie shoe with a semirigid sole.
- Provide an obstacle free, well-lit environment.
- Raise chair heights and seat heights; add arm rests.
- Prescribe physical therapy as indicated.
- Counsel avoidance of quick position change and to perform multiple foot flex maneuvers before trying to move from supine to stand or sit to stand.
- Treat for any concomitant conditions associated with increased fall risk.

DISCUSSION SOURCES

Merck Manual of Geriatrics. Orthostatic hypotension. Available at: www.merckmanuals.com/professional/cardiovascular_disorders/symptoms_of_cardiovascular_disorders/orthostatic_hypotension.html?qt=&sc=&alt.
Patient Safety Authority. Medication assessment: One determinant of falls risk. Available at: www.patientsafetyauthority.org/ADVISORIES/AdvisoryLibrary/2008/Mar5(1)/Pages/16.aspx.

TABLE 16-5
Medication Use Associated With Increased Fall Risk in Older Adults

Medication Class	Example	Comment
Anxiolytics and hypnotics	Benzodiazepines, long-acting and shorter acting, including lorazepam, oxazepam, alprazolam, temazepam, triazolam. Nonbenzodiazepines including zolpidem	In particular, gait issues most likely to arise with onset and peak of medication's action, usually ½–2 hr after benzodiazepine or hypnotic is taken.
Antidepressants	Tricyclic antidepressants (TCAs), such as amitriptyline; selective serotonin reuptake inhibitors (SSRIs), such as sertraline, citalopram	Orthostatic hypotension risk, typically worse with TCA compared with SSRI use.
Neuroleptics and antipsychotics including atypical or second-generation antipsychotics (SGA)	Neuroleptics, including haloperidol; SGA including risperidone	Orthostatic hypotension and dizziness risk significant and extrapyramidal movement risk.
Opioid analgesics/antagonists	Meperidine, morphine, codeine	Risk of sedation; meperidine particularly problematic. Pain should be appropriately and adequately treated and opioids used if benefit outweighs risk and with careful monitoring.
Insulin, oral hypoglycemics	Insulins, short-acting and longer acting; sulfonylureas, such as glyburide, glipizide	Fall risk most often seen in presence of drug-induced hypoglycemia. If this occurs, it is most likely noted at drug's peak of action. Glyburide use in the older adult is not advised due to higher rate of adverse effects with its use when compared to other sulfonylureas.
Cardiac medications	Antihypertensives including diuretics, calcium channel blockers (CCBs), high-dose beta blockers, and nitrates	Fall risk increases with excessive diuretic use because of circulating volume constriction or peripheral vasodilation related to CCB or nitrate use. With high-dose beta blocker use, normative heart rate increase with position change can be blunted, resulting in dizziness.

Note: This list is not intended to include all medications associated with increased fall risk in older adults but rather to highlight products with well-documented risk.
Source: Patient Safety Authority. Medication assessment: One determinant of falls risk. Available at: www.patientsafetyauthority.org/ADVISORIES/AdvisoryLibrary/2008/Mar5(1)/Pages/16.aspx.

Incontinence

70. Factors that contribute to stress incontinence include:
    A. detrusor overactivity.
    B. pelvic floor weakness.
    C. urethral stricture.
    D. urinary tract infection (UTI).

71. Factors that contribute to urge incontinence include:
    A. detrusor overactivity.
    B. pelvic floor weakness.
    C. urethral stricture.
    D. UTI.

72. An 82-year-old man presents with his caretaker who reports new-onset urinary incontinence occurring in the past 3 days. Diagnostic evaluation should include:
    A. PSA testing.
    B. urine culture with susceptibility testing.
    C. ultrasound of the bladder.
    D. urine stream flow assessment.

73. Pharmacological intervention for patients with urge incontinence includes the use of:
    A. doxazosin (Cardura).
    B. tolterodine (Detrol).
    C. finasteride (Proscar).
    D. pseudoephedrine (Sudafed).

386 CHAPTER 16 ■ Older Adults

74. Intervention for patients with stress incontinence includes:
    A. establishing a voiding schedule.
    B. gentle bladder-stretching exercises.
    C. periurethral bulking agent injection.
    D. restricting fluid intake.

75. Which form of urinary incontinence is most common in older adults?
    A. stress
    B. urge
    C. iatrogenic
    D. overflow

76. Medications used to treat urge incontinence and overactive bladder usually have anticholinergic and antimuscarinic effects that can lead to problems in older adults including:
    A. tachycardia and hypertension.
    B. sedation and dry mouth.
    C. agitation and excessive saliva production.
    D. loose stools and loss of appetite.

77. Poorly controlled diabetes mellitus is a potential cause of reversible urinary incontinence primarily caused by which of the following mechanisms?
    A. increased urinary volume
    B. increased UTI risk
    C. irritating effect of increased glucose in the urine
    D. decreased ability to perceive need to void

78. A 78-year-old woman who has osteoarthritis affecting both knees but no current problems with urinary incontinence is placed on a loop diuretic. She is now at increased risk for _____ urinary incontinence.
    A. overflow
    B. urge
    C. functional
    D. idiopathic

79. The diagnosis of _____ should be considered in an older adult with new-onset urinary incontinence coupled with an acute change in mental status.
    A. dementia
    B. spinal cord compression
    C. bladder stone
    D. delirium

Answers

70. B.	74. C.	78. C.
71. A.	75. B.	79. D.
72. B.	76. B.	
73. B.	77. A.	

Urinary incontinence is the involuntary loss of urine in sufficient amounts to be a problem. This condition is often thought by many elderly adults, women in particular, to be a normal part of aging. In reality, numerous treatment options are available after the cause of urinary incontinence is established (Table 16–6). In all cases, urinalysis and urine culture and susceptibility should be obtained. If UTI is present, treatment with an appropriate antimicrobial is indicated. Further diagnostic testing should be directed by patient presentation.

Urge incontinence is the most common form of urinary incontinence in elderly persons. Behavioral therapy, including a voiding schedule and gentle bladder stretching, are helpful. Pharmacological intervention is indicated in conjunction with behavioral therapy (Table 16–6). Medication such as tolterodine (Detrol) and solifenacin succinate (VESIcare) are selective muscarinic receptor antagonists that block bladder receptors and limit bladder contraction. Helpful in the treatment of urge incontinence, the use of these products is associated with a decrease in the numbers of micturitions and of incontinent episodes, along with an increase in voiding volume. Oxybutynin (Ditropan) is a nonselective muscarinic receptor antagonist that blocks receptors in the bladder and oral cavity, with activity similar to that of tolterodine; adverse effects include dry mouth and constipation with increased risk for fecal impaction. An over-the-counter oxybutynin transdermal patch (Oxytrol for Women, 3.9 mg/day) is available for use in women only with overactive bladder. Darifenacin (Enablex) and fesoterodine fumarate (Toviaz) are newer anticholinergic agents approved for urge incontinence. Compared with older agents, darifenacin is associated with fewer adverse effects, such as confusion, and may be more helpful in older patients with underlying dementia. Mirabegron (Myrbetriq), a beta-3 adrenoceptor agonist, has been shown to be effective in treatment-naïve patients as well as those who fail therapy with anticholinergic agents. Botulinum toxin injections in the bladder have also been approved and can be effective for those who fail or are intolerant of pharmacological treatment. Common to virtually all medications with systemic anticholinergic effect is the risk of sedation and alteration in sensorium (Table 16–7). Among the treatments used for urinary incontinence, oxybutynin tends to have the greatest anticholinergic effects that can impact the tolerability in older adults.

Numerous conditions can contribute to urinary incontinence transiently or permanently. Potentially treatable causes of urinary incontinence are represented in the *DIAPPERS* mnemonic:

Delirium
Infection (urinary tract)
Atrophic urethritis and vaginitis
Pharmaceuticals (diuretics, others)
Psychological disorders (depression)
Excessive urine output (heart failure, hyperglycemia)
Restricted mobility
Stool impaction

DISCUSSION SOURCES

Katzung B. Special aspects in geriatric pharmacology. In: Katzung B. *Basic and Clinical Pharmacology*, ed. 12. New York: McGraw Medical; 2011 pp 1051-1060.

Vasavada SP. Urinary incontinence. Available at: http://emedicine.medscape.com/article/452289-overview.

Resnick NM. Urinary incontinence in the elderly. *Medical Grand Rounds* 3:281–290, 1984.

Weiss B. Selecting medications for the treatment of urinary incontinence. *Am Fam Physician* 71(2):315–322, 2005. Available at: www.aafp.org/afp/20050115/315.html.

Vaugan CP, Goode PS, Burgio KL, Markland AD. Urinary incontinence in older adults. *Mt Sinai J Med* 78:558–570, 2011.

Driving Issues in Older Adults

80. Which of the following is a true statement with regard to driving and the elderly?
A. The number of elderly drivers will decrease over the next decade.
B. Crashes with elderly drivers tend to involve diminished speed of visual processing.
C. There is a greater incidence of accidents involving right-hand turns compared with left-hand turns.
D. There is no evidence to suggest, if the elder's health is preserved, that the skills needed for safe driving deteriorate with age.

81. Which of the following is a false statement with regard to driving and Alzheimer's-type dementia (AD)?
A. Patients with AD typically continue to drive for at least 3 years following the diagnosis.
B. Those with mild-to-moderate AD have an eight-fold increase in the number of accidents.
C. Those at early stages of AD can continue to drive safely, though driving should be monitored regularly.
D. The National Transportation and Safety Board recommends surrendering the driver's license for all individuals with an AD diagnosis.

82. Common driving errors observed with older drivers include all of the following except:
A. difficulty backing up and making turns.
B. delayed glare recovery when driving at night.
C. bumping into curbs and objects.
D. tailgating.

83. When counseling an older driver, you recommend all of the following except:
A. reviewing current medications for potential adverse effects.
B. that having the radio on to an enjoyable talk show enhances driving skills.
C. predetermining the route before driving.
D. driving during the day and in good weather.

Answers

80. B.   **81.** D.   **82.** D.   **83.** B.

With the aging of the population, there are more elderly drivers on the roads. Census data predict that by 2020, there will be 53 million persons in the United States more than the age of 65 years, and approximately 40 million will be licensed drivers. Though being older does not necessarily turn a person into an unsafe driver, it is important to note that age-related changes can affect driving skills. These changes not only include diminished vision and hearing but also musculoskeletal changes that can increase the time to react to changes on the road or the ability to immediately hit the brakes when necessary. Cognitive changes can decrease the attention span of older drivers who often become more easily distracted. Those with Alzheimer's-type dementia (AD) can have a changed way of thinking and behaving. This can include forgetting familiar routes or how to drive safely and can lead to more driving mistakes or "close calls." Though people at early stages of AD are often able to drive safely for a period of time, driving ability will be affected as the disease worsens and caregivers should monitor driving behavior. Patients with AD typically do not stop driving for at least 3 years after the initial diagnosis. There is an eight-fold increase in accidents by drivers with mild-to-moderate AD.

Older driver accidents tend to be related to diminished speed of visual processing and often involve multiple vehicle events that occur at intersections and involve left-hand turns. Common driving errors made by older adults include:
- Difficulty backing up and making turns
- Not seeing traffic signs and other cars quickly enough
- Difficulty in locating and retrieving information from dashboard displays and traffic signs
- Delayed glare recovery when driving at night
- Not checking rearview mirrors and blind spots
- Bumping into curbs and objects
- Not yielding to oncoming traffic and right-of-way vehicles
- Irregular or slow vehicle speeds
- Difficulty with situations requiring quick decision making

Unfortunately, there are no reliable objective measures available to assess driving competency in older adults. Neuropsychiatric testing cannot be used to indicate the level of impairment at which patients are not fit to drive. Additionally, the Folstein Mini-Mental Status Examination (MMSE) has not been demonstrated to reliably predict driver risk. The Clinical Dementia Rating (CDR) can be helpful but is impractical for routine screening practice. The American Academy of Neurology advocates on-road testing for dementia patients with a CDR score of 0.5 or higher. The American Medical Association recommends two tools for screening older drivers. First, the Physician's Guide to Assessing and Counseling Older Drivers can help healthcare providers identify patients at risk for crashes, help enhance their driving safety, and ease the transition to driving retirement if and when it becomes necessary. Second, the National Highway Traffic and Safety Administration: Part B of the Trail Making Test and the Clock Drawing Test can be used to assess driving skills. There is a significant correlation with misplacement of the minute hand with the incidence of crashes, straddling of lanes during driving, and total hazardous errors.

When counseling older adults on driver safety, several steps can be taken to improve safety:

- Exercise regularly to increase strength and flexibility.
- Review prescription and OTC medications to reduce adverse effects that can impair driving.
- Have eyes checked annually and wear glasses or corrective lenses as needed.
- Drive during daylight and good weather.
- Plan the route before you drive.
- Find the safest route with well-lit streets and ample, easy to locate parking.
- Maintain a large following distance behind the car in front.
- Avoid distractions in the car, such as a radio other than soft, background music, talking on the cell phone, texting, and eating.
- Consider potential alternatives to driving, such as riding with a friend or using public transit.

DISCUSSION SOURCES

AMA Physician's Guide to Assessing and Counseling Older Drivers. Available at: www.ama-assn.org//ama/pub/physician-resources/public-health/promoting-healthy-lifestyles/geriatric-health/older-driver-safety/assessing-counseling-older-drivers.

Illness Assessment and Atypical Presentations

84. Which of the following is a true statement with regard to disease presentation in older adults?
    A. Normal age-related changes do not alter the way an illness presents.
    B. Diseases in the elderly are usually more difficult to treat because they present at later stages.
    C. A mild decline in memory and information processing is not a normal age-related change.
    D. Diseases usually present at earlier stages due to impaired compensatory systems.

85. When evaluating illness symptoms in older patients, the disease often presents in a manner different from younger adults due to:
    A. polypharmacy.
    B. increased physiological responses to illness.
    C. normal age-related decline.
    D. increased compensatory mechanisms.

86. In older adults, heart failure can be precipitated by:
    A. mild hypothyroidism.
    B. hyperparathyroidism.
    C. mild hyperkalemia.
    D. mild hyponatremia.

Answers

84. D.   85. C.   86. A.

Although the mechanics of illness assessment are similar when evaluating younger and older adults, certain principles must be remembered to ensure accurate interpretation of history and physical examination findings in older adults. Normal age-related changes must be differentiated from indicators of illness. Examples of age-related changes include an increased anterior–posterior chest diameter, the presence of a corneal ring, and decreased skin turgor.

Specific organ systems can be particularly affected by age-related decline, most notably neurological, cardiovascular, musculoskeletal, and lower urinary tract systems. Because of the weakness in these four organ systems, the strain of illness or disease in any body system will tend to manifest in one of these four. Therefore, in the older patient, the organ system associated with a particular abnormality or clinical finding is less likely to be the source of the symptoms when compared with a younger patient. Some common symptoms observed in older patients that can indicate a more serious illness include acute confusion, depression, falls, incontinence, and syncope. Some common disease presentations include:

- UTI presents as confusion and/or urinary incontinence.
- Myocardial infarction presents as confusion.
- Pneumonia presents as a falling episode.

When assessing disease in the elderly, it is also important to consider that diseases usually present at an earlier stage when compared with younger patients. This is a result of normal, age-related decline in compensatory mechanisms. As a result, these conditions are generally easier to treat.

Atypical presentations frequently observed in the elderly include:

- Heart failure can be precipitated by mild hypothyroidism
- Mild hyperparathyroidism can result in significant cognitive dysfunction
- Mild prostate hypertrophy can result in urinary retention
- Mild glucose intolerance can result in nonketotic coma

DISCUSSION SOURCES

Merck Manual of Geriatrics: Evaluation of the Elderly Patient, available at http://www.merckmanuals.com/professional/geriatrics/approach_to_the_geriatric_patient/evaluation_of_the_elderly_patient.html.

Katzung B. Special aspects in geriatric pharmacology. In: Katzung B. *Basic and Clinical Pharmacology*, ed. 12. New York: McGraw Medical; 2011, pp 1051-1060.

Pressure Ulcers

87. Risk factors for pressure ulcers include all of the following except:
    A. malnutrition.
    B. dehydration.
    C. smoking.
    D. weight gain.

88. Complications of pressure ulcers include all of the following except:
   A. squamous cell carcinoma.
   B. osteoporosis.
   C. bone and joint infections.
   D. cellulitis.

89. A pressure ulcer that exhibits full-thickness skin loss with a crater-like appearance can be categorized as:
   A. stage 1.
   B. stage 2.
   C. stage 3
   D. stage 4.

90. Appropriate treatment of a stage 1 pressure ulcer can include all of the following except:
   A. ensuring proper nutrition and hydration of the patient.
   B. regular repositioning of the patient.
   C. debridement of non-vital skin.
   D. special padding for vulnerable skin areas.

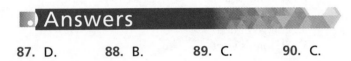

Answers

87. D.   **88. B.**   **89. C.**   **90. C.**

Pressure ulcers (also known as bedsores or pressure sores) are injuries to the skin that result from prolonged pressure on the skin. Normally, there is a balance between pressure intensity and duration with tissue tolerability. Pressure ulcers occur when vascular pressure inhibits adequate supply of blood to the skin and underlying tissue. Significant contributing factors include sustained pressure, friction, shear, and nutritional debilitation. Pressure ulcers are most commonly observed in individuals who have medical conditions that limit their ability to change positions, require the use of a wheelchair, or are confined to a bed for prolonged periods. Other risk factors include high moisture, advanced age, low blood pressure, smoking, elevated body temperature, lack of sensory perception, weight loss, urinary or fecal incontinence, decreased mental awareness, and dehydration. Some conditions can mimic pressure ulcers and should be considered during evaluation, such as fungal and yeast infection, malignancy, venous and arterial ulcers, and neuropathic ulcers. Complications of pressure ulcers include sepsis, cellulitis, and bone and joint infections. Chronic, nonhealing wounds can also increase the risk of an aggressive type of squamous cell carcinoma (Marjolin's ulcer).

Prevention of pressure ulcers requires routine evaluation of patients at risk. This evaluation can involve using the Braden scale or Norton scale that measures the physical and mental condition of the patient, as well as the state of nutrition, mobility, and continence. Regular nutritional and hydration assessment is also important to evaluate risk for pressure ulcers. Position changes are critical in prevention. For patients confined to a bed, repositioning should be done every 2 hours. Special cushions, foam mattress pads, and air- or water-filled mattresses can be helpful in keeping a patient in a certain position and relieve pressure on vulnerable skin. The head of the bed should be elevated no more than 30 degrees to prevent shearing. Those in wheelchairs should change position as much as possible on their own every 15 minutes and should have assistance with changing positions every hour.

Pressure ulcers are categorized into four categories based on their severity.

- Stage 1: a nonblanchable erythema is present on intact skin (induration may be present)
- Stage 2: presence of epidermal or dermal skin loss; can appear as an intact blister
- Stage 3: full-thickness skin loss with exposure of some amount of fat; ulcer has a crater-like appearance
- Stage 4: full-thickness skin and tissue loss; wound exposes muscle, bone, and tendons

Stage 1 and stage 2 pressure ulcers can usually heal within several weeks to months of general care that manages risks for pressure ulcers. Stage 3 and stage 4 ulcers are more difficult to treat and efforts may primarily focus on managing pain rather than complete healing of the wound. Debridement can be used to remove dead tissue, and regular cleaning and dressing the wounds are needed to promote healing and prevent infection.

DISCUSSION SOURCES

Jaul E. Assessment and management of pressure ulcers in the elderly: Current strategies. *Drugs Aging* 27:311–325, 2010.

Delirium, Dementia, and Depression

91 to 95. Identify the following as most likely associated with delirium or dementia.

____ **91.** Insidious onset over months to years

____ **92.** Acute onset of change in mental status

____ **93.** Associated with use of medications with anticholinergic effect

____ **94.** Mental status potentially returns to pre illness baseline

____ **95.** No perceptual disturbances (i.e., hallucinations) until later disease

96. The most common trigger for delirium is:
   A. alcohol withdrawal.
   B. fecal impaction.
   C. head trauma.
   D. acute infection.

97. The most common etiology of dementia is:
    A. vascular disease.
    B. Alzheimer's disease.
    C. traumatic head injury.
    D. drug-drug interaction induced.

98. Medications that commonly contribute to delirium include all of the following except:
    A. first-generation antihistamines.
    B. cardioselective beta-adrenergic antagonists.
    C. opioids.
    D. benzodiazepines.

99. Which of the following electrolyte disorders is commonly associated with delirium?
    A. hyponatremia.
    B. hypernatremia.
    C. hyperkalemia.
    D. hypophosphatemia.

100. Older adults are at greater risk of subdural hematoma, even with minor head trauma, due to:
    A. lower bone density in the skull.
    B. relatively fragile blood vessels.
    C. decreased adipose tissue reserves.
    D. age-related reduction in circulating clotting factors.

101. When discussing the use of a cholinesterase inhibitor with a 72-year-old woman with a recent diagnosis of Alzheimer's-type dementia and her family, you report that:
    A. this medication will help return memory to her pre-illness baseline.
    B. the risk associated with the use of this medication outweighs its benefits.
    C. this medication will likely afford clear, although minor and time-limited, benefits.
    D. the medication should have been started earlier to help prevent any change in cognition.

102. When managing dementia, cholinesterase inhibitors offer the greatest benefit:
    A. for prevention of Alzheimer's-type dementia.
    B. in patients with mild cognitive impairment.
    C. in patients with mild-to-moderate AD.
    D. in patients with severe AD.

103. When assessing a 76-year-old man with new-onset mental status change, all of the following diagnostic tests are essential except:
    A. serum glucose.
    B. PET scan.
    C. CBC with white blood cell differential.
    D. ECG.

104. A 81-year-old man who was recently diagnosed with Alzheimer's-type dementia is accompanied by his granddaughter for an office visit. The granddaughter reports that her grandfather often acts erratic with angry outbursts that can soon be followed by a more "normal" demeanor. She reports that the grandfather recently moved in with her, and she would like for this to continue as long as possible. In counseling the granddaughter, you consider all of the following except:
    A. behavioral difficulties often arise in patients with AD if their usual routine is disrupted.
    B. treatment with a cholinesterase inhibitor will likely improve his mental status to a point similar to his pre-dementia baseline.
    C. a home safety evaluation should be conducted and appropriate modification performed.
    D. any sudden change in mental status should be reported to the healthcare provider as soon as possible.

105. Which of the following supplements is used to potentially slow cognitive decline in AD?
    A. vitamin B12
    B. vitamin E
    C. ginkgo biloba
    D. St. John's wort

106. The NMDA receptor antagonist memantine works via:
    A. slowing the death of neurons in the brain.
    B. creating an environment that allows for storage and retrieval of information.
    C. promoting more rapid transduction of nerve signals.
    D. a largely unknown mechanism.

107. Potential noncognitive reasons for behavioral issues observed in older adults include all of the following except:
    A. ADHD.
    B. pain.
    C. infection.
    D. depression.

108 to 110. Match the term with its correct definition.
    108. Aphasia   A. failure to recognize objects despite intact sensory function
    109. Apraxia
    110. Agnosia   B. language disturbance
                      C. impairment of motor activities despite intact motor function

111. The use of antipsychotic medications in older adults is associated with an increased risk for:
    A. stroke and cardiovascular events.
    B. hypoglycemia.
    C. delirium.
    D. hypertension.

112. Dementia syndrome or cognitive impairment that is associated with severe depression is called:
    A. delirium.
    B. pseudodementia.
    C. Alzheimer's disease.
    D. bipolar disorder.

113. When managing depression in older adults, all of the following should be considered except:
   A. start at the highest dose possible of antidepressant and then titrate down once symptoms resolve.
   B. encourage psychotherapy in addition to pharmacotherapy.
   C. utilize electroconvulsive therapy for severe depression.
   D. conduct a medication review to minimize potential drug-drug interactions.

Answers

91.	Dementia	99.	A.	107.	A.
92.	Delirium.	100.	B.	108.	B.
93.	Delirium.	101.	C.	109.	C.
94.	Delirium.	102.	C.	110.	A.
95.	Dementia	103.	B.	111.	A.
96.	D.	104.	B.	112.	B.
97.	B.	105.	B.	113.	A.
98.	B.	106.	B.		

Delirium is a condition in which the patient exhibits an acute onset, over hours to a few days, of reduced ability to maintain attention to external stimuli and shift attention appropriately to new stimuli. The result is disorganized thinking. Two or more of the following are usually noted: an altered level of consciousness from baseline; memory impairment; perceptual disturbance, such as hallucinations; altered sleep; change in psychomotor activity; and disorientation to time, place, and person. Delirium is not a diagnosis but rather a clinical state caused by an underlying health problem. Following is the *DELIRIUMS* mnemonic, which can serve as a helpful memory aid regarding the most common causes of delirium.

- *D*rugs—When any medication is added or dose is adjusted. Particularly problematic medications include anticholinergics (tricyclic antidepressants [TCAs], first-generation antihistamines), neuroleptics (haloperidol, others), opioids (in particular, meperidine), long-acting benzodiazepines (diazepam, clonazepam), and alcohol.
- *E*motional (mood disorders, loss); *E*lectrolyte disturbance, especially hyponatremia.
- *L*ow PO2 (hypoxemia from CAP, COPD, PE, MI); *L*ack of drugs (withdrawal from alcohol, other habituating substances).
- *I*nfection—Urinary tract infection and community-acquired pneumonia (the most common delirium trigger).
- *R*etention of urine or feces; *R*educed sensory input (blindness, deafness, darkness, change in surroundings).
- *I*ctal or postictal state—Alcohol withdrawal is a common reason for an isolated first seizure in an older adult.
- *U*nder-nutrition—Protein/calorie, vitamin B12, or folate deficiency, dehydration including postoperative volume disturbance.

- *M*etabolic (poorly controlled diabetes mellitus, under-treated or untreated hypothyroidism or hyperthyroidism); *M*yocardial problems (myocardial infarction, heart failure, dysrhythmia).
- *S*ubdural hematoma—Can be as a result of relatively minor head trauma to brain atrophy, fragile vessels.

The evaluation of a patient with delirium should be focused on defining the underlying cause. A thorough health history, including social and home assessment, and a physical examination should be conducted. A standardized evaluation of mental status must be included in the evaluation. The evaluation of the patient with mental status change starts with a comprehensive health history and physical examination. Diagnostic testing should be focused to reveal the diagnosis of the underlying etiology with potentially reversible conditions (Table 16–6).

Delirium treatment is aimed at assessing patients at greatest risk to help avoid its occurrence. When delirium occurs, treatment is focused on the condition's underlying cause. Mental status should return to baseline with recovery, although ongoing research suggests that perhaps this recovery is incomplete in some individuals. In about two-thirds of all patients with delirium, the condition resolves within 1 week of onset.

Dementia is defined by a chronic loss of intellectual or cognitive function of sufficient severity to interfere with social or occupational function; this condition is a symptom of an underlying diagnosis (Table 16–7). In dementia, mental status changes can evolve insidiously over months or years with a gradually worsening course. The most common causes of dementia are Alzheimer's-type and multi-infarct or vascular

TABLE 16-6
Evaluation of the Person With Mental Status Change

The evaluation of the patient with mental status change starts with a comprehensive health history and physical examination. Diagnostic testing should be focused to reveal the underlying etiology with potentially reversible conditions.

Definite	As Directed by Patient Presentation
BUN, Cr	Brain imaging (CT vs. MRI)
Glucose	PET scan
Calcium	Toxic screen
Sodium	CXR
Hepatic enzymes	ESR
Vitamin B12/folate	HIV
TSH	Additional studies as needed
RPR	
CBC with WBC differential	
UA, U C & S	
ECG	

TABLE 16-7
Dementia Etiology

Dementia Type	Comment
Alzheimer's-type	60%–80%
Vascular (multi-infarct) dementia	10%–20%
Parkinson disease	5%
Miscellaneous causes	HIV, dialysis encephalopathy, neurosyphilis, normal pressure hydrocephalus, others

(language disturbance); apraxia (impairment of motor activities despite intact motor function); agnosia (failure to recognize objects despite intact sensory function); and executive functioning disturbance (planning, organizing, sequencing, abstracting). The deficits cause a significant impairment that represents a considerable decline from previous level of function.

In addition to behavior and supportive therapies, patients with dementia often benefit from the use of a cholinesterase inhibitor, such as donepezil (Aricept), tacrine (Cognex), rivastigmine (Exelon), galantamine (Razadyne), or a NMDA-receptor antagonist, such as memantine (Namenda). These classes of medications have different mechanisms of action and can be given together and have a demonstrated, although minor and time-limited, effect in dementia care (Table 16–9); the use of these products to prevent dementia is currently not supported.

Pseudodementia is a dementia syndrome or cognitive impairment that is associated with severe depression. Its onset is often well demarcated as compared with the gradual and insidious development of dementia. Patients with pseudodementia

dementia. The evaluation of a person with suspected dementia is similar to assessment in delirium; the two conditions often overlap and can mimic each other (Table 16–8). Diagnosis of Alzheimer's-type dementia (AD) requires a gradual onset of memory impairment plus one or more of the following: aphasia

TABLE 16-8
Delirium versus Dementia

	Delirium	Dementia
DEFINED	A sudden state of rapid changes in brain function reflected in confusion, changes in cognition, activity, and level of consciousness	A slowly developing impairment of intellectual or cognitive function that is progressive and interferes with normal functioning
ETIOLOGY	Precipitated by acute underlying cause, such as an acute illness	Various causes
ONSET	Abrupt onset, over hours to days, usually a precise date, rapidly progressive change in mental status	Insidious onset that cannot be related to a precise date, gradual change in mental status
MEMORY	Impaired by variable recall	Memory loss, especially for recent events
DURATION	Duration hours to days	Duration months to years
REVERSIBLE?	Usually reversible to baseline mental status when underlying illness resolved	Chronically progressive and irreversible
SLEEP DISTURBANCE	Disturbed sleep-wake cycle, with hour-to-hour variability, often worse as the day progresses	Disturbed sleep-wake cycle but lacks hour-to-hour variability, often day-night reversal
PSYCHOMOTOR	Change in psychomotor activity, either hyperkinetic (25%), hypoactive (25%), or mixed (35%); no change in motor activity in approximately 15%	No psychomotor changes until later in disease
PERCEPTUAL DISTURBANCES	Perceptual disturbances including hallucinations	No perceptual disturbances until later disease.
SPEECH	Speech content incoherent, confused with a wide variety of often inappropriately used words such as misnamed persons and items	Speech content sparse, progressing to sparse speech content; mute in later disease

Note: Delirium and dementia often coexist. The diagnosis of delirium must be considered in the presence of a sudden-onset change in mental status in the individual with dementia.

Sources: Merck Manual: Overview of Delirium and Dementia. Available at: www.merckmanuals.com/professional/neurologic_disorders/delirium_and_dementia/overview_of_delirium_and_dementia.html#v1036234.

TABLE 16-9

American Academy of Neurology Standards for Care in Alzheimer's-type Dementia (AD)

Strategy	Comment
To slow decline in AD.	Vitamin E 1000 IU twice daily or selegiline 5 mg twice daily. No added benefit to using both products. The use of NSAIDs and postmenopausal hormone therapy has not been supported for this purpose.
In mild to moderate stage disease, the use of cholinesterase inhibitors is considered to be the mainstay of treatment. The use of these products in mild cognitive impairment, early AD, and severe AD is not supported though study on these issues is ongoing.	Cholinesterase inhibitors (donepezil [Aricept], rivastigmine [Exelon], galantamine [Razadyne]) have clear, although minor and time-limited benefits by increasing availability of cholinesterase. This small effect is clinically significant.
In moderate to severe AD, further studies of multiple interventions are needed.	Approved for use in moderate-to-severe AD, NMDA receptor antagonist memantine (Namenda). Through its effect on glutamate, helps to create an environment that allows for storage and retrieval of information. Also used in earlier disease with cholinesterase inhibitor. Donepezil also approved for use in more advanced disease.
Treat agitation and depression.	Approximately 40% of individuals with dementia will also have depression. SSRIs, select tricyclic antidepressants, and MAOIs (monoamine oxidase inhibitors) are appropriate treatment options, bearing in mind potential drug-drug and drug-food interactions.
Consider reasons (noncognitive) not related to AD for behavioral issues, such as behavioral disturbances.	Evaluate for depression, pain, infection, and other clinical conditions commonly found in older adults.
If environmental manipulation fails to eliminate agitation or psychosis in the person with dementia, consider treatment with psychotropic medication.	Antipsychotics best studied for this indication, recognizing the increased risk of stroke and cardiovascular events associated with the use of this drug class in older adults with dementia.

Source: Doody RS, et al. Practice parameter: Management of dementia (an evidence-based review): Report of the Quality Standards Subcommittee of the American Academy of Neurology. *Neurology* 56:1154–1166, 2001. Available at: www.neurology.org/content/56/9/1154.full.pdf.

can take increased effort to complete a mental status exam (MSE) but often do better on MSE questions with some encouragement and coaching. Neurocognitive testing may be needed to differentiate between pseudodementia and dementia. Treating the depression often improves cognition in these patients.

Depression in older adults is common but should not be considered a normal part of aging. Some estimates of major depression in older adults range from 1% to 5% for persons living in the community but rises to 13.5% for those who require home healthcare. Depression is also more common in those who have comorbid conditions (e.g., heart disease, cancer). Signs of depression in the elderly can be wide and varied:

- Feelings of hopelessness and/or pessimism
- Feelings of guilt, worthlessness, and/or helplessness
- Irritability and/or restlessness
- Loss of interest in activities or hobbies that were once pleasurable
- Fatigue and decreased energy
- Difficulty concentrating, remembering details, and making decisions
- Insomnia, early-morning wakefulness, or excessive sleeping

- Overeating or appetite loss
- Thoughts of suicide or suicide attempts
- Persistent aches and pains, headaches, cramps, or digestive problems that do not resolve, even with treatment

For those suspected of depression, several screening tools are available to aid in the diagnosis or indicate when further investigation is needed (Table 16–10). When considering treatment for depression, the patient should be encouraged to undergo psychotherapy in addition to any pharmacological treatment in order to work on building skills needed to help manage this usually long-term health problem. There are several types of antidepressant medications that can be used to treat depression, including SSRIs, SNRIs, tricyclic antidepressants (TCAs), and monoamine oxidase inhibitors (MAOIs). The type and degree of depression as well as the adverse effect profile must be considered when selecting an appropriate antidepressant. Some patients are candidates for other forms of intervention, particularly if there is an inadequate response to pharmacotherapy and/or psychotherapy; one option is electroconvulsive therapy (ECT). ECT is safe and effective for all older adults with severe depression,

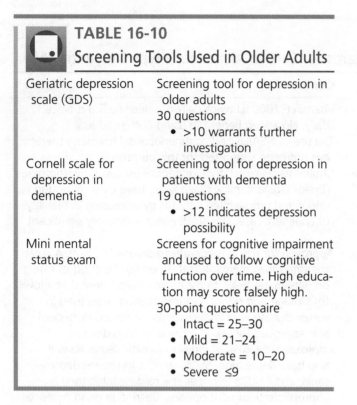

TABLE 16-10

Screening Tools Used in Older Adults

Geriatric depression scale (GDS)	Screening tool for depression in older adults 30 questions • >10 warrants further investigation
Cornell scale for depression in dementia	Screening tool for depression in patients with dementia 19 questions • >12 indicates depression possibility
Mini mental status exam	Screens for cognitive impairment and used to follow cognitive function over time. High education may score falsely high. 30-point questionnaire • Intact = 25–30 • Mild = 21–24 • Moderate = 10–20 • Severe ≤9

particularly in the presence of a psychosis and/or nutritional compromise.

When initiating pharmacotherapy for a variety of conditions, including mood disorders in older adults, it is important to start low, go slow, but get to goal. The latter point is important as there is a tendency to undertreat. As polypharmacy is frequent in older adults, healthcare providers must consider any potential drug-drug interactions; routine monitoring of renal and hepatic function is also recommended.

DISCUSSION SOURCES

Merck Manual: Overview of Delirium and Dementia. Available at: www.merckmanuals.com/professional/neurologic_disorders/del irium_and_dementia/overview_of_delirium_and_dementia.ht ml#v1036234.

Bottino CM, et al. Treatment of depression in older adults. *Curr Psychiatry Rep* 14:289–297, 2012.

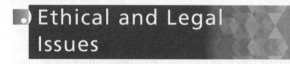

Ethical and Legal Issues

114. Which of the following statements is true with regard to decision making for the impaired patient?
A. Only a court or close family member can declare a person incompetent.
B. Impaired judgment can be used to declare a person incompetent.
C. Healthcare providers have the ability to determine whether a patient can provide informed consent.
D. Informed consent does not necessarily require disclosing the diagnosis to the patient.

115. The use of physical restraints in older adults is appropriate:
A. as a form of discipline.
B. when needed to meet a healthcare need.
C. to prevent wandering outside an institution.
D. under no circumstances.

116. When considering end-of-life decisions, which of the following statements is false?
A. Advanced directives include living wills and do not resuscitate (DNR) orders.
B. A videotaped or audiotaped discussion may include advanced directives.
C. Advanced directives are legally binding in all states.
D. Advanced directives are only recognized when the patient is hopelessly and terminally ill.

Answers

114. C.   **115.** B.   **116.** C.

When caring for older adults, there are particular legal and ethical issues that must be considered by healthcare providers. Due to age-related diminished cognitive function in many older adults, there is the issue of patient competence to make informed decisions. The law presumes that all adults are competent to make their own decisions regarding their healthcare. Only a court can declare a person incompetent and appoint a guardian to make decisions for them. It is important to remember that impaired judgment does not make a person incompetent. Healthcare providers have the ability to determine whether or not a patient has the ability to provide informed consent. When obtaining informed consent for healthcare treatment, it is essential that the patient has knowledge of the diagnosis, understands the nature and purpose of the procedure, understands the risks, benefits, and adverse effects of the procedure, and understands reasonable alternatives, if available.

Despite many older adults being physically and mentally active, they are often subjected to ageism. This is defined as the process of stereotyping, prejudice, or discrimination for or against the elderly. Ageism can diminish choice, independence, and dignity and can negatively impact quality of life. Common ageism stereotypes include the association of various physical or mental illnesses or disabilities with older age (e.g., memory loss or slow to understand things) as well as a lack of knowledge of new technologies or culture (e.g., computers, social media, etc.). The consequences of ageism on an individual can be substantial, including depression, employment discrimination, lower socioeconomic status, and conforming to the stereotyped image.

Physical restraints are commonly used in elderly patients in nonpsychiatric care settings, with one estimate of between 25% and 43% of residents in long-term care facilities being restrained at least once. The Omnibus Reconciliation Act of 1987 provides that every resident of long-term care facilities has the right to be free from physical or chemical restraints imposed for the purpose of discipline or convenience and not required to treat healthcare needs. Restraints are often seen as the only practical way to protect the safety of elderly patients and reduce the potential for liability if they injure themselves. However, when injury occurs to unrestrained individuals in the institutional setting, successful lawsuits are typically not the result of failure to restrain but a failure to meet reasonable standards of care—that is, there was negligence in duty to provide care for a wandering patient or alarm systems were not functional at the institution. Common alternatives for restraints include the use of alarms, using beds or chairs that are close to the floor, and/or ensuring the unit/floor/facility is equipped to care for a patient with known behaviors. If restraints are needed for patient safety, it is important for healthcare providers to have a thorough understanding of the risks and benefits of using restraints. This will be important in explaining the need for restraints to family members, who may see their use in a negative manner. Adverse effects of restraints include falls, pressure sores, depression, aggression, and even death. Physical restraints can also be a source of aggravation to the patient under restraint.

End-of-life decision making has become an important aspect of healthcare as technology has changed the circumstances of death, providing options on when, where, and how a patient dies. When considering end-of-life decisions for a terminally ill patient who cannot communicate, several approaches can be used. Often, an appointed person can make the decision based on the patient's past wishes and values. A rational approach can make the decision based on what a "rational" person would do under the circumstances. A substituted judgment approach attempts to determine what decision the patient would make if he/she was able.

Advanced directives are durable statements of intent based on the patient's last written wishes and can be used to help make end-of-life decisions. Advanced directives can exist in several forms. *Living wills* and *do not resuscitate* (DNR) orders are contracts between the patient and healthcare provider that specify wishes for end-of-life care in terminal events. A *durable power of attorney for healthcare* authorizes another person to make decisions regarding healthcare when the patient is no longer able (not to be confused with a *durable power of attorney*, which covers decisions regarding property and financial matters). Alternatively, a *values history* can be a written, videotaped, or audiotaped personal discussion that can contain advanced directives that can be taken into consideration when making end-of-life decisions. It is important to note that advanced directives are not legally binding and not all states recognize them in a legal sense. States that do recognize advanced directives only do so when the patient is, in the opinion of the healthcare provider, hopelessly and terminally ill.

DISCUSSION SOURCES

Ziglar SP. Physical restraints in the elderly: To use or not to use. http://nursing.advanceweb.com/Article/Physical-Restraints-in-the-Elderly-To-Use-or-Not-to-Use.aspx.

National Institute on Aging. End of life: Helping with comfort and care. www.nia.nih.gov/health/publication/end-life-helping-comfort-and-care/planning-end-life-care-decisions.

Author's Note

Please see Index for information on commonly encountered problems in older adults, including urinary tract infection, male and female genitourinary problems, endocrine disorders, pneumonia, chronic obstructive pulmonary disease, heart failure, and others.

Dr. Sally Miller's assistance in the development of this chapter is gratefully acknowledged.

Pediatrics

17

Breastfeeding

1. Which of the following is appropriate advice to give to a mother who is breastfeeding her 10-day-old infant?
   A. "Your milk will come in today."
   B. "To minimize breast tenderness, the baby should not be kept on either breast for more than 5 to 10 minutes."
   C. "A clicking sound made by the baby during feedings signifies a good latch and suck."
   D. "The baby's urine should be light or colorless."

2. Which of the following is appropriate advice to give to a mother who is breastfeeding her 12-hour-old infant?
   A. "You will likely have enough milk to feed the baby within a few hours of birth."
   B. "The baby might need to be awakened to be fed."
   C. "Supplemental feeding is needed unless the baby has at least four wet diapers in the first day of life."
   D. "The baby will likely have a seedy yellow bowel movement today."

3. Compared with the use of infant formula, advantages for the baby of breastfeeding include all of the following except:
   A. lower incidence of diarrheal illness.
   B. greater weight gain in the first few weeks of life.
   C. reduced risk of allergic disorders.
   D. lower occurrence of constipation.

4. At 3 weeks of age, the average-weight, formula-fed infant should be expected to take: mL
   A. 2 to 3 oz, or 60 to 90 mL, every 2 to 3 hours.
   B. 2 to 3 oz, or 60 to 90 mL, every 3 to 4 hours.
   C. 3 to 4 oz, or 90 to 118 mL, every 2 to 3 hours.
   D. 3 to 4 oz, or 90 to 118 mL, every 3 to 4 hours.

5. In infants, solid foods are best introduced no earlier than:
   A. 1 to 3 months.
   B. 3 to 5 months.
   C. 4 to 6 months.
   D. 6 to 8 months.

6. Nursing infants generally maximally receive about which percentage of the maternal dose of a drug?
   A. 1%
   B. 3%
   C. 5%
   D. 10%

7. Most drugs pass into breast milk through:
   A. active transport.
   B. facilitated transfer.
   C. simple diffusion.
   D. creation of a pH gradient.

8. To remove a drug from breast milk through "pump and dump," the nursing mother should refrain from taking the offending medication and the process must be continued for:
   A. two infant feeding cycles.
   B. approximately 8 hours.
   C. three to five half-lives of the drug.
   D. a period of time that is highly unpredictable.

9. When counseling a breastfeeding woman about alcohol use during lactation, you relate that:
   A. drinking a glass of wine or beer will enhance the let-down reflex.
   B. because of its high molecular weight, relatively little alcohol is passed into breast milk.
   C. maternal alcohol use causes a reduction in the amount of milk ingested by the infant.
   D. infant intoxication can be seen with mother's having as few as one to two alcoholic drinks.

10. A 23-year-old woman is breastfeeding her healthy newborn. She wishes to start using hormonal contraception. Which of the following represents the best regimen?
    A. combined oral contraception initiated at 2 weeks
    B. progesterone-only oral contraception initiated at 3 weeks
    C. medroxyprogesterone acetate (Depo-Provera) given day 1 postpartum
    D. use of all forms of hormonal contraception is discouraged during lactation

11. Guidelines recommend that a breastfeeding mother waits until breastfeeding is well established for approximately 6 months before using combined oral contraceptives (COC) because:
    A. in early breastfeeding, the amount of hormone in COC could cause significant harm to the nursing infant.
    B. efficacy of COC could be compromised by breastfeeding.
    C. milk flow could be compromised by COC.
    D. COC oral contraceptive use could affect mother's sleep patterns.

12. At what point after childbirth can a combined oral contraceptive be started without other risk factors for venous thrombosis in a woman who is not breastfeeding?
    A. 1 day
    B. 1 week
    C. 3 weeks
    D. 6 weeks

13. The anticipated average daily weight gain during the first 3 months of life is approximately:
    A. 15 g or 0.53 oz.
    B. 20 g or 0.7 oz.
    C. 25 g or 0.88 oz.
    D. 30 g or 1 oz.

14. The average required caloric intake in an infant from age 0 to 3 months is usually:
    A. 40 to 60 kcal/kg/d.
    B. 60 to 80 kcal/kg/d.
    C. 80 to 100 kcal/kg/d.
    D. 100 to 120 kcal/kg/d.

_____ 15. Regarding physiologic jaundice in the newborn, select all that are correct:
    A. It occurs between the first 12 and 24 hours of life.
    B. It progresses from the abdomen toward the head of the infant.
    C. Unconjugated bilirubin is elevated.
    D. Risk of development of hyperbilirubinemia can be reduced in a breastfed infant with frequent breastfeeding every 2 to 3 hours per 24 hours.
    E. It can be avoided by supplemental water and dextrose feedings between breastfeeding in the first 3 to 4 days of life to increase infant hydration while awaiting mother's milk to come in.

● Answers

1. D.	6. A.	11. C.
2. B.	7. C.	12. C.
3. B.	8. C.	13. D.
4. A.	9. C.	14. D.
5. C.	10. B.	15. C and D.

Breastfeeding provides the ideal form of nutrition during infancy. According to the Centers for Disease Control and Prevention (CDC), in the United States, approximately 77% of all infants are breastfed at birth, with about 49% of all infants continuing at age 6 months. Healthcare providers can help influence successful breastfeeding. Although the content of commercially prepared formula available in the developed world continues to be improved with composition closer to breast milk, infant formula continues to lack critically important components. Breast milk contains immunoactive factors that help protect infants against infectious disease and may reduce the frequency of allergic disorders. Human milk transfers the mother's antibodies to disease to the infant. About 80% of the cells in breast milk are macrophages, cells that kill bacteria, fungi, and viruses. In contrast to formula-fed infants, a breastfed infant's digestive tract contains large amounts of *Lactobacillus bifidus,* beneficial bacteria that prevent the growth of harmful organisms.

To promote milk production and reduce the risk of developing physiologic jaundice, a new mother should be advised to keep well hydrated and breastfeed a minimum of 8, preferably 12, times per 24 hours. Supplementing feeding with dextrose and water or formula should be avoided because this will interfere with the newborn's hunger drive to breastfeed and will delay and reduce breast milk production. Physiologic jaundice usually presents between days 3 and 5 and results from to the normal breakdown of fetal hemoglobin and immature liver metabolism. Unconjugated bilirubin is elevated in this process. If there is an increase in conjugated bilirubin or jaundice occurs in the first 24 hours of life, pathological etiologies need to be considered, such as an ABO incompatibility, familial Gilbert syndrome, or other anomaly.

If an infant is formula fed, the parents and caregivers should be encouraged to hold the infant during feeding to have the interaction inherent in breastfeeding. Questions about frequency, amount, and type of feedings are often asked during well-baby visits. Counseling should be offered to help ensure optimal nutrition (Box 17–1 and Table 17–1).

If a nursing mother becomes ill or has a chronic health problem, she is often erroneously advised to discontinue breastfeeding on the basis of the healthcare provider's incorrect assumption by that most medications are harmful to the infant. Most medications can be used during lactation, but the benefit of improved maternal health should be balanced against the risk of exposing an infant to medication.

Postpartum contraception is usually an important concern of new mothers. Some women opt not to breastfeed, fearing an inability to access reliable hormonal contraception while lactating. Many options are available, however, including the progestin-only pill (POP) and medroxyprogesterone acetate (Depo-Provera, Depo-SubQ Provera 104). For lactating women who wish to use an oral hormonal contraceptive, POP is highly effective and does not alter the quality or quantity of breast milk. One significant disadvantage of POP use is bleeding irregularity, ranging from prolonged flow to amenorrhea. Medroxyprogesterone acetate in a depot injection given every 90 days is a highly reliable form of contraception with 99.7%

BOX 17-1

Guidelines for Nutrition in the First Months of Life

■ Frequency of feeding during months 1 and 2
  Breastfed infants: A minimum of 10 minutes at each
    breast every 1.5 to 3 hours
  Bottle-fed infants: 2–3 oz (60–90 mL) every 2 to
    3 hours
■ Fluoride supplementation is advisable for breastfed
  infants or if formula is not mixed with fluoridated
  water in formula-fed infants
■ Solid foods are best introduced no sooner than age
  4 to 6 months
■ Signs that an infant is ready for solid food
  Doubled birth weight and at least 4 to 6 months
    of age
  Eats more than 32 oz (946 mL) formula per day or
    more than 8 to 10 feedings (breast or bottle) per day

Source: Nemours Foundation, http://kidshealth.org/parent
/nutrition_fit/nutrition/feednewborn.html, Feeding your newborn.

TABLE 17-1

Anticipated Weight Gain and Caloric Requirements in the First 3 Years of Life

Age	Anticipated Average Weight Gain per Day (g)	Required Kilocalorie per Kilogram per Day
0–3 mo	26–31	100–120 kcal
3–6 mo	17–18	105–115 kcal
6–9 mo	12–13	100–105 kcal
9–12 mo	9	100–105 kcal
1–3 yr	7–9	100 kcal

efficacy. Progestin-only oral contraceptive options can be started immediately postpartum if the woman is not breast-feeding and as early as 3 weeks postpartum if she is breast-feeding. A progestin-only implant (Nexplanon or Implanon) is also an option. Earlier use, starting less than 3 weeks postpartum, could diminish the quantity, but not quality, of breast milk. Nonsystemic contraceptive methods, such as barrier methods, intrauterine devices, and levonorgestrel intrauterine systems, are also acceptable.

Combined oral contraceptives, which utilize both estrogen and progesterone, could affect milk flow early postpartum and thus ideally should be avoided until the baby has been nursing for 6 months or longer and breastfeeding is well established. It is known that combined oral contraceptives can increase thromboembolic risk in women with

other risk factors for venous thrombosis (VTE), including aged 35 or older, history of VTE, thrombophilia, immobility, transfusion at delivery, a body mass index (BMI) of ≥30 kg/m². postpartum hemorrhage, postcesarean delivery, preeclampsia, or smoking. In women with lower VTE risk and not breastfeeding, COCs can be started as soon as 21 days postpartum.

Nearly all breastfeeding mothers use some type of medication (most often analgesic agents such as nonsteroidal anti-inflammatory drugs, acetaminophen, opioids, or antibiotics) in the first 2 weeks after giving birth. About 25% need to use medication intermittently to manage episodic disease. Such medications usually include analgesics, antihistamines, decongestants, and antibiotics.

About 5% of breastfeeding women have a chronic health problem necessitating daily use of a medication; the most common long-term medications used are for treating asthma, mental health problems, seizure disorder, and hypertension. Nursing infants usually get about 1%, often less, of the maternal dose, and only a few drugs are contraindicated.

The "pump-and-dump" procedure is not an effective means to reduce drug levels in a mother's milk because it creates an area of lower drug concentration in the empty breast. This enables the drug to diffuse from the area of high concentration (maternal serum) to the area of low concentration (breast milk). If the mother takes a medication that may be problematic for the nursing infant, she need to immediately stop taking the medication. Pumping and discarding the milk needs to continue for three to five drug-free half-lives of the medication.

Alcohol has a low molecular weight and is highly lipid soluble; both of these characteristics allow it to have easy passage into breast milk. Even in small amounts, alcohol ingestion by a nursing mother can cause a smaller amount of milk to be produced, reduction in the let-down reflex, and less rhythmic and frequent sucking by the infant, resulting in a smaller volume of milk ingested. Cigarette smoking is similarly problematic. Nicotine, a highly lipid-soluble substance with a low molecular weight, passes easily into breast milk. Maternal cigarette smoking can reduce milk supply and expose an infant to passive smoke. Infant crankiness, diarrhea, tachycardia, and vomiting have been reported with high maternal nicotine intake.

DISCUSSION SOURCES

Centers for Disease Control and Prevention Press Release: U.S. breastfeeding rates continue to rise, http://content.govdelivery.com/accounts/USCDC/bulletins/858447

Summary of Classifications for Hormonal Contraceptive Methods and Intrauterine Devices: Appendix L. *MMWR* 59:76–81, 2010.

Update to CDC's Medical Eligibility Criteria for Contraceptive Use, 2010. Revised Recommendations for the Use of Contraceptive Methods During Postpartum Period. *MMRW* 60: 878–883, 2011.

Briggs G, Freeman R, Yaffe S. *Drugs in Pregnancy and Lactation*, ed. 9. Philadelphia: Lippincott Williams & Wilkins, 2011.

Hale T. *Medications and Mothers' Milk, 2012*, ed. 76. Amarillo, TX: Pharmasoft Medical Publishers, 2012.

American Association of Clinical Chemistry Clinical Laboratory Notes June 2010: Bilirubin, http://aacc.org/publications/cln/2010 /june/pages/seriesarticle.aspx

Early Childhood Development

16. Which of the following is most consistent with a normal developmental examination for a 3-month-old infant born at 40 weeks' gestation?
    A. sitting briefly with support
    B. experimenting with sound
    C. rolling over
    D. having a social smile

17. Which of the following is most consistent with a normal developmental examination for a thriving 5-month-old infant born at 32 weeks' gestation?
    A. sitting briefly with support
    B. experimenting with sound
    C. rolling over
    D. performing hand-to-hand transfers

18. A healthy full-term infant at age 3 to 5 months should be able to:
    A. gesture to an object.
    B. bring hands together.
    C. reach for an object with one hand.
    D. feed self a biscuit.

19. A healthy infant at age 9 to 11 months is expected to:
    A. roll from back to stomach.
    B. imitate "bye-bye."
    C. play peek-a-boo.
    D. hand toy on request.

20. A healthy 2-year-old child is able to:
    A. speak in phrases of two or more words.
    B. throw a ball at a target.
    C. scribble spontaneously.
    D. ride a tricycle.

21. At which age would a child likely start to imitate housework?
    A. 18 months
    B. 24 months
    C. 30 months
    D. 36 months

22. A healthy 3-year-old child is expected to:
    A. give his or her first and last name.
    B. use pronouns.
    C. kick a ball.
    D. name a best friend.

23. A healthy 6- to 7-month-old infant is able to:
    A. roll from back to stomach.
    B. confidently feed self a cracker.
    C. reach for an object.
    D. crawl on abdomen.

24. You examine a healthy 9-month-old infant from a full-term pregnancy and expect to find that the infant:
    A. sits without support.
    B. cruises.
    C. has the ability to recognize his or her own name.
    D. imitates a razzing noise.

25. A healthy 3-year-old child is in your office for well-child care. You expect this child to be able to:
    A. name five colors.
    B. alternate feet when climbing stairs.
    C. speak in two-word phrases.
    D. tie shoelaces.

26. Which of the following would not be found in newborns?
    A. best vision at a range of 8 to 12 inches
    B. presence of red reflex
    C. light-sensitive eyes
    D. lack of defensive blink

27. Which of the following do you expect to find in an examination of a 2-week-old infant?
    A. a visual preference for the human face
    B. a preference for low-pitched voices
    C. indifference to the cry of other neonates
    D. poorly developed sense of smell

28. Which of the following is the most appropriate response in a developmental examination of a healthy 5-year-old child?
    A. being able to name a best friend
    B. giving gender appropriately
    C. naming an intended career
    D. hopping on one foot

29. You are examining an 18-month-old boy who is not speaking any discernible words. Mom tells you he has not said "mama or dada" yet or babbled or smiled responsively. You:
    A. encourage the mother to enroll her son in daycare to increase his socialization.
    B. conduct further evaluation of milestone attainment.
    C. reassure the parent that delayed speech is common in boys.
    D. order audiogram and tympanometry.

30. The following benchmarks indicate normal development by a healthy child born at term who is now 12-months of age (choose all that apply):
    A. talking in two-word sentences.
    B. pointing to a desired object.
    C. reaching to a desired object.
    D. walking backward.

31. It is considered a developmental "red flag" if a child does not respond to his or her name by nine months of age.
    A. true
    B. false

32. A child needs to demonstrate more than one developmental "red flag" to warrant further evaluation.
A. true
B. false

33. The presumptive diagnosis of fragile X syndrome can be confirmed by a blood test.
A. true
B. false

34. The following chromosomal syndrome is a common etiology of social and verbal developmental delays in boys:
A. Tay-Sachs disease.
B. cystic fibrosis.
C. fragile X.
D. trisomy 18.

35. One physical sign of fragile X syndrome in males includes:
A. large eyes.
B. large forehead.
C. small head.
D. recessive jaw.

36. Klinefelter syndrome is most commonly marked by:
A. language impairment in males.
B. fine motor delay in males.
C. hip and breast enlargement in women.
D. attention deficit disorder in males.

37. Klinefelter syndrome and risk for having a child with this condition can be accurately identified by (choose all that apply):
A. urine test.
B. literacy assessment.
C. amniocentesis.
D. blood testing for carrier state.

Answers

16. B.	24. C.	32. B.
17. B.	25. B.	33. A.
18. B.	26. D.	34. C.
19. C.	27. A.	35. B.
20. A.	28. A.	36. A.
21. A.	29. B.	37. C and D.
22. A.	30. B and C.	
23. A.	31. B.	

Performing a developmental assessment is one of the most important parts of providing pediatric primary care. Surveillance of growth and development and determining potential lags is essential to care of the child. Initiation of early intervention measures improves outcomes. The American Academy of Pediatrics (AAP) recommends routine screening for autism between 18 and 24 months (Table 17–2).

Table 17-2

Developmental "Red Flags" in the Young Child.

Persistent presence of ≥1 of the indicators warrants further evaluation.

- **By 6 months:** No big smiles or other warm, joyful expressions
- **By 9 months:** No back-and-forth sharing of sounds, smiles, or other facial expressions
- **By 12 months:** Lack of response to name
- **By 12 months:** No babbling or "baby talk"
- **By 12 months:** No back-and-forth gestures, such as pointing, showing, reaching, or waving
- **By 16 months:** No spoken words
- **By 24 months:** No meaningful two-word phrases that don't involve imitating or repeating

Source: First Signs; Available at www.firstsigns.org. Additional resource for screening, please see M-CHAT, www2.gsu.edu/~psydlr/Diana_L._Robins,_Ph.D._files/M-CHAT_new.pdf.

In addition to providing a marker for evaluating the child, the assessment also affords an important learning tool for the parents. Pointing out milestones to be achieved in the near future and their impact on safety can help the family prepare appropriately (Table 17–3).

An additional portion of primary care is to assess the child with altered development. Often, this is a result of a chromosomal abnormality. Fragile X syndrome, a chromosomal alteration, is the most common known cause of autism in either gender and occurs in all racial and ethnic groups. Another chromosomal anomaly, Klinefelter syndrome (XXY male), also is associated with developmental issues, mainly verbal in nature (Table 17–4).

DISCUSSION SOURCE

Burns, CE, et al. *Pediatric Primary Care*, ed. 5. Philadelphia: Elsevier Saunders, 2012.

Developmental Benchmarks and Anticipatory Guidance

38. At which of the following ages in an infant's life is parental anticipatory guidance about teething most helpful?
A. 1 to 2 months
B. 2 to 4 months
C. 4 to 6 months
D. 8 to 10 months

TABLE 17-3
Anticipated Early Childhood Developmental Milestones

Age	Able to Be Observed During Office Visit	Reported by Parent or Caregiver

Newborn	• Moves all extremities
	• Spontaneous stepping
	• Reacts to sound by blinking, turning
	• Responds to cries of other neonates
	• Well-developed sense of smell
	• Cries when uncomfortable
	• Preference for higher pitched voices
	• Primitive reflexes
	  • Tonic neck
	  • Palmar grasp
	  • Babinski response
	  • Rooting awake and asleep
	  • Sucking
		• Able to be calmed by feeding, cuddling
		• Reinforces presence of developmental tasks seen in examination room

1–2 mo	• Lifts head • Holds head erect • Regards face • Follows objects through visual field • Moro and palmar grasp reflexes fading	• Social smile • Recognizes parents
3–4 mo	• Grasps cube • Reaches for objects • Brings objects to mouth • Raspberry sound	• Laughs, squeals, vocalizes in response to others • Recognizes food by sight • Rolls back to side
5 mo	• Back straight when pulled to sitting • Bears weight on legs when standing • Plays with feet • Sits with support	• Imitates others • Repeats interesting actions • Coughs, snorts to attract attention
6–8 mo	• Sits without support • Scoops small object with rake grip; some thumb use • Hand-to-hand transfer • Imitates "bye-bye" • Stranger and separation anxiety begins (6 mo) and increases during this time period • Pulls feet into mouth	• Closes lips in response to dislike of food • Rolls back to stomach and stomach to back • Recognizes "no" • Chains together syllables (dada, papa, mama) but does not have meaning
9–11 mo	• Crawls, pulling self forward by hands, then creeps with abdomen off floor • Stands initially by holding onto furniture, later stands solo • Imitates peek-a-boo and pat-a-cake • Picks up small object with thumb and index finger	• Cruises • Follows simple command, such as "Come here." Assigns meaning to words such as "mama, papa, dada"
12–15 mo	• Initially walks with help, progresses to walking solo • Neat pincer grasp • Places cube in cup • Hands over objects on request • Builds tower of two bricks	• Says one to two words • Indicates wants by pointing • Scribbles spontaneously • Imitates animal sounds
15–20 mo	• Points to several body parts • Throws a ball overhand • Seats self in chair • Climbs	• Uses a spoon with little spilling • Walks up and down steps with help • Understands two-step commands • Feeds self

TABLE 17-3

Anticipated Early Childhood Developmental Milestones—cont'd

Age	Able to Be Observed During Office Visit	Reported by Parent or Caregiver
		• Carries and hugs doll
		• Imitates housework
		• Speech: 4–6 words by 15 mo, increases to ≥10 words by 18 mo
		• Scribbles vigorously
		• Builds tower three cubes tall
24 mo	• Speaks in sentences of ≥2 words	• Runs
	• Kicks ball on request	• Copies vertical and horizontal lines
	• Jumps with both feet	• Has up to a 300-word vocabulary
	• Uses pronouns	• Washes and dries hands
	• Is developing handedness	• Engages in parallel play
		• Puts on simple clothing
30 mo	• Walks backward	• Gives first and last name
	• Hops on one foot	• Uses plurals
	• Copies circle	• Usually separates easily from parents
36 mo	• Holds crayons with fingers	• Walks down stairs alternating steps
	• Nearly all speech intelligible to people not in daily contact with child	• Rides tricycle
	• Three-word sentences	• Copies circles
		• Dresses with supervision
3–4 yr	• Responds to command to place object in, on, or under a table	• Takes off jacket and shoes
	• Knows gender	• Washes and dries face
	• Draws circle when one is shown	• Engages in cooperative play
		• Speech includes plurals, personal pronouns, verbs
		• Skips
		• Asks many questions
4–5 yr	• Runs and turns while maintaining balance	• Buttons clothes
	• Stands on one foot for at least 10 seconds	• Dresses self (not including tying shoelaces)
	• Counts to four	• Can play without adult input for about 30 min
	• Draws a person without torso	
	• Copies (1) by imitation	
	• Verbalizes activities to do when cold, hungry, tired	
5–6 yr	• Catches ball	• Able to complete simple chores
	• Knows age	• Understands concept of 10 items; likely counts higher by rote
	• Knows right from left hand	• Has sense of gender
	• Draws person with six to eight parts, including torso	
	• Identifies best friend	
	• Likes teacher	
6–7 yr	• Copies triangle shape	• Ties shoelaces
	• Draws person with at least 12 parts	• Counts to ≥30
	• Prints name	• Able to differentiate morning from later in day
	• Reads multiple single-syllable words	• Generally plays well with peers
		• No significant behavioral problems in school
		• Can name intended career
7–8 yr	• Copies diamond shape	• Ties shoelaces
	• Reads simple sentences	• Knows day of the week
	• Draws person with at least 16 parts	

Continued

TABLE 17-3

Anticipated Early Childhood Developmental Milestones—cont'd

Age	Able to Be Observed During Office Visit	Reported by Parent or Caregiver
8–9 yr	• Able to give response to question such as what to do if an object is accidentally broken	• Able to add, subtract, borrow, carry • Understands concept of working as a team
9–10 yr	• Knows month, day, year • Gives months of the year in sequence	• Able to multiply and do complex subtraction • Has increased reading fluency
10–12 yr	• Beginning of pubertal changes for many children	• Able to perform simple division • Has complex reading skills

Source: Burns CE, Dunn AM, Brady MA, et al. *Pediatric Primary Care*, ed. 5. Philadelphia: Elsevier Saunders, 2012.

Table 17-4

Findings of Fragile X and Klinefelter Syndrome

Diagnosis	Findings
FRAGILE X SYNDROME	In males: Large testicles (macroorchidism) after the beginning of puberty, large body habitus, learning and behavioral differences (hyperactivity, developmental disability common), large forehead, ears, prominent jaw, tendency to avoid eye contact In females: Significantly less common with fewer prominent findings, usually with less severe developmental issues Most common known cause of autism in either gender, 1 in 4000 males and 1 in 8000 females, and occurs in all racial and ethnic groups. Blood testing available for carrier state (genetic risk for having a child with fragile X syndrome) or for diagnosis of the condition. Antenatal diagnosis possible.
KLINEFELTER SYNDROME XXY MALE	Only males affected, with developmental issues, most commonly language impairment. Physical habitus = low testicular volume, hip and breast enlargement. Blood testing available for carrier state (genetic risk for having a child with Klinefelter syndrome) or for diagnosis of the condition. Antenatal diagnosis possible.

Sources: The National Fragile X Syndrome Society: Fragile X Syndrome Checklist, www.fragilex.org/fragile-x-associated-disorders/fragile-x-syndrome.
National Institutes of Health: Klinefelter Syndrome, www.ghr.nlm.nih.gov/condition/klinefelter-syndrome.

39. At which of the following ages in a young child's life is parental anticipatory guidance about temper tantrums most helpful?
A. 8 to 10 months
B. 10 to 12 months
C. 12 to 14 months
D. 14 to 16 months

40. At which of the following ages in a young child's life is parental anticipatory guidance about using "time out" as a discipline method most helpful?
A. 12 to 18 months
B. 18 to 24 months
C. 24 to 30 months
D. 30 to 36 months

41. At which of the following ages in a young child's life is parental anticipatory guidance about protection from falls most helpful?
A. birth
B. 2 months
C. 4 months
D. 6 months

42. At which of the following ages in a young child's life is parental anticipatory guidance about toilet-training readiness most helpful?
A. 12 months
B. 15 months
C. 18 months
D. 24 months

43. At which of the following ages in a young child's life is parental anticipatory guidance about infant sleep position most helpful?
A. birth
B. 2 weeks
C. 2 months
D. 4 months

38. C.   40. B.   42. C.
39. B.   41. A.   43. A.

Developmental Benchmarks

Providing health advice to the growing family is a critical role of the NP. During anticipatory guidance counseling, the NP should review the normal developmental landmarks that the child is expected to reach in the near future and offer advice about how parents can cope with, adapt to, and avoid problems with these changes. This guidance is tailored to meet the needs of the family but typically follows a developmental framework and should continue through adolescence.

DISCUSSION SOURCE

American Academy of Pediatrics Bright Futures Tool and Resource Kit, http://brightfutures.aap.org/tool_and_resource_kit.html

Hypertension, Type 2 Diabetes, and Dyslipidemia in Children

44. The following are risk factors for hypertension in children and teens (choose all that apply):
A. being obese.
B. drinking whole milk.
C. being exposed to second-hand smoke.
D. watching 2 or more hours of television per day.

45. Fruit juice intake is acceptable in children 6 months and older per the following recommendation (choose all that apply):
A. The juice is mixed in small amounts to flavor water.
B. Only 100% juice is used.
C. Juice replaces no more than one serving of milk.
D. The juice is consumed in the morning with breakfast.
E. No more than 6 oz (177 mL) per day is recommended for children 6 months to 5 years.

46. In evaluating a 9-year-old child with a healthy BMI during a well visit, a comprehensive cardiovascular evaluation should be conducted by the following methods (choose all that apply):
A. Obtain fasting lipid profile.
B. Screen for type 2 diabetes mellitus by measuring HbA1c.
C. Assess for family history of thyroid disease.
D. Assess diet and physical activity.

47. At what age is it appropriate to recommend dietary changes to parents if overweight or obesity is a concern?
A. 12 months old
B. 5 years old
C. 10 years old
D. 18 years old

48. The following are risk factors for type 2 diabetes mellitus in children and teens (choose all that apply):
A. hyperinsulinemia.
B. abnormal weight-to-height ratio.
C. onset of nonorganic failure to thrive in the toddler years.
D. Native American ancestry.

49. Screening children with a known risk factor for type 2 diabetes mellitus is recommended at age 10 or at onset of puberty, and should be repeated how often?
A. every other year.
B. every year.
C. every six months.
D. if child presents with a body mass index in the 85th percentile or higher.

50. Prediabetes in children is defined as (choose all that apply):
A. impaired fasting glucose (glucose level ≥100 mg/dL or 6.2 mmol/L) but ≤125 mg/dL or 7 mmol/L).
B. impaired glucose tolerance (2-hour postprandial ≥140–199 mg/dL or 7.8 mmol/L–11 mmol/L).
C. body mass index in the 85th percentile or higher.
D. body mass index in the 60th percentile or higher.

51. Risk factors for dyslipidemia in children include (choose all that apply):
A. blood pressure at the 70th to 80th percentile for age.
B. breastfeeding into the toddler years.
C. family history of lipid abnormalities.
D. family history of type 2 diabetes mellitus.

52. Screening cholesterol levels in children with one or more risk factors begins at what age?
   A. birth
   B. 2 years
   C. 5 years
   D. 10 years

53. An acceptable level of total cholesterol (mg/dL) in children and teens is:
   A. <170 mg/dL or 9.4 mmol/L.
   B. <130 mg/dL or 7.2 mmol/L.
   C. 110–130 mg/dL or 6.2 mmol/L–7.2 mmol/L.
   D. 130–199 mg/dL or 7.2 mmol/L–11 mmol/L.

Answers

44. A and C.	48. A, B, D.	52. B.
45. A, B, E.	49. A.	53. A.
46. A and D.	50. A and B.	
47. A.	51. C and D.	

Prevalence of hypertension, type 2 diabetes mellitus, and dyslipidemia has increased in recent years in association with the rise in childhood obesity. Appropriate screening for these conditions in children and teens can result in earlier diagnosis and treatment, potentially reducing the risk for adult disease and its complications.

Risk factors for hypertension in children and teens include a family history of heart disease, high blood pressure, elevated lipid levels, exposure to tobacco smoke, a diet low in daily recommended intake of nutrients, obesity, type 2 diabetes, and lack of physical activity. Risk factors for type 2 diabetes in children include obesity, sedentary lifestyle, race/ethnicity, family history, augmentation of growth hormone (GH) and insulin-like growth factor (IGF) secretion during puberty, polycystic ovary syndrome (PCOS), hyperandrogenism, intrauterine exposure to maternal diabetes, low birth weight, and poor infant growth. Risk factors for dyslipidemia in children include family history of lipid abnormalities and type 2 diabetes.

Prediabetes in children is defined as impaired fasting glucose (glucose level ≥100 mg/dL or 5.6 mmol/L but ≤125 mg/dL or 7 mmol/L) or impaired glucose tolerance (2-hour postprandial ≥140–199 mg/dL or 7.8 mmol/L–11 mmol/L) or an A1C of 5.7% to 6.4%. Diagnosis of type 2 diabetes is confirmed if random plasma glucose level is ≥200 mg/dL or 11.1 mmol/L in conjunction with symptoms of 2 diabetes or an A1C ≥6.5%. Screening for type 2 diabetes begins at age 10 or at onset of puberty and continues every 2 years until adulthood; at that point, the adult guidelines should be followed. Criteria for screening includes a BMI greater than 85th percentile for age and sex, weight-for-height greater than 85% percentile, or weight of more than 120% of ideal for height, plus any two or more of the aforementioned risk factors.

The AAP screening guidelines for total cholesterol levels in children and adolescents aged 2 to 19 years old are as follows: acceptable level is <170 mg/dL (<9.4 mmol/L), borderline is 170–199 mg/dL (9.4 mmol/L–11 mmol/L), and high is >200 mg/dL (≥11.1 mmol/L) (Table 17–5). Definitions for elevated low-density lipoprotein (LDL), high-density lipoprotein (HDL), and triglyceride-specific levels in children and teens depend on age, gender, and percentile of height. Children should be screened for family history of cardiovascular disease (CVD) beginning at age 3 and should be periodically updated annually or as required by risk factors during non-urgent health visits. As family history and/or risk factors for CVD are identified, the NP should evaluate the child's family for risk factors, including parents, grandparents, aunts, and uncles (Table 17–5). For at-risk children, fasting lipid levels should be tested after 2 years of age (but no later than 10 years of age) and should be retested in 3–5 years if the values fall within the reference range.

According to CVD screening guidelines, a child's family history for obesity should be reviewed beginning at birth. Weight-for-height tracking, growth chart, and healthy diet should be discussed with the parents. The NP should encourage parents to promote physical activity from the child's birth. At age 2, encourage active play and recommend limiting television and other screen time, including video games, to no more than total of 2 hours or less per day. A smoke-free home should be encouraged and smoking cessation assistance offered to parents. Beginning between ages 9 to 11 years, smoking status of the child should be assessed and anti-smoking counseling offered at each visit. Smoking cessation assistance or referral should be offered when needed.

CVD screening guidelines state that the child's diet should be evaluated at every visit. At birth, the mother should be encouraged to breastfeed at least until the infant is 12 months of age. If the mother is not breastfeeding, iron-fortified infant formula is recommended for the first 12 months; the majority of the child's caloric intake in the first year of life should come from breast milk or iron-fortified infant formula. From 12 to 24 months of age, drinking whole cows' milk is recommended. After 24 months, children should switch to skim or 1% milk. After 12 months, limit milk to a total of 16 to 24 ounces (480–720 mL) a day. Fruit juice should contain 100% juice without added sugar if possible, should not replace breast milk or formula, and should be introduced no earlier than 6 months of age. Intake should be limited to 6 ounces a day for children 6 months to 5 years old. Parents and caregivers should be encouraged to use small amounts of fruit juice to flavor water, therefore increasing fluid intake while minimizing excessive juice intake. If vitamin C intake from fresh fruit is adequate, fruit juice does not need to be part of the child's diet. Dietary guidelines for children should be recommended and reinforced throughout childhood.

Body mass index (BMI) should be measured beginning at age 2. For children between 12 months and 2 years of age for whom overweight or obesity is a concern, the use of reduced-fat milk would be appropriate. Beginning at age 5, if BMI is ≥85th percentile, intensify dietary and activity changes to the parent. The National Diabetes Education Program provides

Table 17-5

Lipid Screening and Cardiovascular Health in Childhood

1. The population approach to a healthful diet should be recommended to all children older than 2 years, according to Dietary Guidelines for Americans. This approach includes the use of low-fat dairy products. For children between 12 months and 2 years of age for whom overweight or obesity is a concern or who have a family history of obesity, dyslipidemia, or cardiovascular disease (CVD), the use of reduced-fat milk would be appropriate.

2. The individual approach for children and adolescents at higher risk for CVD and with a high concentration of low-density lipoprotein (LDL) includes recommended changes in diet with nutritional counseling and other lifestyle interventions such as increased physical activity.

3. The most current recommendation is to screen children and adolescents with a positive family history of dyslipidemia or premature (≤55 years of age for men and ≤65 years of age for women) CVD or dyslipidemia. It is also recommended that pediatric patients for whom family history is not known or those with other CVD risk factors, such as overweight (body mass index [BMI] ≥85th percentile, <95th percentile), obesity (BMI ≥95th percentile), hypertension (blood pressure ≥95th percentile), cigarette smoking, or diabetes mellitus, be screened with a fasting lipid profile.

4. For these children, the first screening should take place after 2 years of age but no later than 10 years of age. Screening before 2 years of age is not recommended.

5. A fasting lipid profile is the recommended approach to screening because there is no currently available noninvasive method to assess atherosclerotic CVD in children. This screening should occur in the context of well-child and health-maintenance visits. If values are within the reference range on initial screening, the patient should be retested in 3 to 5 years.

6. For pediatric patients who are overweight or obese and have a high triglyceride concentration or low HDL concentration, weight management is the primary treatment, which includes improvement of diet with nutritional counseling and increased physical activity to produce improved energy balance.

7. For patients 8 years and older with an LDL concentration of ≥190 mg/dL/10.6 mmol/L (or ≥160 mg/dL/8.9 mmol/L with a family history of early heart disease or ≥2 additional risk factors present or ≥130 mg/dL/7.2 mmol/L if diabetes mellitus is present), pharmacologic intervention should be considered. The initial goal is to lower LDL concentration to <160 mg/dL/8.9 mmol/L. However, targets as low as 130 mg/dL/7.2 mmol/L or even 110 mg/dL/6.2 mmol/L may be warranted when there is a strong family history of CVD, especially with other risk factors including obesity, diabetes mellitus, the metabolic syndrome, and other higher risk situations.

Source: Daniels SR, Greer FR, and the Committee on Nutrition. Lipid screening and cardiovascular health in childhood. *Pediatrics* 122;1:198–208, 2008.

guidelines for healthy eating choices. A diet high in nutrients, protein, and complex carbohydrates and low in sugar and saturated fat is recommended.

In the well child, check blood pressure annually beginning at age 3 years and chart for age, gender, and history. Refer to National Institutes of Health guidelines when screening pediatric patients for elevated blood pressure because definitions for elevated systolic and diastolic blood pressure vary with age, gender, and percentile of height. Blood pressure should be measured in the first 12 months only if child has a renal, urologic, or cardiac diagnosis or a history of being hospitalized in the neonatal intensive care unit.

Nonpharmacologic interventions in children and adolescents diagnosed with dyslipidemia, type 2 diabetes, hypertension, or more than one of these conditions include eating well; attaining or maintaining a healthy weight; increasing physical activity. If cholesterol, glucose, and/or blood pressure goals are not reached using nonpharmacologic methods, medication use is an option. Refer children to appropriate resources for treatment as needed.

DISCUSSION SOURCES

Halpern A, Mancini MC, Magalhães MC, et al. Metabolic syndrome, dyslipidemia, hypertension and type 2 diabetes in youth: From diagnosis to treatment. *Diabetol Metab Syndr* 2:55, 2010.

National Institutes of Health Expert Panel on Integrated Guidelines for Cardiovascular Health and Risk Reduction in Children and Adolescents: Summary Report, http://www.nhlbi.nih.gov/guidelines/cvd_ped/summary.htm#chap3.

National Institutes of Health: Blood Pressure Tables for Children and Adolescents, http://www.nhlbi.nih.gov/guidelines/hypertension/child_tbl.htm.

Rodbard HW. Diabetes screening, diagnosis, and therapy in pediatric patients with type 2 diabetes. *Medscape J Med* 10:184, 2008.

The Committee on Nutrition. Lipid Screening and Cardiovascular Health in Childhood. *Pediatrics* 122;1:198–208, 2008.

American Heart Association; Children and Cholesterol, http://www.heart.org/HEARTORG/Conditions/Cholesterol/Understand-YourRiskforHighCholesterol/Children-and-Cholesterol_UCM_305567_Article.jsp.

National Diabetes Education Program: Healthy Lifestyle Choices, http://ndep.nih.gov/teens/MakeHealthyFoodChoices.aspx.

Measles, Mumps, and Rubella

54. When considering a person's risk for measles, mumps, and rubella, the NP considers the following:
    A. Children should have two doses of the measles, mumps, and rubella (MMR) vaccine before their sixth birthday.
    B. Considerable mortality and morbidity occur with all three diseases.
    C. Most cases in the United States occur in infants.
    D. The use of the vaccine is often associated with protracted arthralgia.

55. Which of the following is true about the MMR vaccine?
    A. This vaccine contains live virus.
    B. Its use is contraindicated in persons with a history of egg allergy.
    C. Revaccination of an immune person is associated with risk of allergic reaction.
    D. One dose is recommended for young adults who have not been previously immunized.

56. How many doses of the MMR vaccine should a child 6 to 11 months of age receive before traveling outside of the United States?
    A. none
    B. one dose
    C. two doses
    D. depends on where the child is traveling

57. A 9-year-old child with no documentation of vaccinations comes in for an MMR immunization update. Her parent states that child has received "some" vaccinations, but no documentation is available. How many doses of MMR should the child receive and at what frequency?
    A. one MMR dose
    B. two MMR doses together at the same time
    C. two MMR doses 1 month apart
    D. no MMR immunization is needed

58. Which of the following viruses is a potent teratogen?
    A. measles
    B. mumps
    C. rubella
    D. influenza

59. Evidence demonstrates that the MMR virus acquired via vaccine can be shed into the body during lactation.
    A true
    B. false

60. In whom is serological documentation of immunity to rubella advised?
    A. school-aged children
    B. government employees
    C. pregnant women and women of childbearing age who could become pregnant
    D. healthcare workers

Answers

54. A.	57. C.	60. C.
55. A.	58. C.	
56. B.	59. B.	

The MMR vaccine is a live, attenuated vaccine. The recommended schedule for early childhood immunization is two doses of MMR vaccine, one given between age 12 and 15 months and one between 4 and 6 years (Fig.17–1). Infants traveling abroad are at risk of contracting measles because the disease is still common in many foreign countries. The CDC recommends giving one dose of MMR to infants 6 through 11 months of age if traveling outside of the United States, regardless of the country. Two immunizations 1 month apart are recommended for older children who were not immunized earlier in life. As with other immunizations, giving additional doses to individuals with an unclear immunization history is safe.

Rubella, also known as German measles, typically causes a relatively mild, 3- to 5-day illness with little risk of complication for the person infected. However, rubella is a potent teratogen. If rubella is contracted during pregnancy, the effects on the fetus can be devastating. Immunizing the entire population against rubella protects unborn children from the risk of congenital rubella syndrome. Measles can cause severe illness with serious sequelae, including encephalitis and pneumonia. Sequelae of mumps include orchitis.

The MMR vaccine is safe to use during lactation, but its use in pregnant women is discouraged because of the possible risk of passing the virus on to the unborn child; this risk exists in theory but has not been noted in ongoing observation. The live attenuated virus is not shed into the breast milk or other body fluids. The MMR vaccine is well tolerated, with rare reports of mild, transient adverse reactions such as rash and sore throat. Systemic reaction to the MMR vaccine is rare.

Verify immunity to measles, mumps, or rubella by the following methods: documentation of vaccination, laboratory evidence of disease, birth date before 1957, or laboratory evidence of immune markers. Sufficient levels of immunoglobulin G (IgG) in serum provide laboratory evidence of immunity for measles, mumps, or rubella. Documentation of immunity is needed for children who are school-aged and for those traveling internationally. Pregnant women and women of childbearing age who could become pregnant should be tested for rubella immunity.

DISCUSSION SOURCES

Centers for Disease Control and Prevention. Vaccine Preventable Childhood Diseases, http://www.cdc.gov/vaccines/schedules/hcp/child-adolescent.html

Centers for Disease Control and Prevention. Birth–18 Years and "Catch-Up" Immunization Schedules—United States 2014. http://www.cdc.gov/vaccines/schedules/hcp/child-adolescent.html

McLean HQ, Fiebelkorn AP, Temte JL, et al. Prevention of measles, rubella, congenital rubella syndrome, and mumps, 2013: Summary recommendations of the Advisory Committee on Immunization Practices. *MMRW* 62:1–34, 2013.

(Text continued on page 415)

Recommended Immunization Schedules for Persons Aged 0 Through 18 Years
UNITED STATES, 2014

This schedule includes recommendations in effect as of January 1, 2014. Any dose not administered at the recommended age should be administered at a subsequent visit, when indicated and feasible. The use of a combination vaccine generally is preferred over separate injections of its equivalent component vaccines. Vaccination providers should consult the relevant Advisory Committee on Immunization Practices (ACIP) statement for detailed recommendations, available online at http://www.cdc.gov/vaccines/hcp/acip-recs/index.html. Clinically significant adverse events that follow vaccination should be reported to the Vaccine Adverse Event Reporting System (VAERS) online (http://www.vaers.hhs.gov) or by telephone (800-822-7967).

The Recommended Immunization Schedules for Persons Aged 0 Through 18 Years are approved by the

Advisory Committee on Immunization Practices
(http://www.cdc.gov/vaccines/acip)

American Academy of Pediatrics
(http://www.aap.org)

American Academy of Family Physicians
(http://www.aafp.org)

American College of Obstetricians and Gynecologists
(http://www.acog.org)

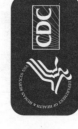

U.S. Department of Health and Human Services
Centers for Disease Control and Prevention

Continued

Figure 17-1 Birth–18 Years & "Catch-up" Immunization Schedules United States, 2013 (CDC Guidelines). Available at http://www.cdc.gov/vaccines/schedules/hcp/child-adolescent.html; accessed 10/16/13.

Figure 1. Recommended immunization schedule for persons aged 0 through 18 years – United States, 2014. (FOR THOSE WHO FALL BEHIND OR START LATE, SEE THE CATCH-UP SCHEDULE [FIGURE 2]).

These recommendations must be read with the footnotes that follow. For those who fall behind or start late, provide catch-up vaccination at the earliest opportunity as indicated by the blue bars in Figure 1. To determine minimum intervals between doses, see the catch-up schedule (Figure 2). School entry and adolescent vaccine age groups are in bold.

Vaccine	Birth	1 mo	2 mos	4 mos	6 mos	9 mos	12 mos	15 mos	18 mos	19–23 mos	2–3 yrs	4–6 yrs	7–10 yrs	11–12 yrs	13–15 yrs	16–18 yrs
Hepatitis B[1] (HepB)	1st dose	←—— 2nd dose ——→			←——————— 3rd dose ———————→											
Rotavirus[2] (RV) RV1 (2-dose series); RV5 (3-dose series)			1st dose	2nd dose	See footnote 2											
Diphtheria, tetanus, & acellular pertussis[3] (DTaP: <7 yrs)			1st dose	2nd dose	3rd dose		←———— 4th dose ————→					5th dose				
Tetanus, diphtheria, & acellular pertussis[4] (Tdap: ≥7 yrs)														(Tdap)		
Haemophilus influenzae type b[5] (Hib)			1st dose	2nd dose	See footnote 5		3rd or 4th dose, See footnote 5									
Pneumococcal conjugate[6] (PCV13)			1st dose	2nd dose	3rd dose		←—— 4th dose ——→									
Pneumococcal polysaccharide[6] (PPSV23)																
Inactivated poliovirus[7] (IPV) (<18 yrs)			1st dose	2nd dose	←——————— 3rd dose ———————→							4th dose				
Influenza[8] (IIV; LAIV) 2 doses for some: See footnote 8					Annual vaccination (IIV only)							Annual vaccination (IIV or LAIV)				
Measles, mumps, rubella[9] (MMR)							←—— 1st dose ——→					2nd dose				
Varicella[10] (VAR)							←—— 1st dose ——→					2nd dose				
Hepatitis A[11] (HepA)							←——————————— 2-dose series, See footnote 11 ———————————→									
Human papillomavirus[12] (HPV2: females only; HPV4: males and females)														(3-dose series)		
Meningococcal[13] (Hib-Men-CY ≥6 weeks; MenACWY-D ≥9 mos; MenACWY-CRM ≥2 mos)														1st dose		Booster

Legend:
- Range of recommended ages for all children
- Range of recommended ages for catch-up immunization
- Range of recommended ages for certain high-risk groups
- Range of recommended ages during which catch-up is encouraged and for certain high-risk groups
- Not routinely recommended

This schedule includes recommendations in effect as of January 1, 2014. Any dose not administered at the recommended age should be administered at a subsequent visit, when indicated and feasible. The use of a combination vaccine generally is preferred over separate injections of its equivalent component vaccines. Vaccination providers should consult the relevant Advisory Committee on Immunization Practices (ACIP) statement for detailed recommendations, available online at http://www.cdc.gov/vaccines/hcp/acip-recs/index.html. Clinically significant adverse events that follow vaccination should be reported to the Vaccine Adverse Event Reporting System (VAERS) online (http://www.vaers.hhs.gov) or by telephone (800-822-7967). Suspected cases of vaccine-preventable diseases should be reported to the state or local health department. Additional information, including precautions and contraindications for vaccination, is available from CDC online (http://www.cdc.gov/vaccines/recs/vac-admin/contraindications.htm) or by telephone (800-CDC-INFO [800-232-4636]).

This schedule is approved by the Advisory Committee on Immunization Practices (http//www.cdc.gov/vaccines/acip), the American Academy of Pediatrics (http://www.aap.org), the American Academy of Family Physicians (http://www.aafp.org), and the American College of Obstetricians and Gynecologists (http://www.acog.org).

NOTE: The above recommendations must be read along with the footnotes of this schedule.

FIGURE 2. Catch-up immunization schedule for persons aged 4 months through 18 years who start late or who are more than 1 month behind —United States, 2014.

The figure below provides catch-up schedules and minimum intervals between doses for children whose vaccinations have been delayed. A vaccine series does not need to be restarted, regardless of the time that has elapsed between doses. Use the section appropriate for the child's age. Always use this table in conjunction with Figure 1 and the footnotes that follow.

Vaccine	Minimum Age for Dose 1	Minimum Interval Between Doses			
		Dose 1 to dose 2	Dose 2 to dose 3	Dose 3 to dose 4	Dose 4 to dose 5
Persons aged 4 months through 6 years					
Hepatitis B[1]	Birth	4 weeks	8 weeks and at least 16 weeks after first dose; minimum age for the final dose is 24 weeks		
Rotavirus[2]	6 weeks	4 weeks	4 weeks[2]		
Diphtheria, tetanus, & acellular pertussis[3]	6 weeks	4 weeks	4 weeks	6 months	6 months[3]
Haemophilus influenzae type b[5]	6 weeks	4 weeks if first dose administered at younger than age 12 months / 8 weeks (as final dose) if first dose administered at age 12 through 14 months / No further doses needed if first dose administered at age 15 months or older	4 weeks[5] if current age is younger than 12 months and first dose administered at < 7 months old / 8 weeks and age 12 months through 59 months (as final dose)[5] if current age is younger than 12 months and first dose administered between 7 through 11 months (regardless of Hib vaccine [PRP-T or PRP-OMP] used for first dose); OR if current age is 12 through 59 months and first dose administered at younger than age 12 months; OR first 2 doses were PRP-OMP and administered at younger than 12 months. / No further doses needed if previous dose administered at age 15 months or older	8 weeks (as final dose) / This dose only necessary for children aged 12 through 59 months who received 3 (PRP-T) doses before age 12 months and started the primary series before age 7 months	
Pneumococcal[6]	6 weeks	4 weeks if first dose administered at younger than age 12 months / 8 weeks (as final dose for healthy children) if first dose administered at age 12 months or older / No further doses needed for healthy children if first dose administered at age 24 months or older	4 weeks if current age is younger than 12 months / 8 weeks (as final dose for healthy children) if current age is 12 months or older / No further doses needed for healthy children if previous dose administered at age 24 months or older	8 weeks (as final dose) / This dose only necessary for children aged 12 through 59 months who received 3 doses before age 12 months or for children at high risk who received 3 doses at any age	
Inactivated poliovirus[7]	6 weeks	4 weeks[7]	4 weeks[7]	6 months[7] minimum age 4 years for final dose	
Meningococcal[13]	6 weeks	8 weeks[13]	See footnote 13	See footnote 13	
Measles, mumps, rubella[9]	12 months	4 weeks			
Varicella[10]	12 months	3 months			
Hepatitis A[11]	12 months	6 months			
Persons aged 7 through 18 years					
Tetanus, diphtheria; tetanus, diphtheria, & acellular pertussis[4]	7 years[4]	4 weeks	4 weeks if first dose of DTaP/DT administered at younger than age 12 months / 6 months if first dose of DTaP/DT administered at age 12 months or older and then no further doses needed for catch-up	6 months if first dose of DTaP/DT administered at younger than age 12 months	
Human papillomavirus[12]	9 years	Routine dosing intervals are recommended[12]			
Hepatitis A[11]	12 months	6 months			
Hepatitis B[1]	Birth	4 weeks	8 weeks (and at least 16 weeks after first dose)		
Inactivated poliovirus[7]	6 weeks	4 weeks	4 weeks[7]	6 months[7]	
Meningococcal[13]	6 weeks	8 weeks[13]	See footnote 13		
Measles, mumps, rubella[9]	12 months	4 weeks			
Varicella[10]	12 months	3 months if person is younger than age 13 years / 4 weeks if person is aged 13 years or older			

NOTE: The above recommendations must be read along with the footnotes of this schedule.

Figure 17-1 —cont'd

Continued

Footnotes — Recommended immunization schedule for persons aged 0 through 18 years—United States, 2014

For further guidance on the use of the vaccines mentioned below, see: http://www.cdc.gov/vaccines/hcp/acip-recs/index.html.
For vaccine recommendations for persons 19 years of age and older, see the adult immunization schedule.

Additional information

- For contraindications and precautions to use of a vaccine and for additional information regarding that vaccine, vaccination providers should consult the relevant ACIP statement available online at http://www.cdc.gov/vaccines/hcp/acip-recs/index.html.
- For purposes of calculating intervals between doses, 4 weeks = 28 days. Intervals of 4 months or greater are determined by calendar months.
- Vaccine doses administered 4 days or less before the minimum interval or minimum age should not be counted as valid doses and should be repeated as age-appropriate. The repeat dose should be spaced after the invalid dose by the recommended minimum interval. For further details, see *MMWR, General Recommendations on Immunization and Reports / Vol. 60 / No. 2; Table 1. Recommended and minimum ages and intervals between vaccine doses available online at* http://www.cdc.gov/mmwr/pdf/rr/rr6002.pdf.
- Information on travel vaccine requirements and recommendations is available at http://wwwnc.cdc.gov/travel/destinations/list.
- For vaccination of persons with primary and secondary immunodeficiencies, see Table 13, "Vaccination of persons with primary and secondary immunodeficiencies," in General Recommendations on Immunization (ACIP), available at http://www.cdc.gov/mmwr/pdf/rr/rr6002.pdf.; and American Academy of Pediatrics. Immunization in Special Clinical Circumstances, in Pickering LK, Baker CJ, Kimberlin DW, Long SS. eds. *Red Book: 2012 report of the Committee on Infectious Diseases. 29th ed.* Elk Grove Village, IL: American Academy of Pediatrics.

1. **Hepatitis B (HepB) vaccine. (Minimum age: birth)**

   Routine vaccination:

   At birth:
   - Administer monovalent HepB vaccine to all newborns before hospital discharge.
   - For infants born to hepatitis B surface antigen (HBsAg)-positive mothers, administer HepB vaccine and 0.5 mL of hepatitis B immune globulin (HBIG) within 12 hours of birth. These infants should be tested for HBsAg and antibody to HBsAg (anti-HBs) 1 to 2 months after completion of the HepB series, at age 9 through 18 months (preferably at the next well-child visit).
   - If mother's HBsAg status is unknown, within 12 hours of birth administer HepB vaccine regardless of birth weight. For infants weighing less than 2,000 grams, administer HBIG in addition to HepB vaccine within 12 hours of birth. Determine mother's HBsAg status as soon as possible and, if mother is HBsAg-positive, also administer HBIG for infants weighing 2,000 grams or more as soon as possible, but no later than age 7 days.

   Doses following the birth dose:
   - The second dose should be administered at age 1 or 2 months. Monovalent HepB vaccine should be used for doses administered before age 6 weeks.
   - Infants who did not receive a birth dose should receive 3 doses of a HepB-containing vaccine on a schedule of 0, 1 to 2 months, and 6 months starting as soon as feasible. See Figure 2.
   - The second dose should be administered 1 to 2 months after the first dose (minimum interval of 4 weeks), the third dose at least 8 weeks after the second dose AND at least 16 weeks after the <u>first</u> dose. The final (third or fourth) dose in the HepB vaccine series should be administered <u>no earlier than age 24 weeks.</u>
   - Administration of a total of 4 doses of HepB vaccine is permitted when a combination vaccine containing HepB is administered after the birth dose.

   Catch-up vaccination:
   - Unvaccinated persons should complete a 3-dose series.
   - A 2-dose series (doses separated by at least 4 months) of adult formulation Recombivax HB is licensed for use in children aged 11 through 15 years.
   - For other catch-up guidance, see Figure 2.

2. **Rotavirus (RV) vaccines. (Minimum age: 6 weeks for both RV1 [Rotarix] and RV5 [RotaTeq])**

   Routine vaccination:

   Administer a series of RV vaccine to all infants as follows:
   1. If Rotarix is used, administer a 2-dose series at 2 and 4 months of age.
   2. If RotaTeq is used, administer a 3-dose series at ages 2, 4, and 6 months.
   3. If any dose in the series was RotaTeq or vaccine product is unknown for any dose in the series, a total of 3 doses of RV vaccine should be administered.

   Catch-up vaccination:
   - The maximum age for the first dose in the series is 14 weeks, 6 days; vaccination should not be initiated for infants aged 15 weeks, 0 days or older.
   - The maximum age for the final dose in the series is 8 months, 0 days.
   - For other catch-up guidance, see Figure 2.

3. **Diphtheria and tetanus toxoids and acellular pertussis (DTaP) vaccine. (Minimum age: 6 weeks.**
   Exception: DTaP-IPV [Kinrix]: 4 years)

   Routine vaccination:
   - Administer a 5-dose series of DTaP vaccine at ages 2, 4, 6, 15 through 18 months, and 4 through 6 years. The fourth dose may be administered as early as age 12 months, provided at least 6 months have elapsed since the third dose.

   Catch-up vaccination:
   - The fifth dose of DTaP vaccine is not necessary if the fourth dose was administered at age 4 years or older.
   - For other catch-up guidance, see Figure 2.

4. **Tetanus and diphtheria toxoids and acellular pertussis (Tdap) vaccine. (Minimum age: 10 years for Boostrix, 11 years for Adacel)**

   Routine vaccination:
   - Administer 1 dose of Tdap vaccine to all adolescents aged 11 through 12 years.
   - Tdap may be administered regardless of the interval since the last tetanus and diphtheria toxoid-containing vaccine.
   - Administer 1 dose of Tdap vaccine to pregnant adolescents during each pregnancy (preferred during 27 through 36 weeks gestation) regardless of time since prior Td or Tdap vaccination.

   Catch-up vaccination:
   - Persons aged 7 years and older who are not fully immunized with DTaP vaccine should receive Tdap vaccine as 1 (preferably the first) dose in the catch-up series; if additional doses are needed, use Td vaccine. For children 7 through 10 years who receive a dose of Tdap as part of the catch-up series, an adolescent Tdap vaccine dose at age 11 through 12 years should NOT be administered. Td should be administered instead 10 years after the Tdap dose.
   - Persons aged 11 through 18 years who have not received Tdap vaccine should receive a dose followed by tetanus and diphtheria toxoids (Td) booster doses every 10 years thereafter.
   - Inadvertent doses of DTaP vaccine:
     - If administered inadvertently to a child aged 7 through 10 years may count as part of the catch-up series. This dose may count as the adolescent Tdap dose, or the child can later receive a Tdap booster dose at age 11 through 12 years.
     - If administered inadvertently to an adolescent aged 11 through 18 years, the dose should be counted as the adolescent Tdap booster.
   - For other catch-up guidance, see Figure 2.

5. **Haemophilus influenzae type b (Hib) conjugate vaccine. (Minimum age: 6 weeks for PRP-T [ACTHIB, DTaP-IPV/Hib (Pentacel) and Hib-MenCY (MenHibrix)], PRP-OMP [PedvaxHIB or COMVAX], 12 months for PRP-T [Hiberix])**

   Routine vaccination:
   - Administer a 2- or 3-dose Hib vaccine primary series and a booster dose (dose 3 or 4 depending on vaccine used in primary series) at age 12 through 15 months to complete a full Hib vaccine series.
   - The primary series with ActHIB, MenHibrix, or Pentacel consists of 3 doses and should be administered at 2, 4, and 6 months of age. The primary series with PedvaxHib or COMVAX consists of 2 doses and should be administered at 2 and 4 months of age; a dose at age 6 months is not indicated.
   - One booster dose (dose 3 or 4 depending on vaccine used in primary series) of any Hib vaccine should be administered at age 12 through 15 months. An exception is Hiberix vaccine. Hiberix should only be used for the booster (final) dose in children aged 12 months through 4 years who have received at least 1 prior dose of Hib-containing vaccine.

Figure 17-1 —cont'd

For further guidance on the use of the vaccines mentioned below, see: http://www.cdc.gov/vaccines/hcp/acip-recs/index.html.

5. Haemophilus influenzae type b (Hib) conjugate vaccine (cont'd)

- For recommendations on the use of MenHibrix in patients at increased risk for meningococcal disease, please refer to the meningococcal vaccine footnotes and also to *MMWR* March 22, 2013; 62(RR02);1–22, available at http://www.cdc.gov/mmwr/pdf/rr/rr6202.pdf.

Catch-up vaccination:

- If dose 1 was administered at ages 12 through 14 months, administer a second (final) dose at least 8 weeks after dose 1, regardless of Hib vaccine used in the primary series.
- If the first 2 doses were PRP-OMP (PedvaxHIB or COMVAX), and were administered at age 11 months or younger, the third (and final) dose should be administered at age 12 through 15 months and at least 8 weeks after the second dose.
- If the first dose was administered at age 7 through 11 months, administer the second dose at least 4 weeks later and a third (and final) dose at age 12 through 15 months or 8 weeks after second dose, whichever is later, regardless of Hib vaccine used for first dose.
- If first dose is administered at younger than 12 months of age and second dose is given between 12 through 14 months of age, a third (and final) dose should be given 8 weeks later.
- For unvaccinated children aged 15 months or older, administer only 1 dose.
- For other catch-up guidance, see Figure 2. For catch-up guidance related to MenHibrix, please see the meningococcal vaccine footnotes and also *MMWR* March 22, 2013; 62(RR02);1–22, available at http://www.cdc.gov/mmwr/pdf/rr/rr6202.pdf.

Vaccination of persons with high-risk conditions:

- Children aged 12 through 59 months who are at increased risk for Hib disease, including chemotherapy recipients and those with anatomic or functional asplenia (including sickle cell disease), human immunodeficiency virus (HIV) infection, immunoglobulin deficiency, or early component complement deficiency, who have received either no doses or only 1 dose of Hib vaccine before 12 months of age, should receive 2 additional doses of Hib vaccine 8 weeks apart; children who received 2 or more doses of Hib vaccine before 12 months of age should receive 1 additional dose.
- For patients younger than 5 years of age undergoing chemotherapy or radiation treatment who received a Hib vaccine dose(s) within 14 days of starting therapy or during therapy, repeat the dose(s) at least 3 months following therapy completion.
- Recipients of hematopoietic stem cell transplant (HSCT) should be revaccinated with a 3-dose regimen of Hib vaccine starting 6 to 12 months after successful transplant, regardless of vaccination history; doses should be administered at least 4 weeks apart.
- A single dose of any Hib-containing vaccine should be administered to unimmunized* children and adolescents 15 months of age and older undergoing an elective splenectomy; if possible, vaccine should be administered at least 14 days before procedure.
- Hib vaccine is not routinely recommended for patients 5 years or older. However, 1 dose of Hib vaccine should be administered to unimmunized* persons aged 5 years or older who have anatomic or functional asplenia (including sickle cell disease) and unvaccinated persons 5 through 18 years of age with human immunodeficiency virus (HIV) infection.
  * Patients who have not received a primary series and booster dose or at least 1 dose of Hib vaccine after 14 months of age are considered unimmunized.

6. Pneumococcal vaccines. (Minimum age: 6 weeks for PCV13, 2 years for PPSV23)

Routine vaccination with PCV13:

- Administer a 4-dose series of PCV13 vaccine at ages 2, 4, and 6 months and at age 12 through 15 months.
- For children aged 14 through 59 months who have received an age-appropriate series of 7-valent PCV (PCV7), administer a single supplemental dose of 13-valent PCV (PCV13).

Catch-up vaccination with PCV13:

- Administer 1 dose of PCV13 to all healthy children aged 24 through 59 months who are not completely vaccinated for their age.
- For other catch-up guidance, see Figure 2.

Vaccination of persons with high-risk conditions with PCV13 and PPSV23:

- All recommended PCV13 doses should be administered prior to PPSV23 vaccination if possible.
1. For children 2 through 5 years of age with any of the following conditions: chronic heart disease (particularly cyanotic congenital heart disease and cardiac failure); chronic lung disease (including asthma if treated with high-dose oral corticosteroid therapy); diabetes mellitus; cerebrospinal fluid leak; cochlear implant; sickle cell disease and other hemoglobinopathies; anatomic or functional asplenia; HIV infection; chronic renal failure; nephrotic syndrome; diseases associated with treatment with immunosuppressive drugs or radiation therapy, including malignant neoplasms, leukemias, lymphomas, and Hodgkin disease; solid organ transplantation; or congenital immunodeficiency:
   1. Administer 1 dose of PCV13 if 3 doses of PCV (PCV7 and/or PCV13) were received previously.
   2. Administer 2 doses of PCV13 at least 8 weeks apart if fewer than 3 doses of PCV (PCV7 and/or PCV13) were received previously.

6. Pneumococcal vaccines (cont'd)

3. Administer 1 supplemental dose of PCV13 if 4 doses of PCV7 or other age-appropriate complete PCV7 series was received previously.
4. The minimum interval between doses of PPSV (PCV7 or PCV13) is 8 weeks.
5. For children with no history of PPSV23 vaccination, administer PPSV23 at least 8 weeks after the most recent dose of PCV13.
- For children aged 6 through 18 years who have cerebrospinal fluid leak; cochlear implant; sickle cell disease and other hemoglobinopathies; anatomic or functional asplenia; congenital or acquired immunodeficiencies; HIV infection; chronic renal failure; nephrotic syndrome; diseases associated with treatment with immunosuppressive drugs or radiation therapy, including malignant neoplasms, leukemias, lymphomas, and Hodgkin disease; generalized malignancy; solid organ transplantation; or multiple myeloma:
1. If neither PCV13 nor PPSV23 has been received previously, administer 1 dose of PCV13 now and 1 dose of PPSV23 at least 8 weeks later.
2. If PCV13 has been received previously but PPSV23 has not, administer 1 dose of PPSV23 at least 8 weeks after the most recent dose of PCV13.
3. If PPSV23 has been received but PCV13 has not, administer 1 dose of PCV13 at least 8 weeks after the most recent dose of PPSV23.
- For children aged 6 through 18 years with chronic heart disease (particularly cyanotic congenital heart disease and cardiac failure), chronic lung disease (including asthma if treated with high-dose oral corticosteroid therapy), diabetes mellitus, alcoholism, or chronic liver disease, who have not received PPSV23, administer 1 dose of PPSV23. If PCV13 has been received previously, then PPSV23 should be administered at least 8 weeks after any prior PCV13 dose.
- A single revaccination with PPSV23 should be administered 5 years after the first dose to children with sickle cell disease or other hemoglobinopathies; anatomic or functional asplenia; congenital or acquired immunodeficiencies; HIV infection; chronic renal failure; nephrotic syndrome; diseases associated with treatment with immunosuppressive drugs or radiation therapy, including malignant neoplasms, leukemias, lymphomas, and Hodgkin disease; generalized malignancy; solid organ transplantation; or multiple myeloma.

7. Inactivated poliovirus vaccine (IPV). (Minimum age: 6 weeks)

Routine vaccination:

- Administer a 4-dose series of IPV at ages 2, 4, 6 through 18 months, and 4 through 6 years. The final dose in the series should be administered on or after the fourth birthday and at least 6 months after the previous dose.

Catch-up vaccination:

- In the first 6 months of life, minimum age and minimum intervals are only recommended if the person is at risk for imminent exposure to circulating poliovirus (i.e., travel to a polio-endemic region or during an outbreak).
- If 4 or more doses are administered before age 4 years, an additional dose should be administered at age 4 through 6 years and at least 6 months after the previous dose.
- A fourth dose is not necessary if the third dose was administered at age 4 years or older and at least 6 months after the previous dose.
- If both OPV and IPV were administered as part of a series, a total of 4 doses should be administered, regardless of the child's current age. IPV is not routinely recommended for U.S. residents aged 18 years or older.
- For other catch-up guidance, see Figure 2.

8. Influenza vaccines. (Minimum age: 6 months for inactivated influenza vaccine [IIV], 2 years for live, attenuated influenza vaccine [LAIV])

Routine vaccination:

- Administer influenza vaccine annually to all children beginning at age 6 months. For most healthy, nonpregnant persons aged 2 through 49 years, either LAIV or IIV may be used. However, LAIV should NOT be administered to some persons, including 1) those with asthma, 2) children 2 through 4 years who had wheezing in the past 12 months, or 3) those who have any other underlying medical conditions that predispose them to influenza complications. For all other contraindications to use of LAIV, see *MMWR* 2013; 62 (No. RR-7):1–43, available at http://www.cdc.gov/mmwr/pdf/rr/rr6207.pdf.

For children aged 6 months through 8 years:

- For the 2013–14 season, administer 2 doses (separated by at least 4 weeks) to children who are receiving influenza vaccine for the first time. Some children in this age group who have been vaccinated previously will also need 2 doses. For additional guidance, follow dosing guidelines in the 2013-14 ACIP influenza vaccine recommendations, *MMWR* 2013; 62 (No. RR-7):1–43, available at http://www.cdc.gov/mmwr/pdf/rr/rr6207.pdf.
- For the 2014–15 season, follow dosing guidelines in the 2014 ACIP influenza vaccine recommendations.

For persons aged 9 years and older:

- Administer 1 dose.

Figure 17-1 —cont'd

Continued

For further guidance on the use of the vaccines mentioned below, see: http://www.cdc.gov/vaccines/hcp/acip-recs/index.html.

9. **Measles, mumps, and rubella (MMR) vaccine. (Minimum age: 12 months for routine vaccination)**

Routine vaccination:

- Administer a 2-dose series of MMR vaccine at ages 12 through 15 months and 4 through 6 years. The second dose may be administered before age 4 years, provided at least 4 weeks have elapsed since the first dose.
- Administer 1 dose of MMR vaccine to infants aged 6 through 11 months before departure from the United States for international travel. These children should be revaccinated with 2 doses of MMR vaccine, the first at age 12 through 15 months (12 months if the child remains in an area where disease risk is high), and the second dose at least 4 weeks later.
- Administer 2 doses of MMR vaccine to children aged 12 months and older before departure from the United States for international travel. The first dose should be administered on or after age 12 months and the second dose at least 4 weeks later.

Catch-up vaccination:

- Ensure that all school-aged children and adolescents have had 2 doses of MMR vaccine; the minimum interval between the 2 doses is 4 weeks.

10. **Varicella (VAR) vaccine. (Minimum age: 12 months)**

Routine vaccination:

- Administer a 2-dose series of VAR vaccine at ages 12 through 15 months and 4 through 6 years. The second dose may be administered before age 4 years, provided at least 3 months have elapsed since the first dose. If the second dose was administered at least 4 weeks after the first dose, it can be accepted as valid.

Catch-up vaccination:

- Ensure that all persons aged 7 through 18 years without evidence of immunity (see MMWR 2007; 56 [No. RR-4], available at http://www.cdc.gov/mmwr/pdf/rr/rr5604.pdf) have 2 doses of varicella vaccine. For children aged 7 through 12 years, the recommended minimum interval between doses is 3 months (if the second dose was administered at least 4 weeks after the first dose, it can be accepted as valid); for persons aged 13 years and older, the minimum interval between doses is 4 weeks.

11. **Hepatitis A (HepA) vaccine. (Minimum age: 12 months)**

Routine vaccination:

- Initiate the 2-dose HepA vaccine series at 12 through 23 months; separate the 2 doses by 6 to 18 months.
- Children who have received 1 dose of HepA vaccine before age 24 months should receive a second dose 6 to 18 months after the first dose.
- For any person aged 2 years and older who has not already received the HepA vaccine series, 2 doses of HepA vaccine separated by 6 to 18 months may be administered if immunity against hepatitis A virus infection is desired.

Catch-up vaccination:

- The minimum interval between the two doses is 6 months.

Special populations:

- Administer 2 doses of HepA vaccine at least 6 months apart to previously unvaccinated persons who live in areas where vaccination programs target older children, or who are at increased risk for infection. This includes persons traveling to or working in countries that have high or intermediate endemicity of infection; men having sex with men; users of injection and non-injection illicit drugs; persons who work with HAV-infected primates or with HAV in a research laboratory; persons with clotting-factor disorders; persons with chronic liver disease; and persons who anticipate close, personal contact (e.g., household or regular babysitting) with an international adoptee during the first 60 days after arrival in the United States from a country with high or intermediate endemicity. The first dose should be administered as soon as the adoption is planned, ideally 2 or more weeks before the arrival of the adoptee.

12. **Human papillomavirus (HPV) vaccines. (Minimum age: 9 years for HPV2 [Cervarix] and HPV4 [Gardasil])**

Routine vaccination:

- Administer a 3-dose series of HPV vaccine on a schedule of 0, 1-2, and 6 months to all adolescents aged 11 through 12 years. Either HPV4 or HPV2 may be used for females, and only HPV4 may be used for males.
- The vaccine series may be started at age 9 years.
- Administer the second dose 1 to 2 months after the first dose (minimum interval of 4 weeks), administer the third dose 24 weeks after the first dose and 16 weeks after the second dose (minimum interval of 12 weeks).

Catch-up vaccination:

- Administer the vaccine series to females (either HPV2 or HPV4) and males (HPV4) at age 13 through 18 years if not previously vaccinated.
- Use recommended routine dosing intervals (see above) for vaccine series catch-up.

13. **Meningococcal conjugate vaccines. (Minimum age: 6 weeks for Hib-MenCY [MenHibrix], 9 months for MenACWY-D [Menactra], 2 months for MenACWY-CRM [Menveo])**

Routine vaccination:

- Administer a single dose of Menactra or Menveo vaccine at age 11 through 12 years, with a booster dose at age 16 years.
- Adolescents aged 11 through 18 years with human immunodeficiency virus (HIV) infection should receive a 2-dose primary series of Menactra or Menveo with at least 8 weeks between doses.
- For children aged 2 months through 18 years with high-risk conditions, see below.

Catch-up vaccination:

- Administer Menactra or Menveo vaccine at age 13 through 18 years if not previously vaccinated.
- If the first dose is administered at age 13 through 15 years, a booster dose should be administered at age 16 through 18 years with a minimum interval of at least 8 weeks between doses.
- If the first dose is administered at age 16 years or older, a booster dose is not needed.
- For other catch-up guidance, see Figure 2.

Vaccination of persons with high-risk conditions and other persons at increased risk of disease:

Children with anatomic or functional asplenia (including sickle cell disease):

1. For children younger than 19 months of age, administer a 4-dose infant series of MenHibrix or Menveo at 2, 4, 6, and 12 through 15 months of age.
2. For children aged 19 through 23 months who have not completed a series of MenHibrix or Menveo, administer 2 primary doses of Menveo at least 3 months apart.
3. For children aged 24 months and older who have not received a complete series of MenHibrix or Menveo or Menactra, administer 2 primary doses of either Menactra or Menveo at least 2 months apart. If Menactra is administered to a child with asplenia (including sickle cell disease), do not administer Menactra until 2 years of age and at least 4 weeks after the completion of all PCV13 doses.

Children with persistent complement component deficiency:

1. For children younger than 19 months of age, administer a 4-dose infant series of either MenHibrix or Menveo at 2, 4, 6, and 12 through 15 months of age.
2. For children 7 through 23 months who have not initiated vaccination, two options exist depending on age and vaccine brand:
    a. For children who initiate vaccination with Menveo at 7 months through 23 months of age, a 2-dose series should be administered with the second dose after 12 months of age and at least 3 months after the first dose.
    b. For children who initiate vaccination with Menactra at 9 months through 23 months of age, a 2-dose series of Menactra should be administered at least 3 months apart.
    c. For children aged 24 months and older who have not received a complete series of MenHibrix, Menveo, or Menactra, administer 2 primary doses of either Menactra or Menveo at least 2 months apart.

- For children who travel to or reside in countries in which meningococcal disease is hyperendemic or epidemic, including countries in the African meningitis belt or the Hajj, administer an age-appropriate formulation and series of Menactra or Menveo for protection against serogroups A and W meningococcal disease. Prior receipt of MenHibrix is not sufficient for children traveling to the meningitis belt or the Hajj because it does not contain serogroups A or W.
- For children at risk during a community outbreak attributable to a vaccine serogroup, administer or complete an age- and formulation-appropriate series of MenHibrix, Menactra, or Menveo.
- For booster doses among persons with high-risk conditions, refer to MMWR 2013; 62(RR02);1-22, available at http://www.cdc.gov/mmwr/preview/mmwrhtml/rr6202a1.htm.

Catch-up recommendations for persons with high-risk conditions:

1. If MenHibrix is administered to achieve protection against meningococcal disease, a complete age-appropriate series of MenHibrix should be administered.
2. If the first dose of MenHibrix is given at or after 12 months of age, a total of 2 doses should be given at least 8 weeks apart to ensure protection against serogroups C and Y meningococcal disease.
3. For children who initiate vaccination with Menveo at 7 months through 9 months of age, a 2-dose series should be administered with the second dose after 12 months of age and at least 3 months after the first dose.
4. For other catch-up recommendations for these persons, refer to MMWR 2013; 62(RR02);1-22, available at http://www.cdc.gov/mmwr/preview/mmwrhtml/rr6202a1.htm.

For complete information on use of meningococcal vaccines, including guidance related to vaccination of persons at increased risk of infection, see MMWR March 22, 2013; 62(RR02);1-22, available at http://www.cdc.gov/mmwr/pdf/rr/rr6202.pdf.

Figure 17-1 —cont'd

American Academy of Pediatrics Bright Futures Practice Guides, http://brightfutures.aap.org/practice_guides_and_other_resources.html

Influenza

61. When advising parents about injectable influenza immunization, the clinician considers the following about the vaccine:
   A. The vaccine is contraindicated with a personal history of an anaphylactic reaction to eggs.
   B. Its use is limited to children older than 2 years.
   C. The vaccine contains live virus.
   D. Its use is recommended for members of households of high-risk patients.

62. A 7-year-old child with type 1 diabetes mellitus is about to receive injectable influenza vaccine. His parents and he should be advised that:
   A. the vaccine is more than 90% effective in preventing influenza.
   B. use of the vaccine is contraindicated during antibiotic therapy.
   C. localized immunization reactions are common.
   D. a short, intense, flu-like syndrome typically occurs after immunization.

63. When giving influenza vaccine to a 7-year-old who has not received this immunization in the past, the NP considers that:
   A. two doses 4 weeks or more apart should be given.
   B. a single dose is adequate.
   C. children in this age group have the highest rate of influenza-related hospitalization.
   D. the vaccine should not be given to a child with shellfish allergy.

64. With regard to seasonal influenza prevention in well children, the NP considers that:
   A. compared with school-aged children, younger children (≤24 months old) have an increased risk of seasonal influenza-related hospitalization.
   B. a full adult dose of seasonal influenza vaccine should be given starting at age 4 years.
   C. the use of the seasonal influenza vaccine in well children is discouraged.
   D. widespread use of the vaccine is likely to increase the risk of eczema and antibiotic allergies.

65. When advising a patient about immunization with the nasal spray flu vaccine, the NP considers the following:
   A. its use is acceptable during pregnancy.
   B. its use is limited to children younger than age 2 years.
   C. it contains live virus.
   D. A potentially harmful virus can be shed to vulnerable household members post vaccination.

66. Which of the following should not receive vaccination against influenza?
   A. a 19 year old with a history of hive-form reaction to eating eggs
   B. A 24-year-old woman who is 8 weeks pregnant
   C. a 4-month-old infant who was born at 32 weeks' gestation
   D. A 28-year-old woman who is breastfeeding a 2 week old

67. The most common mode of influenza virus transmission is via:
   A. contact with a contaminated surface.
   B. respiratory droplet.
   C. saliva contact.
   D. skin-to-skin contact.

Answers

61. D.	64. A.	67. B.
62. C.	65. C.	
63. A.	66. C.	

Influenza is a viral illness that typically causes many days of incapacitation and suffering and the risk of hospitalization and death. Children with influenza commonly have acute otitis media, nausea, and vomiting in addition to the aforementioned signs and symptom. Although the worst symptoms in most uncomplicated cases resolve in about 1 week, the cough and malaise often persist for 2 or more weeks. Individuals with ongoing health problems such as pulmonary or cardiac disease, young children, and pregnant women also have increased risk of influenza-related complications including pneumonia.

Influenza viruses spread from person to person largely via respiratory droplet from an infected person, primarily through a cough or sneeze. Children remain infectious for 10 or more days after the onset of symptoms and can shed the virus before the onset of symptoms. People who are immunocompromised can remain infectious for up to 3 weeks.

Historically, the risks for complications, hospitalizations, and deaths from influenza are higher among adults older than 65 years, young children, and individuals of any age with certain underlying health conditions than among healthy older children and younger adults. In children younger than 5 years, hospitalization rates for influenza-related illness have ranged from approximately 500/100,000 for children with high-risk medical conditions to 100/100,000 for children without high-risk medical conditions. Influenza strains such as H1N1, an influenza A virus also known as swine flu, and H5N1, an influenza A virus also known as avian flu, appear to cause a greater disease burden in younger adults. Considering these factors, influenza is a potentially serious illness with significant morbidity and mortality risk across the life span.

Immunization is considered to be generally effective with rates varying based on type of virus strain, regions of the country, age; it also varies year to year. In general individuals aged 2 through 50 tend to be well protected by the flu vaccine, whereas those on either end of the age spectrum having greater risk. Historically, influenza vaccine has been 70% to 80% effective in preventing or reducing the severity of the influenza A and B viruses.

The CDC recommends that all members of the population age 6 months and older should receive annual immunization against seasonal influenza (Table 17–6). In addition, certain groups at highest risk of influenza complications or transmission should be prioritized for immunization. The optimal time to receive seasonal influenza vaccine is usually in October or November, about 1 month before the anticipated onset of the flu season in the northern hemisphere. When a child younger than 8 years receives influenza vaccine for the first time, two doses 4 or more weeks apart should be given.

Pregnant women should be immunized against influenza; the vaccine can be given regardless of pregnancy trimester. Partly because of the change in the respiratory and immune system normally present during pregnancy, influenza is five times more likely to cause serious disease in a pregnant woman compared with a nonpregnant woman. In addition, women who are immunized against influenza during pregnancy are able to pass a portion of this protection on to the unborn child, providing important protection during the first 6 months of life. Flu vaccine is also safe to give during lactation. Injectable trivalent influenza vaccine (TIV), more commonly called the "flu shot," is available in a variety of forms. These include the standard-dose TIV, given intramuscularly (IM), the low-dose

TIV given intradermally, and the high-dose IM TIV. The standard dose is given to children and teens younger than 18 years old (see Table 17–6). Having a mild illness or taking an antibiotic is not a contraindication to any immunization, including influenza. The injectable vaccine does not contain live virus and is not shed. Injectable influenza vaccine is recommended for household members of high-risk patients to avoid transmission of infection.

The nasal-spray flu vaccine, also known as live attenuated influenza vaccine (LAIV), differs from the injectable influenza vaccine or "flu shot" because it contains weakened live influenza viruses instead of killed viruses and is administered by nasal spray instead of injection. The nasal-spray flu vaccine contains three different influenza viruses that are sufficiently weakened as to be incapable of causing disease but have sufficient strength to stimulate a protective immune response. The viruses in the LAIV are cold adapted and temperature sensitive. As a result, the viruses can grow in the nose and throat but not in the lower respiratory tract, where the temperature is higher. LAIV is currently approved for use in healthy people 2 to 49 years old. Aside from the age restrictions, individuals who should not receive LAIV include those with a health condition that places them at high risk for complications from influenza, including patients with chronic heart or lung disease, such as asthma or reactive airway disease, patients with immunosuppression, children or adolescents receiving long-term aspirin therapy, people with a history of Guillain-Barré syndrome, pregnant women, and people with a history of allergy to any of the components of LAIV. While there is a potential to have virus shed from the nose post LAIV administration, this is not harmful to

---

Table 17-6

Advisory Committee on Immunization Practices (ACIP) Recommendations on Influenza Immunization

Routine influenza vaccination is recommended for all persons aged 6 months and older. Although everyone should get a flu vaccine each flu season, certain patient populations are at high risk of having serious flu-related complications or live with or care for people at high risk for developing flu-related complications. This populations include:

- Pregnant women
- Children younger than 5 years, especially children younger than 2 years old
- Individuals age 50 years of age and older
- Individuals of any age with certain chronic medical conditions
- Residents of nursing homes and other long-term-care facilities
- People who live with or care for those at high risk for complications from flu, including:
  Healthcare workers
  Household contacts of persons at high risk for complications from the flu
  Household contacts and out-of-home caregivers of children younger than 6 months of age (these children are too young to be vaccinated)

All children aged 6 months to 8 years who receive a seasonal influenza vaccine for the first time should receive two doses. Children who received only one dose of a seasonal influenza vaccine in the first influenza season should receive two doses, rather than one, the following influenza season.

Source: Prevention and control of seasonal influenza with vaccines: Recommendations of the Advisory Committee on Immunization Practices (ACIP)—United States, 2013–2014; *MMWR* 62(RR07);1–43, 2013.

close contacts under virtually all circumstances. Adverse effects include nasal irritation and discharge, muscle aches, sore throat, and fever.

Until relatively recently, egg allergy was considered a contraindication to receiving all forms of influenza vaccine. Current recommendations advise that most individuals with an egg allergy can safely receive the influenza vaccine (Table 17–7).

DISCUSSION SOURCES

Centers for Disease Control and Prevention. Vaccine Preventable Childhood Diseases, http://www.cdc.gov/vaccines/schedules /hcp/child-adolescent.html

Centers for Disease Control and Prevention: Influenza: The Basics, available at http://www.cdc.gov/flu/about/disease/index.htm

) Hepatitis B

68. Which of the following statements is true about the hepatitis B virus (HBV) vaccine?
A. The vaccine contains live HBV.
B. Children should have hepatitis B surface antibody (HBsAb, anti-HBs) titers drawn after three doses of vaccine.
C. Hepatitis B immunization series should be offered to all children.
D. Serological testing for HBsAb should be checked before HBV vaccination is initiated in children.

69. You are making rounds in the nursery and examine the neonate of a mother who is HBsAg-positive. Your most appropriate action is to:
A. administer hepatitis B immune globulin (HBIG).
B. isolate the infant.
C. administer hepatitis B immunization.
D. give hepatitis B immunization and HBIG.

70. Without intervention, approximately 40% of infants born to mothers with HBV infection will go on to:
A. develop acute hepatitis B infection.
B. die from chronic liver disease.
C. develop chronic hepatitis B.
D. develop lifelong immunity to the hepatitis B virus.

71. Hepatitis B vaccine should not be given to a child with a history of anaphylactic reaction to:
A. egg.
B. baker's yeast.
C. neomycin.
D. streptomycin.

72. Infants who have been infected perinatally with HBV have an estimated ___% lifetime chance of developing hepatocellular carcinoma or cirrhosis.
A. 10
B. 25
C. 50
D. 75

Table 17-7
Providing Influenza Vaccine With Egg Allergy History

The following recommendations apply when considering influenza vaccination for patients who have or report a history of egg allergy.

1. People who have experienced only hives following exposure to egg should receive influenza vaccine with the following additional measures:
    * Because studies published to date involved use of TIV, TIV (flu shot) rather than LAIV should be used.
    * Vaccine should be administered by a healthcare provider who is familiar with the potential manifestations of egg allergy.
    * Vaccine recipients should be observed for at least 30 minutes for signs of a reaction following administration of each vaccine dose.
    * Other measures, such as dividing and administering the vaccine by a two-step approach and skin testing with vaccine, are not necessary.
2. People who report having had reactions to egg involving angioedema, respiratory distress, lightheadedness, or recurrent emesis, or persons who required epinephrine or other emergency medical intervention, particularly those that occurred immediately or within minutes to hours after egg exposure, are more likely to have a serious systemic or anaphylactic reaction upon re-exposure to egg proteins. Before receipt of vaccine, such persons should be referred to a clinician with expertise in the management of allergic conditions for further risk assessment.
3. Some people who report allergy to egg might not be egg allergic. Those who are able to eat lightly cooked egg (scrambled eggs) without reaction are unlikely to be allergic. Conversely, people with egg allergy might tolerate egg in baked products (bread, cake, other bakery products); tolerance to egg-containing foods does not exclude the possibility of egg allergy. Egg allergy can be confirmed by a consistent medical history of adverse reactions to eggs and egg-containing foods plus skin and/or blood testing for immunoglobulin E antibodies to egg proteins.
4. A previous severe allergic reaction to influenza vaccine, regardless of the component suspected to be responsible for the reaction, is a contraindication to receipt of influenza vaccine.

Source: Prevention and control of seasonal influenza with vaccines: Recommendations of the Advisory Committee on Immunization Practices (ACIP)—United States, 2013–2014; *MMWR* 62(RR07);1–43, 2013.

73. In healthy children, the second and third doses of the HBV vaccine should be separated by at least how much time?
   A. 4 weeks
   B. 8 weeks
   C. 6 months
   D. 1 year

74. Jason is a healthy 18 year old who presents for primary care. According to his immunization record, he received two doses of HBV vaccine 1 month apart at age 14 years. Which of the following best describes his HBV vaccination needs?
   A. He should receive a single dose of HBV vaccine now.
   B. A three-dose HBV vaccine series should be started during today's visit.
   C. He has completed the recommended HBV vaccine series.
   D. He should be tested for HBsAb and further immunization recommendations should be made according to the test results.

75. Universal infant vaccination against HBV was recommended in what year?
   A. 1972
   B. 1978
   C. 1982
   D. 1991

76. Routine adolescent vaccination against HBV was recommended in what year?
   A. 1996
   B. 1991
   C. 1982
   D. 1978

Answers

68. C.	71. B.	74. A.
69. D.	72. B.	75. D.
70. C.	73. B.	76. A.

Hepatitis B virus (HBV) infection is caused by a small, double-stranded DNA virus that contains the inner protein of hepatitis B core antigen and an outer surface of hepatitis B surface antigen. The virus is transmitted through exchange of blood and body fluids. HBV infection can be prevented by limiting exposure to blood and body fluids and through immunization. Recombinant HBV vaccine, which does not contain live virus, is well tolerated but is contraindicated in a person who has a history of anaphylactic reaction to baker's yeast. HBV vaccine is recommended routinely for all infants and is administered in a three-injection series at 0, 1, and 6 months of age. If the vaccine series is interrupted after the first dose, the second dose should be administered as soon as possible. The second pend third doses should be separated by an interval of at least 8 weeks. If only the

third dose is delayed, it should be administered as soon as possible. However, it is not necessary to restart the series if a vaccine dose is missed.

Universal infant vaccination against HBV was recommended in 1991, and routine adolescent vaccination was recommended in 1996. One major at-risk group is adults who have not received the vaccine. As with all vaccines, immunization against HBV should be delayed only in the face of serious or life-threatening illness and not for milder illness. Approximately 90% to 95% of people who receive the vaccine develop HBsAb after three doses, which implies protection from the virus. Routine testing for the presence of HBsAb after immunization is not generally recommended.

Perinatal transmission of HBV is highly efficient and usually occurs during exposure to blood during labor and delivery. Infants who have been infected perinatally with HBV have an estimated 25% lifetime chance of developing hepatocellular carcinoma or cirrhosis. As a result, all pregnant women should undergo screening for hepatitis B surface antigen (HBsAg) at the first prenatal visit, regardless of HBV vaccine history, because the vaccine is not 100% effective and a woman could have been infected with HBV before pregnancy. Women at particularly high risk for new HBV acquisition during pregnancy should be retested for HBsAg in later pregnancy.

During the first 24 hours of life, a neonate born to a mother with HBV should receive HBV vaccine and hepatitis B immune globulin (HBIG) to minimize the risk of perinatal transmission and subsequent development of chronic HBV infection. If maternal HBsAg status is unknown, a situation common in children who have been adopted internationally, consideration should be given to testing the child for evidence of perinatal acquisition of HBV infection.

Without intervention, the risk for chronic HBV infection is 70% to 90% by age 6 months in a newborn infant whose mother is positive for both HBsAg and HBeAg and <10% for infants of women who are HBsAg positive but HBeAg negative. HBV vaccine and one dose of HBIG administered within 24 hours after birth are 85% to 95% effective in preventing both acute HBV infection and chronic infection. HBV vaccine administered alone beginning within 24 hours after birth is 70% to 95% effective in preventing perinatal HBV infection. Infants of infected mothers should then complete the vaccine series, which should be followed by postvaccination serological testing to determine whether the infant has developed immunity or chronic HBV infection. Infants diagnosed with chronic HBV infection should receive appropriate follow-up and treatment.

DISCUSSION SOURCES

Centers for Disease Control and Prevention: Hepatitis B for Healthcare Professionals, http://www.cdc.gov/NCIDOD/DISEASES/hepatitis/b,Viral hepatitis B.

Advisory Committee on Immunization Practices (ACIP) recommended immunization schedule for persons aged 0 through 18 years—United States, 2013. *MMWR* 62:2–8, 2013.

A comprehensive immunization strategy to eliminate transmission of hepatitis B virus infection in the United States—Recommendations

of the Advisory Committee on Immunization Practices (ACIP) —
Part 1: Immunization of infants, children, and adolescents. *MMWR*
54(RR16):1–23, 2005.
A comprehensive immunization strategy to eliminate transmission of
hepatitis B virus infection in the United States—Recommendations
of the Advisory Committee on Immunization Practices (ACIP) —
Part II: Immunization of adults. *MMWR* 55(RR16):1–25, 2006.

Varicella

77. Which of the following statements is correct about the
varicella vaccine?
A. This vaccine contains killed varicella-zoster virus
(VZV).
B. A short febrile illness is common during the first
days after vaccination.
C. Children should have a varicella titer drawn before
receiving the vaccine.
D. Rarely, mild cases of chickenpox have been reported
in immunized patients.

78. Expected outcomes with the use of varicella vaccine
include a reduction in the rate of all of the following
except:
A. shingles.
B. Reye syndrome.
C. aspirin sensitivity.
D. invasive varicella.

79. A parent asks about varicella-zoster immune globulin,
and you reply that it is a:
A. synthetic product that is well tolerated.
B. derived blood product that has been known to
transmit infectious disease.
C. blood product obtained from a single donor.
D. pooled blood product with an excellent safety
profile.

80. A healthy child with no evidence of immunity is ex-
posed to chickenpox at school. How soon after expo-
sure will a dose of the varicella vaccine prevent or
modify the disease in the child?
A. only if given the same day
B. only if given within 2 to 3 days
C. if given within 3 to 5 days
D. if given within 1 week

81. Maria is a 28-year-old well woman who is 6 weeks pregnant and voices her intent to breastfeed her infant for at
least 6 months. Her routine prenatal laboratory testing
reveals she is not immune to varicella. Which of the
following represents the best advice for Maria?
A. She should receive VZV vaccine once she is in her
second pregnancy trimester.
B. Maria should be advised to receive two appropriately timed doses of VZV vaccine after giving birth.
C. Once Maria is no longer breastfeeding, she should
receive one dose of VZV vaccine.
D. A dose of VZIG should be administered now.

82. How is the varicella virus most commonly transmitted?
A. droplet transmission
B. contact with inanimate reservoirs
C. contact transmission
D. waterborne transmission

____ 83. Which groups with no history of varicella infec-
tion or previous immunization should be targeted
for vaccination (choose all that apply)?
A. those born before 1980
B. individuals >8 years old with HIV infection with
CD4+ T-lymphocyte counts ≥200 cells/µL
C. adults and children with a history of anaphylactic
reaction when exposed to neomycin
D. day-care workers

84. Which group is shown to have the highest rate of vari-
cella mortality?
A. children aged 6 and younger
B. teenagers aged 12–19
C. adults aged 30–49
D. health-care workers

Answers

77. D.	80. C.	83. B and D.
78. C.	81. B.	84. C.
79. D.	82. A.	

VZV causes the highly contagious, systemic disease commonly known as chickenpox. Varicella infection usually
confers lifetime immunity. Reinfection may be seen, however,
in patients who are immunocompromised. More often,
re-exposure causes an increase in antibody titers without
causing disease.

VZV can lie dormant in sensory nerve ganglion. Later
reactivation causes shingles, a painful, vesicular-form
rash in a dermatomal pattern. About 15% of people who
have had chickenpox develop shingles at least once during
their lifetime. Shingles rates are markedly reduced in people who have received the varicella vaccine compared with
people who have had chickenpox. The virus is transmitted
via respiratory droplet and contact with open lesions.
Chickenpox can be serious, especially in infants, who are
immunocompromised.

A patient-reported history of varicella is considered a
valid measurement of immunity, with 97% to 99% of persons having serological evidence of immunity. Individuals
born before 1980 also have evidence of immunity. Individuals who are recommended to present evidence of immunity through serologic testing include pregnant women, and
immunocompromised persons. Varicella immunity should
be confirmed through varicella titers, even in the presence
of a positive varicella history, in healthcare workers because
of their risk of exposure and potential transmission of the
disease.

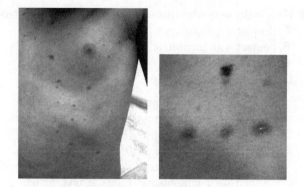

Figure 17-2 Skin Lesions in Varicella.

The varicella vaccine contains live attenuated virus. The vaccine is administered in two doses, one at age 1 year and the second at age 4 to 6 years. Older children and adults with no history of varicella infection or previous immunization should receive two immunizations 4 to 8 weeks apart. In particular, healthcare workers, people >8 years old with HIV and CD4+ T-lymphocyte counts ≥200 cells/μL, family contacts of immunocompromised patients, and daycare workers without evidence of varicella immunity should be targeted for varicella vaccine. In addition, adults who are in environments with a high risk of varicella transmission (e.g., college dormitories, military barracks, long-term-care facilities) should receive the immunization if there is no evidence of varicella immunity.

Pregnant women should be assessed for evidence of varicella immunity. Women who do not have evidence of immunity should receive the first dose of varicella vaccine on completion or termination of pregnancy and before discharge from the healthcare facility. The second dose should be administered 4 to 8 weeks after the first dose.

For healthy children older than 12 months without evidence of immunity, vaccination within 3 to 5 days of exposure to varicella is beneficial in preventing or modifying the disease. Studies have shown that vaccination administered within 3 days of exposure to rash is at least 90% effective in preventing varicella, whereas vaccination within 5 days of exposure to rash is approximately 70% effective in preventing varicella and 100% effective in modifying severe disease.

The vaccine is highly protective against severe, invasive varicella; however, mild forms of chickenpox are occasionally reported after immunization. Varicella immune globulin, as with all forms of immune globulin, provides temporary, passive immunity to infection. Immune globulin is a pooled blood product with an excellent safety profile. Although most cases are seen in children younger than age 18 years, the greatest varicella mortality is found in persons 30 to 49 years old.

DISCUSSION SOURCES

Centers for Disease Control and Prevention. Varicella vaccination: information for healthcare providers, http://www.cdc.gov/vaccines/vpd-vac/varicella/default-hcp.htm

Centers for Disease Control and Prevention. Assessing immunity to varicella, http://www.cdc.gov/chickenpox/hcp/immunity.html

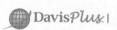
See full color images of this topic on DavisPlus at
http://davisplus.fadavis.com |
Keyword: Fitzgerald

Diphtheria and Tetanus

85. An 11-year-old well child presents with no documented primary tetanus immunization series. Which of the following represents the immunization needed?
   A. three doses of DTaP (diphtheria, tetanus, acellular pertussis) vaccine 2 months apart
   B. tetanus immune globulin now and two doses of tetanus-diphtheria (Td) 1 month apart
   C. one dose of Tdap (tetanus, diphtheria, acellular pertussis vaccine) followed by two doses of Td (tetanus, diphtheria) in 1 and 6 months
   D. Td (tetanus, diphtheria) as a single dose

86. Problems after tetanus immunization typically include:
   A. localized reaction at site of injection
   B. myalgia and malaise
   C. low-grade fever
   D. diffuse rash

87. Which wound presents the greatest risk for tetanus infection?
   A. a puncture wound obtained while playing in a garden
   B. a laceration obtained from a knife used to trim raw beef
   C. a human bite
   D. an abrasion obtained by falling on a sidewalk

88. Infection with *Corynebacterium diphtheriae* usually causes:
   A. a diffuse rash.
   B. meningitis.
   C. pseudomembranous pharyngitis.
   D. a gastroenteritis-like illness.

Answers

85. C.   **86.** A.   **87.** A.   **88.** C.

The tetanus infection is caused by *Clostridium tetani,* an anaerobic, gram-positive, spore-forming rod. This organism is found in soil and is particularly potent in manure. If contracted, it enters the body through a contaminated wound and causes a life-threatening systemic disease characterized by painful muscle weakness and spasm ("lockjaw"). Diphtheria is caused by *C. diphtheriae,* a gram-negative bacillus. This infection is typically transmitted person-to-person or through contaminated liquids such as milk. Diphtheria is characterized by severe respiratory tract infection, including the appearance of pseudomembranous pharyngitis. Pertussis, or whopping cough, is a highly contagious disease that is passed from person to person by droplets from coughing or sneezing. Many infants are infected by older siblings, parents, or caregivers who might be unaware that they have the disease. Symptoms of pertussis usually develop within 7 to 10 days after being exposed, but they may appear up to 6 weeks later. If left untreated, adverse outcomes from pertussis can lead to pneumonia, seizures, brain damage, or death. All three infections are now uncommon because of widespread immunization. The DTaP vaccine is administered to infants and children, and the booster vaccine Tdap is given to adolescents and adults. Children should get five doses of DTaP vaccine, one dose at each of the following ages: 2 months, 4 months, 6 months, 5 to 18 months and 4 to 6 years. A child who has a life-threatening allergic reaction or has suffered a brain or nervous system disease within 7 days after a dose of DTaP should not be given another dose. DT does not contain acellular pertussis and is used as a substitute for DTaP for children who cannot tolerate the pertussis vaccine. The rate of adverse effects with acellular pertussis vaccine is quite low; problems were more commonly noted with the older whole-cell pertussis vaccine form that is no longer in use in North America.

Tetanus and diphtheria immunizations with or without acellular pertussis are well tolerated and produce few adverse reactions. A short-term, localized area of redness and warmth is common and is not predictive of future problems with tetanus immunization.

A single dose of Tdap is recommended for people 11 through 64 years of age. A booster tetanus dose every 10 years is recommended, but protection is likely provided for 20 to 30 years after a primary series. Using the tetanus–diphtheria (Td) vaccine rather than the tetanus toxoid form for the primary series and booster doses in adults also assists in keeping diphtheria immunity.

The use of a single dose of Tdap during adulthood provides additional protection from pertussis, whereas older children (7 through 18 years old) undergoing a "catch-up" immunization schedule should receive one Tdap and two Td doses at the appropriate interval. Women, including teens, should receive Tdap during each of their pregnancies (preferably in the third trimester between the 27th and 36th week).

At the time of a wound-producing injury, tetanus immune globulin may provide temporary protection for individuals who have not received tetanus immunization. The tetanus booster and appropriate antibiotics should also be administered, if needed.

DISCUSSION SOURCES

Centers for Disease Control and Prevention: Diphtheria, http://www.cdc.gov/diphtheria/clinicians.html.
Centers for Disease Control and Prevention: Tetanus, http://www.cdc.gov/vaccines/vpd-vac/tetanus.
Centers for Disease Control and Prevention: Pertussis, http://www.cdc.gov/vaccines/vpd-vac/pertussis/default.htm.

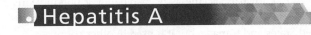

Hepatitis A

89. Which of the following is one of the more common sources of hepatitis A infection in the United States?
    A. receiving blood products
    B. ingestion of raw shellfish
    C. drinking municipally sourced tap water drinking water
    D. exposure to fecally contaminated food

90. When answering questions about hepatitis A vaccine, you consider stating that it:
    A. contains live virus.
    B. should be given to all children unless contraindicated.
    C. frequently causes systemic postimmunization reaction.
    D. is nearly 100% protective after a single injected dose.

91. The hepatitis A vaccine should be administered in childhood per the following schedule:
    A. two doses 3 months apart.
    B. two doses 6 months apart.
    C. two doses 1 year apart.
    D. two doses are not recommended because of efficacy of a single dose.

92. Family members and caregivers of an international adoptee should be given the hepatitis A vaccine per the following schedule:
    A. two doses 6 months apart, one dose before the child arrives.
    B. two doses 3 months apart, one dose before the child arrives.
    C. two doses 1 year apart, one dose before the child arrives.
    D. one dose before the child arrives in the United States.

93. Usual treatment option for a child with hepatitis A includes:
    A. interferon alpha.
    B. ribavirin.
    C. acyclovir.
    D. supportive care.

Answers

89. D.	91. B.	93. D.
90. B.	92. A.	

Hepatitis A infection is caused by hepatitis A virus (HAV), a small RNA virus. It is transmitted primarily by oral–fecal contact, including through sexual and household contact; however, common-source foodborne outbreaks also occur periodically as a result of poor hand-washing by food handlers with HAV infection. The likelihood of having symptoms with HAV infection is related to age; children younger than 6 years of age are likely to have symptoms (>70%), whereas older children and adults are typically asymptomatic. Signs and symptoms typically last <2 months, although 10% to 15% of symptomatic persons have disease lasting up to 6 months. Symptoms, which are not specific to which type of hepatitis, include fever, malaise, anorexia, nausea, abdominal discomfort, dark urine, and jaundice. The only method of diagnosing the type of hepatitis is via laboratory diagnosis.

Hepatitis A is typically a self-limited infection that resolves with supportive care. Acute liver failure can occur in rare (<1%) cases, including among adults age >50 years and in individuals with chronic liver disease. In developing countries with inadequately treated water, most children contract this disease by age 5 years. Since the implementation of universal childhood HAV vaccination in the United States, rates of hepatitis A infection have declined among all age groups. The local public health department should be consulted for advice when a suspected or documented outbreak of hepatitis A infection occurs.

All children at 1 year of age (12–23 months), all children and adolescents age 2 to 18 years in communities with high incidence of HAV, any person traveling to or from countries with intermediate- to high-risk incidence of HAV (such as adoptees), and select high-risk groups (such as injection drug users, men who have sex with men, and persons with chronic liver disease) should be immunized against HAV. HAV vaccination is also recommended for all previously unvaccinated persons who anticipate close personal contact (e.g., household contact or regular babysitting) with an international adoptee from a country of high or intermediate endemicity during the first 60 days following arrival of the adoptee in the United States. The first dose of the two-dose hepatitis A vaccine series (given at 0 and 6 months) should be administered as soon as adoption is planned, ideally 2 or more weeks before the arrival of the adoptee. Two doses of HAV vaccine are recommended (at 0 and 6 months) to ensure an enhanced immunological response. However, the first dose of HAV vaccine is highly efficacious (94%–100%). HAV vaccine, which does not contain live virus, is usually well tolerated without systemic reaction.

DISCUSSION SOURCES

Wasley AF, Bell B. Prevention of Hepatitis A through active or passive immunization: Recommendations of the Advisory Committee on Immunization Practices (ACIP). *MMWR* 55:1–23, 2006.

Updated recommendations from the Advisory Committee on Immunization Practices (ACIP) for use of Hepatitis A vaccine in close contacts of newly arriving international adoptees. *MMWR* 58;1006–1007, 2009.

Polioviruses

94. Which of the following statements is true about oral poliovirus vaccine (OPV)?
    A. It contains killed virus.
    B. It is the preferred method of immunization in North America.
    C. Two doses should be administered by a child's fourth birthday.
    D. After administration of OPV, attenuated live poliovirus can be shed from the stool.

95. Which of the following statements is true about inactivated poliovirus vaccine (IPV)?
    A. It contains live virus.
    B. It is the preferred method of immunization in North America.
    C. Two doses should be administered by a child's fourth birthday.
    D. After administration of IPV, live poliovirus is usually shed from the stool.

96. Which of the following is the route of transmission of the poliovirus?
    A. fecal–oral
    B. droplet
    C. blood and body fluids
    D. skin-to-skin contact

97. Post-polio syndrome is commonly marked by:
    A. muscular hypertrophy.
    B. muscle atrophy
    C. flulike symptoms
    D. increased mortality

Answers

94. D.	95. B.	96. A.	97. B.

Polioviruses are highly contagious and capable of causing paralytic, life-threatening infection. The viral infection is transmitted by the fecal–oral route. Rates of infection among household contacts may be as high as 96%. Most people infected with polio have no symptoms. Between 4% and 8% of those infected have minor symptoms, including fever, fatigue, nausea, headache, flulike symptoms, stiffness in the neck and back, and pain in the limbs, which often resolve. Less than 1% of polio cases result in permanent paralysis of the limbs, usually the legs. Of those paralyzed, 5% to 10% die when the paralysis strikes the respiratory muscles.

Post-polio syndrome (PPS) is a condition that affects polio survivors years after recovery from an initial acute attack of the poliomyelitis virus. Polio survivors may experience gradual weakening of muscles that were affected by the polio infection. The most common symptoms include slowly progressive muscle weakness, generalized and muscular fatigue, and muscle atrophy. Pain from joint degeneration and increasing skeletal deformities such as scoliosis is common and can precede the weakness and muscle atrophy. PPS is rarely life-threatening, but the symptoms can significantly interfere with an individual's quality of life.

Since 1994 North and South America have been declared free of indigenous poliomyelitis, largely because of the efficacy of poliovirus immunization. The vaccine is available in two forms: a live-virus vaccine that is given orally (OPV) and an injectable vaccine that contains inactivated virus (IPV). When OPV is used, a small amount of weakened virus is shed via the stool. This shedding presents household members with possible exposure to poliovirus, resulting in a rare risk of paralytic poliomyelitis, known as vaccine-associated paralytic poliomyelitis (VAPP). Because of VAPP risk, OPV is no longer used in the United States and Canada, but it is used in other countries.

IPV is given as an injection in the leg or arm, depending on the patient's age. Most adults likely received polio vaccine in childhood if fully immunized. Children should be given four doses of IPV at the following ages: 2 months, 4 months, 6 to 18 months, and a booster dose at 4 to 6 years. A child with a life-threatening allergy to any component of IPV, including the antibiotics neomycin, streptomycin, or polymyxin B, should not be given IVP. Children with severe allergic reactions to a dose of IVP should not receive another one. Although adverse effects of IPV have not been documented among pregnant women or their fetuses, vaccination of pregnant women should be avoided, according to CDC guidelines.

DISCUSSION SOURCES

Centers for Disease Control and Prevention: Polio Vaccination. Available at: http://www.cdc.gov/vaccines/vpd-vac/polio/#clinical.

National Institutes of Health: Post-Polio Syndrome Fact Sheet. Available at:http://www.ninds.nih.gov/disorders/post_polio/detail_post_polio.htm.

Lead Poisoning

98. Which of the following children is most likely to have lead poisoning?
    A. a developmentally disabled 5-year-old child who lives in a 15-year-old house in poor repair
    B. an infant who lives in a 5-year-old home with copper plumbing
    C. a toddler who lives in an 85-year-old home
    D. a preschooler who lives nears an electric generating plant

99. Sources of lead that can contribute to plumbism include select traditional remedies such as azarcon and greta.
    A. true.
    B. false.

____ 100. A diet low in the following nutrients encourages lead absorption (choose all that apply):
    A. protein.
    B. carbohydrates.
    C. zinc.
    D. magnesium.

101. You are devising a program to screen preschoolers for lead poisoning. The most sensitive component of this campaign is:
    A. environmental history.
    B. physical examination.
    C. hematocrit level.
    D. hemoglobin electrophoresis.

102. Patients with plumbism present with which kind of anemia?
    A. macrocytic, hyperchromic
    B. normocytic, normochromic
    C. hemolytic
    D. microcytic, hypochromic

103. At which of the following ages should screening begin for a child who has significant risk of lead poisoning?
    A. 3 months
    B. 6 months
    C. 1 year
    D. 2 years

104. Intervention for a child with a lead level of 5 to 44 mcg/dL usually includes all of the following except:
    A. removal from the lead source.
    B. iron supplementation.
    C. chelation therapy.
    D. encouraging a diet high in vitamin C.

105. Intervention for a child with a lead level of 40 to 50 mcg/dL usually includes:
    A. chelation therapy.
    B. calcium supplementation.
    C. exchange transfusion.
    D. iron depletion therapy.

Answers

98. C.	101. A.	104. C.
99. A.	102. D.	105. A.
100. C and D	103. B.	

Lead poisoning, or plumbism, remains a significant public health problem. More than 12 million children in the United States have levels above the acceptable threshold, which is estimated to cost billions of dollars in lifetime productivity associated with this exposure. Ingested lead inactivates heme synthesis by inhibiting the insertion of iron into the protoporphyrin ring. This leads to the development of a microcytic, hypochromic anemia; basophilic stippling is often noted on red blood cell morphology. In addition, lead is significantly toxic to the solid organs, bones, and nervous system. Long-term complications of lead poisoning include behavior or attention problems, poor academic performance, hearing problems, kidney damage, reduced IQ, and slowed body growth.

Lead poisoning is caused by exposure to lead in the environment. The major source in children is lead-based paint. This paint has not been available for household use in the United States for more than 35 years. Unless deleading procedures have been performed, however, most homes built before 1957 contain lead-based paint. A diet low in calcium, iron, zinc, magnesium, and copper and high in fat, which is a typical diet for children living in poverty, enhances oral lead absorption.

For lead poisoning to occur, there must be an intersection between the environmental hazard and the child. In older homes, the point of greatest risk is the window because the windowsills and putty have high lead concentration. Because toddlers (age 2 to 3) are the ideal height to reach windowsills and are often drawn to open windows, they are at greatest risk and summer is the riskiest season. Children can ingest lead by inhaling paint chips, house dust, and soil contaminated by leaded paint. Inhalation of paint dust is a potent lead source for infants and for children with lead levels of less than 45 mcg/dL, although toddlers and children with lead levels of more than 45 mcg/dL are typically poisoned by also eating paint chips. The question often arises as to why children would eat a nonfood substance such as a paint chip; these chips are reported to have a slightly sweet taste. In addition to paint, other household products contain lead hazards, including traditional home health remedies such as azarcon and greta, which are used for upset stomach or indigestion in the Hispanic and other ethnic communities, and select imported products including candies, toys, jewelry, cosmetics, pottery, and ceramics. Additional sources include drinking water contaminated by lead leaching from lead pipes, solder, brass fixtures, or valves and consumer products, including tea kettles and vinyl blinds.

Clinical manifestation of lead poisoning is usually not apparent until a child's lead level is markedly elevated. Symptoms of elevated lead levels include abdominal pain and cramping, aggressive behavior, anemia, constipation, difficulty sleeping, headaches, irritability, loss of previous developmental skills in young children, low appetite and energy, and reduced sensations. Very high levels of lead can result in vomiting, staggering walk, muscle weakness, seizures, or coma. Because most children have low-level exposure or chronic lead exposure with few or no symptoms, periodic screening of all children is recommended. Primary prevention of lead poisoning should be the goal to reduce risk for all children. After lead risk is identified, removing the child or limiting exposure is vital.

A measure of 5 mcg/dL is now used to identify children with elevated blood lead levels. This value is in the highest 2.5% for children aged 1 to 5 years in the U.S. population. In the past, blood lead levels of 10 mcg/dL were defined as elevated. This lower value is being used to identify more children likely to have lead exposure, allowing parents, healthcare providers, public health officials, and communities to take action earlier to reduce future exposure to lead. Most children with lead levels of 5–44 mcg/dL are treated with removal from the source, improved nutrition, and iron therapy. Those with lead levels of 45–50 mcg/dL are treated with a chelation agent such as succimer, in addition to the previously listed interventions. For children with lead levels of greater than 51 mcg/dL, hospital admission with expert evaluation is likely the most prudent course to avoid serious problems (including encephalopathy) associated with markedly elevated lead levels.

DISCUSSION SOURCES

Centers for Disease Control and Prevention. Healthy Homes and Lead Poisoning Prevention Program, http://www.cdc.gov/nceh/lead/about/program.htm.
Centers for Disease Control and Prevention: Blood Lead Levels, http://www.cdc.gov/nceh/lead/ACCLPP/blood_lead_levels.htm.
National Institutes of Health: Lead Poisoning, http://nlm.nih.gov/medlineplus/ency/article/002473.htm.

Bronchiolitis

106. Bronchiolitis most commonly occurs in the United States during the warm weather months.
   A. true
   B. false

107. The rate of bronchiolitis is highest in which age group:
   A. toddlers.
   B. school-aged children.
   C. preschool children.
   D. infants younger than age 2 years.

108. The most common causative organism of bronchiolitis is:
   A. *Haemophilus influenzae.*
   B. parainfluenza virus.
   C. respiratory syncytial virus.
   D. coxsackievirus.

109. One of the most prominent clinical features of bronchiolitis is:
   A. fever.
   B. vomiting.
   C. wheezing.
   D. conjunctival inflammation.

110. Which of the following laboratory tests can identify the causative organism of bronchiolitis?
   A. nasal washing antigen test
   B. antibody test via blood sample
   C. urine culture
   D. a laboratory test is not available

111. In most children with bronchiolitis, intervention includes:
   A. aerosolized ribavirin therapy.
   B. supportive care.
   C. oral theophylline therapy.
   D. oral corticoid steroid therapy.

112. Common clinical findings in a young child with bronchiolitis include all of the following except:
   A. pharyngitis.
   B. tachypnea.
   C. bradycardia.
   D. conjunctivitis.

Answers

106. B.	109. C.	112. C.
107. D.	110. A.	
108. C.	111. B.	

Bronchiolitis is a common illness in early childhood; the peak incidence is in children younger than 2 years, with more than 90% of episodes occurring between November and April. The most likely causative organism is respiratory syncytial virus (RSV); it is less often caused by parainfluenza, influenza, or adenovirus. During the acute stage of infection, bronchiolar respiratory and ciliated epithelial cell function is altered, producing increased mucus secretion, cell death, and sloughing. This stage is followed by peribronchiolar lymphocytic infiltrate and submucosal edema; the end result is narrowing and obstruction of small airways with resulting cough and wheezing.

Additional findings include tachypnea, mild fever, conjunctivitis, and pharyngitis. Bronchiolitis is usually diagnosed by clinical findings; rapid antigen tests of nasal washings provide rapid, accurate RSV detection, which can be supplemented with cell culture. Early detection can be particularly helpful in the setting of an outbreak in a daycare or other similar setting. According to the CDC, these tests are 80% to 90% sensitive and are most reliable in young children and less accurate in older children or adults.

Infants and children infected with RSV usually show symptoms within 4 to 6 days of infection. Infants with a lower respiratory tract infection typically have rhinorrhea and a decrease in appetite. Cough usually develops 1 to 3 days later, followed by sneezing, fever, and/or wheezing. In very young infants (<3 months) irritability, decreased activity, and apnea may be the only symptoms of infection. In most children, bronchiolitis runs a course of 2 to 3 weeks. These findings resolve as ciliary function returns. Younger infants and children with weakened immune systems can be contagious for as long as 3 weeks.

Supportive therapy is usually sufficient. In infants younger than 3 months and in children with chronic health problems, hypoxemia or hypercapnia may necessitate hospital admission for hydration and oxygenation. The use of corticosteroids, ribavirin, and bronchodilators, including beta$_2$-agonists, remains controversial with little evidence of efficacy, although standard asthma therapies are effective in children who also have underlying reactive airway disease. Long-term sequelae of bronchiolitis often include recurrent airway reactivity.

DISCUSSION SOURCES

Centers of Disease Control and Prevention: Respiratory Syncytial Virus Infection, http://www.cdc.gov/rsv/.
National Institutes of Health: Bronchiolitis, http://www.nlm.nih.gov/medlineplus/ency/article/000975.htm.

Dermatology Conditions in Younger Children

113. You examine a newborn with a capillary hemangioma on her thigh. You advise her parents that this lesion:
A. is likely to increase in size over the first year of life.
B. should be treated to avoid malignancy.
C. usually resolves within the first months of life.
D. is likely to develop a superimposed lichenification.

114. You examine a 2-month-old infant with a port-wine lesion over her right cheek. You advise the parents that this lesion:
A. needs to be surgically excised.
B. grows proportionally with the child.
C. becomes lighter over time.
D. can become malignant.

115. An infant is born with port-wine stain and Sturge-Weber syndrome. The two conditions are unlikely to be related.
A. true
B. false

116. A 10-day-old child presents with multiple raised lesions resembling flea bites over the trunk and nape of the neck. The infant is nursing well and has no fever or exposure to animals. These lesions likely represent:
A. erythema toxicum neonatorum.
B. milia.
C. acne neonatorum.
D. staphylococcal skin infection.

117. Milia is usually marked by white pinpoint papular lesions found:
A. on the back and buttocks.
B. across the chest.
C. in the underarms.
D. on the nose and cheeks.

118. Milia is typically caused by:
A. low levels of androgen.
B. enlarged sebaceous glands.
C. excessive oil production in the skin follicles.
D. an unknown etiology.

119. Milia are treated by the following method:
A. no special skin care.
B. a topical retinoid.
C. cryotherapy.
D. a topical antimicrobial.

120. Typical distribution of acne neonatorum consists of open and closed comedones and pustules:
A. on the hands and wrists.
B. on the neck and chest.
C. on the forehead and cheeks.
D. on the neck and ears.

121. Acne neonatorum treatment options include which of the following (more than one can apply)?
A. no special skin care is needed because these lesions are self-resolving
B. topical retinoids
C. oral antibiotic
D. low-dose benzoyl peroxide

122. An Asian couple comes in with their 4-week-old infant, who has blue–black macules scattered over the buttocks. These most likely represent:
A. benign mottling.
B. mongolian spots.
C. ecchymosis.
D. hemangioma.

123. The clinician anticipates that a child with mongolian spots will cry out because of discomfort when the area is gently pressed or palpated.
A. true
B. false

124. Eczema is thought to be caused by:
   A. overactive mucous glands.
   B. allergic reaction.
   C. degradation of mast cells.
   D. dry air.

125. The most important aspect of skin care for children with eczema is:
   A. frequent bathing with antibacterial soap.
   B. consistent use of medium- to high-potency topical steroids.
   C. application of lubricants.
   D. treatment of dermatophytes.

126. A common site for eczema in infants is the:
   A. dorsum of the hand.
   B. face.
   C. neck.
   D. flexor surfaces.

Answers

113. A.	118. B.	123. B.
114. B.	119. A.	124. C.
115. B.	120. C.	125. C.
116. A.	121. A, D.	126. B.
117. D.	122. B.	

Numerous dermatologic conditions are found in infancy and early childhood. Parents understandably have concerns about these lesions. It is important for the NP to have a thorough knowledge of common conditions (Table 17–8).

Capillary, or strawberry, hemangioma is a congenital vascular malformation. Such lesions are rarely present at birth but become evident in the first weeks of life, growing rapidly in the first year, then plateauing in size, and eventually regressing. About 90% disappear by age 9, usually leaving bluish vascularity over the area. If the lesion is large or involves a vital organ such as the eye or extremity, treatment by an expert in the condition is indicated. Oral propranolol is commonly used for treatment; current recommendations provide formulation, target dose, and frequency of dosing. Other treatment options include systemic corticosteroids and, less commonly, interferon alpha. Vincristine, injected corticosteroids, and laser therapy are used rarely for severe cases.

A port-wine stain is a flat hemangioma with a stable course. These lesions usually appear on the face and are usually present at birth. Port-wine stains tend to deepen in color as time goes on and grow proportionally with the child. Although not malignant, the lesions are often cosmetically challenging and can be minimized or occasionally eliminated through the use of laser therapy. Port-wine stain is occasionally associated with other congenital or genetic syndromes (Sturge-Weber or arteriovenous [AV] malformation syndrome).

The typical presentation of milia is as white pinpoint papular lesions caused by sebaceous hyperplasia. The usual distribution is over the nose, cheeks, and other areas with an abundance of sebaceous glands. The cause is likely the maternal androgenic effect on the sebaceous glands. Benign in nature, milia resolve without special therapy by 4 weeks to 6 months of life. The infant's parents and caregivers should be advised to avoid attempting to remove or open milia as this could result in scarring.

Erythema toxicum neonatorum is a benign rash of unknown etiology that occurs in about 50% of full-term infants. Usually beginning in the first 10 days of life, the lesions look like flea bites and are widely distributed; the palms and soles are spared. The lesions usually fade by 5 to 7 days after eruption without specific treatment and do not seem to bother the infant.

Mongolian spots occur in about 90% of children of African and Asian ancestries and in less than 10% of children of European ancestry. The distribution is usually over the lower back and buttocks but can occur over a wider area. Caused by an accumulation of melanocytes, these are benign lesions that typically fade by age 7 without special therapy. Uninformed providers can misinterpret this normal finding as an ecchymotic area, raising the suspicion of child abuse. In contrast to an area of bruising or ecchymosis, when a mongolian spot is pressed or palpated, there is no discomfort.

Acne neonatorum consists of open and closed comedones and pustules over the forehead and cheeks, similar to the adolescent version of the condition. The etiology is likely the effect of maternal androgens on the infant's skin. It usually resolves in about 4 to 8 weeks but occasionally persists up to age 1 year. Low-dose benzoyl peroxide can be used as therapy, although the lesions typically resolve without intervention.

Eczema or atopic dermatitis is a manifestation of a Type I hypersensitivity reaction. This type of reaction is caused when immunoglobulin E antibodies occupy receptor sites on mast cells, causing a degradation of the mast cells and subsequent release of histamine, vasodilation, mucous gland stimulation, and tissue swelling. There are two subgroups of type I hypersensitivity reactions: atopy and anaphylaxis.

The atopy subgroup comprises numerous common clinical conditions, such as allergic rhinitis, atopic dermatitis, allergic gastroenteropathy, and allergy-based asthma. Atopic diseases have a strong familial component and tend to cause localized rather than systemic reactions. Individuals with atopic disease are often able to identify allergy-inducing agents.

Treatment for atopic disease of eczema includes avoiding offending agents, minimizing skin dryness by limiting soap and water exposure, and consistently using lubricants. The NP should explain to the patient that the skin tends to be sensitive and needs to be treated with some care. When flares occur, the skin eruption is largely caused by histamine release. Antihistamines and topical corticosteroids can be used to control eczema flares. With an acute flare of eczema or with contact dermatitis in the older child, a topical corticosteroid with intermediate potency is likely needed to control acute symptoms. After this control is achieved, the lowest potency topical corticosteroid that yields the desired effect should be used. For eczema or contact dermatitis on the face of infants and children 3 months and older, the lowest potency (class 7) corticosteroid cream may be used, such as 1% hydrocortisone. Over-the-counter nonsteroid moisturizing and healing ointment is recommended for frequent use.

Table 17-8
Common Infant Dermatological Conditions

Condition	Pathophysiology	Presentation	Management	Comments
HEMANGIOMA	Benign tumors of endothelium; local proliferative process that affects endothelial cells; perhaps genetic mutation of epithelial regulation	Often not present at birth, rapid growth from first days of life to 6 months, slow proliferation 6–12 months, then involution phase from 12 months to age 3–6 years; one-third present at birth as light port wine stain	Treatment dependent on location, risk of complication, scarring, ulceration; options to slow growth = oral propranolol, systemic corticosteroids. Additional options = vincristine, interferon alpha. Uncommonly used = injected corticosteroids, laser therapy	Active nonintervention for superficial lesions in low function areas (i.e., thigh, upper arm)—watchful waiting; will involute slowly through early childhood
PORT WINE LESION	Disorder of dermal capillaries and post-capillary venules. Occasionally associated with other congenital or genetic syndromes (Sturge-Weber or AV malformation syndrome)	Present from birth. Blanchable from red to dark pink, grows proportionally with child. Will darken and often becomes nodular as child grows and will not regress. Lesions on face tend to follow branches of trigeminal nerve	Pulse dye laser therapy is standard; lightens lesion but does not remove. Referral to ophthalmology if on eyelids; associated with glaucoma. Referral to neurology if facial lesions and seizures	Important to consider genetic and congenital syndrome when these are present
SEBORRHEA DERMATITIS INFANTS—CRADLE CAP	Usually in areas of dense sebaceous glands (scalp, face, groin, underarms). Thought to be over-stimulation of sebum production; possibly lipid-dependent yeast	Erythematous plaque; appears greasy with yellow scales. Commonly seen in infants but can be present through life	Infant scalp treatment: Apply emollient (petrolatum, vegetable or mineral oil) overnight, then remove plaque with soft brush. For other parts of body, ketoconazole 2% cream once daily for 1 week or low-dose hydrocortisone 1% daily for 1 week	Common from 3 weeks to 12 months. 10% of cases present before 1 month of age. 70% present by 3 months. Steadily decreases in prevalence at 7% in 1–2 year olds

Sources: Habif, T. *Skin Disease*, ed. 3. St. Louis: Elsevier Health Sciences, 2011.
Habif T. *Dermatology DDxDeck*, ed. 2. St. Louis: Elsevier Health Sciences, 2012.

DISCUSSION SOURCES

Habif T. *Skin Disease*, ed. 3. St. Louis: Elsevier Health Sciences, 2011.

Drolet BA, Frommelt PC, Chamlin SL, et al. Initiation and use of propranolol for infantile hemangioma: Report of a consensus conference. *Pediatrics* 131:128–140, 2013.

Medscape: Capillary Malformation, http://emedicine.medscape.com/article/1084479-overview.

Medscape: Infantile Hemangioma, http://emedicine.medscape.com/article/1083849-overview.

National Eczema Association. Topical Steroids, http://www.nationaleczema.org/eczema-treatments/topical-corticosteroids.

Acute Otitis Media

127. Which of the following is the most prudent first-line treatment choice for an otherwise well toddler with acute otitis media (AOM) who requires antimicrobial therapy?
A. ceftibuten
B. amoxicillin
C. cefuroxime
D. azithromycin

128. Most AOM is caused by:
A. certain gram-positive and gram-negative bacteria and respiratory viruses.
B. atypical bacteria and pathogenic fungi.
C. rhinovirus and methicillin-resistant *Staphylococcus aureus*.
D. predominately beta-lactamase–producing organisms.

129. The incidence of AOM has decreased in the past decade in part because of:
A. earlier detection and treatment.
B. more effective treatment options.
C. an increase in select vaccination use.
D. lower rates of viral infections.

130. Which of the following represents the best choice of clinical agents for a child who has had a history of penicillin allergy who requires antimicrobial therapy?
A. ciprofloxacin
B. cefdinir
C. amoxicillin
D. trimethoprim-sulfamethoxazole (TMP-SMX)

131. Which of the following does not represent a risk factor for recurrent AOM in younger children?
A. pacifier use after age 10 months
B. history of first episode of AOM before age 3 months
C. exposure to second-hand smoke
D. beta-lactam allergy

132. The main risk factor for AOM in infants is:
A. undiagnosed dairy allergy.
B. eustachian tube dysfunction.
C. cigarette smoke exposure.
D. use of soy-based infant formula.

133. In the treatment of acute otitis media in the child, which of the following antimicrobial agents affords the most effective activity against *Streptococcus pneumoniae*?
A. nitrofurantoin
B. cefixime
C. trimethoprim-sulfamethoxazole (TMP-SMX)
D. cefuroxime

134. A 3-year-old boy with AOM continues to have otalgia and fever (≥39°C [≥102.2°F]) after 3 days of amoxicillin 80 mg/kg/d with an appropriate dose of clavulanate (Augmentin) therapy. Which of the following is recommended?
A. Watch and wait while using analgesics.
B. Start antimicrobial therapy with oral azithromycin.
C. Initiate therapy with oral clindamycin.
D. Administer intramuscular ceftriaxone.

135. Which of the following must be present for the diagnosis of AOM? More than one can apply.
A. bulging of the tympanic membrane (TM)
B. TM retraction
C. otalgia
D. anterior cervical lymphadenopathy

136. Which of the following signs indicates possible AOM diagnosis in a preverbal child?
A. loss of appetite
B. colic
C. tugging on the ear
D. fever

137. Which of the following is usually absent in otitis media with effusion (OME)?
A. fluid in the middle ear
B. otalgia
C. fever
D. itch

138. The following criteria should be met for a child to be treated for AOM with observation and analgesia but no antimicrobial therapy (choose all that apply):
A. age greater than 6 months.
B. bilateral infection.
C. moderate illness.
D. presumptively caused by bacterial infection.

139. Treatment of otitis media with effusion usually includes:
A. symptomatic therapy.
B. antimicrobial therapy.
C. an antihistamine.
D. a mucolytic.

140. Characteristics of *M. catarrhalis* include:
A. high rate of beta-lactamase production.
B. antimicrobial resistance because of altered protein binding sites.
C. difficult to eradicate even with antimicrobial therapy.
D. gram-positive organism.

141. Characteristics of *H. influenzae* include:
   A. rare beta-lactamase production.
   B. antimicrobial resistance because of altered protein binding sites.
   C. organism most commonly isolated from mucoid middle ear effusion.
   D. gram-positive organism.

142. Characteristics of *S. pneumoniae* include:
   A. beta-lactamase production common.
   B. antimicrobial resistance because of altered protein binding sites.
   C. causative organism of skin infection associated with acute otitis media.
   D. gram-negative organism.

Answers

127. B.	133. D.	139. A.
128. A.	134. D.	140. A.
129. C.	135. A and C.	141. C.
130. B.	136. C.	142. B
131. D.	137. C.	
132. B.	138. A and C.	

Acute otitis media (AOM) is among the most frequent diagnoses noted in office visits in children younger than age 15 years. Almost all cases of AOM are found to be caused either by bacteria and viruses together (66%), bacteria alone (27%), or virus alone (4%). *Streptococcus pneumonia* (49%), *Haemophilus influenza* (29%), *Moraxella catarrhalis* (28%), and various respiratory tract viruses contribute to the infectious and inflammatory processes of the middle ear. Nearly two-thirds of all children have at least one episode by their second birthday; one-third have more than three episodes. Although AOM remains the most common childhood condition for which antibiotics are prescribed, the incidence of AOM and the resulting antimicrobial prescriptions have decreased over the past decade as a result of many factors, including increased rates of pneumococcal and influenza vaccination.

The eustachian tubes provide drainage of middle ear secretions and protection of the middle ear from pharyngeal secretions and bacterial contaminants. As a result, conditions that cause eustachian tube dysfunction or eustachian tube obstruction, such as allergic rhinitis, upper respiratory infection, and craniofacial abnormalities, encourage status of secretions and allow aspiration of pharyngeal flora into the middle ear, resulting in AOM. Eustachian tube obstruction caused by an upper respiratory viral illness remains the most common predisposing factor for developing AOM. Passive cigarette smoke exposure, feeding in a supine position, and pacifier use beyond age 10 months likely also predispose a child to AOM secondary to eustachian tube dysfunction or eustachian tube obstruction. Because children in daycare settings typically have more upper respiratory infections, attendance at group child care is also a risk factor for nasopharyngeal carriage of bacteria implicated in AOM. Bottle-feeding is a risk factor for AOM, with rates significantly lower among infants who were breastfed for the first 6 to 12 months of life; boys and children of Native American ancestry are also noted to be at increased risk. An additional intervention to reduce AOM risk includes universal childhood pneumococcal and influenza immunization.

S. pneumoniae causes 49% of AOM (Table 17–9); it is the least likely of the three major causative bacteria to resolve without antimicrobial intervention and causes the most significant symptoms. This organism has exhibited resistance more recently to numerous antibiotic agents, including amoxicillin, cephalosporins, and macrolides. The mechanism of resistance is an alteration of intracellular protein-binding sites, which can typically be overcome by using higher doses of amoxicillin and certain cephalosporins; on rare occasions,

Table 17-9

Causative Organisms in Acute Bacterial Otitis Media (AOM)

Overall pathogens in AOM = No pathogen (4%), virus (70%), bacteria plus virus (66%)

Organism	Comment
S. pneumoniae (gram-positive diplococci) (49%) **Treatment target in AOM**	Consider drug-resistant *S. pneumoniae* risk Mechanism of resistance—Alter binding sites within bacterial cells Low rate (~10%–20%) of spontaneous resolution without antimicrobial therapy
H. influenzae (gram-negative bacillus) (29%)	Resistance via beta-lactamase production Moderate rate (~50%) of spontaneous resolution without antimicrobial therapy
M. catarrhalis (gram-negative cocci) (28%)	Resistance via beta-lactamase production Nearly all spontaneously resolve without antimicrobial therapy

Source: Sanford Guide 2014: Otitis Media, Acute Empiric Therapy, webedition.sanfordguide.com/sanford-guide-online/disease-clinical-condition/otitis-media?searchterm=otitis+media.

clindamycin is also used. The pneumococcal conjugate vaccine is effective in reducing risk of invasive pneumococcal disease and in minimizing AOM risk when caused by serotypes included in the vaccine.

H. influenzae (29%) and *M. catarrhalis* (28%) are gram-negative organisms capable of producing beta-lactamase. Although these two organisms have relatively high rates of spontaneous resolution (50% and 90% respectively), without antimicrobial intervention, *H. influenzae* is the organism most commonly isolated from mucoid and serious middle ear effusion, conditions often noted in recurrent AOM.

Beta-lactamase production by organisms probably contributes less to AOM treatment failure than to prescribing an inadequate dosing of amoxicillin needed to eradicate drug-resistant *S. pneumoniae*. Respiratory syncytial virus is commonly isolated from the middle ear fluid in children with AOM. Other common viral agents include human rhinovirus and coronavirus. AOM caused by these viral agents usually resolves in 7 to 10 days with supportive care alone.

Appropriate assessment is critical to the diagnosis of AOM (Table 17–10). The AOM treatment guidelines emphasize proper diagnosis based on strict definitions of AOM and

Table 17-10
Diagnosis and Management of Acute Otitis Media (AOM) in Children

DIAGNOSIS OF AOM IN CHILDREN	Moderate or severe bulging of tympanic membrane (TM) *OR* new onset of otorrhea not related to otitis externa (OE) with otalgia • Mild bulging of TM *AND* recent (≤48 hrs) onset of ear pain (in nonverbal child—tugging, holding, rubbing) *OR* intense TM erythema with otalgia
MANAGEMENT OF AOM SHOULD INCLUDE ASSESSMENT OF PAIN AND, IF PRESENT, CLINICIAN SHOULD RECOMMEND TREATMENT FOR PAIN MANAGEMENT	Analgesics: Acetaminophen or ibuprofen is recommended Topical anesthetic agent can provide short-term (approximately 30 minutes) pain relief
WATCHFUL WAITING, CONSISTING OF ANALGESIA WITHOUT ANTIMICROBIAL THERAPY, IS AN ACCEPTABLE TREATMENT OPTION IN AOM	In the otherwise well child, rationale for not immediately initiation antibiotic therapy • Low risk for adverse outcome without antimicrobial therapy • High rate of spontaneous AOM resolution without antimicrobial therapy or worsening of symptoms • Watchful waiting is only appropriate for the child ≥6 months with nonsevere illness based on joint decision-making with parents/caregivers for unilateral AOM • If watchful waiting is used, the follow-up must be ensured with ability to start antibiotic therapy within 48–72 hours if symptoms do not improve or worsen
NONSEVERE VS. SEVERE ILLNESS	Nonsevere illness: • Mild otalgia for <48 hours *Or* • Fever <39°C (<102.2°F) in the past 24 hours Severe illness: • Moderate to severe otalgia *Or* • Otalgia for >48 hours *Or* Fever ≥39°C (≥102.2°F)
TREATMENT OPTIONS INITIAL TREATMENT	Antibiotic therapy at time of AOM diagnosis in the following. • Nonsevere or severe illness whether unilateral or bilateral AOM in children younger than 6 months • Severe illness with unilateral or bilateral AOM in children ≥6 months • Nonsevere illness with bilateral AOM in young children (6–23 months) Either prescribe antibiotic therapy OR offer observation with close follow-up of AOM in children ≥6 months with nonsevere illness based on joint decision-making with parents/caregivers for unilateral AOM If observation is used, follow-up must be ensured with ability to start antibiotic therapy within 48–72 hours if symptoms do not improve or worsen

Source: Lieberthal, AS, Carroll AE, Chonmaitree T, et al. The diagnosis and management of acute otitis media. *Pediatrics* 31(3):e964–e999, 2013.

decisions regarding initial treatment. Management of AOM should include assessment of pain, and if present, clinician should recommend treatment for pain management. Acetaminophen or ibuprofen can be used as analgesics. Topical anesthetic agent can provide short-term (approximately 30 minutes) pain relief. The components of AOM include objective findings such as a bulging, erythematous tympanic membrane (TM) with limited or absent mobility on insufflation, or otorrhea unrelated to otitis externa. Presentation can also include bulging of TM and recent (≤48 hours) onset of ear pain (seen as tugging, holding, rubbing in nonverbal child) or intense TM erythema with otalgia. Distinct otalgia with discomfort clearly referable to the ear results in interference with or precludes normal activity or sleep. With recovery, TM mobility returns in about 1 to 2 weeks, but middle ear effusion typically persists for 4 to 6 weeks and often up to 3 months.

The AOM evaluation and treatment recommendations apply only to otherwise healthy children without underlying conditions that could alter the natural course of AOM, including anatomic abnormalities such as cleft palate, certain genetic conditions such as Down syndrome, immunodeficiencies, presence of cochlear implants, and recurrent AOM.

Observation as initial treatment is only appropriate if child is >6 months, has nonsevere illness, and infection is unilateral. Placebo-controlled trials of AOM conducted during more

three decades have shown consistently that selected children who meet the criteria for observation do well, without adverse sequelae, without antibacterial therapy. Observation should include assurance of follow-up, and appropriate analgesia should be provided (Table 17–11).

Amoxicillin remains the first-line antimicrobial for AOM treatment for the majority of children who do not have PCN allergy. Given the wide therapeutic index of this medication and the prevalence of drug-resistant *S. pneumoniae*, 80 to 90 mg/kg/d is the recommended dose; in the overweight or obese child, the dose should not exceed the adult dose. Amoxicillin/clavulanate (Augmentin), 80 to 90 mg/kg/d, is recommended as first-line therapy in select situations.

Children younger than 3 months old with AOM should be seen in 1 to 2 days because of increased risk of treatment failure. In a child older than 3 months, otalgia, fever, and other symptoms that persist beyond 48 to 72 hours of therapy can indicate treatment failure, and repeat evaluation is in order and a change in therapy is recommended.

Otitis media with effusion (OME), formerly known as serous otitis media, is defined as the presence of fluid in the middle ear in the absence of signs or symptoms of acute infection. With OME, 80% of children clear the middle ear by 8 weeks. If OME persists beyond 8 weeks, the presence of communication problems and other symptoms dictates the need for further evaluation and treatment (Table 17–12). If

Table 17-11
Recommended Acute Otitis Media (AOM) Treatment Options

Length of therapy unless otherwise specified: Younger than age 2 years = 10 days, 2–6 years = 7 days, ≥6 years = 5–7 days

	Recommended	With PCN allergy
FIRST-LINE TREATMENT	Amoxicillin (80–90 mg/kg/day in 2 divided doses) OR Amoxicillin-clavulanate (90 mg/kg per day of amoxicillin, with 6.4 mg/kg/day of clavulanate in 2 divided doses)	Cefdinir (14 mg/kg/day in 1 or 2 doses) OR Cefuroxime (30 mg/kg/day in 2 divided doses) OR Cefpodoxime (10 mg/kg/day in 2 divided doses) OR Ceftriaxone (50 mg IM or IV/day for 1 or 3 d)
ANTIBIOTIC TREATMENT AFTER 48–72 H OF FAILURE OF INITIAL ANTIBIOTIC TREATMENT	Amoxicillin-clavulanate (90 mg/kg/day of amoxicillin, with 6.4 mg/kg/day of clavulanate in 2 divided doses) OR Ceftriaxone (50 mg IM/IV for 3 d)	Ceftriaxone × 3 d (as above) OR Clindamycin (30–40 mg/kg/day in 3 divided doses) with or without a third-generation cephalosporin Tympanocentesis Referral to specialist

Sources: Lieberthal, AS, Carroll AE, Chonmaitree T, et al. The diagnosis and management of acute otitis media. *Pediatrics* 31(3):e964–e999, 2013.
Fitzgerald M. How would you prescribe cephalosporins to patients with penicillin allergies? *FHEA News,* 2012, p. 13, http://fhea.com/main/content/Newsletter/fheanews_volume12_issue8.pdf.

TABLE 17-12
Otitis Media with Effusion (OME)

DEFINED	Fluid in middle ear without signs or symptoms of ear infection
FIRST-LINE INTERVENTION	Watchful waiting in most 75%–90% resolve within 3 mo without specific treatment
SELECT INTERVENTION IN AT-RISK CHILDREN	Tympanostomy if chronic bilateral OME (3 months or longer) with documented hearing difficulty and recurrent AOM with unilateral or bilateral middle ear effusion

Sources: Otitis media with effusion. *Pediatrics* 113:1412–1429, 2004.
Rosenfeld RM, Schwartz SR, Pynnonnen MA, et al. Clinical practice guideline: Tympanostomy tubes in children—Executive Summary. *OTO-HNS* 149:8–16, 2013.

persistent effusion is accompanied by language delay or suspected or documented hearing loss, intervention by tympanostomy (ventilating tube) is warranted. Current guidelines recommend that clinicians should only offer tympanostomy to children with chronic bilateral OME (3 months or longer) with documented hearing difficulty and to those with recurrent AOM who have unilateral or bilateral MEE. Routine retreatment with an antimicrobial is not indicated for OME (Table 17–12). When a child is seen for AOM, measures to reduce AOM risk should be reviewed and reinforced.

DISCUSSION SOURCES

Lieberthal SA, Carroll AE, Chonmaitree T, et al. The diagnosis and management of acute otitis media. *Pediatrics* 131:E964–E999, 2013.
Wald ER, Applegate KE, Bordley C, et al. Clinical practice guideline for the diagnosis and management of acute bacterial sinusitis in children aged 1 to 18 years. *Pediatrics* 132:E262–E280, 2013.
Rosenfeld RM, Schwartz SR, Pynnonnen MA, et al. Clinical practice guideline: Tympanostomy tubes in children—Executive summary. *Oto-Hns* 149:8–16, 2013.
Otitis media with effusion. *Pediatrics* 113:1412–1429, 2004.

Acute Bacterial Rhinosinusitis

143. Which of the following findings is most consistent with the diagnosis of acute bacterial rhinosinusitis (ABRS) in children?
   A. upper respiratory tract infection symptoms persisting beyond 10 days
   B. nasal discharge progresses from clear to purulent to clear without antibiotics
   C. headaches and myalgias that resolve in 24 to 48 hours as the respiratory symptoms worsen
   D. persistent cough

144. Double sickening is defined as (choose all that apply):
   A. nasal discharge progressing from clear to purulent to clear without antibiotic use.
   B. acute worsening of respiratory symptoms.
   C. new fever occurring 6 to 7 days after signs of upper respiratory infection (URI).
   D. persistent cough.

145. The most common causative bacterial pathogen in ABRS is:
   A. *M. pneumoniae.*
   B. *S. pneumoniae.*
   C. *M. catarrhalis.*
   D. unidentified virus.

146. Risk factors for ABRS include all of the following except:
   A. viral infection.
   B. environmental allergies.
   C. tobacco smoke exposure.
   D. beta-thalassemia minor.

147. Which of the following is a first-line therapy option for the treatment of ABRS in an otherwise well child?
   A. amoxicillin-clavulanate
   B. clindamycin with cefixime
   C. doxycycline
   D. levofloxacin

148. Which of the following represents a therapeutic option for ABRS in an otherwise well 7-year-old child who has not had significant clinical improvement but is not worse after 72 hours of observation?
   A. continued observation
   B. oral levofloxacin
   C. oral clindamycin and cefixime
   D. injectable ceftriaxone

149. A 5-year-old girl presents with ABRS. She has a penicillin allergy but is otherwise well and is going to be treated with an antimicrobial. You prescribe:
   A. no medication; continue observation.
   B. cefdinir.
   C. levofloxacin.
   D. amoxicillin.

Answers

143. A.	146. D.	149. B.
144. B and C.	147. A.	
145. B.	148. C.	

Acute bacterial rhinosinusitis (ABRS) is a clinical condition resulting from inflammation of the lining of the membranes of the paranasal sinuses caused by bacterial infection. Risk factors include any condition that alters the normal cleansing mechanism of the sinuses, including viral infection, allergies, secondhand tobacco smoke exposure, and abnormalities in sinus structure. Inhaled tobacco smoke disturbs normal sinus mucociliary action and drainage, causing secretions to pool, and increases the risk of superimposed bacterial infection. In addition, viral upper respiratory infections (URI) and poorly controlled allergic rhinitis cause similar dysfunction, increasing ABRS risk.

Only a minority (6%–7%) of children presenting with symptoms of URI will meet criteria for persistence and therefore ABRS risk. It is important to differentiate between sequential episodes of uncomplicated viral URI from the onset of acute bacterial sinusitis with persistent symptoms and establish whether the symptoms are clearly not improving. Further, because ABRS is a clinical diagnosis based on the child's presentation, with findings also reported in children with a viral URI, the problem arises as to how to differentiate between these two common conditions. Uncomplicated viral URI in children is marked by nasal symptoms and/or cough; nasal discharge progresses from clear to purulent to clear without antibiotics, usually within 10 days, and fever early in the illness is associated with constitutional symptoms such as headaches and myalgias that resolve in 24 to 48 hours as the respiratory symptoms worsen (Table 17–13). ABRS in children should only be considered if at least one of the following criteria are observed: worsening URI course such as double sickening, defined as acute worsening of respiratory symptoms or new fever at day 6 or 7 of URI, persistence of URI-like symptoms without improvement after 7 to 10 days, including nasal discharge, daytime cough, fetid breath odor, fatigue, headache, decreased appetite, acute onset of a temperature of >102.2°F (39°C), and purulent nasal discharge, or acutely ill appearing for 3-4 days (Table 17–13).

According the ABRS practice guidelines developed by the American Academy of Pediatrics, *S. pneumoniae* (30%) is the causative organism in most childhood ABRS; this pathogen is also the least likely of the three major causative bacteria to resolve without antimicrobial intervention, and it causes the most significant symptoms. This organism exhibits resistance to numerous antibiotic agents, including lower dose amoxicillin, certain cephalosporins, and macrolides. The mechanism of resistance is alteration of intracellular protein-binding sites, which can typically be overcome by using higher doses of amoxicillin, certain cephalosporins, and respiratory fluoroquinolones (levofloxacin [Levaquin, not FDA approved for use in <18 years but has a long history of safety in this age group]). Recent antimicrobial use is the major risk for infection with drug-resistant *S. pneumoniae*.

H. influenzae (30%) and *M. catarrhalis* (20%) are gram-negative organisms capable of producing beta-lactamase; the presence of this enzyme renders the penicillins ineffective. Although these two organisms have relatively high rates of spontaneous resolution without antimicrobial intervention in AOM, infections caused by these pathogens seldom resolve without antimicrobial therapy in ABRS. Empirical antimicrobial therapy in ABRS should be aimed at choosing an agent with significant activity against gram-positive (*S. pneumoniae*) and gram-negative organisms (*H. influenzae, M. catarrhalis*), with consideration for drug-resistant *S. pneumoniae* risk and possible need for stability in the presence of beta-lactamase. Of childhood sinusitis cases, 25% are sterile wherein the cause is likely viral.

Initial treatment options for ABRS include observation, amoxicillin 80–90 mg/kg/day, or high-dose amoxicillin (Table 17–14).If no improvement is seen in 3 days, treatment options include continued observation, antibiotic therapy, high-dose amoxicillin, or change to clindamycin and cefixime or linezolid and cefixime or levofloxacin only depending on initial treatment. If symptoms worsen in 3 days, amoxicillin 80–90 mg/kg/day with or without clavulanate or high-dose amoxicillin or clindamycin and cefixime or linezolid and cefixime or levofloxacin only should be given depending on prior treatment (Table 17–14). Children who have a penicillin allergy can safely be treated with cefdinir, cefuroxime, or cefpodoxime.

Acute URI with persistent illness (nasal discharge of any quality) or daytime cough for >10 days without improvement should be treated with antibiotics or 3-day observation. Worsening course or new onset of nasal discharge, daytime cough or fever after initial improvement, or severe onset and concurrent fever (102.2°F [39°C]) and purulent nasal discharge >3 consecutive days should be treated with antibiotics.

DISCUSSION SOURCE

Wald ER, Applegate KE, Bordley C, et al. Clinical practice guideline for the diagnosis and management of acute bacterial sinusitis in children aged 1 to 18 years. *Pediatrics* 132:e262–280, 2013.

Urinary Tract Infection

150. Rates of urinary tract infection (UTI) among uncircumcised infant boys are how much higher than those in circumcised boys?
    A. as much as 10%
    B. as much as 20%
    C. as much as 30%
    D. less than 10%

151. Which of the following is most likely to be part of the clinical presentation of UTI in a 20-month-old child?
    A. urinary frequency and urgency
    B. fever
    C. suprapubic tenderness
    D. nausea and vomiting

152. Which of the following is the most common UTI organism in children?
    A. *Pseudomonas aeruginosa*
    B. *Escherichia coli*
    C. *Klebsiella pneumonia*
    D. *Proteus mirabilis*

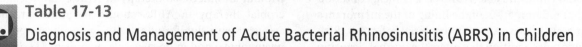

Table 17-13
Diagnosis and Management of Acute Bacterial Rhinosinusitis (ABRS) in Children

Exclusions from these recommendations include children <1 year of age including neonates and children with subacute and chronic sinusitis, anatomic abnormalities of the sinuses, immunodeficiencies, cystic fibrosis, and/or primary ciliary dyskinesia

DIFFERENTIATE BETWEEN ACUTE URI AND ABRS DIAGNOSTIC CRITERIA	• Uncomplicated viral upper respiratory infection (URI) course Nasal symptoms and/or cough, nasal discharge progresses from clear to purulent to clear without antibiotics, usually within 10 days Fever early in the illness associated with constitutional symptoms such as headaches and myalgias that resolve in 24–48 hours as the respiratory symptoms worsen • ABRS should be considered only in the setting of ≥1 of the following. Worsening URI course such as double sickening, defined as acute worsening of respiratory symptoms or new fever at day 6–7 of URI Persistence of URI-like symptoms without improvement after 7–10 days, including nasal discharge, daytime cough, bad breath, fatigue, headache, decreased appetite Acute onset: Temperature >102.2°F (>39°C), purulent nasal discharge, ill appearing for 3–4 days

TREATMENT OPTIONS	Acute URI with
	• Persistent illness (nasal discharge of any quality) or daytime cough for >10 days without improvement
	  Option: Antibiotic treatment or 3-day observation
	• Worsening course or new onset of nasal discharge, daytime cough, or fever after initial improvement
	  Option: Antibiotic treatment
	• Severe onset/concurrent fever (>102.2°F [>39°C]) and purulent nasal discharge >3 consecutive days.
	  Option: Antibiotic treatment

RADIOGRAPHIC RECOMMENDATIONS	• In children with uncomplicated ABRS imaging is not necessary to differentiate viral from bacterial sinusitis. • Contrast CT of paranasal sinuses and/or MRI with contrast should be obtained whenever a child is suspected of having orbital or central nervous system complications
LIKELY PATHOGENS	*S. pneumoniae* = 30% Decreased second to pneumococcal vaccine • Nontypeable *H. influenzae* = 30% • *M. catarrhalis* = 20% • Sterile (no pathogen isolated, likely viral) = 25%

153. All of the following uropathogens are capable of reducing urinary nitrates to nitrites except:
    A. *E. coli.*
    B. *Proteus* species.
    C. *K. pneumoniae.*
    D. *S. saprophyticus.*

154. Which of the following is considered the ideal method for obtaining a urine sample for culture and sensitivity in an 18-month-old-old girl with suspected UTI?
    A. suprapubic aspiration
    B. transurethral bladder catheterization
    C. bag collection
    D. diaper sample

155. When choosing an antimicrobial agent for the treatment of UTI in a febrile female child who is 16 months old, the NP considers that:
    A. gram-positive organisms are the most likely cause of infection.
    B. a parenteral aminoglycoside is the preferred treatment choice.
    C. the use of an oral third-generation cephalosporin is acceptable if gastrointestinal function is intact.
    D. nitrofurantoin use is considered first-line therapy.

156. When evaluating the urinalysis of a 10-month-old infant with UTI, the NP considers that:
    A. leukocytes would be consistently noted.
    B. proteinuria is usually absent.
    C. the presence of urobilinogen is commonly noted.
    D. 20% of urinalyses can be normal.

Table 17-14
Acute Bacterial Rhinosinusitis (ABRS) Treatment in Children

Initial Treatment	No Improvement in 72 Hours	Worse at 72 Hours
Observation	Additional observation OR antibiotic therapy	Amoxicillin 80-90 mg/kg/day with or without clavulanate
Amoxicillin* 80–90 mg/kg/day	Additional observation OR HD amoxicillin/clavulanate	HD amoxicillin/clavulanate
HD amoxicillin/clavulanate	Continue high dose amoxicillin/clavulanate or change to clindamycin AND cefixime OR linezolid AND cefixime OR levofloxacin	Clindamycin AND cefixime OR linezolid AND cefixime OR levofloxacin

*In the case of PCN allergy, both non-type 1 reaction (delayed or late, >72) and Type 1 (immediate, severe reaction) can safely be treated with cefdinir, cefuroxime, or cefpodoxime. Consider allergy testing for PCN and cephalosporin in both cases prior to initiation of treatment.
Source: Wald ER, Applegate KE, Bordley C, et al. Clinical practice guideline for the diagnosis and management of acute bacterial sinusitis in children aged 1 to 18 years. *Pediatrics* 132;e262, 2013.

157. In children 2 months to 2 years old with UTI, antimicrobial therapy should be prescribed for:
   A. 3 to 5 days.
   B. 5 to 10 days.
   C. 7 to 14 days.
   D. 14 to 21 days.

158. A 12-month-old boy with fever who has a suspected UTI who has vomited 5 times in the past 7 hours. His last wet diaper was approximately 6 hours ago. He is accompanied by his parents. The following action should be taken:
   A. Recommend continued observation at home.
   B. Recommend antimicrobial therapy.
   C. Conduct renal ultrasound.
   D. Arrange for the child to be admitted to the hospital.

159. The preferred urinary tract imaging study for a 22-month-old girl with first-time febrile UTI is:
   A. renal-bladder ultrasound (RBUS).
   B. renal scan.
   C. voiding cystogram (VCUG).
   D. none unless a second UTI occurs.

160. Which of the following is the most compelling reason to use RBUS instead of VCUG?
   A. This is a noninvasive test.
   B. Results are available more rapidly.
   C. The test is less technically demanding.
   D. RBUS is less expensive.

161. VCUG is indicated:
   A. after UTI diagnosis is confirmed to determine course of antimicrobial therapy.
   B. when UTI is recurrent.
   C. to confirm high-grade reflux.
   D. as an alternative to RBUS to assure accurate detection of scarring.

162. The urinary tract abnormality most often associated with UTI in younger children is:
   A. bladder neck stricture.
   B. ureteral stenosis.
   C. urethral stricture.
   D. vesicoureteral reflux.

Answers

150. B.	155. C.	160. A.
151. B.	156. D.	161. B.
152. B.	157. C.	162. D.
153. D.	158. D.	
154. A.	159. A.	

Although often thought of as a problem primarily of women during the reproductive years, UTIs do occur in early childhood. Rates in girls younger than 1 year are about 6.5% and at 1 to 2 years are 8.1%. The rates are lower in boys: 3.3% at younger than 1 year and 1.9% at 1 to 2 years. Uncircumcised boys can have rates of UTI many times higher than that in circumcised boys, but this difference decreases dramatically when normal penile growth loosens the foreskin, usually occurring by the time the boy is 1 to 2 years old. However, this potential health issue is not considered to be an indication for routine circumcision.

The clinical presentation of UTI in children can be without the classic symptoms such as frequency, dysuria, or flank pain. In younger children, UTI often manifests as irritability, lethargy, and fever with no obvious focal infectious source. Older children often present with abdominal pain, unexplained fever, or both; as children approach puberty, flank pain becomes more common. UTI should be considered in infants and young children 2 months to 2 years old with unexplained fever, particularly in boys younger than 6 months and girls younger than 2 years who have a temperature greater than or equal to 39°C (≥102.2°F).

A urinalysis should be obtained in a child with unexplained fever or symptoms that suggest a UTI; however, 20% of urinalyses from UTI cases return a false-negative result. Any of the following findings are suggestive, although not diagnostic, of UTI: positive leukocyte esterase, positive nitrite, more than five white blood cells (WBCs) per high-power field in spun specimen, and bacteria present in unspun Gram-stained specimen. An evaluation for sepsis should also be initiated if clinical presentation warrants.

The method of obtaining a urinalysis in younger children (generally younger than 5 or 6 years old) has been long debated. Suprapubic bladder aspiration yields the specimen that is least likely to be contaminated; for the parent and child this method can be fraught with fear and it requires special provider skill. The next acceptable method is transurethral bladder catheterization. An unacceptable method because of the high rate of skin and fecal contamination in a urine specimen collection via bag or from the diaper.

Urinary tract abnormality is a major risk factor for pediatric UTI, with vesicoureteral reflux noted in 30% to 50% of cases. Reflux nephropathy increases the risk of ascending infection that can cause pyelonephritis and renal scarring. This is a risk factor for renal failure but is largely avoidable with early reflux recognition and proper treatment. Little difference is usually found in the clinical presentation and laboratory findings of cystitis or pyelonephritis in a febrile child, and determining whether a UTI is limited to the lower urinary tract or involves the soft tissue of the kidney is not clinically significant. The management of a UTI in a child is dictated by the clinical severity of the illness, rather than by the specific site of infection in the urinary tract. As a result, a single documented UTI in a child must be taken seriously. If an infant or young child 2 months to 2 years old with suspected UTI is assessed as toxic, dehydrated, or unable to retain oral intake, hospitalization is advised. In this circumstance, initial antimicrobial therapy should be administered parenterally, usually with a second- or third-generation cephalosporin. An aminoglycoside such as gentamicin can be used if there is a history of severe penicillin allergy. For a child who is well hydrated and able to take an antimicrobial and fluids orally, home-based care is reasonable. Oral amoxicillin, TMP-SMX, or a second- or third-generation cephalosporin is recommended as options for initial therapy; the use of TMP-SMX has a small risk of treatment failure. Current evidence-based practice recommendations indicate a 7- to 14-day course of antibiotics because the outcomes are superior to a 1- to 3-day course in preventing spread of infection and subsequent renal scarring. Close clinical follow-up of the child and instruction of parents regarding prompt attention to recurrence of symptoms is highly recommended. Routine antimicrobial treatment for prophylaxis of recurrent infection is not recommended for children without verified urinary tract abnormalities. Although fluoroquinolone antibiotics have not been widely used in children, ciprofloxacin is approved by the U.S. Food and Drug Administration (FDA) for use in pediatric

patients for the treatment of UTI; this use is approved starting at age 1 year.

Urinary tract imaging should be considered for all children with UTI, particularly if this occurs before toilet training. The two mainstays for imaging in young children are renal-bladder ultrasound (RBUS) and voiding cystourethrography (VCUG). RBUS is an easily obtained, noninvasive test but can miss a small number of high-grade reflux cases. The benefits of this imaging (no radiation exposure, non-invasive, minimal discomfort for child and parents), however, outweigh the slight increase in specificity of VCUG. A renal scan is useful for detecting renal scarring, a finding present after infection, but is not recommended for routine, initial evaluation of young child with their first febrile UTI. VCUG only is indicated if RBUS reveals hydronephrosis, scarring, or other findings that would suggest either high-grade vesicoureteral reflux (VUR) or obstructive uropathy, as well as other atypical or complex clinical circumstances. VCUG may also be performed if febrile UTI is recurrent. However, some parents may want to avoid VCUG even after the second UTI. These preferences should be considered. Only if high-grade (Grade V) VUR or other urinary tract abnormality is noted on imaging should antimicrobial prophylaxis be continued until the abnormality is corrected. Current studies do not support the use of antimicrobial prophylaxis to prevent febrile recurrent UTI in infants with Grade I to IV VUR.

DISCUSSION SOURCES

Steering Committee on Quality Improvement and Management, Subcommittee on Urinary Tract Infection. Urinary Tract Infection: Clinical Practice Guideline for the Diagnosis and Management of the Initial UTI in Febrile Infants and Children 2 to 24 Months. *Pediatrics* 128;3:595–610, 2011.

Medscape: Pediatric Urinary Tract Infection Medication, http://emedicine.medscape.com/article/969643-medication#2/

Common Childhood Febrile Illness With Skin Alterations

163. You examine a 10-year-old boy with suspected streptococcal pharyngitis. His mother asks if he can get a "shot of penicillin." Which of the following statements is/are true regarding the use of intramuscular (IM) penicillin (PCN) (select all that apply)?
    A. Injectable benzathine PCN, oral amoxicillin, and cephalexin are each strongly recommended for as treatment of *Streptococcus pyogenes* (GAS) pharyngitis
    B. Injectable benzathine PCN would be indicated for treatment of GAS if poor adherence to recommended therapy or inability to take full course of oral antibiotics is anticipated.
    C. The risk of severe allergic reaction with IM products is similar to that of oral preparations.
    D. Injectable penicillin has a superior spectrum of antimicrobial coverage compared with the oral form of the drug.

164. You examine a 15-year-old presenting with a 1-day history of sore throat, low-grade fever, maculopapular rash, and posterior cervical and occipital lymphadenopathy. The most likely diagnosis is:
A. scarlet fever.
B. roseola.
C. rubella.
D. rubeola.

165. A 4-year-old child presents with fever; exudative pharyngitis; anterior cervical lymphadenopathy; and a fine, raised, pink rash. The most likely diagnosis is:
A. scarlet fever.
B. roseola.
C. rubella.
D. rubeola.

166. An 18-year-old woman has a chief complaint of "a sore throat and swollen glands" for the past 3 days. Her physical examination reveals exudative pharyngitis, minimally tender anterior and posterior cervical lymphadenopathy, and maculopapular rash. Abdominal examination reveals right and left upper quadrant abdominal tenderness. The most likely diagnosis is:
A. group A beta-hemolytic streptococcal pharyngitis.
B. infectious mononucleosis.
C. rubella.
D. scarlet fever.

167. Which of the following is most likely to be found in the laboratory data of a child who has infectious mononucleosis?
A. neutrophilia
B. lymphocytosis
C. positive antinuclear antibody
D. macrocytic anemia

168. You examine a 15-year-old boy who has infectious mononucleosis with marked tonsillar hypertrophy, exudative pharyngitis, significantly difficulty swallowing, and a patent airway. You consider prescribing a course of oral:
A. amoxicillin.
B. prednisone.
C. ibuprofen.
D. acyclovir.

169. A 2-year-old girl presents with pustular, ulcerating lesions on the hands and feet and oral ulcers. The child is cranky, well hydrated, and afebrile. The most likely diagnosis is:
A. hand-foot-and-mouth disease.
B. aphthous stomatitis.
C. herpetic gingivostomatitis.
D. Vincent angina.

170. A 6-year-old boy presents with a 1-day history of a fiery red, maculopapular facial rash concentrated on the cheeks. He has had mild headache and myalgia for the past week. The most likely diagnosis is:
A. erythema infectiosum.
B. roseola.
C. rubella.
D. scarlet fever.

171. The incubation period for measles caused by the rubeola virus is:
A. 7–10 days.
B. 10–14 days.
C. 1–2 weeks.
D. 2–3 weeks.

172. Most cases of roseola caused by human herpesvirus-6 occur in:
A. newborns who contracted the virus *in utero*.
B. infants younger than 3 months old.
C. children younger than 24 months old.
D. children older than 2 years.

173. The following symptom indicates possible acute human immunodeficiency virus (HIV) infection:
A. pustular lesions in a scattered pattern.
B. red wheals that begins on the face and spreads to the truck and extremities.
C. vesicular-form skin lesion.
D. maculopapular rash.

174. Kawasaki disease most commonly occurs in what age group?
A. infants
B. children aged 2 to 3 years.
C. children approaching puberty
D. children aged 1 to 8 years

Answers

163. A and B.	167. B.	171. B.
164. C.	168. B.	172. C.
165. A.	169. A.	173. D.
166. B.	170. A.	174. D.

Developing an accurate diagnosis of an acute febrile illness with associated rash or skin lesion can be a daunting task. Knowledge of the infectious agent, its incubation period, its mode of transmission, and its common clinical presentation can be helpful (Table 17–15).

DISCUSSION SOURCES

Shulman ST, Bisno AL, Clegg HW, et al. Clinical practice guideline for the diagnosis and management of group A streptococcal pharyngitis: 2012 update by the Infectious Diseases Society of America. *Clin Infect Dis* 55:e86–e102, 2012.

Habif T, Campbell J, Chapman, MS, et al. *Skin Disease: Diagnosis and Treatment*, ed. 3. Philadelphia: Elsevier, 2011.

Table 17-15
Rash-Producing Febrile Illness

Condition with Causative Agent	Presentation	Comments
Scarlet fever Agent: *S. pyogenes* (group A beta hemolytic streptococci)	Scarlatina-form or sandpaper-like rash with exudative pharyngitis, fever, headache, tender, localized anterior cervical lymphadenopathy. Rash usually erupts on day 2 of pharyngitis and often peels a few days later.	Presence of rash does not imply a more severe or serious disease or greater risk of contagion. Treatment = Identical to streptococcus pharyngitis, penicillin as first-line therapy, macrolide (azithro-, clarithro-, erythromycin) only in PCN allergy
Roseola Agent: Human herpesvirus-6 (HHV-6)	Discrete rosy-pink macular or maculopapular rash lasting hours to 3 days that follows a 3-7 day period of fever, often quite high.	90% of cases seen in children <2 years Febrile seizures in 10% of children affected. Supportive treatment
Rubella Agent: Rubella virus	Mild symptoms; fever, sore throat, malaise, nasal discharge, diffuse maculopapular rash lasting about 3 days. Posterior cervical and postauricular lymphadenopathy 5-10 days prior to onset of rash. Arthralgia in about 25% (most common in women).	Incubation period about 14–21 days with disease transmissible for ~1 week prior to onset of rash to ~2 weeks after rash appears. Generally a mild self-limiting illness. Greatest risk is effect of virus on the unborn child, especially with 1st trimester exposure (~80% rate congenital rubella syndrome). ***Vaccine-preventable disease.*** Notifiable disease, usually to the state and/or public health authorities,* laboratory confirmation by presence of serum rubella IgM.
Measles Agent: Rubeola virus	Usually acute presentation with fever, nasal discharge, cough, generalized lymphadenopathy, conjunctivitis (copious clear discharge), photophobia, Koplik spots (appear ~2 days prior to onset of rash as white spots with blue rings held within red spots in oral mucosa in ~1/3). Pharyngitis is usually mild without exudate. Maculopapular rash onset 3-4 days after onset of symptoms, may coalesce to generalized erythema.	Incubation period about 10-14 days with disease transmissible for ~1 week prior to onset of rash to ~2-3 weeks after rash appears. CNS and respiratory tract complications common. Permanent neurologic impairment or death possible. Supportive treatment as well as intervention for complications. ***Vaccine-preventable disease.*** Notifiable disease usually to the state and/or public health authorities,* laboratory confirmation by presence of serum rubeola IgM.
Infectious mononucleosis (IM) Agent: Epstein-Barr virus (human herpesvirus 4)	Rash: Maculopapular rash in ~20%, rare petechial rash Fever, "shaggy" purple-white exudative pharyngitis, malaise, marked diffuse	Incubation period 20-50 days >90% will develop a rash if given amoxicillin or ampicillin during the illness. Potential for respiratory distress when enlarged

Table 17-15

Rash-Producing Febrile Illness—cont'd

Condition with Causative Agent	Presentation	Comments
	lymphadenopathy, hepatic and splenic tenderness, occasionally enlarged. Diagnostic testing: Heterophil antibody test (Monospot), leukopenia with lymphocytosis and atypical lymphocytes.	tonsils and lymphoid tissue impinges on the upper airway; corticosteroids may be helpful. Splenomegaly most often occurs between day 6 and 21 after the onset of the illness. Avoid contact sports for ≥1 month due to risk of splenic rupture.
Hand-foot-and-mouth disease Agent: Coxsackie virus A16 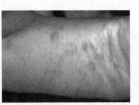 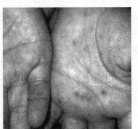	Fever, malaise, sore mouth, anorexia; 1-2 days later, lesions; also can cause conjunctivitis, pharyngitis. Duration of illness: 2-7 days.	Transmission via oral-fecal or droplet. Highly contagious with incubation periods of 2-6 weeks. Supportive treatment, analgesia important.
	See full color images of this topic on DavisPlus at http://davisplus.fadavis.com | Keyword: Fitzgerald	
Fifth disease Agent: Human parvovirus B19	3-4 days of mild flu-like illness followed by 7-10 days of red rash that begins on face with slapped cheek appearance, spreads to trunk and extremities. Rash onset corresponds with disease immunity with patient. Viremic and contagious prior but not after onset of rash.	Droplet transmission; leukopenia common. Risk of hydrops fetalis with resulting pregnancy loss when contracted by woman during pregnancy. Supportive treatment.
Acute HIV infection Agent: Human immunodeficiency virus	Maculopapular rash, fever, mild pharyngitis, ulcerating oral lesions, diarrhea, diffuse lymphadenopathy.	Most likely to occur in response to infection with large viral load. Consult with HIV specialist concerning initiation of antiretroviral therapy.
Kawasaki disease Agent: Unknown	For acute phase illness (usually lasts about 11 days), fever with T≥104°F (40°C) lasting≥5 days, polymorphous exanthem on trunk, flexor regions, and perineum, erythema of the oral cavity ("strawberry tongue") with extensively chapped lips, bilateral conjunctivitis usually without eye discharge, cervical lymphadenopathy, edema and erythema of the hands and feet with peeling skin (late finding, usually 1-2 weeks after onset of fever), no other illness accountable for the findings.	Usually in children age 1-8 years Treatment with IV immunoglobulin and PO aspirin during the acute phase is associated with a reduction in rate of coronary abnormalities such as coronary artery dilatation and coronary aneurysm. Expert consultation and treatment advice about aspirin use and ongoing monitoring warranted.

*A notifiable disease is one for which regular, frequent, and timely information regarding individual cases is considered necessary for the prevention and control of the disease. Check with state public health department to receive direction on notification.

Sources: Summary of notifiable diseases—United States, 2011. *MMWR* 60(53):1–117, 2013.

▶ Asthma

175. Which of the following best describes the pathophysiology and resulting clinical presentation of asthma?
A. intermittent airway inflammation with occasional bronchospasm
B. a disease of bronchospasm leading to airway inflammation
C. chronic airway inflammation with superimposed bronchospasm
D. relatively fixed airway constriction

176. A 6-year-old boy has a 1-year history of moderate persistent asthma that is normally well controlled with budesonide via dry powder inhaler (DPI) twice a day and the use of albuterol once or twice a week as needed for wheezing. Three days ago, he developed a sore throat, clear nasal discharge, and a dry cough. In the past 24 hours, he has had intermittent wheezing, necessitating the use of albuterol two puffs with use of an age-appropriate spacer every 3 hours) with partial relief. Your next most appropriate action is to obtain:
A. a chest radiograph.
B. an oxygen saturation measurement.
C. a peak expiratory flow (PEF) measurement.
D. a sputum smear for WBCs.

177. You see a 4-year-old girl who has a 2-day history of signs and symptoms of an acute asthma flare resulting from viral upper respiratory tract infection. She is using inhaled budesonide and albuterol as directed and continues to have difficulty with increased occurrence of coughing and wheezing. Her respiratory rate is within 50% of upper limits of normal for her age. Her medication regimen should be adjusted to include:
A. oral theophylline.
B. inhaled salmeterol (Serevent).
C. oral prednisolone.
D. oral montelukast (Singulair).

178. Which of the following is inconsistent with the diagnosis of asthma?
A. a troublesome nocturnal cough
B. cough or wheeze after exercise
C. morning sputum production
D. colds "go to the chest" or take more than 10 days to clear

179. Celeste is a 9-year-old girl with moderate persistent asthma. She is not taking a prescribed inhaled corticosteroid but is using albuterol PRN to relieve her cough and wheeze. According to her mother, she currently uses about six albuterol doses per day, in particular for cough and wheeze after active play. You consider that:
A. albuterol use can continue at this level.
B. excessive albuterol use is a risk factor for asthma death.
C. she should also use salmeterol (Serevent) to reduce her albuterol use.
D. active play should be limited to avoid triggering cough and wheeze.

180. In the treatment of asthma, leukotriene modifiers should be used as:
A. long-acting bronchodilators.
B. an inflammatory inhibitor.
C. a rescue drug.
D. intervention in acute inflammation.

181. Which of the following is not a risk factor for asthma death?
A. hospitalization or an emergency department visit for asthma in the past month.
B. current use of systemic corticosteroids or recent withdrawal from systemic corticosteroids.
C. difficulty perceiving airflow obstruction or its severity.
D. rural residence.

182. A middle-school student presents, asking for a letter stating that he should not participate in gym class because he has asthma. The most appropriate response is to:
A. write the note because gym class participation could trigger an asthma flare.
B. excuse him from outdoor activities only to avoid pollen exposure.
C. remind him that with appropriate asthma care, he should be capable of participating in gym class.
D. excuse him from indoor activities only to avoid dust mite exposure.

183. After inhaled corticosteroid or leukotriene modifier therapy is initiated, clinical effects are seen:
A. immediately.
B. within the first week.
C. in about 1 to 2 weeks.
D. in about 1 to 2 months.

184. Compared with albuterol, levalbuterol (Xopenex):
A. has a different mechanism of action.
B. has the ability to provide greater bronchodilation with a lower dose.
C. has an anti-inflammatory effect similar to an inhaled corticosteroid.
D. is contraindicated for use in children.

185. In caring for a child with an acute asthma flare, the NP considers that, according to the National Asthma Education and Prevention Program, Expert Panel Report 3 guidelines, antibiotic use is recommended:
A. routinely.
B. with evidence of concomitant bacterial infection.
C. when asthma flares are frequent.
D. with sputum production.

186. Poorly controlled asthma in children can lead to:
A. attenuated lung development.
B. chronic tracheitis.
C. sleep apnea.
D. alveolar destruction.

175. C.	179. B.	183. C.
176. C.	180. B.	184. B.
177. C.	181. D.	185. B.
178. C.	182. C.	186. A.

Asthma is a common chronic disorder of the airways that is complex and characterized by variable and recurring symptoms, airflow obstruction, bronchial hyperresponsiveness, underlying inflammation, and a resulting decrease in the ratio of forced expiratory volume in 1 second to forced vital capacity. Although the condition ranks second after allergic rhinitis as the most common chronic respiratory disease in North America, many children and adults with asthma continue to be undiagnosed and untreated.

Guidelines for classifying asthma severity and initiating treatment differ for children aged 0 to 4 years (Fig. 17–3) and those aged 5 to 11 years (Fig. 17–4). Asthma symptoms typically follow a circadian rhythm in which bronchospasm is worse during the nighttime sleep hours. A marker of effective airway inflammation control is minimal nocturnal symptoms. With young children, parents often report awakening to the child's repeated cough while the child continues to sleep. Conversely, asthma flares are often harder to control during the nighttime hours.

When airway inflammatory control is poor, children with asthma typically use emergency services for treatment of frequent acute flares. With appropriate asthma family teaching to help with management of acute and chronic

Components of Severity		Classification of Asthma Severity (0–4 years of age)			
			Persistent		
		Intermittent	Mild	Moderate	Severe
Impairment	Symptoms	≤2 days/week	>2 days/week but not daily	Daily	Throughout the day
	Nighttime awakenings	0	1–2x/month	3–4x/month	>1x/week
	Short-acting beta₂-agonist use for symptom control (not prevention of EIB)	≤2 days/week	>2 days/week but not daily	Daily	Several times per day
	Interference with normal activity	None	Minor limitation	Some limitation	Extremely limited
Risk	Exacerbations requiring oral systemic corticosteroids	0–1/year	≥2 exacerbations in 6 months requiring oral systemic corticosteroids, or ≥4 wheezing episodes/1 year lasting >1 day AND risk factors for persistent asthma		
		Consider severity and interval since last exacerbation. Frequency and severity may fluctuate over time. ⟵ ⟶ Exacerbations of any severity may occur in patients in any severity category.			
Recommended Step for Initiating Therapy (See figure 4–1a for treatment steps.)		Step 1	Step 2	Step 3 and consider short course of oral systemic corticosteroids	
		In 2–6 weeks, depending on severity, evaluate level of asthma control that is achieved. If no clear benefit is observed in 4–6 weeks, consider adjusting therapy or alternative diagnoses.			

Key: EIB, exercise-induced bronchospasm

Notes:

• The stepwise approach is meant to assist, not replace, the clinical decisionmaking required to meet individual patient needs.

• Level of severity is determined by both impairment and risk. Assess impairment domain by patient's/caregiver's recall of previous 2–4 weeks. Symptom assessment for longer periods should reflect a global assessment such as inquiring whether the patient's asthma is better or worse since the last visit. Assign severity to the most severe category in which any feature occurs.

• At present, there are inadequate data to correspond frequencies of exacerbations with different levels of asthma severity. For treatment purposes, patients who had 2 exacerbations requiring oral systemic corticosteroids in the past 6 months, or ≥4 wheezing episodes in the past year, and who have risk factors for persistent asthma may be considered the same as patients who have persistent asthma, even in the absence of impairment levels consistent with persistent asthma.

Figure 17-3 Stepwise Approach to Managing Asthma in Children 0–4 Years of Age
Source: National Institutes of Health: Guidelines for the Diagnosis and Management of Asthma; Available at: http://www.nhlbi.nih.gov/guidelines/asthma/asthgdln.htm.

Components of Severity		Classification of Asthma Severity (5–11 years of age)			
		Intermittent	Persistent		
			Mild	Moderate	Severe
Impairment	Symptoms	≤2 days/week	>2 days/week but not daily	Daily	Throughout the day
	Nighttime awakenings	≤2x/month	3–4x/month	>1x/week but not nightly	Often 7x/week
	Short-acting beta₂-agonist use for symptom control (not prevention of EIB)	≤2 days/week	>2 days/week but not daily	Daily	Several times per day
	Interference with normal activity	None	Minor limitation	Some limitation	Extremely limited
	Lung function	• Normal FEV₁ between exacerbations • FEV₁ >80% predicted • FEV₁/FVC >85%	• FEV₁ ≥ 80% predicted • FEV₁/FVC >80%	• FEV₁ = 60–80% predicted • FEV₁/FVC = 75–80%	• FEV₁ <60% predicted • FEV₁/FVC <75%
Risk	Exacerbations requiring oral systemic corticosteroids	0–1/year (see note)	≥2/year (see note) →→→→→→		
		Consider severity and interval since last exacerbation. ←———→ Frequency and severity may fluctuate over time for patients in any severity category.			
		Relative annual risk of exacerbations may be related to FEV₁.			
Recommended Step for Initiating Therapy (See figure 4–1b for treatment steps.)		Step 1	Step 2	Step 3, medium-dose ICS option and consider short course of oral systemic corticosteroids	Step 3, medium-dose ICS option, or step 4
		In 2–6 weeks, evaluate level of asthma control that is achieved, and adjust therapy accordingly.			

Key: EIB, exercise-induced bronchospasm; FEV1, forced expiratory volume in 1 second; FVC, forced vital capacity; ICS, inhaled corticosteroids

Notes:
• The stepwise approach is meant to assist, not replace, the clinical decisionmaking required to meet individual patient needs.
• Level of severity is determined by both impairment and risk. Assess impairment domain by patient's/caregiver's recall of the previous 2–4 weeks and spirometry. Assign severity to the most severe category in which any feature occurs.
• At present, there are inadequate data to correspond frequencies of exacerbations with different levels of asthma severity. In general, more frequent and intense exacerbations (e.g., requiring urgent, unscheduled care, hospitalization, or ICU admission) indicate greater underlying disease severity. For treatment purposes, patients who had ≥2 exacerbations requiring oral systemic corticosteroids in the past year may be considered the same as patients who have persistent asthma, even in the absence of impairment levels consistent with persistent asthma.

Figure 17-4 Classifying Asthma Severity and Initiating Treatment in Children 5–11 Years of Age
Source: National Institutes of Health: Guidelines for the Diagnosis and Management of Asthma; Available at: http://www.nhlbi.nih.gov/guidelines/asthma/asthgdln.htm.

airway inflammation and its resulting symptoms, emergency visits can be minimized or eliminated.

Asthma is a disease of airway inflammation with superimposed bronchospasm. The need for a short-acting beta₂-agonist as a rescue drug should be viewed as failure to provide adequate airway inflammatory control. Excessive beta₂-agonist use is a risk factor for asthma death.

When airway inflammation is inadequate, asthma symptoms such as cough or wheeze can accompany or immediately follow physical activity. A child with well-controlled asthma should be able and encouraged to participate in fitness and leisure activities.

With asthma treatment that focuses on the prevention of airway inflammation and bronchospasm, the peak expiratory flow (PEF) can be normal or near normal. The body's normal circadian rhythm provides a variation of awakening to late-evening PEF of 10% to 15%. With asthma, this variation increases to more than 15%, reflecting the nocturnal bronchospasm that is a part of the disease. Usually a child younger than 4 or 5 has some difficulty with obtaining a peak flow.

The approach to managing asthma is differentiated into two age groups: those aged 0 to 4 (Fig. 17–5) and those aged 5 to 11 years (Fig. 17–6). Because of the wide range of asthma medications currently available, the NP, patient, and family can work together to find an age-specific lifestyle and treatment regimen that provides optimal care with minimal to few adverse medication effects.

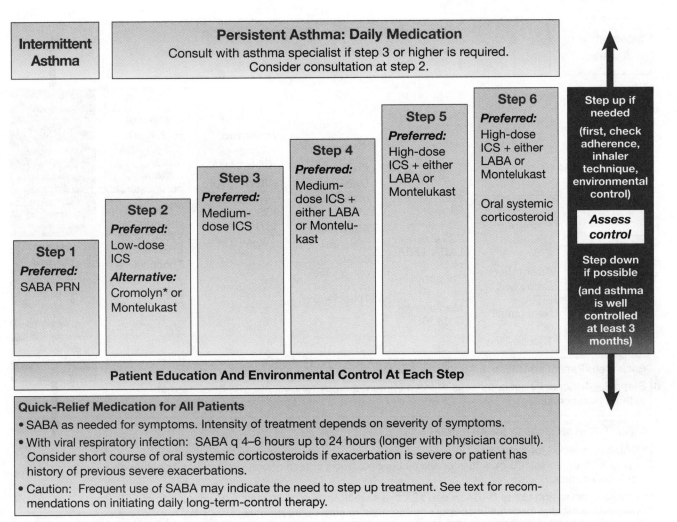

Intermittent Asthma	Persistent Asthma: Daily Medication Consult with asthma specialist if step 3 or higher is required. Consider consultation at step 2.

Step 1
Preferred:
SABA PRN

Step 2
Preferred:
Low-dose ICS
Alternative:
Cromolyn* or Montelukast

Step 3
Preferred:
Medium-dose ICS

Step 4
Preferred:
Medium-dose ICS + either LABA or Montelukast

Step 5
Preferred:
High-dose ICS + either LABA or Montelukast

Step 6
Preferred:
High-dose ICS + either LABA or Montelukast

Oral systemic corticosteroid

Step up if needed
(first, check adherence, inhaler technique, environmental control)

Assess control

Step down if possible
(and asthma is well controlled at least 3 months)

Patient Education And Environmental Control At Each Step

Quick-Relief Medication for All Patients
- SABA as needed for symptoms. Intensity of treatment depends on severity of symptoms.
- With viral respiratory infection: SABA q 4–6 hours up to 24 hours (longer with physician consult). Consider short course of oral systemic corticosteroids if exacerbation is severe or patient has history of previous severe exacerbations.
- Caution: Frequent use of SABA may indicate the need to step up treatment. See text for recommendations on initiating daily long-term-control therapy.

Key: Alphabetical order is used when more than one treatment option is listed within either preferred or alternative therapy. ICS, inhaled corticosteroid; LABA, inhaled long-acting beta₂-agonist, LTRA, leukotriene receptor antagonist; SABA, inhaled short-acting beta₂-agonist.

Notes:
- The stepwise approach is meant to assist, not replace, the clinical decisionmaking required to meet individual patient needs.
- If alternative treatment is used and response is inadequate, discontinue it and use the preferred treatment before stepping up.
- Theophylline is a less desirable alternative due to the need to monitor serum concentration levels.
- If clear benefit is not observed within 4–6 weeks and patient/family medication technique and adherence are satisfactory, consider adjusting therapy or alternative diagnosis.
- Studies on children 0–4 years of age are limited. Step 2 preferred therapy is based on Evidence A. All other recommendations are based on expert opinion and extrapolation from studies in older children.

* Cromolyn no longer availabe in US but remains mentioned in guidelines.

Figure 17-5 Estimated Comparative Daily Dosages for ICS in Children 0–4 Years of Age
Source: National Institutes of Health: Guidelines for the Diagnosis and Management of Asthma; Available at: http://www.nhlbi.nih.gov/guidelines/asthma/asthgdln.htm.

The formerly held concept in asthma was that no matter how severe the airway obstruction, the process was fully reversible. The newer disease model acknowledges that continued airway inflammation contributes to significant and potentially permanent airway remodeling and fixed obstruction. In addition, there is evidence that poorly controlled asthma can contribute to overall attenuated lung development in children.

The backbone of therapy for mild persistent, moderate persistent, or severe persistent asthma is the use of an inflammatory controller drug, such as an inhaled corticosteroid; an additional option includes a leukotriene modifier such as montelukast. Although all these products have anti-inflammatory capability, inhaled corticosteroids have proved to be the most effective in preventing airway inflammation and are recognized as the preferred asthma controller drug. Dosing should be based on age and strength needed to control symptoms (Figs. 17–7 and 17–8). Adding a leukotriene modifier to an inhaled corticosteroid (ICS) or increasing the dosage of the inhaled corticosteroid also improves asthma outcome. The clinical effects of inhaled corticosteroid and leukotriene modifier take at least 1 to 2 weeks to be seen.

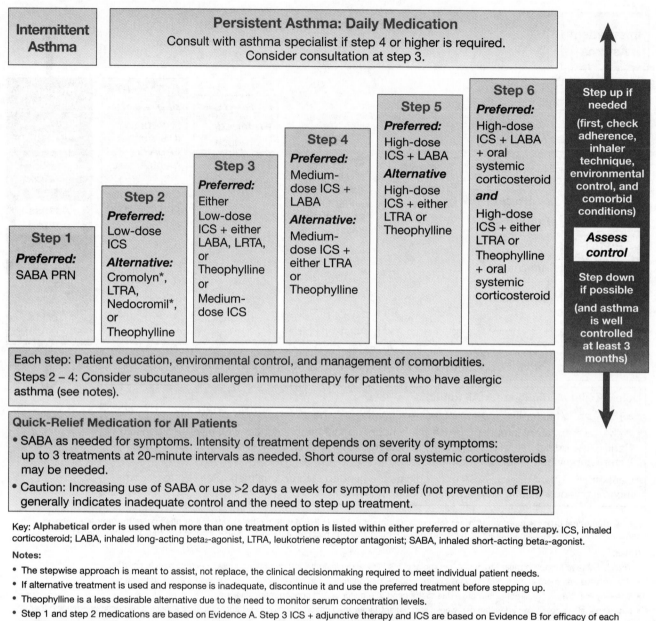

Figure 17-6 Stepwise Approach to Managing Asthma in Children 5–11 Years of Age
Source: National Institutes of Health: Guidelines for the Diagnosis and Management of Asthma; Available at: http://www.nhlbi.nih.gov/guidelines/asthma/asthgdln.htm.

Adding a long-acting beta₂-agonist (LABA) such as salmeterol or formoterol is also an option when ICS therapy is insufficient but should be prescribed only with the understanding of the boxed warning related to the small but significant increased asthma death risk with use. Just as in the adult population, a LABA should never be used as monotherapy for a child and is only be used in combination with an ICS for prevention of symptoms in moderate–severe persistent asthma. Although the inhaled mast cell stabilizers including

nedocromil and cromolyn continue to be mentioned as a controller option, these products are no longer available.

Medications for asthma in children should be age and symptom-specific (Table 17–16). Theophylline, a modestly effective bronchodilator, remains an option in preventing bronchospasm in children ≥5 years of age. Although inexpensive, the cost of using this medication is significant because of the required laboratory monitoring with its use. Theophylline has a narrow therapeutic index, but the dose must be

Estimated Comparative Daily Dosages for ICS in Children Age 0 to 4 years

Drug	Low Daily Dose	Medium Daily Dose	High Daily Dose
Budesonide inhalation suspension for nebulization (child dose)	0.25–0.5mg	0.5–1.0mg	>1.0mg
Fluticasone HFA MDI: 44, 110, or 220 mcg/puff	176 mcg	176 –352 mcg	352 mcg

Available at: http://www.nhlbi.nih.gov/guidelines/asthma/asthma_qrg.pdf

Figure 17-7 Estimated Comparative Daily Dosages for ICS in Children 0–4 Years of Age
Source: National Institutes of Health: Guidelines for the Diagnosis and Management of Asthma; Available at: http://www.nhlbi.nih.gov/guidelines/asthma/asthgdln.htm.

closely titrated and monitored with serial serum drug levels, a particularly problematic issue in children. Rescue medications that relieve acute superimposed bronchospasm include short-acting beta$_2$-agonists, such as albuterol, levalbuterol, and pirbuterol. Compared with albuterol and pirbuterol, one of the therapeutic advantages of levalbuterol includes greater bronchodilation with fewer side effects and at a lower dosage.

When acute asthma flare is present with increased symptoms and objective measurement of airflow obstruction, rapidly acting higher potency anti-inflammatory therapy with an oral corticosteroid is needed. Because asthma is a lower airway disease, a child with asthma has more of a problem with expiration, or getting air out, than with inspiration, or getting air in. This condition leads to findings characteristic of air trapping, such as decreased PEF rate, prolonged expiratory phase, thoracic hyperresonance on percussion, and hyperinflation seen on chest radiographs. Oxygen desaturation is a late finding in an acute asthma flare.

DISCUSSION SOURCES

National Institutes of Health: National Asthma Education and Prevention Program, Expert Panel Report 3. Guidelines for the Diagnosis and Management of Asthma, http://www.nhlbi.nih.gov/guidelines/asthma/asthgdln.pdf.
National Institutes of Health: Guidelines for the Diagnosis and Management of Asthma, http://www.nhlbi.nih.gov/guidelines/asthma/asthgdln.htm.

▶ Gastroenteritis

187. Hydration status can be determined by evaluating (choose all that apply):
A. blood pressure.
B. heart rate.
C. skin turgor.
D. presence of dry lips and oral mucosa.

188. Signs of severe dehydration include (choose all that apply):
A. anuria.
B. tears absent.
C. capillary refill of approximately 3 seconds.
D. elevated blood pressure.

189. What advice should you give to a breastfeeding mother whose 4-month-old has gastroenteritis and reports 2 loose stools and 2 episodes of vomiting within the past 4 hours?
A. Switch to soy-based formula.
B. Give the infant oral rehydration solution only.
C. Continue breastfeeding.
D. Supplement with a sugar water solution.

190. What advice should you give to the parents of a toddler with gastroenteritis?
A. Give the child sips of room temperature cola.
B. Give the child sips of an oral rehydration solution.
C. Give the child sips of a sports drink such as Gatorade.
D. Try sips of apple juice mixed 1:1 with tap water.

Estimated Comparative Daily Dosages for ICS in Children Age 5 to 11 years

Drug	Low Daily Dose	Medium Daily Dose	High Daily Dose
Beclomethasone HFA 40 or 80 mcg/puff	80–160 mcg	>160–320 mcg	>320 mcg
Budesonide DPI 90, 180 mcg/inhalation	200–400 mcg	>400–800 mcg	>800 mcg
Budesonide inhalation suspension for nebulization (child dose)	0.5 mg	1.0 mg	2.0 mg
Fluticasone HFA MDI: 44, 110, or 220 mcg/puff	88–176 mcg	>176–352 mcg	>352 mcg
Fluticasone DPI: 50, 100, or 250 mcg/inhalation	100–200 mcg	200–400 mcg	>400 mcg

NA = not approved and no data available for children less than 12 years of age.

Available at: http://www.nhlbi.nih.gov/guidelines/asthma/asthma_qrg.pdf

Figure 17-8 Estimated Comparative Daily Dosages for ICS in Children 5–11 Years of Age
Source: National Institutes of Health: Guidelines for the Diagnosis and Management of Asthma; Available at: http://www.nhlbi.nih.gov/guidelines/asthma/asthgdln.htm.

TABLE 17-16

Pediatric Asthma Medications

Medication	Mechanism of Action	Indication	Comment
Inhaled corticosteroids	Inhibit eosinophilic action and other inflammatory mediators, potentate effects of beta$_2$-agonists	Controller drug, prevention of inflammation	Need consistent use to be helpful
Leukotriene modifier Leukotriene antagonists (montelukast [Singulair], zafirlukast [Accolate])	Inhibits action of inflammatory mediator, leukotriene, by blocking select receptor sites	Controller drug, prevention of inflammation	Likely less effective than inhaled corticosteroids. Particularly effective add-on medication when disease control inadequate with inhaled corticosteroid, when asthma complicated by allergic rhinitis
Oral corticosteroids	Inhibit eosinophilic action and other inflammatory mediators	Treatment of acute inflammation such as in asthma flare	• Indicated in treatment of acute asthma flare to reduce inflammation • In higher dose and with longer therapy • No taper needed if use is short-term Potential for causing gastropathy, particularly gastric ulcer and gastritis
Beta$_2$-agonist Albuterol (Ventolin, Proventil), pirbuterol (Maxair), levalbuterol (Xopenex)	Bronchodilation via stimulation of beta-2 receptor site	Rescue drugs for treatment of acute bronchospasm	• Onset of action 15 min • Duration of action 4–6 hr
Long-acting beta$_2$-agonists (salmeterol [Serevent], formoterol [Foradil])	Beta$_2$-agonist; bronchodilation via stimulation of beta-2 receptor site	Prevention of bronchospasm	Example: Salmeterol • Onset of action 1 hr • Duration of action 12 hr • Indicated for prevention rather than treatment of bronchospasm Patient should also have short-acting beta$_2$-agonist as rescue drug • Onset of action 15–30 hr • Duration of action 12 hr • Indicated for prevention rather than treatment of bronchospasm • Patient should also have short-acting beta$_2$-agonist as rescue drug
Theophylline	Mild bronchodilator, helps with diaphragmatic contraction	Prevention of bronchospasm, mild anti-inflammatory	• Narrow therapeutic index drug with numerous drug interactions • Monitor carefully for toxicity by checking drug levels and clinical presentation

191. The onset of symptoms of food poisoning caused by *Staphylococcus* species is typically how many hours after the ingestion of the offending substance?
    A. 0.5 to 1
    B. 1 to 4
    C. 4 to 8
    D. 8 to 12

192. The onset of symptoms in food poisoning caused by *Salmonella* species is typically how many hours after the ingestion of the offending substance?
    A. 2 to 8
    B. 8 to 12
    C. 12 to 24
    D. 24 to 36

193. To obtain the most accurate hydration status in a child with acute gastroenteritis, the NP should ask about:
    A. the time of last urination.
    B. thirst.
    C. quantity of liquids taken.
    D. number of episodes of vomiting and diarrhea.

194. What percentage of body weight is typically lost in a child with moderate dehydration?
    A. 2% to 3%
    B. 3% to 5%
    C. 6% to 10%
    D. 11% to 15%

195. Clinical features of shigellosis include all of the following except:
    A. bloody diarrhea.
    B. high fever.
    C. malaise.
    D. vomiting.

Answers

187. A, B, C,	190. B.	194. C.
D.	191. B.	195. D.
188. A, B, C.	192. C.	
189. C.	193. A.	

Acute gastroenteritis is a common episodic disease of childhood, usually viral in nature. A child presents with short-duration vomiting and diarrhea; the vomitus and stool are free of blood, and the stool is free of pus. In addition, the child usually does not have a fever. Given that these viral illnesses are highly contagious and easily transmitted person to person, usually there is a history of contacts with children or adults who have similar symptoms. The duration of illness is usually short, usually fewer than 3 to 5 days and often as short as 24 hours.

An important part of the assessment of a child with acute gastroenteritis is determining hydration status. Asking about the last urination is a helpful way of evaluating this. If the child has voided within the previous few hours, the degree of dehydration is minimal. Many other clinical parameters are helpful in assessing for dehydration (Table 17–17). Although mild dehydration can usually be managed with frequent small-volume feedings of commercially prepared oral rehydration solutions such as Pedialyte™, a child with moderate to severe dehydration likely needs parenteral fluids in addition to small amounts of fluids orally as tolerated (Table 17–18). Because they contain inappropriate glucose and electrolyte composition, sports drinks such as Gatorade (tm), soda, and most fruit juices are inappropriate for rehydration. The use of antidiarrheal agents is usually discouraged because of the risk of increasing the severity of illness if toxin-producing bacteria are the causative agent. Warning signs

Table 17-17
Assessment Criteria for Hydration Status

Parameter	Mild 3%–5%	Moderate 6%–9%	Severe ≥10%
Blood pressure	Normal	Normal to decreased	Weak, thready, impalpable
Pulse quality	Normal	Normal to slightly decreased	Moderately decreased
Heart rate	Normal	Normal to increased	Increased (sometimes bradycardia)
Turgor	Normal	Recoil <2 seconds	Recoil >2 seconds, tenting
Fontanels	Normal	Slightly depressed	Depressed
Mucous membranes	Slightly dry lips, thick saliva	Dry lips and oral mucosa	Very dry lips, oral mucosa
Eyes	Normal, tears present	Slightly sunken, tears decreased	Deeply sunken, tears absent
Capillary refill	Normal (<2 seconds)	Prolonged	Minimal
Mental status	Normal	Normal, fatigued, restless, irritable	Apathetic, lethargic, unconscious
Urine output	Slightly decreased	Decreased	Minimal
Thirst	Normal, to slightly increased	Moderately increased	Very thirsty or too lethargic to assess

Medscape: Pediatric Dehydration Clinical Presentation, http://emedicine.medscape.com/article/801012-clinical#a0256.

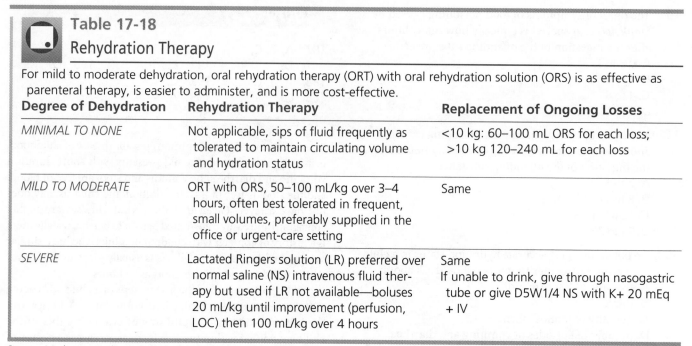

Table 17-18

Rehydration Therapy

For mild to moderate dehydration, oral rehydration therapy (ORT) with oral rehydration solution (ORS) is as effective as parenteral therapy, is easier to administer, and is more cost-effective.

Degree of Dehydration	Rehydration Therapy	Replacement of Ongoing Losses
MINIMAL TO NONE	Not applicable, sips of fluid frequently as tolerated to maintain circulating volume and hydration status	<10 kg: 60–100 mL ORS for each loss; >10 kg 120–240 mL for each loss
MILD TO MODERATE	ORT with ORS, 50–100 mL/kg over 3–4 hours, often best tolerated in frequent, small volumes, preferably supplied in the office or urgent-care setting	Same
SEVERE	Lactated Ringers solution (LR) preferred over normal saline (NS) intravenous fluid therapy but used if LR not available—boluses 20 mL/kg until improvement (perfusion, LOC) then 100 mL/kg over 4 hours	Same If unable to drink, give through nasogastric tube or give D5W1/4 NS with K+ 20 mEq + IV

Source: Medscape: Pediatric Dehydration Treatment & Management, http://emedicine.medscape.com/article/801012-treatment#aw2aab6b6b4.

during acute gastroenteritis include fever coupled with bloody or pus-filled stools. If these are present, a bacterial source of infection such as shigellosis should be considered. Stool culture should be obtained, and appropriate antimicrobial therapy should be initiated.

Improperly handled food is a common source of the gastrointestinal infection commonly known as food poisoning. A child typically presents, often along with family members and caregivers who ate the same food, with a history of sudden onset of abdominal pain, nausea, and vomiting. Knowledge of the timing of the onset of symptoms is helpful when attempting to discern the offending organism. Most food poisoning episodes are short and self-limiting, resolving over a few hours to days without special intervention.

DISCUSSION SOURCES

King, KC, Glass R, Bresee JS. Managing acute gastroenteritis among children. *MMRW* 2;RR16:1–16, 2003.

Medscape. Pediatric Dehydration Overview, http://emedicine.medscape.com/article/801012-overview.

Alterations in Puberty

196. The most common reason for precocious puberty in girls is:
A. ovarian tumor.
B. adrenal tumor.
C. exogenous estrogen.
D. early onset of normal puberty.

197. The most common reason for precocious puberty in boys is:
A. testicular tumor.
B. a select number of relatively uncommon health problems.
C. exogenous testosterone.
D. early onset of normal puberty.

198. Which of the following is noted in a child with premature thelarche?
A. breast enlargement.
B. accelerated linear growth.
C. pubic hair.
D. body odor.

199. Which of the following is noted in a child with premature adrenarche?
A. breast development.
B. accelerated linear growth.
C. pubic hair.
D. menstruation.

200. Girls typically grow to their adult height by:
A. menarche.
B. 1 year before menarche.
C. 1 year after onset of menstruation.
D. by their sixteenth birthday.

201. A 15-year-old male is found to be at Tanner stage 1 on exam. The least likely cause of this finding is:
A. a variation of normal based on ethnicity or familial factors.
B. human growth hormone abnormality.
C. Klinefelter syndrome.
D. nutritional factors.

202. Which is not a reason for the delayed onset of puberty in a 13-year-old boy?
A. report of a high level of physical activity
B. Kallmann syndrome
C. familial trait
D. history of radiation exposure

203. Which is possible reason for delayed onset of puberty in a 13-year-old girl?
A. history of abdominal irradiation
B. obesity
C. report of a high level of physical activity
D. Turner syndrome

Answers

196. D.	199. C.	202. A.
197. B.	200. C.	203. D.
198. A.	201. A.	

Precocious puberty in girls has long been defined as the onset of secondary sexual characteristics before the child's eighth birthday. A more recent study reveals that there is likely a group of girls who have the onset of slowly developing secondary sexual characteristics between ages 6 and 8 years as a benign normal variant. In particular, thelarche (the isolated appearance of breast development) is common as early as age 7 and pubarche (the appearance of pubic hair without other signs of puberty) as early as age 8 in otherwise healthy girls. Consequently, the most common reason for precocious puberty in girls is early onset of normal puberty.

A subset of girls, particularly girls with pubertal changes noted before their sixth birthday, often has significant health problems, however, such as ovarian or adrenal tumors. Expert evaluation and referral is indicated in these children. Evaluation typically includes measuring bone age, level of follicle-stimulating hormone, and level of luteinizing hormone; performing abdominal ultrasound; and conducting other studies warranted by clinical presentation. Treatment depends on the cause. In the absence of an adrenal or ovarian tumor or other secondary cause, counseling about the nature of the process of early puberty should be discussed with the child and family.

Because girls typically achieve nearly all of their adult height 1 year after the first menstrual period (menarche), a girl achieving menarche at a premature age often has short stature. If the child and family wish to attempt to halt the onset of puberty, a gonadotropin-releasing hormone analogue and additional therapies can be given to counteract the effects of endogenous hormones. This therapy is provided with expert consultation and family informed consent.

Premature thelarche is a relatively common, benign process in which breast development is noted in female toddlers. Usually present unilaterally or bilaterally, the child has no other signs of puberty including accelerated linear growth. Reassurance and ongoing monitoring are the typical course of treatment. In premature adrenarche, a parent usually reports that

a child 5 to 6 years old has body odor, pubic hair, and (rarely) axillary hair. The child has no other signs of puberty, including accelerated linear growth. Reassurance and ongoing monitoring constitute the typical course of treatment.

In boys, precocious puberty is defined as the onset of secondary sexual characteristics before his ninth birthday. Overall, this condition is less common in boys than in girls and is unlikely to be a benign normal variation. Gonadal and adrenal tumors and a select number of genetically based diseases are the most likely causes. Prompt referral to expert care is indicated.

Delayed puberty is defined as no evidence of sexual maturation (Tanner stage 1) in girls older than age 13 and in boys older than age 14. Delayed onset of puberty is multifactorial in both boys and girls. This delay can occur because the child is healthy but maturing more slowly when compared with same-age peers, a condition called constitutional delay of puberty, which often runs in families. However, delay in puberty can be caused by hypogonadism, in which the gonads (the testes in males and the ovaries in females) produce few or no hormones. Numerous medical conditions can result in hypogonadism, including certain autoimmune disorders, developmental disorders, history of radiation exposure and/or chemotherapy, infection, surgery, or brain or pituitary tumors. Chromosomal anomalies can also result in hypogonadism, such as Kallmann syndrome (occurring more often in boys than girls), Turner syndrome in girls (XO female), and Klinefelter syndrome in boys (XXY male). For both genders, poor diet lacking in the daily recommended values of nutrients can also contribute to delayed onset. Occasionally, young girls who undergo intense physical training for a sport, such as running or gymnastics, experience delayed puberty, largely as a result of low body weight; this is not noted in males with a similar level of activity.

DISCUSSION SOURCES

Medscape: Precocious Puberty, http://emedicine.medscape.com/article/924002-overview#a0104.

National Institutes of Health: What Causes Normal Puberty, Precocious Puberty, & Delayed Puberty? http://nichd.nih.gov/health/topics/puberty/conditioninfo/Pages/causes.aspx.

Heart Murmur

204. An innocent heart murmur has which of the following characteristics?
A. occurs late in systole
B. has localized area of auscultation
C. becomes softer when the patient moves from supine to standing position
D. frequently obliterates the second heart sound (S_2)

205. The murmur of atrial septal defect is usually:
A. found in children with symptoms of cardiac disease.
B. first found on a 2- to 6-month well-baby examination.
C. found with mitral valve prolapse.
D. presystolic in timing.

206. A Still murmur:
- A. is heard in the presence of cardiac pathology.
- B. has a humming or vibratory quality.
- C. is a reason for denying sports participation clearance.
- D. can become louder when the patient is standing.

❯ Answers

204. C.   **205.** B.   **206.** B.

The ability to appropriately assess children with a heart murmur is an important part of the role of an NP. Knowledge of the most common murmurs, the clinical presentation of the murmurs, etiology of the murmur, and the impact on a child's health is critical to appropriate assessment. It is also necessary to be able to determine the need for specialty referral (Table 17–19).

DISCUSSION SOURCE

Park M. *Pediatric Cardiology for Practitioners*, ed. 5. St. Louis: Mosby, 2007.

TABLE 17-19
Differential Diagnosis of Common Heart Murmurs in Children

When evaluating a child with cardiac murmur:
- Ask about major symptoms of heart disease: chest pain, congestive heart failure symptoms, palpitations, syncope, activity intolerance, poor growth and development
- The bell of the stethoscope is most helpful for auscultating lower pitched sounds, and the diaphragm is better for higher pitched sounds
- Systolic murmurs are graded on a 1 to 6 scale, from barely audible to audible with stethoscope off the chest. Diastolic murmurs are usually graded on the same scale, but abbreviated to grades 1 to 4 because these murmurs are not loud enough to reach grades 5 and 6.
- A critical part of the evaluation of a child with a heart murmur is the decision to offer antimicrobial prophylaxis. No prophylaxis is needed with benign murmurs. Refer to the American Heart Association's Guidelines for the latest advice.

Murmur	Important Cardiac Examination Findings	Additional Findings	Comments
Newborn	Grade 1–2/6 early systolic, vibratory, heard best at left lower sternal border (LLSB) with little radiation Pulses intact, otherwise well neonate	Subsides or disappears when pressure applied to abdomen	Heard in first few days of life; disappears in 2–3 weeks Benign condition
Still (vibratory innocent murmur)	Grade 1–3/6 early systolic ejection, musical or vibratory, short, often buzzing, heard best midway between apex and LLSB	Softens or disappears when sitting, when standing, or with Valsalva maneuver Louder when supine or with fever or tachycardia	Usual onset age 2–6 years; may persist through adolescence Benign condition
Hemic	Grade 1–2/6 systolic ejection, high-pitched, heard best in pulmonic and aortic areas	Heard only in presence of increased cardiac output, such as fever, anemia, stress	Disappears when underlying condition resolves Usually seen without cardiac disease Most often heard in children and younger adults with thin chest walls
Venous hum	Grade 1–2/6 continuous musical hum heard best at upper right sternal border (URSB) and upper left sternal border (ULS) and the lower neck	Disappears in supine position, when jugular vein is compressed Common after age 3 years.	Believed to be produced by turbulence in subclavian and jugular veins Benign condition

TABLE 17-19

Differential Diagnosis of Common Heart Murmurs in Children—cont'd

Murmur	Important Cardiac Examination Findings	Additional Findings	Comments
Pulmonary outflow ejection murmur	Grade 1–2/6 soft, short, systolic ejection murmur, heard best at LLSB, usually localized	Softens or disappears when sitting, when standing, or with Valsalva maneuver Louder when supine	Heard throughout childhood Benign condition but has qualities similar to murmurs caused by pathological condition such as atrial septal defect (ASD), coarctation of the aorta (COA), pulmonic stenosis (PS)
Patent ductus arteriosus	Grade 2–4/6 continuous murmur heard best at ULSB and left infraclavicular area	In premature newborns, seen with active precordium; in older children, seen with full pulses	Normal ductus closure occurs by day 4 of life Often isolated finding but may be seen with COA, ventricular septal defect (VSD) Accounts for ±12% of all congenital heart disease Twice as common in girls In preterm infants <1500 g, rate 20%–60%
Atrial septal defect	Grade 1–3/6 systolic ejection murmur, heard best at ULSB with widely split fixed S_2	Accompanying mid-diastolic murmur heard at fourth intercostal space (ICS) left sternal border (LSB); commonly caused by increased flow across tricuspid valve	Two times as common in girls Child is often entirely well or present with heart failure Often missed in the first few months of life or even entire childhood Watch for children with easy fatigability Cyanosis rare
Ventricular septal defect	Grade 2–5/6 regurgitant systolic murmur heard best at LLSB Occasionally holosystolic, usually localized	Thrill may be present and a loud P_2 with large left-to-right shunt	Usually without cyanosis Children with small- to moderate-sized left-to-right shunt without pulmonary hypertension likely to have minimal symptoms Larger shunts may result in CHF with onset in infancy
Aortic stenosis	Grade 2–5/6 systolic ejection murmur heard best in upper left sternal border (ULSB) or second right ICS, possibly with paradoxically split S_2	Ejection click at apex, third left ICS, second right ICS Radiation or thrill to the carotid arteries	More common in boys than girls In children, usually caused by unicuspid (if noted in infancy) or bicuspid (if noted in childhood) valve Mild exercise intolerance common

Continued

TABLE 17–19

Differential Diagnosis of Common Heart Murmurs in Children—cont'd

Murmur	Important Cardiac Examination Findings	Additional Findings	Comments
Coarctation of aorta	Grade 1–5/6 systolic ejection murmur heard best at ULSB and left interscapular area (on back)	Weak or absent femoral pulses, hypertension in arms	Often seen with aortic stenosis (AS), mitral regurgitation (MR) Presence of dorsalis pedis pulse in child essentially rules out this condition
Mitral valve prolapsed	Grade 1–3/6 mid-systolic click followed by late systolic murmur heard best at the apex	Murmur heard earlier in systole and often louder with standing or squatting	Often with pectus excavatum, straight back (>85%)
Pulmonic valve stenosis	Grade 2–5/6 heard best at ULSB, ejection click at second left ICS	Radiates to back S_2 may be widely split	No symptoms with mild to moderate disease Usually a fusion of valvular cusps

Source: Park M. *Pediatric Cardiology for Practitioners*, ed. 5. St. Louis: Mosby, 2007.

Acute Febrile Illness

207. Which of the following is not consistently performed as part of the workup for sepsis?
A. CBC with WBC differential
B. stool culture
C. blood culture
D. urine culture

208. Rates of sepsis in children have lowered in recent years mainly because of:
A. more stringent screening and diagnosis of febrile illness.
B. increased use of antipyretics.
C. longer observation period in children with febrile illness.
D. higher rates of select immunization.

209. The mechanism of action in fever includes which of the following?
A. an increase in systematic vascular resistance
B. endogenous pyrogens increase prostaglandin synthesis
C. immature neutrophil forms in circulation
D. atypical or reactive lymphocytes

210. When assessing a febrile child, the NP considers that:
A. even minor temperature elevation is potentially harmful.
B. nuchal rigidity is usually not found in early childhood meningitis.
C. fever-related seizures usually occur at the peak of the temperature.
D. most children with temperatures of 38.3°C to 40°C (101°F to 104°F) have a potentially serious bacterial infection.

211. Which of the following is not seen during body temperature increase found in fever?
A. lower rate of viral replication
B. toxic effect on select bacteria
C. negative effect on *S. pneumoniae* growth
D. increased rate of atypical pneumonia pathogen replication

212. When providing care for a febrile patient, the NP bears in mind that all of the following are true except that:
A. the use of antipyretics is potentially associated with prolonged illness.
B. consistent use of an antipyretic provides a helpful way to shorten the course of infectious illnesses.
C. fever increases metabolic demand.
D. in a pregnant woman, increased body temperature is a potential first-trimester teratogen.

213. Concerning the use of antipyretics in a febrile young child, which of the following statements is false?
A. A child with a serious bacterial infection usually does not have fever reduction with an antipyretic.
B. The degree of temperature reduction in response to antipyretic therapy is not predictive of presence or absence of bacteremia.
C. Compared with ibuprofen, acetaminophen has a shorter duration of antipyretic action.
D. Ibuprofen should not be used if a child is also taking a macrolide antimicrobial.

214. When counseling the family of an otherwise healthy 2-year-old child who just had a febrile seizure, you consider the following regarding whether the child is at risk for future febrile seizures (choose all that apply):
    A. The occurrence of one febrile seizure is predictive of having another.
    B. Intermittent diazepam can be used prophylactically during febrile illness to reduce risk of recurrence.
    C. A milder temperature elevation in a child with a history of a febrile seizure poses significant risk for future recurrent febrile and nonfebrile seizures.
    D. Consistent use of antipyretics during a febrile illness will significantly reduce the risk of a future febrile seizure.

215. When evaluating a child who has bacterial meningitis, the NP expects to find cerebrospinal fluid (CSF) results of:
    A. low protein.
    B. predominance of lymphocytes.
    C. glucose at about 30% of serum levels.
    D. low opening pressure.

216. When evaluating a child who has aseptic or viral meningitis, the NP expects to find CSF results of:
    A. low protein.
    B. predominance of lymphocytes.
    C. glucose at about 30% of serum levels.
    D. low opening pressure.

217. Sepsis is defined as the:
    A. clinical manifestation of systemic infection.
    B. presence of bacteria in the blood.
    C. circulation of pathogens.
    D. allergenic response to infection.

218. Gina is 2 years old and presents with a 3-day history of fever, crankiness, and congested cough. Her respiratory rate is more than 50% of the upper limits of normal for age. Tubular breath sounds are noted at the right lung base. Skin turgor is normal, and she is wearing a wet diaper. She is alert, is resisting the examination as age appropriate, and engages in eye contact. Temperature is 38.3°C (101°F). Gina's diagnostic evaluation should include:
    A. chest x-ray.
    B. urine culture and sensitivity measurement.
    C. lumbar puncture.
    D. sputum culture.

219. An early indicator of hypoperfusion is:
    A. an elevation in total white blood cell count.
    B. dehydration.
    C. capillary refill of >2 seconds.
    D. nonresponsive child.

220. As part of the evaluation in a febrile 3-year-old boy, the following white blood cell count with differential is obtained:
    WBCs = 22,100/mm^3
    Neutrophils = 75% (normal 40% to 70%) with toxic granulation
    Bands = 15% (normal 0% to 4%)
    Lymphocytes = 4% (normal 30% to 40%)
    Which of the following best describes the WBC with differential results?
    A. leukocytosis with neutrophilia
    B. leukopenia with lymphocytosis
    C. lymphopenia with neutropenia
    D. leukopenia with neutropenia

221. These results increase the likelihood that the cause of the above-mentioned child's infection is:
    A. viral.
    B. parasitic.
    C. fungal.
    D. bacterial.

222. Which of the following is the most appropriate way to relieve fever and discomfort in a child with varicella?
    A. ibuprofen
    B. aspirin
    C. acetaminophen
    D. cold bath

223. Potential adverse events of acetaminophen in a child with fever and mild dehydration include:
    A. seizure.
    B. hepatotoxicity.
    C. petechial rash.
    D. gastric ulcer.

Answers

207. B.	213. D.	219. C.
208. D.	214. A and B.	220. A.
209. B.	215. C.	221. D.
210. B.	216. B.	222. C.
211. A.	217. A.	223. B.
212. B.	218. A.	

Most young children with an acute febrile illness do not have a serious bacterial infection and recover fully without sequelae. On rare occasion, however, febrile young children with no obvious source of infection have serious sequelae including sepsis and death. The risk of serious illness in the presence of fever is now significantly reduced in the advent of immunization against *H. influenzae* type B and *S. pneumoniae*. Nonetheless, the evaluation and treatment of a febrile child are an important part of providing pediatric healthcare. The NP needs to ascertain the febrile child's immunization status, including where in a particular series the child is or if any immunizations are missing, because this is an essential component of assessing risk of possible pathogens. Unfortunately, as more parents chose not to immunize their children, a resurgence of serious, potentially life-threatening vaccine-preventable diseases is inevitable.

Fever is a complex physiological reaction that occurs when exogenous pyrogens (microorganisms and their products, drugs, incompatible blood products) are introduced to the body. This triggers the production of endogenous pyrogens (polypeptides produced by host cells such as monocytes, macrophages, and interleukin-1). Prostaglandins activate thermoregulatory neurons and alter the hypothalamic set point. Vasomotor center reactions increase heat conservation and heat production.

Although most parents and healthcare providers usually treat fever with antipyretics and other options, in the otherwise well child, an increase in body temperature has benefits. During fever, viral replication rate is reduced. Increased body temperature is toxic to encapsulated bacteria, particularly *S. pneumoniae*. In animal models and clinical trials in humans, the presence of fever has been associated with lower rates of morbidity and mortality associated with infectious diseases. Also, the use of antipyretics including acetaminophen and ibuprofen has been associated with prolonged illness, especially when viral in origin. Conversely, a child with fever is often uncomfortable and cranky, which reinforces the perception that this is a condition that warrants treatment. Fever also increases metabolic demands, a potential problem in a child or adult with a chronic health problem; in pregnancy, fever is potentially teratogenic in the first trimester and increases metabolic demands throughout pregnancy.

Fear of febrile seizure also contributes to the propensity to treat fever aggressively, with the thought that if the body temperature is reduced, seizure risk is reduced. The cause of febrile seizures is unclear but likely involves a relationship between endogenous pyrogens or cytokines and fever. Febrile seizures occur in young children when their seizure threshold is lowest. A simple febrile seizure actually is most likely to occur as fever is increasing rather than at its peak; however, there is no evidence that the rapidity of the rate of increase is associated with febrile seizures. A familial tendency has been noted with febrile seizure, but the condition is not predictive of the development of epilepsy. A simple febrile seizure is a benign, although frightening, common event in children 6 months to 5 years old; a child who has had one seizure is at increased risk for a recurrence. The majority of children with febrile seizures do not need to be treated with medication. Although effective therapies including phenobarbital and valproate, which need to be taken daily, reduce risk and could prevent the occurrence of additional simple febrile seizures, the potential adverse effects of these therapies outweigh the potential benefit in this self-limiting condition. In situations in which parental anxiety about febrile seizures is severe, intermittent oral diazepam (Valium) at the onset of febrile

illness is likely helpful in preventing recurrence. Although use of antipyretics may improve the comfort of the child, these agents do not prevent febrile seizures.

In the first 2 years of life, most children average four to six acute febrile episodes per year, with healthcare sought in about two-thirds of cases. Of these younger children with temperatures lower than 39°C (<102.2°F), most have a viral or obvious bacterial source, and less than 10% have no obvious source for fever. The most common causes of fever in young children are viruses and bacteria, with fungi, parasites, neoplasms, collagen vascular disease, and factitious disease being important but less common. Before pneumococcal conjugate vaccine (PCV13 [Prevnar]) became available, *S. pneumoniae* was implicated in approximately 90% of cases of occult bacteremia in febrile infants and young children. This vaccine provides activity against the most common pneumococcal serotypes implicated in invasive pneumococcal disease and dramatically reduces, but does not eliminate, the risk of invasive pneumococcal disease. Rapid testing for influenza and other viruses can help reduce the need for more invasive studies.

In a previously well, febrile child who is alert, able to tolerate oral fluids, age 3 months to 3 years old, without an identifiable source of fever and temperature lower than 39°C (<102.2°F), the evaluation for the source of fever should start with a careful history and physical examination. Urine testing is indicated in those with unexplained fever because of an increase in the incidence of urinary tract infections in children. If the child is alert, the child's caregivers should be advised about the judicious use of antipyretics, increased fluid intake, and signs of deteriorating condition. Follow-up in 48 hours is prudent if fever persists; follow-up should be sooner if the child's condition worsens.

Advising the child's caregivers about the appropriate choice and use of antipyretics is an important part of providing care for a child with a non–life-threatening illness and fever. As previously mentioned, fever plays an important role in controlling infection. If a child with fever appears fairly comfortable, no treatment is needed. Even a cranky child usually is not harmed and may be helped by allowing the fever to run its course. If the child is uncomfortable with fever, common-sense measures include dressing the child lightly and increasing fluid intake. A cooling bath should not be used because the resulting shivering would drive up body temperature.

The choice of an antipyretic is dictated by numerous factors, including the length of time for onset of action of the product (ideally, less than half an hour) and the duration of action (ideally, 4 to 8 hours), with no or few major reported adverse effects. Ibuprofen and acetaminophen are the most commonly prescribed antipyretics; both have onset of action within half an hour of the dose. The duration of action of acetaminophen is about 4 hours, whereas the duration of ibuprofen is around 6 hours. The antipyretic potential of acetaminophen is equal to that of ibuprofen. Acetaminophen has an excellent gastrointestinal adverse event profile but can be hepatotoxic with excessive use and high dose. Ibuprofen is usually well tolerated but does have the potential to cause gastric ulcer and gastritis, albeit usually with long-term high-dose use. Aspirin should not be prescribed to a child with a febrile illness because of its association with Reye syndrome. Ibuprofen should not be prescribed for varicella because its use is implicated in necrotizing fasciitis.

A young child with a high fever (>39.4°C [>102.9°F]) is more likely to be bacteremic than a child with a temperature equal to or lower than 39.3°C (<102.8°F); this risk is most pronounced in children who have not received immunization against *S. pneumoniae* and *H. influenzae* type B. The degree of temperature reduction in response to antipyretic therapy is not predictive of presence or absence of bacteremia. In one major study among infants with bacteremia but without meningitis, differences in children without bacteremia were detected in clinical appearance before fever reduction but not after defervescence. All children with meningitis appeared seriously ill before and after defervescence.

An early indicator of hypoperfusion is a capillary refill of >2 seconds. Decreased perfusion of the skin is associated with an increase in systematic vascular resistance, which occurs early in an infant with hypovolemia.

When sepsis is suspected, a septic work-up should be initiated (Table 17–20) in an appropriate urgent or emergent setting. Empirical antimicrobial therapy with supportive care is prudent, pending the outcome of evaluation. An antiviral such as acyclovir also may be indicated. The child can be managed at home if the following conditions are met: the child is intact neurologically, adequate hydration can be maintained via the oral route, the caregiver is willing and able to provide the needed close attention to the child, and follow-up and emergency care are easily accessible.

A total WBC count with differential is obtained as part of the evaluation of a child with suspected sepsis. The most typical WBC pattern found in severe bacterial infection is the "left shift." A "left shift" is usually seen in the presence of severe bacterial infection, such as appendicitis and pneumonia. The following is typically noted:

- Leukocytosis: An elevation in the total WBC count.
- Neutrophilia: An elevation in the number of neutrophils in circulation, defined as more than 10,000 neutrophils/mm³. Neutrophils are also known as polys or segs, both referring to the polymorph shape of the segmented nucleus of this WBC.
- Bandemia: An elevation in the number of bands or young neutrophils in circulation. Usually, less than 4% of the total WBCs in circulation are bands. When this percentage is exceeded and the absolute band counts exceed 500/mm³, bandemia is present. This finding indicates that the body has called up as many mature neutrophils that were available in storage pool and is now accessing less mature forms. Bandemia further reinforces the potential seriousness of the infection.
- Toxic granulation: Often reported on WBC morphologic study.
- Other neutrophil forms do not belong in circulation even with severe infection; these include myelocytes and metamyelocytes, immature neutrophil forms that are typically found in granulopoiesis pool. The presence of these cells in the circulation is an ominous marker for life-threatening bacterial infection.
- In viral infection, the total WBC count can be elevated but is often normal or slightly depressed (leukopenia). Lymphocytes, the leukocytes most active in viral infection, predominate. Atypical or reactive lymphocytes are often reported on WBC morphology.
- To eliminate or support the diagnosis of meningitis, lumbar puncture with cerebrospinal fluid (CSF) evaluation should be part of the evaluation of a febrile younger child who has an altered neurological examination. Pleocytosis, defined as a CSF WBC count of more than 5 cells/mm³, is

TABLE 17-20
Evaluation of Young Child With Suspected Sepsis

Evaluation	Rationale
Complete blood count with white blood cell (WBC) differential	Identify viral versus bacterial shifts, general leukocytic response
Blood culture	Potentially identify causative organism in sepsis
Urinalysis and urine culture via transurethral catheter or suprapubic tap	Evaluate for urinary tract infection including pyelonephritis, particularly important in child ≤2 years old
Lumbar puncture with cerebrospinal fluid analysis	Evaluate for bacterial or viral meningitis, particularly important if alterations in neurological examination
Chest x-ray	Rule in or out pneumonia or other respiratory tract condition that can contribute to sepsis, particularly important if dyspnea, tachypnea, decreased breath sounds, WBC (20,000 mm³, or other findings suggestive of lower respiratory tract infection
Stool culture, fecal WBC count	Only if diarrhea present, to evaluate for possible focus of infection

Source: Medscape: Sepsis. Available at: http://emedicine.medscape.com/article/978352-overview.

an expected finding in meningitis caused by bacterial, viral, tubercular, fungal, or protozoan infection. An elevated CSF opening pressure is also a nearly universal finding. Typical CSF response in bacterial meningitis includes a median WBC count of 1200 cells/mm³ with 90% to 95% neutrophils; additional findings are a reduction in CSF glucose below the normal level of about 60% of the plasma level and an elevated CSF protein level. CSF results in viral or aseptic meningitis include normal glucose level, normal to slightly elevated protein level, and lymphocytosis. Further testing to ascertain the causative organism is warranted. Measurement of serum lactate as well as some inflammatory markers and acute-phase reactants can aid in the early identification and management of pediatric sepsis. These include erythrocyte sedimentation rate (ESR), C-reactive protein (CRP), interleukin (IL)-1b, IL-6, IL-8, tumor necrosis factor-alpha (TNF-α), leukotriene B4, and procalcitonin.

- Treatment of a child with meningitis includes supportive care and use of the appropriate anti-infective agent. Acyclovir is an option in aseptic meningitis, pending identification of the offending virus. Ceftriaxone with vancomycin is usually the initial treatment of choice in suspected bacterial meningitis, pending bacterial sensitivity results. Treatment of other forms of sepsis in a younger child depends on its cause. Prudent practitioners should seek expert help in evaluating and treating a child with suspected or documented sepsis.

DISCUSSION SOURCES

National Institutes of Health: Feverish Illness in Children: Assessment and Initial Management in Children Younger Than 5 Years, http://www.ncbi.nlm.nih.gov/books/NBK45971.

National Institutes of Health: Febrile Seizures, http://www.ninds.nih.gov/disorders/febrile_seizures/detail_febrile_seizures.htm.

Hamilton JL, John SP. Evaluation of fever in infants and young children. *Am Fam Physician* 87:254–260, 2013.

Pneumonia

224. When treating a 3-year-old well child with community-acquired pneumonia (CAP), the NP realizes that the most likely causative pathogen is:
    A. *Mycoplasma pneumoniae.*
    B. a respiratory virus.
    C. *H. influenzae.*
    D. *S. pneumoniae.*

225. Which of the following is the most appropriate antimicrobial for treatment of CAP in a 2 year old who is clinically stable and able to be treated in the outpatient setting?
    A. amoxicillin
    B. doxycycline
    C. TMP-SMX
    D. levofloxacin

226. Which of the following is most likely to be noted in a 3 year old with CAP?
    A. complaint of pleuritic chest pain
    B. sputum production
    C. report of dyspnea
    D. tachypnea

227. What percentage of children have an episode of pneumonia before the age of age 5?
    A. 18% to 20%
    B. 9% to 10%
    C. 3% to 4%
    D. 20% to 30%

228. Which of the following antimicrobials provides effective activity against atypical pathogens?
    A. amoxicillin
    B. cefprozil
    C. ceftriaxone
    D. clarithromycin

Answers

224. B.	226. D.	228. D.
225. A.	227. C.	

In all age groups, pneumonia is the most common cause of death from infectious disease worldwide and results in 20% of all deaths in children younger than age 5 years. In the developed world, the annual incidence of pneumonia is 3 to 4 cases per 100 children <5 years old. Most often caused by bacteria or viruses, pneumonia is an acute lower respiratory tract infection involving lung parenchyma, interstitial tissues, and alveolar spaces. The term community-acquired pneumonia (CAP) is used to describe the onset of the disease in an individual who resides within the community, not in a nursing home or other care facility, with no recent (within 2 weeks) hospitalization.

Most children with pneumonia present with cough. Tachypnea is the most sensitive, although not specific, finding. In particular, the diagnosis of lower respiratory tract disease should be considered with a respiratory rate exceeding 50/min in children younger than 1 year and a rate exceeding 40/min in children older than 1 year. Pulse oximetry is also informative but less so than respiratory rate. Compared with an adult with pneumonia, a child is less likely to complain of dyspnea, produce sputum, or report pleuritic chest pain. Diagnostic evaluation of a child with CAP usually includes a chest x-ray; further evaluation for invasive disease (sepsis) should be dictated by clinical presentation.

Although numerous organisms are implicated in CAP in children, few are seen with significant frequency. Respiratory viruses are the causes in most; *S. pneumoniae* and the atypical pathogens including *M. pneumoniae* and *C. pneumoniae* are also implicated. As with adults with CAP, in children with CAP, sputum specimens are usually unobtainable, and the results are unreliable; the choice of an antimicrobial is largely empirically based.

Successful community-based care of a child with CAP requires many factors. The child must have intact gastrointestinal function and be able to take and tolerate oral medications and adequate amounts of fluids. A competent caregiver must be available. Also, the child should be able to return for follow-up examination and evaluation.

As previously mentioned and consistent with CAP treatment in adults, antimicrobial therapy in children with pneumonia is chosen empirically (Table 17–21). In adequate dosages, amoxicillin or a cephalosporin provides activity against *S. pneumoniae* but is ineffective against the atypical pathogens. A macrolide such as azithromycin or clarithromycin provides activity against nonresistant *S. pneumoniae* and the atypical pathogens. Treatment failure is possible when a macrolide is used and drug-resistant *S. pneumoniae* is the causative organism, in which case high-dose amoxicillin can be used. Tetracyclines, including doxycycline, are a treatment option in adult CAP and provide coverage for *S. pneumoniae* and atypical pathogens; their use in children younger than age 8 is not advised due to the risk of permanent tooth staining. Presumed influenza pneumonia can be treated with oseltamivir in children ≤5 and with oseltamivir or zanamivir for those <7 years. Because most childhood CAP is viral in origin, watchful waiting can also be used, whereby the child is not placed on an antimicrobial regimen, but rather is observed to see whether the illness improves over a few days.

Table 17-21

Empiric Therapy for Pediatric Community-Acquired Pneumonia (CAP) in the Outpatient Setting in Children Age 3 Months to 17 Years

	Presumed Bacterial Pneumonia	Presumed Atypical Pneumonia	Presumed Influenza Pneumonia
<5 years old (preschool)	Amoxicillin, oral (90 mg/kg/day in 2 doses) Alternative: Oral amoxicillin clavulanate (amoxicillin component, 90 mg/kg/day in 2 doses)	Azithromycin oral (10 mg/kg on day 1, followed by 5 mg/kg/day once daily on days 2–5) Alternatives: Oral clarithromycin (15 mg/kg/day in 2 doses for 7–14 days) or oral erythromycin (40 mg/kg/day in 4 doses)	Oseltamivir
≥5 years old	Oral amoxicillin (90 mg/kg/day in 2 doses to a maximum of 4 g/day); for children with presumed bacterial CAP who do not have clinical, laboratory, or radiographic evidence that distinguishes bacterial CAP from atypical CAP, a macrolide can be added to a beta-lactam antibiotic for empiric therapy Alternative: Oral amoxicillin clavulanate (amoxicillin component, 90 mg/kg/day in 2 doses to a maximum dose of 4000 mg/day, e.g., one 2000-mg tablet twice daily)	Oral azithromycin (10 mg/kg on day 1, followed by 5 mg/kg/day once daily on days 2–5 to a maximum of 500 mg on day 1, followed by 250 mg on days 2–5) Alternatives: Oral clarithromycin (15 mg/kg/day in 2 doses to a maximum of 1 g/day); erythromycin, doxycycline for children >7 years old	Oseltamivir or zanamivir (for children 7 years and older) Alternatives: Peramivir, oseltamivir, and zanamivir (all intravenous) are under clinical investigation in children Intravenous zanamivir available

For children with a history of possible, nonserious allergic reactions to amoxicillin, treatment is not well defined and should be individualized. Options include a trial of amoxicillin under clinical observation; a trial of an oral cephalosporin that has substantial activity against *S. pneumoniae*, such as cefpodoxime, cefprozil, or cefuroxime, can be provided under clinical supervision. Additional options for the child with a penicillin allergy include levofloxacin, linezolid, clindamycin, or a macrolide; close clinical follow-up and full knowledge of the use of all of these medications in children is needed.

Source: Bradley JS, Byington CL, Shah SS, et al. The management of community-acquired pneumonia in infants and children older than 3 months of age: Clinical practice guidelines by the Pediatric Infectious Diseases Society and the Infectious Diseases Society of America. *Clin Infect Dis* 53(7):e25–76, 2011.

NPs are ideally positioned to help minimize risk for pneumonia through immunization and hygienic measures. Nearly two-thirds of all fatal pneumonia is caused by *S. pneumoniae*, the pneumococcal organism. Pneumococcal conjugate vaccine is recommended for all children, starting in infancy, to minimize the risk of invasive pneumococcal disease. The use of influenza vaccine can help minimize the risk of postinfluenza pneumonia. Ensuring adequate ventilation, reinforcing cough hygiene, and proper hand washing can help minimize pneumonia risk.

DISCUSSION SOURCES

Gilbert D, Moerlling R, Eliopoulos G, Chambers H, Saag M. *The Sanford Guide to Antimicrobial Therapy*, ed. 42. Sperryville, VA: Antimicrobial Therapy, Inc., 2014.

Bradley JS, Byington CL, Shah SS, et al. The management of community-acquired pneumonia in infants and children older than 3 months of age: Clinical Practice Guidelines by the Pediatric Infectious Diseases Society and the Infectious Diseases Society of America. *Clin Infect Dis* 53(7):e25–76, 2011.

Kawasaki Disease

229. Sam is a 4-year-old boy who presents with a 1-week history of intermittent fever, rash, and "watery, red eyes." Clinical presentation is of an alert child who is cooperative with examination but irritable, with a temperature of 38°C (100.4°F), pulse rate of 132 bpm, and respiratory rate of 38/min. Physical examination findings include nasal crusting; dry, erythematous, cracked lips; red, enlarged tonsils without exudate; and elevated tongue papillae. The diagnosis of Kawasaki disease is being considered. Additional findings are likely to include:
    A. vesicular-form rash.
    B. purulent conjunctivitis.
    C. peeling hands.
    D. occipital lymphadenopathy.

230. Laboratory findings in Kawasaki disease include all of the following except:
    A. sterile pyuria.
    B. elevated liver enzyme levels.
    C. blood cultures positive for offending bacterial pathogen.
    D. elevated erythrocyte sedimentation rate.

231. Long-term consequences of Kawasaki disease include:
    A. renal insufficiency.
    B. coronary artery obstruction.
    C. hepatic failure.
    D. hypothyroidism.

232. The cause of Kawasaki disease is:
    A. fungal.
    B. viral.
    C. bacterial.
    D. unknown.

233. An important part of the treatment of Kawasaki disease includes the use of:
    A. antibiotics.
    B. antivirals.
    C. immune globulin.
    D. antifungals.

Answers

229. C.	231. B.	233. C.
230. C.	232. D.	

Kawasaki disease, also known as Kawasaki syndrome, is a typically self-limited vasculitis of unknown etiology, although an infectious or immunological basis is suggested. Clinical presentation includes fever lasting 5 or more days and presence of at least four of the following five symptoms: skin rash, bilateral conjuctival injection, cervical lymphadenopathy, swelling of the hands and feet, and mucocutaneous lesion. Disease implications include myocarditis (early disease stage) and development of coronary artery aneurysms (later disease stage; Table 17–22).

Occurring primarily in the late winter and spring at 3-year intervals, Kawasaki disease is more frequent among children of Asian ancestry, twice as common in boys than in girls, and now surpasses rheumatic fever as the leading cause of acquired heart disease in the United States among children younger than 5 years. The development of coronary artery aneurysms can lead to coronary artery obstruction, myocarditis, heart failure, pericarditis, mitral or aortic insufficiency, and dysrhythmias. Risk of aneurysm is increased in patients who have fever for

---

TABLE 17-22

Diagnostic Criteria for Kawasaki Disease

- Fever ≥5 days in duration, usually abrupt in onset, symptoms with no response to antibiotic therapy; if given, usually with irritability out of proportion to degree of fever or other signs
- In addition to fever lasting at least 5 days, ≥4 of the following should be present:
    - Changes in extremities (erythema, edema, desquamation), usually with discomfort so that child may refuse to bear weight
    - Bilateral, nonexudative conjunctivitis
    - Polymorphous rash
    - Cervical lymphadenopathy
    - Changes in lips and oral cavity (pharyngeal edema, dry/fissured or swollen lips, strawberry tongue)

Note: If fever is present with fewer than four of the above symptoms, the diagnosis is established with echocardiogram to evaluate the coronary arteries to support or exclude the disease.

Source: Centers for Disease Control and Prevention. Kawasaki Syndrome, http://www.cdc.gov/kawasaki, accessed 4/25/14.

more than 16 days, have recurrence of fever after an afebrile period of at least 48 hours, are male, are younger than 1 year, and have cardiomegaly at the time of diagnosis. Some patients who do not fulfill the criteria for Kawasaki disease have been diagnosed as having "incomplete" or "atypical" Kawasaki disease, a diagnosis that often is based on echocardiographic findings of coronary artery abnormalities.

Although no specific laboratory test for Kawasaki disease exists, the presence of certain laboratory findings can support the diagnosis when coupled with clinical presentation. Blood test often detects mild anemia, elevated white blood cell count, elevated sedimentation rate, and sharp increase in the number of platelets. Urine test often reveals the presence of albumin and white blood cells. In the acute stage (days 1 to 11), leukocytosis with a left shift and elevated erythrocyte sedimentation rate are found; both are neither sensitive nor specific for the condition. In the subacute stage (days 11 to 21), the platelet count is often markedly elevated, with a measurement of more than 1 million/mm³ being common. These values begin to normalize during the convalescent stage (days 21 to 60) but may not reach baseline values for 8 weeks.

During the acute stage of Kawasaki disease, or if the diagnosis is in question, an echocardiogram should be obtained. If tests reveal an aneurysm or other heart or blood vessel abnormality, repeated echocardiograms or other tests are usually necessary for several years. In children who return to completely normal activity after the acute phase of the illness, the study should be repeated in the second or third week of disease and repeated 1 month after laboratory tests have resolved.

Treatment of Kawasaki disease includes consultation with experts in managing this condition and the use of intravenous immune globulin and aspirin. Confirmation of the diagnosis and treatment are likely to involve consultation with a specialist in this disease. Long-term prognosis is generally related to the degree of permanent cardiac involvement.

DISCUSSION SOURCES

Centers for Disease Control and Prevention. Kawasaki Syndrome, http://www.cdc.gov/kawasaki.
Baker AN, Newburger JW. Kawasaki disease. *Circulation* 118:e110–e112, 2008.

Car Seat Guidelines

234. A young child should use a rear-facing car seat until at least age ____.
A. 12 months
B. 18 months
C. 24 months
D. 30 months

235. You anticipate that adult car seat belts fit correctly when a child is approximately _____ tall and is ____ old.
A. 51 inches (129.5 cm), 6 to 8 years
B. 53 inches (134.6 cm), 5 to 7 years
C. 57 inches (144.8 cm), 8 to 12 years
D. 59 inches (150 cm), 12 to 14 years

236. In general, children should ride in the back seat of the car until age:
A. 10 years.
B. 11 years.
C. 12 years.
D. 13 years.

Answers

234. C.   **235.** C.   **236.** D.

Knowledge of appropriate child car seat restraint is an important part of providing pediatric primary care (Table 17–23).

DISCUSSION SOURCE

American Academy of Pediatrics: Updates Recommendations on Car Seats, www.aap.org/advocacy/releases/carseat2011.htm.

Pertussis

237. At which age is a child at greatest risk of death from pertussis?
A. <1 year
B. 2-4 years
C. 5-10 years
D. >10 years

238. Common signs and symptoms of pertussis in a 3-year-old child include all of the following except:
A. uncontrollable cough.
B. vomiting.
C. fatigue.
D. diffuse rash.

239. The most helpful tests to support the diagnosis of pertussis include which of the following? More than one can apply.
A. chest x-ray.
B. nasopharyngeal culture.
C. blood culture
D. polymerase chain reaction (PCR) testing

240. Which of the following can be used to differentiate pertussis from acute bronchitis or asthma exacerbation?
A. presence of fever
B. PCR assay
C. presence of productive cough
D. evidence of consolidation on chest x-ray

241. The preferred treatment option for a 6-year-old boy with pertussis is:
A. amoxicillin.
B. ceftriaxone.
C. azithromycin.
D. levofloxacin.

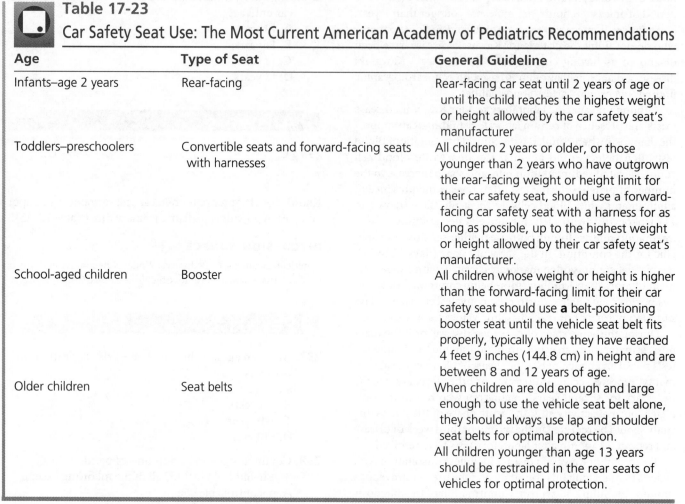

Table 17-23

Car Safety Seat Use: The Most Current American Academy of Pediatrics Recommendations

Age	Type of Seat	General Guideline
Infants–age 2 years	Rear-facing	Rear-facing car seat until 2 years of age or until the child reaches the highest weight or height allowed by the car safety seat's manufacturer
Toddlers–preschoolers	Convertible seats and forward-facing seats with harnesses	All children 2 years or older, or those younger than 2 years who have outgrown the rear-facing weight or height limit for their car safety seat, should use a forward-facing car safety seat with a harness for as long as possible, up to the highest weight or height allowed by their car safety seat's manufacturer.
School-aged children	Booster	All children whose weight or height is higher than the forward-facing limit for their car safety seat should use **a** belt-positioning booster seat until the vehicle seat belt fits properly, typically when they have reached 4 feet 9 inches (144.8 cm) in height and are between 8 and 12 years of age.
Older children	Seat belts	When children are old enough and large enough to use the vehicle seat belt alone, they should always use lap and shoulder seat belts for optimal protection. All children younger than age 13 years should be restrained in the rear seats of vehicles for optimal protection.

Source: American Academy of Pediatrics: Updates Recommendations on Car Seats, www.aap.org/advocacy/releases/carseat2011.htm, accessed 4/25/14.

Answers

237. A.   **239.** B and D.   **241.** C.
238. D.   **240.** B.

Pertussis, also known as whooping cough, is a highly contagious respiratory disease caused by the bacterium *Bordetella pertussis*. The infection is characterized by a paroxysmal cough (a series of severe, vigorous coughs during a single expiration) that often makes it difficult to breathe. Following a coughing fit, the child often needs to take deep breaths resulting in the high-pitched "whooping" sound. Pertussis most often affects infants and young children and can be fatal, particularly in infants less than 1 year old. Following infection, it can take 1 to 3 weeks for signs and symptoms to appear. Early signs resemble the common cold and include runny nose, nasal congestion, sneezing, a mild fever, and mild cough. Symptoms worsen over the next week or two to include thick mucus accumulating in the airways causing uncontrollable coughing. Prolonged coughing episodes can provoke vomiting and result in a red or blue face and cause

extreme fatigue. Many do not develop the characteristic whoop. A persistent hacking cough may be the only sign for the presence of pertussis. Positive culture results from a nose or throat specimens is considered the gold standard when diagnosing pertussis. However, the bacteria can be difficult to grow and can take as long as 2 weeks for a positive result. PCR testing of nasopharyngeal secretions offers a faster and more sensitive assay to detect the bacteria, though there is no standardized PCR protocol available. Direct fluorescent antibody (DFA) testing of nasopharyngeal specimens can also offer a rapid screening test for pertussis, though sensitivity is low. The CDC recommends a combination of culture and PCR assay if a patient has a cough lasting more than 3 weeks to confirm a diagnosis. A blood sample can be used to check for infection by the presence of elevated WBC. In infants, the absolute lymphocyte count often exceeds 20,000 cells/mm^3. A chest x-ray can be used to detect abnormalities in the lungs including the chest-x-ray in perihilar infiltrates or edema; additional findings can usually noted when pneumonia complicates pertussis. These diagnostic techniques, along with the characteristic paroxysmal cough and whoop, can help to differentiate pertussis from other similar respiratory conditions, such as acute bronchitis or asthma. Additionally, viral acute bronchitis typically has an incubation period of 1–3 days compared to up to 3 weeks for pertussis. Asthma is characterized by variable and recurring symptoms, wheezing, airflow obstruction, and underlying inflammation and will generally lack signs of many other types of infection (e.g., elevated WBC with neutrophilia, fever). Pertussis should also be suspected if there is an outbreak in the area and/or the patient had close contact with another person diagnosed with pertussis.

Infants with pertussis are often hospitalized for treatment due to an increased risk of death. Older children can usually be treated at home. Antimicrobial treatment can include a macrolide with azithromycin being the preferred agent. Clarithromycin and erythromycin are not recommended in infants younger than 1 month due to a risk of infantile hypertrophic pyloric stenosis (IHPS). Children older than 2 months who exhibit hypersensitivity to macrolides can be treated with TMP-SMX. Antimicrobial prophylaxis should be considered for household or close contacts of children diagnosed with pertussis.

Immunization against pertussis remains the most effective method to prevent these infections. A 5-dose series of the DTaP (diphtheria and tetanus toxoids and acellular pertussis) is given at ages 2, 4, 6, 15–18 months, and 4–6 years of age. One dose of the Tdap vaccine is given to all adolescents aged 11 through 12 years. In addition, women during pregnancy are recommended to have a Tdap dose with each pregnancy, regardless of previous Td or Tdap history, in order to provide protection to her unborn child. Prior to the baby's birth, all household members and anyone who will be in regular close contact with the newborn should have updated pertussis immunization.

DISCUSSION SOURCES

Centers for Disease Control and Prevention: Pertussis, http://www.cdc.gov/vaccines/pubs/pinkbook/pert.html#diagnosis.
Bocka JJ. Pertussis. http://emedicine.medscape.com/article/967268-overview.

Childbearing

18

Stages of Pregnancy

1–4. Match the stage of pregnancy with the appropriate term.

_____ **1.** Fertilized ovum

_____ **2.** Up to 2 weeks postconception

_____ **3.** Up to 8 to 10 weeks

_____ **4.** 10 weeks to term

A. Embryo
B. Fetus
C. Blastocyst
D. Zygote

Answers

1. D.   **2.** C.   **3.** A.   **4.** B.

Knowledge of appropriate terminology is a critical component to providing prenatal care (Table 18–1).

Uterine Size During Pregnancy

5–10. Match uterine size with stage of pregnancy.

_____ **5.** Nongravid

_____ **6.** 8 weeks

_____ **7.** 10 weeks

_____ **8.** 12 weeks

_____ **9.** 16 weeks

_____ **10.** 20 weeks

A. Size of a baseball

B. Size of a softball or grapefruit

C. Size of a large lemon

D. Size of a tennis ball or orange

E. Uterine fundus at umbilicus

F. Uterine fundus halfway between symphysis pubis and umbilicus

11–13. Match each sign with its correct characteristic.

_____ **11.** Hegar sign

_____ **12.** Goodell sign

_____ **13.** Chadwick sign

A. blue–violet vaginal color

B. softening of uterus isthmus

C. softening of vaginal portion of the cervix

Answers

5. C.   **8.** B.   **11.** B .
6. D.   **9.** F.   **12.** C.
7. A.   **10.** E.   **13.** A.

Knowledge of normal pregnancy development is a critical component to providing prenatal care (Table 18–2).

Nutritional Requirements, Prenatal Counseling and Monitoring

14. Approximately ___% of fetuses are in vertex position by the 36th week of pregnancy.
A. 30
B. 50
C. 75
D. 95

TABLE 18-1
Stages of Human Pregnancy

Period	Stage
At fertilization	Zygote
Up to 2 weeks	Blastocyst
2–8 weeks	Embryo
8–12 weeks to term	Fetus
Born between 37 weeks 0 days and 38 weeks 6 days	Early term
Born between 39 weeks 0 days and 40 weeks 6 days	Full term
Born between 41 weeks 0 days and 41 weeks 6 days	Late term
Born after 42 weeks 0 days	Post-term

Source: American College of Obstetricians and Gynecologists. Committee Opinion No. 579. November 2013, http://www.acog.org/Resources_And_Publications/Committee_Opinions/Committee_on_Obstetric_Practice/Definition_of_Term_Pregnancy.

TABLE 18-2
Uterine Size During Pregnancy

Stage of Pregnancy	Uterine Size	Comment
Nongravid	Lemon	Mobile, firm, nontender
8 weeks	Tennis ball or orange	Hegar sign (softening of uterine isthmus), Goodell sign (softening of vaginal portion of the cervix), and Chadwick sign (blue–violet vaginal color) often present by this time
10 weeks	Baseball	First fetal heart tone via abdominal Doppler at 10–12 weeks
12 weeks	Softball or grapefruit	Rising above symphysis pubis, uterine fundus palpable through abdominal wall
16 weeks	Halfway between symphysis pubis and umbilicus	Quickening first noted in woman who has been pregnant before (second trimester or beyond) during 16–17 weeks, at ~18 weeks with first pregnancy
20–36 weeks	~1-cm gain in fundal height per week	Uterine fundus at the umbilicus at 20 weeks. Usually concordant with gestational age, plus or minus 1 cm
At term	Uterus dips into pelvis with fetal head engagement, fundal height decreases	Vertex position (cephalic) in 95% by 36 weeks

15. The recommended weight gain during pregnancy for a woman with a desirable or healthy pre-pregnancy body mass index (BMI) is:
   A. 15 to 20 lb (6.8 to 9.1 kg)
   B. 20 to 30 lb (9.1 to 13.6 kg)
   C. 25 to 35 lb (11.3 to 15.9 kg)
   D. 35 to 45 lb (15.9 to 20.4 kg)

16. For a healthy woman with a desirable or healthy pre-pregnancy BMI, daily caloric requirements during pregnancy are typical baseline caloric needs plus ___ kcal.
   A. 100
   B. 300
   C. 600
   D. 1000

17. For a healthy woman with a healthy or desirable pre-pregnancy BMI, daily caloric requirements during lactation are typical baseline caloric needs plus ___ kcal.
   A. 250
   B. 500
   C. 750
   D. 1000

18. Recommended calcium intake for a woman during pregnancy is _____ mg of elemental calcium per day.
   A. 400 to 600
   B. 600 to 800
   C. 800 to 1000
   D. 1000 to 1300

19. Increased folic acid intake before conception is likely to reduce the risk of which of the following birth defects?
    A. congenital cataract
    B. pyloric stenosis
    C. clubfoot
    D. open neural tube defects

20. Maternal iron requirements are greatest during what part of pregnancy?
    A. first trimester
    B. second and third trimesters
    C. equal throughout pregnancy
    D. preconception

21. The most common form of acquired anemia during pregnancy is:
    A. iron deficiency.
    B. folate deficiency.
    C. vitamin B12 deficiency.
    D. primary hypoproliferative.

22. Concerning the use of alcohol during pregnancy, which of the following statements is most accurate?
    A. Although potentially problematic, maternal alcohol intake does not increase the risk of miscarriage.
    B. Risk to the fetus from alcohol exposure is greatest in the third trimester.
    C. No level or time of exposure is considered to be safe.
    D. Risk of fetal alcohol syndrome is present only if alcohol exposure has occurred throughout the pregnancy.

23. Pica (ingestion of nonfood substances) during pregnancy should be considered:
    A. a harmless practice common in certain ethnic groups.
    B. problematic only if more nutritious food sources are left out of the diet and are replaced by the nonfood substance.
    C. a way of providing select micronutrients not usually found in food products.
    D. potentially dangerous because of contaminants in the nonfood substance.

24. Examples of neural tube defects include all of the following except:
    A. anencephaly.
    B. spina bifida.
    C. encephalocele.
    D. omphalocele.

Answers

14. D.	18. D.	22. C.
15. C.	19. D.	23. D.
16. B.	20. B.	24. D.
17. B.	21. A.	

The clinician should have knowledge of nutritional requirements during pregnancy to provide appropriate counseling. Folic acid deficiency is a teratogenic state, leading to an increased risk of neural tube defects (NTDs) and other defects in the developing pregnancy. NTDs are common serious fetal malformations, affecting approximately 3000 pregnancies each year in the United States. Examples of NTDs include anencephaly, spina bifida, and encephalocele. Correcting folic acid deficiency before pregnancy by increased dietary and supplement intake dramatically reduces this risk, and continuing this increased intake throughout pregnancy minimizes the mother's risk of developing folate-deficiency anemia. Dietary-associated folic acid deficiency is rare unless severe malnutrition is present. A genetic contribution to NTDs is likely and is thought to be the result of a complex interaction of environment and heredity. As a result, if a woman has carried a pregnancy with an NTD, or there is a family history of NTD, recommended folic acid intake increases to 4 mg/d 1 month before pregnancy and during the first 3 months of gestation. Most prescription prenatal multivitamins contain 1 mg of folic acid.

Increased calcium intake is important to the development of bones and teeth; the required amount can usually be met by ensuring three to four servings of high-quality dairy products per day. Examples of a single dairy serving include 8 oz (240 mL) of milk, 1–1.5 oz (28–43 g) of cheese, 1 cup (240 mL) of yogurt, or 1 cup (240 mL) of calcium-fortified juice. Although dietary sources of calcium are best, supplementation is sometimes required if a woman is lactose intolerant or is otherwise unable to meet these goals. The recommended daily intake of calcium for women 19–50 years of age is 1000 mg. Women 14–18 years of age have an increased calcium requirement of 1300 mg daily.

Maternal iron requirements increase in the second and third trimesters of pregnancy, in part because of the fetus's need to build iron stores. Iron deficiency is the most common form of anemia during pregnancy, with most cases occurring because the woman enters pregnancy with iron deficiency, rather than develops this problem because of increased iron requirements. Pregnancy-related iron requirements, given in terms of elemental iron, are as follows: in the absence of iron deficiency, 30 mg/d; with iron deficiency or in a multiple-gestation pregnancy, 60 to 100 mg/d. A 325-mg ferrous sulfate tablet contains 65 mg of elemental iron, whereas most prescription prenatal vitamins contain 30 to 65 mg.

Fetal alcohol syndrome (FAS) has most often been noted in the offspring of women who drank heavily throughout pregnancy. More commonly, infants whose mothers drink lightly or moderately are born with lesser degrees of alcohol-related problems. Given that FAS is the leading preventable cause of developmental disability and can be eliminated by avoiding alcohol consumption throughout pregnancy, no level of maternal alcohol intake during pregnancy is deemed safe. Maternal alcohol intake also increases the risk of miscarriage. Less is known about fetal risks when exposed to other recreational drugs, such as marijuana, a substance often considered more benign and "natural" compared with alcohol. A safe level of maternal ingestion during pregnancy for marijuana and other intoxicating substances has not been established, and abstinence should be encouraged.

Pica is the ingestion of nonfood substances, such as clay, cornstarch, laundry starch, dry milk of magnesia, paraffin, coffee grounds, or ice. Although usually noted to be more common in select ethnic groups, pica is found in all socioeconomic groups. Certain pica habits are likely harmless, such as sucking on ice chips, but do little to replace intake of more nutritious substances. Most other pica forms contain potential risk, however, because nonfood substances are taken in preferably over more nutritious food sources. With the ingestion of clay, starches, and paraffin, there is risk of constipation, bowel obstruction, and nutritional deficiency. In particular, many common pica substances can be contaminated with heavy metals such as lead or mercury and other industrial pollutants that are particularly toxic to the mother and the developing fetus. The issue of pica should be raised with all pregnant women. Some women believe that pica is normal, or are encouraged to eat substances such as clay by well-meaning friends and family members as a way of relieving tension. Recognize this, but inform the woman about the potential risks of pica.

DISCUSSION SOURCES

Nutritional Facts During Pregnancy, http://www.womenshealth.gov/pregnancy/you-are-pregnant/staying-healthy-safe.cfm

March of Dimes, http://www.marchofdimes.com/pregnancy/eating-and-nutrition.aspx

National Clinical Clearinghouse, http://www.guideline.gov/content.aspx?id=14306&search=prenatal+care, Routine prenatal and postnatal care, 2011

Physiological Changes

25 to 37. Identify the following changes in a normal pregnancy as true (normal, anticipated finding) or false (not associated with normal pregnancy)

_____ **25.** Blood volume increases by 40% to 50%, peaking at week 32.

_____ **26.** Decrease in diastolic blood pressure most notable during second trimester.

_____ **27.** S_1 heart sound becomes louder.

_____ **28.** Physiologic systolic ejection murmur usually evident.

_____ **29.** Dilation of renal collecting system.

_____ **30.** Physiologic glucosuria and proteinuria common.

_____ **31.** Decrease in transverse thoracic diameter and diaphragmatic contraction.

_____ **32.** Lower esophageal sphincter more relaxed.

_____ **33.** Increased intestinal motility.

_____ **34.** Gallbladder doubles in size.

_____ **35.** Insulin levels increase by 2-fold to 10-fold over pre-pregnancy levels.

_____ **36.** Fasting plasma glucose increases slightly.

_____ **37.** Thyroid decreases in size.

Answers

25. True	**30.** True	**35.** True
26. True	**31.** False	**36.** False
27. True	**32.** True	**37.** False
28. True	**33.** False	
29. True	**34.** True	

A woman's body changes dramatically throughout pregnancy. Knowledge of these normal physiological changes in pregnancy is crucial to providing safe and competent prenatal care (Table 18–3).

DISCUSSION SOURCE

Datta S, Kodali BS, Segal S. Maternal physiologic changes during pregnancy, labor, and the postpartum period. In: Datta S, Kodali BS, Segal S. (eds.). *Obstetric Anesthesia Handbook*, ed. 5. New York: Springer, 2010, pp. 1–14.

Prenatal Care and Screening

38. The recommended frequency of prenatal visits in weeks 28 to 32 of pregnancy is every:
A. 1 week.
B. 2 weeks.
C. 3 weeks.
D. 4 weeks.

39. Testing for sexually transmitted infection should be initially obtained:
A. as early as possible in pregnancy.
B. during the second trimester.
C. during the third trimester.
D. as close to the anticipated date of birth as possible.

40. Which of the following is a diagnostic test?
A. cell free fetal DNA test
B. serum alpha-fetoprotein
C. serum inhibin-A
D. amniocentesis

41. The "quad screen" should be obtained at about _____ weeks of pregnancy.
A. 6 to 10
B. 11 to 15
C. 16 to 20
D. 21 to 25

42. Aneuploidy is defined as:
A. a physical malformation of the fetus of unknown origin.
B. a birth defect originating from the use of a teratogenic drug.
C. the presence of an abnormal number of chromosomes.
D. a birth defect originating from a nutritional deficiency.

TABLE 18-3
Physiological Adaptations During Pregnancy

Body Area	Physiological Adaptation
Uterus	Size increases from ~10-mL capacity and 70-g weight pre-pregnancy to 5000-mL capacity and 1100-g weight at term. The uterine isthmus becomes soft and compressible (Hegar sign).
Cervix	Its color and texture change, becoming cyanotic (Chadwick sign) and less firm (Goodell sign).
Skin	Striae (stretch marks) in ~50%, melasma (pregnancy mask). Linea nigra (hyperpigmented line on abdomen) appears or darkens as melanocytes are stimulated.
Breast	Nipples and areolae darken and increase in size. Venous congestion noted. Breast tissue becomes more nodular because of proliferation of lactiferous glands
Blood	Blood volume increases by 40%–50%, peaking at week 32. Red blood cell production increases by 33% but still results in dilutional physiological anemia of pregnancy.
Cardiovascular	Decrease in systolic blood pressure throughout pregnancy, with decrease in diastolic blood pressure most notable during second trimester. Cardiac output dependent on maternal position, with a noted decrease if in supine position because of reduced venous return caused by vena cava compression to an increase of 30%–50% with lateral recumbent position. S_1 heart sound becomes louder, and physiological systolic ejection murmur is usually evident. Heart is displaced, resulting in a left axis deviation that resolves post birth.
Renal	Increased renal blood flow, glomerular filtration rate, and dilation of renal collecting system occur. Physiologic glucosuria and proteinuria occur partly because of increase in glomerular filtration rate and resulting inability of renal tubules to reabsorb glucose and protein.
Respiratory	Partly because of increased abdominal content, there is an increase in transverse thoracic diameter and diaphragmatic contraction, and costal angle widens. Tidal volume increases with reduced residual volume in later pregnancy.
Digestive	Lower esophageal sphincter are more relaxed while corresponding pressures increase, resulting in increased esophageal reflux. Decreased stomach and intestinal motility is seen, allowing for greater nutrient absorption but increased risk for constipation. (Increased progesterone levels influence aforementioned changes.) Gallbladder doubles in size with more dilute bile and less soluble cholesterol, increasing risk of stones.
Metabolic/endocrine	Insulin levels increase by 2-fold to 10-fold over pre-pregnancy levels. Fasting plasma glucose decreases slightly. Thyroid and pituitary increase in size. Maternal weight changes account for weight gain in the first half of pregnancy, whereas uterine contents account for most weight gain in second half.

43. The "quad screen" is used to help detect increased risk for which of the following conditions in the fetus?
    A. trisomy 21 and open neural tube defects
    B. cystic fibrosis and Angelman syndrome
    C. Tay-Sachs disease and trisomy 18
    D. sickle cell anemia and beta-thalassemia major

44. Prenatal assessment for aneuploidy should be offered to:
    A. only women older than 35 years of age.
    B. only women younger than 21 years of age.
    C. only women either younger than 21 years or older than 35 years of age.
    D. all women regardless of age.

45. Tina is a 26-year-old woman who is pregnant and has an abnormal "quad screen." When sharing this information with Tina, you consider that:
    A. this testing is diagnostic of specific conditions.
    B. further testing is recommended.
    C. the testing should be repeated.
    D. no further testing is required.

46. The rate of spontaneous fetal loss related to amniocentesis that is done at a facility that performs these procedures on a regular basis is approximately 1 in _____ procedures
    A. 75
    B. 200
    C. 400
    D. 800

47. Women at high risk for aneuploidy include all of the following except:
A. maternal age 35 years and older at delivery.
B. history of prior pregnancy with trisomy.
C. fetal ultrasonographic findings indicating an increased risk of aneuploidy.
D. history of multiparity.

48. All of the following can cause an elevated maternal alpha-fetoprotein (AFP) except:
A. underestimated gestational age.
B. open neural tube defect.
C. meningomyelocele.
D. Down syndrome.

49. Edwards syndrome is the clinical manifestation of trisomy ____.
A. 13
B. 15
C. 18
D. 21

50. In Edwards syndrome, which of the following statements is true?
A. Edwards syndrome is more common than Down syndrome.
B. Most affected infants with Edwards syndrome die during the first year of life.
C. Edwards syndrome is unlikely to cause developmental disability.
D. Edwards syndrome is associated with elevated AFP.

51. In Down syndrome, which of the following is true?
A. Most infants affected with Down syndrome are born to women older than age 35 years.
B. Down syndrome is noted in about 1 in 10,000 live births.
C. Down syndrome is associated with decreased maternal serum AFP level.
D. Antenatal serum analysis is sufficient to make the diagnosis.

52. Down syndrome is the clinical manifestation of trisomy ____.
A. 13
B. 15
C. 18
D. 21

53. Components of the antenatal screening test known as the "quad screen" include all of the following except:
A. AFP.
B. hCG.
C. unconjugated estriol.
D. progesterone.

54. Elevated inhibin-A is noted when a pregnant woman is at increased risk of having an infant with:
A. Down syndrome.
B. Edwards syndrome.
C. open neural tube defect.
D. hemolytic anemia.

55. A 25-year-old woman presents in the 10th week of gestation requesting antenatal screening for Down syndrome. What advice should the NP give?
A. Because of her age, no specific testing is recommended.
B. She should be referred for second-trimester ultrasound.
C. Screening that combines nuchal translucency measurement and biochemical testing is available.
D. She should be referred to a genetic counselor.

56 to 58. Match the following at-risk ethnic groups for the following genetically based conditions.

____ **56.** Tay-Sachs disease A. Ashkenazi Jewish ancestry
____ **57.** Cystic fibrosis B. Northern European ancestry
____ **58.** Sickle cell trait C. African ancestry

Answers

38. B.	45. B.	52. D.
39. A.	46. C.	53. D.
40. D.	47. D.	54. A.
41. C.	48. D.	55. C.
42. C.	49. C.	56. A.
43. A.	50. B.	57. B.
44. D.	51. C.	58. C.

Numerous recommendations exist regarding frequency of prenatal care and associated laboratory and other testing (Table 18–4). These are simply guidelines for the care that is needed for a well woman with a pregnancy with low physiological and psychosocial risk. More frequent visits and testing are often indicated, but a minimum of 8 to 10 visits should be scheduled.

According to the Centers for Disease Control and Prevention (CDC), 1 out of 33 infants in the United States are born with a birth defect. Prenatal screening and diagnostic procedures constitute an important clinical issue, although one that is often confusing, emotionally charged, and marked by disagreement among healthcare providers and patients. One point of confusion is the difference between

TABLE 18-4
Frequency of Prenatal Visits

Time in Pregnancy	Frequency of Visits
Up to 28 weeks	Every 4 weeks
28–36 weeks	Every 2 weeks
≥36 weeks	Every week

Source: Institute for Clinical Systems Improvement (ICSI). Healthcare Guideline: Routine prenatal care, https://www.icsi.org/_asset/13n9y4/Prenatal.pdf.

screening and diagnostic tests. Commonly offered prenatal tests include maternal serum analysis for alpha-fetoprotein (AFP), human chorionic gonadotropin (hCG), inhibin-A, and unconjugated estriol levels, also known as the "quad (quadruple) screen." When the amounts of these substances are analyzed, increased risk of open neural tube defects (NTDs), trisomy 21 (Down syndrome), and trisomy 18 (Edwards syndrome) can be detected. An abnormal "quad screen" result is not diagnostic of any condition, however, and further testing is recommended, including amniocentesis and level II ultrasound. Consultation with a perinatology specialist is also indicated.

Fetal aneuploidy is defined as an abnormal number of chromosomes present in the fetus. A single additional chromosome is called trisomy and is an important cause of congenital malformations and mental impairments. Down syndrome (trisomy 21), Edwards syndrome (trisomy 18), and Patau syndrome (trisomy 13) are the most common types. Initially, screening for fetal aneuploidy involved offering amniocentesis to higher risk mothers. However, noninvasive methods are now available for initial screening. All women regardless of age should be offered prenatal assessment for aneuploidy either by screening or invasive prenatal diagnosis techniques. In addition to the quad screen, the cell free fetal DNA test that assesses fetal DNA derived from the plasma of pregnant women offers a convenient method to screen for fetal aneuploidy. The cell free fetal DNA test can be used as a primary screening test in women at increased risk of aneuploidy. These risks include: (1) maternal age 35 years and older at delivery; (2) fetal ultrasonographic findings indicating an increased risk of aneuploidy; (3) history of a prior pregnancy with a trisomy; (4) positive test result for aneuploidy, including first trimester, sequential, or integrated screen, or a quad screen; or (5) parental balanced robertsonian translocation with increased risk of fetal trisomy 13 or trisomy 21. Women should be counseled on the limitations of the cell free fetal DNA test, which should include a discussion that this test may not be as accurate as diagnostic tests, such as amniocentesis or chorionic villi sampling.

Down syndrome is associated with developmental disability and an increased risk for cardiac and gastrointestinal malformation and early-onset Alzheimer disease. The risk of Down syndrome is approximately 1 in 1000 live births, with this number increasing to 1 in 270 in women 35 to 40 years old and 1 in 100 in women older than 40 years; increased maternal age is a well-known risk factor for Down syndrome and other genetically-based congenital anomalies. Although historically only pregnant women who would be 35 or older at the time of childbirth were offered the opportunity for prenatal diagnosis with amniocentesis or chorionic villus sampling, newer recommendations advise that all pregnant women, regardless of age, be offered the option of antenatal diagnostic testing, including evaluation for Down syndrome. One of the factors leading to this recommendation is the finding that approximately 75% of all infants with Down syndrome are born to mothers younger than age 35. This finding results in part from

the fact that women in this age group are more likely to give birth compared with older women and because of the lower rate of antenatal diagnostic testing such as amniocentesis being performed in younger women giving birth.

Edwards syndrome is much less common than Down syndrome, occurring in 1 in every 6000 births. Edwards syndrome is associated with low birth weight; developmental disability; and cranial, cardiac, and renal malformations. The complexity and severity of these problems are such that most affected infants die within the first year of life; stillbirth or death in the first week of life is sadly quite common.

NTDs are second only to cardiac defects in frequency, with an incidence of NTDs of 1.2 for every 1000 births. Open NTDs such as meningomyelocele, anencephaly, and spina bifida carry risk of significant disability and the potential for a shortened life span.

Alpha-fetoprotein is synthesized in the fetal yolk sac, gastrointestinal tract, and liver. Maternal levels can be elevated for many reasons, including an open NTD such as meningomyelocele, anencephaly, or spina bifida; fetal nephrosis; cystic hygroma; fetal gastrointestinal obstruction; omphalocele; intrauterine growth restriction; multiple fetuses; or fetal demise. Underestimated gestational age can also lead to a misinterpreted test because maternal AFP is higher in earlier pregnancy. The placenta, from precursors provided by the fetal adrenal glands, and the liver produce unconjugated estriol; maternal levels are decreased in trisomy 21 and trisomy 18. hCG is produced by trophoblast shortly after implantation into the uterine wall, with levels increasing rapidly in the first 8 weeks of pregnancy, then steadily decreasing until week 20, when levels plateau. An increased hCG level appears to be a relatively sensitive marker for detecting trisomy 21, whereas a low hCG level is associated with trisomy 18. The hCG levels are typically normal in the presence of NTDs. Inhibin-A is a hormone produced by the placenta; levels of hCG and inhibin-A are higher than normal when a woman has an increased risk of carrying a fetus with Down syndrome. Lower than normal levels of estriol can also indicate that a woman is at high risk for carrying a fetus with Down syndrome

Interpreting the results of a "quad screen" requires knowledge of numerous factors, including the risk of false-positive and false-negative results, the significance of the results, and the woman's individual risk of having an affected pregnancy. In addition, all antenatal testing must be offered to a woman in a manner that allows her to make an informed decision to have or decline the test. Part of informed consent includes the information that the "quad screen" is simply that, a screening test that identifies higher risk situations but is not diagnostic for the condition. With abnormal results, further testing is indicated; results that are normal do not ensure that no problem will occur with the pregnancy, but the risk is minimized.

As previously mentioned, if a "quad screen" yields abnormal results, further testing is indicated. For the detection of a genetic abnormality such as trisomy 18 or 21, the most commonly used test is amniocentesis, a procedure that carries a rate of spontaneous fetal loss of about 1 in every 200 to 400 procedures; the rate is closer to 1 in every 400 procedures when done in facilities where it is performed on a regular basis. The overall pregnancy loss after chorionic villi sampling is higher at approximately 1%, or 1 out of every 100 procedures. If a woman chooses not to have invasive testing, noninvasive follow-up evaluation after an abnormal "quad screen" often includes a level II ultrasound, a high-resolution study that can reveal fetal abnormalities such as an open NTD or increased nuchal folds and other anomalies often found in Down syndrome. Ultrasound can assist with diagnosis but does not take the place of genetically based studies. When first-trimester testing is desired, screening using nuchal translucency as detected by ultrasound and serological testing for decreased pregnancy-associated plasma protein-A and increased free beta-hCG is effective in the general population and is more effective than nuchal translucency alone. Women found to be at increased risk of having an infant with Down syndrome with first-trimester screening should be offered genetic counseling and the option of chorionic villi sampling or mid-trimester amniocentesis.

DISCUSSION SOURCES

American College of Obstetrics and Gynecology. Practice Bulletin #77: Screening for fetal chromosomal abnormalities. *Obstet Gynecol* 109:217–228, 2007.

American Pregnancy Association, http://americanpregnancy.org/?s=cvs.

American Pregnancy Association, http://americanpregnancy.org/?s=quad+screen.

March of Dimes. Quick fact sheet: Amniocentesis, http://www.marchofdimes.com/professionals/14332_1164.asp.

Centers for Disease Control and Prevention. Treating for two: Safer medication use in pregnancy, http://www.cdc.gov/ncbddd/birthdefects/documents/ncbddd_birth-defects_medicationuseonepager_cdcrole.pdf.

Akkerman D, Cleland L, Croft G, et al. *Routine Prenatal Care.* Bloomington, MN: Institute for Clinical Systems Improvement (ICSI), 2012, http://www.guideline.gov/content.aspx?id=38256&search=antenatal+care+and+prenatal.

■) Medication Use During Pregnancy

59. Medications most commonly pass through the placenta via:
A. facilitated transport.
B. passive diffusion.
C. capillary pump action.
D. mechanical carrier state.

60. During pregnancy, the most intense organogenesis occurs how many days following the last menstrual period (LMP)?
A. 12–30 days
B. 31–81 days
C. 92–120 days
D. 121–150 days

61. A drug with demonstrated safety for use in all trimesters of pregnancy is categorized as U.S. Food and Drug Administration (FDA) risk category:
A. A.
B. B.
C. C.
D. D.

62. A drug shown to cause teratogenic effects in human study, but the benefit of which could outweigh the risk of use in a life-threatening situation, is assigned FDA risk category:
A. A.
B. B.
C. C.
D. D.

63. A drug that has not been shown to be harmful to the fetus in animal studies, but for which no human study is available, is assigned FDA risk category:
A. A.
B. B.
C. C.
D. D.

64. A drug shown to cause teratogenic effect in animal studies, but for which no human study is available, is assigned FDA risk category:
A. A.
B. B.
C. C.
D. D.

65. Prior to day 31 post-LMP, the embryo is best described as:
A. a single, undifferentiated cell.
B. a group of poorly differentiated cells.
C. a conglomerate of highly differentiated cells and primitive organs.
D. a small fetus with developed organs.

66. What is the molecular weight requirement for a drug to easily pass through the placental barrier?
A. <250 daltons
B. <500 daltons
C. <1000 daltons
D. <5000 daltons

67. What is the molecular weight requirement for a drug to be unable to pass through the placental barrier?
A. >250 daltons
B. >500 daltons
C. >1000 daltons
D. >5000 daltons

68. When treating a woman with a urinary tract infection who is 28 weeks pregnant, the NP considers prescribing:
A. trimethoprim-sulfamethoxazole (TMP-SMX).
B. cephalexin.
C. ciprofloxacin.
D. doxycycline.

69. According to Hale's Lactation Risk Category, a medication in which there is no controlled study on its use during lactation, or controlled study shows minimal, non–life-threatening risk, is listed as category:
A. L2.
B. L3.
C. L4.
D. L5.

70. According to Hale's Lactation Risk Category, a medication in which there is evidence of risk for its use in lactation, but it can be used if there is a maternal life-threatening situation, is listed as category:
A. L2.
B. L3.
C. L4.
D. L5.

71. In a pregnant woman with asthma, in what part of her pregnancy do symptoms and bronchospasm often worsen?
A. 6 to 14 weeks
B. 15 to 23 weeks
C. 24 to 33 weeks
D. 29 to 36 weeks

72. In treating a pregnant woman with acute bacterial rhinosinusitis, the NP would likely avoid prescribing:
A. amoxicillin.
B. cefuroxime.
C. cefpodoxime.
D. levofloxacin.

73. The duration of antimicrobial therapy for treatment of symptomatic urinary tract infection in a pregnant woman is:
A. 3 days.
B. 5 days.
C. 7 days.
D. 10 days.

74. Selective serotonin reuptake inhibitor (SSRI) withdrawal syndrome is best characterized as:
A. bothersome but not life-threatening.
B. potentially life-threatening.
C. most often seen with medications with a longer half-life.
D. associated with seizure risk.

75. The placenta is best described as:
A. poorly permeable.
B. an effective drug barrier.
C. able to transport lipophilic substances.
D. capable of impeding substances with molecular weight ≤than 300 daltons.

76. Preferred treatment options for a pregnant woman in the second trimester with migraine include:
A. sumatriptan.
B. codeine.
C. aspirin.
D. acetaminophen.

77. In counseling women about SSRI use during pregnancy, the NP considers that studies reveal:
A. a clear teratogenic pattern has been identified for all drugs in this class.
B. the drugs have a negative effect on intellectual development.
C. the use of paroxetine during pregnancy is associated with an increase in risk for congenital cardiac defect.
D. an increased rate of seizure disorder in exposed offspring.

78. All of the following SSRIs are pregnancy risk category C except:
A. paroxetine
B. fluoxetine
C. citalopram
D. sertraline

79. Among the most commonly used medications by women in the first trimester of pregnancy are:
A. antiepileptic drugs.
B. antibiotics.
C. antihypertensives.
D. opioids.

80. Benzodiazepine withdrawal syndrome is best characterized as:
A. bothersome but not life-threatening.
B. not observed during pregnancy.
C. most often seen with agents that have a long half-life.
D. associated with seizure risk.

81. The cornerstone controller therapy for moderate persistent asthma during pregnancy is the use of:
A. oral theophylline.
B. mast cell stabilizers.
C. leukotriene receptor antagonist.
D. inhaled corticosteroids.

82. You examine a 24-year-old woman with mild intermittent asthma who is 24 weeks pregnant and has an acute asthma flare. Her medication regimen should be adjusted to include:
A. titration to a therapeutic theophylline level.
B. addition of timed salmeterol (Serevent) use.
C. a short course of oral prednisone.
D. use of montelukast (Singulair) on a regular basis.

83. For a pregnant woman with asthma, bronchospasm symptoms are often reported to improve during _____weeks of gestation.
A. 8 to 13
B. 20 to 26
C. 29 to 36
D. 36 to 40

84. Most SNRI are FDA pregnancy risk category:
A. B.
B. C.
C. D.
D. X.

85. The benzodiazepines are FDA pregnancy risk category:
    A. B.
    B. C.
    C. D.
    D. X.

86. Bupropion is FDA pregnancy risk category:
    A. B.
    B. C.
    C. D.
    D. X.

87. Most tricyclic antidepressants are FDA pregnancy risk category:
    A. A or B.
    B. C. or D
    C. X.
    D. Unrated as these are older medications.

88. The use of NSAIDs during pregnancy can potentially increase the risk for:
    A. premature birth.
    B. neural tube defects.
    C. premature closure of ductus arteriosis.
    D. ventricular septal defects.

89. A 26-year-old woman has been taking an SSRI for depression during the entire course of her pregnancy. She gives birth to a full-term healthy girl. Five days after the birth, she reports that the baby is irritable with protracted periods of crying. This is likely a result of:
    A. increased intracranial pressure from *en utero* SSRI exposure.
    B. SSRI withdrawal.
    C. colic.
    D. impending sepsis.

90. An example of an antimicrobial that is FDA pregnancy risk category B is:
    A. clarithromycin.
    B. doxycycline.
    C. erythromycin.
    D. ofloxacin.

91. An antimicrobial that is FDA pregnancy risk category D is:
    A. amoxicillin.
    B. levofloxacin.
    C. doxycycline.
    D. TMP-SMX.

92. The penicillins are ranked as FDA pregnancy risk category:
    A. B.
    B. C.
    C. D.
    D. X.

93. All of the following uropathogens are capable of reducing urinary nitrates to nitrites except:
    A. *Escherichia coli.*
    B. *Proteus species.*
    C. *Klebsiella pneumoniae.*
    D. *Staphylococcus saprophyticus.*

94. Which of the following is FDA pregnancy risk category B until the 36th week of pregnancy?
    A. gentamicin
    B. nitrofurantoin
    C. clarithromycin
    D. ciprofloxacin

95. In a pregnant woman, asymptomatic bacteruria:
    A. should be treated only if bladder instrumentation or surgery is planned.
    B. needs to be treated to avoid complicated urinary tract infection (UTI).
    C. is a common, benign finding.
    D. is a risk factor for the development of hypertension.

96. Which of the following is the most common UTI organism in pregnant women?
    A. *Pseudomonas aeruginosa*
    B. *E. coli*
    C. *K. pneumoniae*
    D. *Proteus mirabilis*

97. Recommended length of antimicrobial therapy for a pregnant woman with asymptomatic bacteruria is:
    A. 1 to 3 days.
    B. 3 to 7 days.
    C. 8 to 10 days.
    D. 2 weeks.

98. Postpartum "baby blues" typically begin:
    A. 1–2 weeks prior to the birth.
    B. within a few days following the birth.
    C. 1–2 weeks following the birth.
    D. approximately 1 month following the birth.

99. Risk factors for postpartum depression include all of the following except:
    A. history of depression.
    B. financial problems.
    C. history of caring two or more pregnancies to term.
    D. unplanned pregnancy.

100. Symptoms of postpartum depression include all of the following except:
    A. hallucinations.
    B. overwhelming fatigue.
    C. insomnia.
    D. severe mood swings.

101. Treatment of postpartum depression can typically include all of the following except:
    A. counseling.
    B. antidepressants.
    C. electroconvulsive therapy.
    D. hormone therapy.

102. The risk of infanticide is greatest in a woman with which of the following conditions?
    A. postpartum depression
    B. postpartum "baby blues"
    C. postpartum psychosis
    D. There is little risk of infanticide with any of the above conditions.

103. A risk factor for postpartum psychosis is:
    A. history of depression.
    B. multiple births (i.e., twins, triplets, etc.).
    C. history of bipolar disorder.
    D. illegal drug use.

104. Treatment of postpartum psychosis typically includes all of the following except:
    A. hospitalization.
    B. estrogen replacement therapy.
    C. antipsychotic therapy.
    D. electroconvulsive therapy.

Answers

59.	B.	75.	C.	91.	C.
60.	B.	76.	D.	92.	A.
61.	A.	77.	C.	93.	D.
62.	D.	78.	A.	94.	B.
63.	B.	79.	B.	95.	B.
64.	C.	80.	D.	96.	B.
65.	B.	81.	D.	97.	B.
66.	B.	82.	C.	98.	B.
67.	C.	83.	D.	99.	C.
68.	B.	84.	B.	100.	A.
69.	B.	85.	C.	101.	C.
70.	C.	86.	B.	102.	C.
71.	D.	87.	B.	103.	C.
72.	D.	88.	C.	104.	B.
73.	C.	89.	B.		
74.	A.	90.	C.		

According to the CDC, 90% of American women take at least one medication during their pregnancy and about 70% take at least one prescription medication. Certain medications are potentially teratogenic, or capable of inducing birth defects, and should be avoided or used with great caution during pregnancy. By definition, a teratogenic drug is a substance that has the potential to create a characteristic set of malformations in the fetus. The classic teratogenic period occurs in a specific time of fetal development, usually between day 31 and day 81 following the last menstrual period when organogenesis is occurring. For a teratogen to exert its effect, the product must be taken at the point in the pregnancy when the affected organ system is developing. For example, lithium can cause a characteristic teratogenic cardiac defect when taken as the cardiac tube is forming; taken earlier or later in the organ development process, the drug likely has no effect on the heart. Fetal liver maturity also plays a role because 40% to 60% of fetal blood circulation goes through the liver. With increasing maturity, the fetus's hepatic enzymes become more capable of metabolizing drugs.

Before day 31 post-LMP, the pregnancy exists as a group of poorly differentiated cells with no discrete organ systems to damage. A teratogen could be taken at that point and no damage would result because there are no organ systems to disrupt. After day 81 post-LMP, the organs are formed but are still growing and developing. The likelihood of a substance exerting a teratogenic effect decreases.

Many factors influence drug transfer across the placenta, including the molecular weight of the substance, lipid solubility, and duration of exposure. Medications usually pass by passive diffusion, where the maternal drug level is greater than that of the fetus; more drug is passed when maternal levels are greatest. The degree of diffusion is influenced by many factors besides maternal drug levels including the drug's molecular weight and degree of lipophilicity. Drugs with a low molecular weight (≤500 daltons) cross the placental barrier more easily than drugs with a molecular weight greater than 500 daltons, whereas drugs with a molecular weight greater than 1000 daltons cross the placenta infrequently. The lower the molecular weight, the greater the potential for passage of the drug through the placenta. Alcohol and cocaine have low molecular weights (≤100 daltons) and are easily passed. Insulin and heparin (molecular weight greater than 5000 daltons) are examples of drugs that are poorly transported to the fetus and can be given with relative safety in pregnancy. Most oral over-the-counter and prescription medications have molecular weights of less than 500 daltons and pass easily through the placenta. The placenta preferentially allows highly lipophilic drugs to pass through.

Not all drugs with the same therapeutic endpoint have the same lipid solubility. Diphenhydramine (Benadryl) is a highly lipophilic antihistamine and penetrates the placenta and maternal central nervous system easily, causing sedation. In contrast, loratadine (Claritin) is more hydrophilic and has fewer fetal or maternal effects. Drugs with a long half-life or with extended-release formulations are usually held in maternal circulation for protracted periods and have the potential to have a greater effect on the fetus than similar drugs with shorter half-lives or drugs metabolized more rapidly.

Table 18–5 describes the U.S. Food and Drug Administration (FDA) risk categories and provides examples for each. A quick way to remember the categories is as follows:
Category B for Best because very few products are category A.
Category C for Caution because these products have been shown to have risk in animal models.
Category D for Danger because these products have been shown to have risk when used in human pregnancy but are used occasionally in life-threatening maternal disease.
Category X for "Cross these drugs off the list" because these products have shown teratogenic risk and have no therapeutic indication for use during human pregnancy.

Pregnant women have similar incidence of acute and chronic illnesses to age-matched women who are not pregnant. Up to 8% of pregnant women have asthma, with a documented increase in maternal morbidity and mortality during pregnancy for women with the most severe asthma before conception. Most pregnant women with asthma have no change in their symptoms or experience an improvement in symptoms.

TABLE 18-5
Medication Use During Pregnancy

An FDA risk category is assigned to all drugs based on risk of drug exposure to the human fetus: A–X. New drugs undergo animal studies and perhaps a small number of inadvertent human exposures during clinical trials are considered.

Risk Category	Outcomes	Example
Category A	Well-controlled human study: No fetal risk in first trimester No evidence of risk in second and third trimesters Risk to fetus appears remote	Vitamins at RDA • Vitamin A caution (risk factor X in doses 8000 IU/d or more) Levothyroxine
Category B B: Best because nothing is A	Animal studies do not show fetal risk, but no controlled study in humans, or Animal studies show adverse effect not shown in human study	Beta-lactam antimicrobials • Penicillins, cephalosporins Select macrolides • Azithromycin, erythromycin Acetaminophen
Category C C: Caution	No controlled study in humans available Animal studies reveal adverse fetal effects	~Two-thirds of all prescription medications Select antimicrobials • Clarithromycin • Fluoroquinolones ("-floxacin" suffix) • TMP-SMX Commonly prescribed medications • Most SSRIs, corticosteroids, antihypertensives, others
Category D D: Danger	Positive evidence of human fetal risk Use in pregnant women occasionally acceptable despite risk	Gentamicin ACEI ("-pril" suffix), ARB ("-sartan" suffix) Tetracyclines • Doxycycline, minocycline Paroxetine
Category X Cross these off your list	Animal or human studies show fetal abnormality Evidence of fetal risk based on human study No therapeutic indication in pregnancy	Isotretinoin (Accutane), misoprostol (Cytotec), thalidomide

Source: Briggs G, Freeman R, Yaffee S. *Drugs in Pregnancy and Lactation*, ed. 9. Philadelphia: Lippincott Williams & Wilkins, 2011.

Bronchospasm symptoms are usually worse between 29 and 36 weeks of gestation because of esophageal irritation from gastroesophageal reflux disease. Symptoms usually improve late in gestation when gradual fetal descent occurs. Lifestyle changes that help improve symptoms of gastroesophageal reflux disease help with asthma management. Generally, the risk of fetal hypoxia is greater than the risk of medication exposure, so standard asthma medications should be continued. Most inhaled corticosteroids are FDA risk category C (with budesonide [Pulmicort] being the exception as risk category B), a designation that is based on high oral or parenteral doses given to laboratory animals, but seems to have little applicability in human use, which involves inhaled medications that have low rates of systemic absorption. Oral corticosteroids have the same

designation but should be used only to treat an asthma flare. Beta$_2$-agonist bronchodilators are also category C, based on studies on high oral doses in laboratory animals, and should be prescribed as a rescue drug for a pregnant woman with asthma. Leukotriene modifiers have not been studied as extensively in pregnant women and carry a risk category B or C.

Nausea and vomiting in pregnancy often are complicated by preexisting conditions such as gastritis. The presence of *Helicobacter pylori* infection can worsen nausea and vomiting. Preconceptual evaluation and, if positive, treatment of *H. pylori* should be considered for women with history of a pregnancy complicated by severe nausea and vomiting or of recurrent gastrointestinal problems. Management is targeted toward relieving nausea by increasing rest and decreasing stress. Patients can make their own ginger or lemon aromatherapy "kit" by placing five ginger or lemon teabags in an airtight plastic tub. When nausea occurs, the patient opens the tub and sniffs the vapors. Treating the concomitant gastritis that often accompanies severe nausea and vomiting during pregnancy with a chewable calcium antacid tablet every 2 hours for 2 to 3 days can be helpful. Taking vitamin B_6, 25 mg twice a day, has been noted to prevent future nausea and vomiting. A 5-HT_3-receptor antagonist, such as ondansetron (Zofran, pregnancy risk category B), can offer an effective therapeutic option for preventing severe morning sickness but is not effective in managing acute symptoms.

Among women with a migraine history, most note fewer and less intense headaches during pregnancy; however, about 5% to 10% have worsening headaches. Treatment options are limited and include acetaminophen. Nonsteroidal anti-inflammatory drugs (NSAIDs) are category C and their use during pregnancy is controversial. NSAIDs are generally avoided after 30 to 32 weeks of pregnancy because of a potential for rare serious fetal abnormalities (i.e., premature closure of ductus arteriosis and persistent fetal circulation). Triptans are risk category C, partly because of the theoretical risk of vasoconstriction, but no teratogenic effect in human pregnancy has been noted to date. Lidocaine 4% used as a nasal spray, applied to the nostril on the affected side of the head, can help attenuate headache symptoms with minimal system drug absorption.

Women are twice as likely as men to experience major depressive disorder. Consequently, many women enter pregnancy in a depressed state or develop depression during the course of the pregnancy. Therapy for any mood disorder usually includes lifestyle changes, counseling, and drug therapy. Mood disorder treatment options include serotonin, norepinephrine, and dopamine receptor modulators, tricyclic antidepressants, and benzodiazepines. Although selective serotonin receptor inhibitors (SSRIs) are in risk category C (with the exception of paroxetine, which is risk category D), long-term observational study of children born to women who took these medications during pregnancy has failed to note significant differences compared with nonexposed matched controls. Bupropion is a dopamine receptor modulator and is also pregnancy risk category C. Serotonin-norepinephrine reuptake inhibitors such as venlafaxine (Effexor) and duloxetine (Cymbalta) are risk category C. Although few clinical studies have investigated the effects of these drugs during pregnancy, safety surveillance studies indicate the frequency of abnormal outcomes while taking these agents during pregnancy is consistent with historic rates in the general population.

If a patient wishes to discontinue antidepressant therapy during pregnancy, she should be counseled about the risk of depression recurrence. A slow taper of approximately 25% of the total dose per week is required to avoid SSRI withdrawal syndrome. The withdrawal syndrome is bothersome, but not life-threatening. Symptoms include jitteriness, nausea, and sleep disturbance and is more severe with SSRIs with a shorter half-life such as paroxetine (half-life 26 hours) and less severe with SSRIs with a longer half-life such as fluoxetine (half-life 24 to 72 hours and metabolite half-life up to 26 hours). If SSRIs are used late in the third trimester, fetal withdrawal can also occur, which is the reason for the common recommendation to taper a pregnant woman's SSRI dose over the last month of pregnancy. Neonatal effects are similar to maternal withdrawal and include irritability, protracted crying, and shivering; the timing of the onset of neonatal SSRI withdrawal symptoms is related to the drug's half-life and can occur within days to weeks of birth.

In an FDA advisory, results of domestic and European studies revealed that women who took paroxetine in early pregnancy had an approximately two-fold increased risk for having an infant with a cardiac defect compared with the risk in the general population. The risk of a cardiac defect was about 2% in infants exposed to paroxetine versus 1% among all infants in one study, whereas a 1.5-fold increased risk for cardiac malformations and a 1.8-fold increased risk for congenital malformations overall in the infants exposed to paroxetine was noted in another study. Most of the cardiac defects reported in these studies were atrial or ventricular septal defects. As a result, paroxetine is pregnancy risk category D.

Tricyclic antidepressants and benzodiazepines are risk category C or D and are rarely prescribed during pregnancy. If an expectant mother has been on long-term benzodiazepine therapy, it is critical to taper doses gradually (25% per week) to avoid a withdrawal syndrome. Rapid withdrawal can lead to tremors, hallucinations, seizures, and a delirium tremens–like state and is most common with the use of products with a shorter half-life. The onset of withdrawal symptoms occurs a few days after the last dose in a benzodiazepine with a shorter half-life (e.g., lorazepam) and up to 3 weeks in one with a longer half-life (e.g., clonazepam).

Postpartum mood and anxiety disorders can include the blues, depression, or psychosis (Table 18–6). Postpartum blues is the most common disorder and generally begins within a few days after giving birth. Symptoms include weepiness or crying for no apparent reason, impatience, irritability, restlessness, anxiety, fatigue, insomnia, sadness, mood changes, and poor concentration. The condition may be linked to hormonal changes that occur during pregnancy and following birth. The symptoms generally lessen within 14 days after delivery. Mothers should receive support, reassurance, and assistance in taking care of the newborn so the mother can get needed rest.

Postpartum depression can occur in up to 20% of new mothers and presents around 2 to 4 months following birth. The signs and symptoms are more intense than the postpartum blues and last longer, which can interfere with the mother's ability to care for the baby. Symptoms include loss of appetite, insomnia, intense irritability and anger, overwhelming fatigue, lack of sexual drive, lack of joy in life, severe mood swings, withdrawal from friends and family, and thoughts of harming themselves or the baby. Risk factors include a history of depression or postpartum

TABLE 18-6

Postpartum Mood Disorders

Disorder	Incidence (%)	Presentation	Treatment
Postpartum blues	26–85	Often begins within a few days of giving birth	Support and reassurance including recruiting helpers so mother can get more rest
Postpartum depression	10–20	Most common at 2–4 months postpartum	Psychotherapy, psychopharmacological, medication therapy as indicated, recognizing all will be secreted in breast milk; hospitalization as needed
Postpartum psychosis	0.2	Early onset usually by day 3 postpartum; characterized by delusions	Hospitalization usually needed for safety of mother and infant. Psychopharmacological medication therapy as indicated (antipsychotics, mood stabilizers, benzodiazepines, antidepressants, others)

Source: Cohen LS, Wang B, Nonacs R, et al. Treatment of mood disorders during pregnancy and postpartum. *Psychiatr Clin North Am* 33(2):273–293, 2010.

depression, experiencing stressful events during the past year, having problems in the relationship with spouse or significant other, a weak support system, financial problems, or pregnancy that was unplanned or unwanted. Treatment usually includes counseling, antidepressants, and/or hormone therapy (e.g., estrogen replacement therapy). With appropriate treatment, postpartum depression usually resolves within a few months.

Postpartum psychosis is a rare condition that typically develops within a few weeks following delivery. Symptoms include confusion and disorientation, hallucinations and delusions, paranoia, and attempts to harm themselves or the baby. Women with bipolar disorder are at higher risk of postpartum psychosis. Those with this disorder require immediate treatment, often in the hospital. Treatment involves a combination of antidepressants, antipsychotics, and mood stabilizers. Electroconvulsive therapy also is commonly used.

Pregnancy-related anatomic changes in the urinary tract, such as pressure on the bladder from the enlarging uterus and increase in the size of the ureters, contribute to urinary reflux. Urinary tract infection (UTI) in a pregnant woman is a significant risk factor for low-birth-weight infants and prematurity.

Asymptomatic bacteriuria occurs in 5% to 9% of nonpregnant and pregnant women. If left untreated in pregnancy, progression of asymptomatic bacteriuria to symptomatic UTI, including acute cystitis and pyelonephritis, occurs in 15% to 45%, or fourfold higher than in nonpregnant women. This progression largely results from the lower interleukin-6 levels and serum antibody responses to *E. coli* antigens that occur during pregnancy, resulting in a less robust immune response.

Because asymptomatic bacteriuria, usually caused by aerobic gram-negative bacilli or *Staphylococcus saprophyticus*, can lead to UTI, a urine culture should be obtained from all women early in pregnancy, even in the absence of UTI symptoms. Approximately 20% to 40% of women with asymptomatic bacteriuria develop UTI during the course of the

pregnancy; only 1% to 2% of women with a negative urine culture develop UTI. Asymptomatic bacteriuria should be treated with a 3- to 7-day course of antimicrobials, which reduces the risk of symptomatic UTI by 80% to 90%. Options for the treatment of asymptomatic bacteriuria and symptomatic UTI during pregnancy are guided by pathogen susceptibility, and preferred antimicrobials include those with FDA pregnancy risk category B. Antimicrobials in pregnancy risk category B include beta-lactams (amoxicillin, cephalexin, cefpodoxime, cefixime, and amoxicillin/clavulanate) and nitrofurantoin. Nitrofurantoin has the advantage of sparing disruption of normal vaginal flora and consistent efficacy against *E. coli* and *S. saprophyticus*. Nitrofurantoin should be avoided after the 36th week of gestation because of the potential (although unlikely) risk for hemolysis if the fetus is glucose-6-phosphate dehydrogenase–deficient and in infections caused by *Proteus mirabilis*. Beta-lactam use usually fails to eradicate the offending pathogen from the periurethral and perivaginal area, increasing the risk of reinfection.

Women with symptomatic UTI during pregnancy should be treated for 7 days. When UTI is documented, monthly screening urine cultures should be obtained for the duration of the pregnancy. Daily antimicrobial prophylaxis with an appropriate agent should be considered with evidence of 2 days of a symptomatic UTI or persistent, unresolved bacteriuria despite effective antimicrobial therapy. Urological evaluation should also be considered to rule out structural abnormality.

DISCUSSION SOURCES

Akkerman D, Cleland L, Croft G, et al. *Routine Prenatal Care*. Bloomington, MN: Institute for Clinical Systems Improvement (ICSI), 2012, https://www.icsi.org/_asset/13n9y4/Prenatal.pdf.

Antonucci R, Zaffanello M, Puxeddu E, et al. Use of non-steroidal anti-inflammatory drugs in pregnancy: impact on the fetus and newborn. *Curr Drug Metab* 13(4):474–490, 2012.

Briggs G, Freeman R, Yaffe S. *Drugs in Pregnancy and Lactation: A Reference for Fetal and Neonatal Risk*, ed. 9. Philadelphia: Lippincott Williams & Wilkins, 2012.

Centers for Disease Control and Prevention. Treating for two: Safer medication use in pregnancy, http://www.cdc.gov/ncbddd/birthdefects/documents/ncbddd_birth-defects_medication useonepager_cdcrole.pdf.

Gilbert DN, Moellering RC, Eliopoulos GM, Chambers HF, Saag MS. *The Sanford Guide to Antimicrobial Therapy*, ed. 43. Sperryville, VA: Antimicrobial Therapy, Inc., 2013.

Ogunyemi DA. Hyperemesis gravidarum, http://emedicine.medscape.com/article/254751-overview#a0156.

Hypertensive Disorders, GBS

105 to 109. Match each hypertensive disorder with its characteristic.

105. Chronic hypertension
106. Gestational hypertension
107. Preeclampsia
108. Eclampsia
109. HELLP syndrome

A. high blood pressure diagnosed after the 20th week of pregnancy
B. presence of tonic-clonic seizures or other alteration in mental status
C. high blood pressure diagnosed before pregnancy
D. preeclampsia accompanied by elevated hepatic enzymes and low platelets
E. high blood pressure diagnosed after the 20th week of pregnancy and accompanied by significant proteinuria

110. Risk factors for preeclampsia include all of the following except:
A. low maternal weight.
B. age younger than 16 years or older than 40 years.
C. collagen vascular disease.
D. first pregnancy with a new partner.

111. For a woman who was normotensive before 20 weeks of gestation, an indication of preeclampsia is blood pressure of more than ___ mm Hg systolic and more than ___ mm Hg diastolic.
A. 130, 80
B. 140, 90
C. 150, 95
D. 160, 100

112. Preeclampsia presentation is noted after the ___ week of pregnancy.
A. 10th
B. 15th
C. 20th
D. 25th

113. The components of HELLP syndrome include all of the following except:
A. hepatic enzyme elevations.
B. thrombocytosis.
C. hemolysis.
D. eclampsia.

114. Which of the following is the most important part of care of a woman with preeclampsia?
A. antihypertensive therapy
B. anticonvulsant therapy
C. prompt recognition of the condition
D. induction of labor

115. Regarding the risk for neonatal group B streptococcus (GBS) disease, the NP considers that:
A. about 50% to 70% of all pregnant women harbor this organism.
B. there is no risk of disease with cesarean birth.
C. the organism is most often acquired by vertical transmission in the second trimester of pregnancy.
D. intrapartum antimicrobials should be given to all women with evidence of GBS colonization.

116. GBS cultures should be obtained from:
A. the cervix.
B. the urethra.
C. urine.
D. the lower vagina and rectum.

Answers

105. C.	**109.** D.	**113.** B.
106. A.	**110.** A.	**114.** C.
107. E.	**111.** B.	**115.** D.
108. B.	**112.** C.	**116.** D.

Hypertensive disorders occur in 12% to 22% of all pregnancies. These disorders are usually divided into the following categories: chronic hypertension, or high blood pressure (BP) diagnosis that predates the pregnancy, and hypertensive disorders acquired during pregnancy. Hypertensive disorders acquired during pregnancy include gestational hypertension, preeclampsia, and eclampsia. Preeclampsia risk factors include age (≥40 years, ≤16 years), first pregnancy or first pregnancy with a new partner, pregestational diabetes mellitus, presence of collagen vascular disease, prepregnancy or primary hypertension, presence of maternal renal disease, a family history of pregnancy-induced hypertension, or multiple gestation pregnancy.

An early or milder case presentation of preeclampsia is usually characterized by an increase in systolic BP of 30 mm Hg, an increase in diastolic BP of 15 mm Hg, or an absolute BP reading of 140 mm Hg/90 mm Hg in a pregnant woman with minimal proteinuria and pathological edema, with presentation after the 20th week of gestation. Additional findings, usually with more severe disease, include right upper quadrant abdominal pain, nausea, and vomiting. A systolic BP greater than 160 mm Hg or a diastolic BP greater than 110 mm Hg with significant proteinuria (≥5 g/d) and evidence of hepatic, renal, or central nervous system end-organ damage indicate severe preeclampsia. Preeclampsia can progress to the syndrome of hemolysis with resulting anemia, elevated liver enzymes indicating hepatocellular damage, and low platelet count and eclampsia; this constellation is known as HELLP and is noted in 5% to 10% of patients with preeclamptic symptoms (Table 18–7).

The most important intervention in preeclampsia is maintaining a high index of suspicion in women with considerable risk and prompt recognition of the condition when it occurs. If preeclampsia is recognized, expert obstetrical consultation should be obtained. Intervention includes rest, ongoing maternal and fetal monitoring, and antihypertensive or anticonvulsant medications or both; all of these measures have only a small effect on outcome. Birth is the definitive intervention and is usually the treatment of choice in later pregnancy.

Prenatal care in later pregnancy should include screening for group B streptococcus (GBS). Neonatal infection with GBS is a leading cause of newborn morbidity and mortality, resulting in an estimated 7,600 cases of neonatal sepsis and approximately 300 neonatal deaths per year. Maternal lower genitourinary tract colonization with this organism is a major risk factor for early-onset, usually in the first week of life, GBS disease. The transmission of the organism from mother to fetus usually occurs after the onset of labor or membrane rupture. The lower gastrointestinal tract is the natural reservoir for this organism; this most likely contributes to GBS vaginal or rectal colonization in about 10% to 30% of pregnant women. GBS colonization is not considered to be a sexually transmitted infection and can be transient, chronic, or intermittent. Intrapartum antimicrobial chemoprophylaxis is currently the most effective intervention to help prevent infant GBS disease. As a result, GBS screening should be performed in all women at 35 to 37 weeks of pregnancy, including women who are to undergo cesarean birth because the organism can cause infection across intact membranes. The culture should be obtained by swabbing the lower vagina and vaginal introitus, followed by the rectum; insertion of the swab into the anal sphincter is needed for optimal results. The patient or healthcare provider can obtain the culture. No vaginal speculum is needed, and cervical cultures should not be obtained because these can be negative in the presence of heavy lower vaginal GBS colonization.

DISCUSSION SOURCES

Akkerman D, Cleland L, Croft G, et al. *Routine Prenatal Care.* Bloomington, MN: Institute for Clinical Systems Improvement (ICSI), 2012, https://www.icsi.org/_asset/13n9y4/Prenatal.pdf.

Lim K-H. Preeclampsia, http://emedicine.medscape.com/article/1476919-overview.

TABLE 18-7
Hypertensive Disorders During Pregnancy

Category of Hypertensive Disorder During Pregnancy	Defining Characteristics of Disorder
Chronic hypertension	High blood pressure diagnosed before pregnancy, present before 20th week of pregnancy or persisting ≥6 weeks postpartum
Gestational hypertension	High blood pressure diagnosed after 20th week of pregnancy, but resolving within 6 weeks postpartum, without significant proteinuria or other signs of preeclampsia
Preeclampsia	High blood pressure diagnosed after 20th week of pregnancy, accompanied by significant proteinuria (≥300 mg protein in 24-hour urine collection) that cannot be attributed to another cause; usually accompanied by increased edema
Eclampsia	Presentation as in preeclampsia with tonic-clonic seizures or other alteration in mental status that cannot be attributed to another cause
HELLP syndrome	Preeclampsia accompanied by elevated hepatic enzymes and low platelets

Source: Akkerman D, Cleland L, Croft G, et al. *Routine Prenatal Care.* Bloomington, MN: Institute for Clinical Systems Improvement (ICSI), 2012, https://www.icsi.org/_asset/13n9y4/Prenatal.pdf.

Domestic Violence

117. You note that a 28-year-old woman who is 4 months pregnant has bruises on her right shoulder. She states, "I fell up against the wall." The bruises appear finger-shaped. She denies that another person injured her. What is your best response to this?
  A. "Your bruises really look as if they were caused by someone grabbing you."
  B. "Was this really an accident?"
  C. "I notice the bruises are in the shape of a hand."
  D. "How did you fall?"

118. Which of the following statements is true concerning domestic violence during pregnancy?
  A. This is found largely among women of lower socioeconomic status.
  B. Women in an abusive relationship usually seek help.
  C. Routine screening is indicated during pregnancy.
  D. A predictable cycle of violent activity followed by a period of calm is the norm.

119 to 121. The following questions should be answered true or false.

_____ **119.** Domestic abuse is uncommon in same-sex relationships.

_____ **120.** Access to a firearm does not increase the rate of fatal episodes of domestic abuse.

_____ **121.** Child abuse is present in about half of all homes where partner mistreatment occurs.

Answers

117. C.	**119.** False	**121.** True
118. C.	**120.** False	

Interpersonal violence among family members (i.e., domestic violence) is found in all socioeconomic and ethnic groups. Because providers working with lower income and certain ethnic groups usually are more vigilant about domestic violence, however, there is often an appearance that the abuse is more of a problem in certain groups.

Domestic partner abuse can take many forms: psychological, financial, emotional, and physical. Acts of violence are typically thought to be against the victim but can include destruction of property, intimidation, and threats. A cycle of tension building including criticism, yelling, and threats followed by violence and then a quieter period of apologies and promises to change is often seen. This cycle usually accelerates over time, with the violence becoming less predictable. Love for the perpetrator, hope that behavior will change, and fear of the consequences of leaving the relationship help to keep the victim in the relationship, particularly when the woman is pregnant with the perpetrator's child and fears abandonment. As a result, the victim often does not ask for help.

As with counseling and screening for other health problems, using objective statements beginning with "I" is helpful. When a patient denies that finger-shaped bruises are caused by intentional injury by another person, the NP can simply state what is seen. This statement reinforces the assessment of abuse and allows the patient to offer more information. In a situation in which a patient is verbally abused in the presence of the NP, the NP should reinforce his or her role as patient advocate by stating that the behavior is unacceptable in any circumstance including in the examination room. Some may fear that this assertive behavior could precipitate another episode of abuse; however, this is unlikely.

It is helpful to apply the BATHE model in framing the problem, forming a therapeutic relationship, and directing intervention. Developed by Stuart and Lieberman, this model provides a guide for gathering information, while helping the patient reflect on the issues at hand. The components of BATHE include the following:

B: Background: How are things at home? At work? Has anything changed? Good or bad? Anything you wish would change?
A: Affect, anxiety: How do you feel about home life? Work? School? Life in general?
T: Trouble: What worries you the most? How stressed are you about this problem?
H: Handling: How are you handling the problems in your life? How much support do you get at home or work? Who gives you support in dealing with problems?
E: Empathy: "That sounds difficult."

You may want to add SOAAP to BATHE:
- **S:** Support
  Normalize problems, but do not minimize.
  "Many people struggle with the same (similar) problem."
  "What supports or resources can you use to help deal with this?"
  Some providers use select self-disclosure when discussing support or resource. Self-disclosure usually works best in crises that are common and not of unusually tragic proportions, such as a timely death of a loved one or job change.
- **O:** Objectivity
  Watch your reactions to the story. Maintain your professional composure without acting stonelike but be mindful of "recoiling" gestures.
  Help client with objectivity.
  "What is the worst thing that can happen?"
  "How likely is that?"
  "Then what would happen?"
- **A:** Acceptance
  Coach the client to personal acceptance.
  "That is an understandable way to feel."
  "I think you have done well, considering the stress."
  "I wonder if you are not being too hard on yourself."
- **A:** Acknowledge client priorities.
  "It sounds like family is more important to you than your work."

Acknowledge readiness or difficulty in making a change.
"Change is hard and sometimes very scary."
"It sounds to me like you are (not) ready to make a change."
- **P**: Present focus
Assist client in focusing on the present without minimizing concerns of the past and future.
"How could you cope better?"
"What could you do differently?"
    After you have gathered this information, you should do the following:
- Negotiate a problem-focused contract for behavioral change:
Repeat after me, "I promise not to harm myself or anyone else in any way between now and my next visit with _____."
Homework assignment with "I" messages:
"I would like more help with the children."
"I feel really unimportant to you when _____."
"I feel angry when _____."
How do you keep this to 15 minutes?
- Focus the client, using open and close-ended questions. Tell the client how much time you have, particularly with a revisit.
"We have ___ (fill in the blank) minutes to chat. What would you like to focus on?"
If the client cannot focus, ask, "If one problem in your life could just disappear, what would you choose?"

Interpersonal violence is likely as common in same-sex relationships as in opposite-sex relationships, but it is not as well studied. Violent behavior by a woman against a male partner is unlikely to result in injury as serious as a man's violence against a woman, partly because of the usual disparity in body size and lower likelihood of weapon use. In all socioeconomic groups, access to a firearm by a perpetrator is associated with increased risk of abuse with serious or fatal injury; this is also a risk for completed suicide. The NP is in an ideal position to direct the couple to appropriate resources for help in domestic violence but should not attempt to provide this counseling because of the complexity of this type of care. Individual treatment is the rule as long as the violent behavior continues. Child abuse is present in about half of all households where there is partner abuse.

DISCUSSION SOURCES

Diagnostic and Statistical Manual of Mental Disorders, ed. 5. Arlington, VA: American Psychiatric Publishing, Inc., 2013.
Stuart M, Lieberman J. *The 15-Minute Hour: Practical Therapeutic Intervention in Primary Care.* ed. 4. Philadelphia: Saunders, 2008.

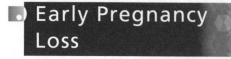

Early Pregnancy Loss

122. Approximately ___% of all clinically recognized pregnancies end in spontaneous abortion.
    A. 10
    B. 20
    C. 30
    D. 40

123. Approximately ___% of spontaneous abortions are associated with chromosomal defects.
    A. 20
    B. 40
    C. 60
    D. 80

124. The classic clinical triad of ectopic pregnancy includes all of the following except:
    A. abdominal pain.
    B. vaginal bleeding.
    C. large-for-gestational-age uterus.
    D. adnexal mass.

125. The classic clinical triad of ectopic pregnancy is found in no more than ___% of women presenting with this condition.
    A. 10
    B. 25
    C. 50
    D. 75

126. In the first weeks of a viable intrauterine pregnancy, serum quantitative hCG levels usually doubles every ___ hours until approximately 10,000-20,000mIU/mL.
    A. 24
    B. 48
    C. 72
    D. 96

127. In ectopic pregnancy, all of the following statements are true except:
    A. hCG is low for gestational age and is not increasing normally.
    B. Ultrasound evaluation fails to reveal abnormality in 20% to 30% of cases.
    C. Location of the pregnancy is often on the ovary or cervix.
    D. Risk factors include current pregnancy via assisted reproduction.

128 to 131. Match the clinical presentation of the following.
____ **128.** Complete abortion
____ **129.** Inevitable abortion
____ **130.** Threatened abortion
____ **131.** Incomplete abortion

    A. Uterine contents include a nonviable pregnancy that is in the process of being expelled.
    B. Some portion of the products of conception remains in the uterus, although the pregnancy is no longer viable.
    C. The products of conception have been completely expelled.
    D. Ultrasound evaluation shows a viable pregnancy, although vaginal bleeding is present.

Answers

122. B.	126. B.	130. D.
123. C.	127. C.	131. B.
124. C.	128. C.	
125. C.	129. A.	

Ectopic pregnancy is defined as any gestation that occurs outside of the uterus. Although reports of cervical, abdominal, and interstitial pregnancies exist, approximately 95% of all ectopic pregnancies are located in a fallopian tube; the term tubal pregnancy is nearly synonymous with ectopic pregnancy. Because the physiological and physical needs of the fetus cannot be met when pregnancy occurs outside the uterus, the pregnancy cannot progress beyond the earliest stages and will be lost. Most ectopic pregnancies resolve without intervention via miscarriage or involution of the gestational sac and reabsorption. Ectopic pregnancies that do not resolve pose a significant risk to the mother.

Risk factors for ectopic pregnancy include factors that can influence normal tubal motility and patency, such as a history of pelvic inflammatory disease, prior ectopic pregnancy, current intrauterine device (IUD) use, pregnancy achieved by means of *in vitro* fertilization or fertility drugs, prior tubal surgery (reconstruction or tubal ligation), and cigarette smoking (Table 18–8). Increased maternal age (35 years of age or greater) is also appears to be a risk factor for ectopic pregnancy.

The classic clinical triad of ectopic pregnancy—abdominal pain, vaginal bleeding, and adnexal mass—is found in only 50% of women with the condition. Consequently, careful clinical assessment to support or disprove the diagnosis is critical. Diagnosis of ectopic pregnancy includes obtaining a quantitative beta hCG value. Urine and serum tests are usually positive, and a negative test rules out the diagnosis. Usually the serum quantity of beta hCG in ectopic pregnancy at gestational weeks 6 to 10, the most common time for clinical presentation, is approximately 1000 to 6000 mIU/mL; this compares with 40,000 mIU/mL or greater for a viable intrauterine pregnancy. The normal rapid increase in serum quantitative beta hCG noted in a viable intrauterine pregnancy is missing, and the value tends to stall. With a positive beta hCG level 1500 mIU/mL or greater, a gestational sac should be identifiable within the uterus on transvaginal ultrasound with an intrauterine pregnancy; the presence of an intrauterine gestational sac effectively excludes the diagnosis of ectopic pregnancy (Tables 18–9 and 18–10).

TABLE 18-8
Risk Factors for Ectopic Pregnancy

Strongest Evidence of Risk	Significant but Less Potent
History of salpingitis (most potent risk factor)	Progestin use
Prior ectopic pregnancy	Current IUD use
Tubal or pelvic surgery	Vaginal douching
Assisted reproduction	Tubal ligation failure (more likely 2 or more years after procedure)
Cigarette smoking	Increased maternal age (35 years of age or greater)

IUD, intrauterine device.

TABLE 18-9
Clinical Presentation in Ectopic Pregnancy

Clinical Presentation	Laboratory Diagnosis	Ultrasound
Abdominal pain (nearly universal, often bilateral)	Serum progesterone (less than 15 mg/mL, found in the majority of ectopic and nonviable intrauterine pregnancies). Low for gestational age serum hCG (IUP less than 6000 mIU/mL, relatively stalled without normal hCG increases)	Consider diagnosis if transvaginal ultrasound fails to identify intrauterine gestational sac and hCG less than 1500 mIU/mL
Adnexal tenderness (75%)		
Menstrual irregularity (75%)		
Uterus size less than anticipated for gestational age (90%)		
Adnexal mass (53%)	Positive urine hCG (99% sensitivity and specificity)	

IUP, intrauterine pregnancy.

TABLE 18-10

Clinical Presentation in Viable Intrauterine Pregnancy (IUP)

Transvaginal ultrasound	Gestational sac visible in viable IUP when hCG greater than 1500 mIU/mL
Transabdominal ultrasound	Gestational sac in viable IUP when hCG greater than 6000 mIU/mL

Of women with ectopic pregnancy, approximately 15% to 26% have a nondiagnostic ultrasound; thus, a normal ultrasound scan does not rule out the condition. If ectopic pregnancy is suspected, a serum progesterone level is often obtained. Progesterone is a hormone produced by the developing chorion. A progesterone level less than 15 ng/mL is seen in only 11% of viable intrauterine pregnancies but is noted in most ectopic pregnancies or with inevitable abortion. Occasionally, pelvic computed tomography or magnetic resonance imaging is indicated, recognizing the limitations of these studies in ectopic pregnancy but their utility in identifying other reasons for abdominal pain.

When the diagnosis of ectopic pregnancy is established, treatment depends on the patient's condition. If the patient is stable, evaluation for a concurrent (heterotopic) intrauterine pregnancy should be done because this can be found in 10% of women presenting with this condition. If the patient is hemodynamically unstable, immediate surgical intervention is warranted. If the patient is stable, surgical or medical intervention is warranted according to the availability of treatment options. Surgical treatments include salpingostomy, in which the tube is opened and the pregnancy contents are removed. The tube is then repaired. Salpingectomy is usually performed when the tubal rupture has occurred or tubal damage is severe, and repair is not possible.

Medical therapy with methotrexate, a medication that inhibits cell division and causes the pregnancy to regress and resolve, is an option when ectopic pregnancy is diagnosed while the tube is intact, the patient is hemodynamically stable, there is no ultrasound evidence of fetal cardiac activity or free fluid in the cul-de-sac, and there are no contraindications for methotrexate use. A quantitative beta hCG of greater than 6,000 mIU/mL, evidence of fetal cardiac activity and free fluid in the cul-de-sac (a common finding in tubal rupture) are all contraindications to methotrexate use. Close follow-up is critical with medical management of ectopic pregnancy to ensure pregnancy resolution; surgical intervention is sometimes needed if this therapy fails. Compared with surgical therapy, tubal patency is usually better preserved with medical management. Regardless of the treatment modality in ectopic pregnancy, considerable emotional support is also needed because the woman has faced a potentially life-threatening illness and the loss of a pregnancy (Table 18–11).

Spontaneous abortion is defined as the natural ending of a pregnancy before 20 weeks of gestation. In about 60% of spontaneous abortions, chromosomal defects of maternal or paternal origin are responsible for the pregnancy loss. Maternal factors such as trauma, illness, or infection lead to the loss in about 15% of cases. In the remaining cases, no obvious cause can be found. With all threatened pregnancy loss, intervention is aimed at maintaining a stable hemodynamic state and providing considerable emotional support.

About 25% to 30% of women experience some vaginal bleeding in the first trimester, and at least 50% of these women have pregnancy loss. Four terms are usually used to modify the condition of spontaneous abortion: threatened, inevitable, incomplete, and complete.

Threatened abortion manifests as vaginal bleeding or brown spotting during early pregnancy with or without cramping but without cervical dilation or change in cervical

TABLE 18-11

Ectopic Pregnancy Management

Many ectopic pregnancies resolve without intervention. No current reliable data are available on predictors of self-resolution.

SURGICAL MANAGEMENT	Salpingostomy, salpingectomy
MEDICAL MANAGEMENT	Methotrexate therapy can be offered if following criteria are met:

- Conceptus less than 3.5-4 cm with no evidence of cardiac activity
- Unruptured tube with no evidence of fluid in cul-de-sac
- Beta hCG level less than 5,000 mIU/mL
- Hemodynamically stable with no signs or symptoms of active bleeding or hemoperitoneum
- Patient is reliable, adherent to therapy, and available for close follow-up care
- *(A beta hCG level >5,000 mIU/mL, fetal cardiac activity, and free fluid in the cul-de-sac are usually considered contraindications for methotrexate therapy.)*

Source: Sepilian VP. Ectopic pregnancy, http://emedicine.medscape.com/article/2041923-overview.

consistency. Ultrasound evaluation shows a viable pregnancy, and serum quantitative beta hCG is consistent with gestational age. Barring other complications, the pregnancy in threatened abortion progresses without problems. Intervention includes a few days of rest, then resumption of normal activities, although even this common-sense treatment likely makes little difference in the pregnancy outcome. Less than one-half of women who have vaginal bleeding during the first trimester proceed to a complete abortion or miscarriage.

In inevitable abortion, the cervix is open, and the uterine contents are in the process of being expelled. The patient has cramping, abdominal pain, and usually brisk vaginal bleeding. Usually the uterine contents are expelled, and no further medical or surgical intervention is needed.

In incomplete abortion, some portion of the products of conception remains in the uterus. The os is usually closed, and minimal cramping is reported. Evacuation of the uterine contents by dilation and aspiration is one option for intervention. Expectant management, or "watch and wait" while the uterus completes the emptying process, and medical therapy to encourage uterine emptying are also appropriate options.

In a complete abortion, pregnancy-related uterine contents have been completely expelled. Quantitative hCG is low for gestational age, and the ultrasound fails to identify a pregnancy. On examination, the patient has minimal cramping, the cervical os is likely still slightly open, and the uterine size is returning to normal. Further medical or surgical intervention is usually not needed. As with all pregnancy loss, considerable emotional support is needed to help the woman and her family deal with this significant event.

DISCUSSION SOURCES

Prine LW, MacNaughton H. Office management of early pregnancy loss. *Am Fam Physician* 84(1):75–82, 2011, http://www.aafp.org/afp/2011/0701/p75.html.
Sepilian V. Ectopic pregnancy, http://emedicine.medscape.com/article/2041923-overview.
Tulandi T. Ectopic (tubal) pregnancy: Beyond the basics, http://www.uptodate.com/contents/ectopic-tubal-pregnancy-beyond-the-basics.

Labor

132. First-time mothers usually have an average of _____ hours of active first-stage labor.
A. 6 to 8
B. 9 to 12
C. 13 to 15
D. 16 to 18

133. For women who have previously given birth vaginally, first-stage and second-stage labor usually lasts a total of _____ hours.
A. 3 to 5
B. 6 to 8
C. 9 to 10
D. 11 to 13

Answers

132. B.   **133. B.**

The NP must have knowledge of the normal process of labor to provide appropriate counseling. Numerous theories exist as to why labor starts. These theories include factors related to placental aging and uterine distention. At the normal pregnancy term, a time between 37 and 42 weeks of gestation, the process of labor begins. Early labor, also called the latent phase of labor, is often the longest part, sometimes lasting 2 to 3 days, and is characterized by mild to moderate contractions that last about 30 to 45 seconds and are 5 to 20 minutes apart, often starting and stopping. The pregnant woman is usually able to be up and around during this period and is often frustrated by the apparent slow progress of labor. During this time, the cervix usually dilates to around 3 cm, and the membranes are intact.

The first stage of active labor starts when the cervix is about 3 to 4 cm dilated and is complete when the cervix is fully dilated. Contractions become closer and more intense, culminating in transition, when contractions occur every 2 to 3 minutes and last 50 to 70 seconds or more. The pregnant woman should be instructed to go to the hospital or birthing center when contractions are every 5 minutes and lasting 1 minute. During active labor, the woman often feels restless and excited by the impending birth but is usually communicative between contractions. In transition, the woman is usually quite focused on getting through the birth process and is often distracted by the comments of others. The presence of a support person is important throughout the birth process.

The second stage of labor is the actual birth, a stage that can last a few minutes or a few hours. The mother often passes through this stage with a variety of emotions, from exhaustion to elation. The third stage of labor occurs when the placenta detaches and is expelled from the uterus.

First-time mothers usually have an average of 9 to 12 hours of first-stage labor, and second-stage labor lasts approximately 30 minutes to 2 hours. For women who have previously given birth, first-stage and second-stage labor usually lasts approximately 6 to 8 hours in total.

The pregnant woman and her labor support person should be encouraged to attend childbirth and infant care class. Referral to these classes usually occurs during the second trimester of pregnancy.

DISCUSSION SOURCES

http://www.womenshealth.gov/pregnancy/childbirth-beyond/labor-birth.html.
American Pregnancy Association. Stage of labor, http://americanpregnancy.org/tag/stage-of-labor.

Professional Issues

19

Medicaid

1. Medicaid is best defined as:
   A. an entitlement program to provide healthcare coverage for unemployed families.
   B. publicly financed health and long-term care coverage for low-income people.
   C. free acute care coverage for those who meet special criteria.
   D. publicly supported healthcare for low-income people under the age of 65 years.

2. A "dual eligible" beneficiary is an individual who receives Medicaid and:
   A. private insurance.
   B. Social Security.
   C. government welfare benefits.
   D. Medicare.

3. Concerning long-term care coverage, Medicaid:
   A. does not provide any coverage of long-term care expenses.
   B. only covers eligible individuals younger than 65 years of age.
   C. finances approximately 40% of all long-term care spending.
   D. provides coverage only for those with physical disabilities.

4. Which of the following statements concerning funding for Medicaid is accurate?
   A. Federal funding of Medicaid for each state is based primarily on the state population size.
   B. The federal government matches at least 50% of state Medicaid spending.
   C. States are not required to provide funding for Medicaid as long as they meet guidelines to receive federal funding.
   D. Federal funding typically accounts for less than 20% of all Medicaid funding.

5. Along with the Children's Health Insurance Program (CHIP), Medicaid provides coverage for approximately what percentage of all children in the United States?
   A. 10%
   B. 20%
   C. 33%
   D. 55%

6. Federal core groups that states must cover to receive federal matching Medicaid funding include all of the following except:
   A. pregnant women.
   B. elderly.
   C. children.
   D. undocumented immigrants.

7. In concerning disabled individuals, Medicaid funding can assist in all of the following except:
   A. fund education opportunities (i.e., tuition).
   B. provide a fuller range of healthcare services.
   C. maximize independent living opportunities.
   D. support participation in the workforce, if possible.

8. What is the impact of the Affordable Care Act (ACA) on Medicaid coverage?
   A. ACA will increase Medicaid coverage for the elderly (more than 65 years of age).
   B. ACA will increase coverage for uninsured adults younger than 65 years of age.
   C. There will be no impact on Medicaid coverage.
   D. More individuals will switch from Medicaid to Medicare coverage.

9. "Mandatory services" defined by federal law for inclusion in Medicaid include all of the following except:
   A. laboratory and x-ray services.
   B. family planning services.
   C. rehabilitation therapy.
   D. nurse practitioner services.

10. Coverage of services from all of the following health-care centers is considered mandatory for inclusion in Medicaid by federal law except:
    A. rural health clinic (RHC).
    B. acute care hospital.
    C. hospice.
    D. federally-qualified health center (FQHC).

11. Which of the following statements is false regarding Medicaid premiums and cost-sharing?
    A. States have limited flexibility to charge Medicaid premiums based on income level.
    B. Preventive services for children are exempt from cost-sharing.
    C. States can terminate Medicaid coverage if premiums are not paid by an individual.
    D. Providers cannot deny care to Medicaid patients even if cost-sharing amounts are not paid.

12. When compared with children with private insurance, those with Medicaid and CHIP are:
    A. comparable in access to healthcare and meeting several core measures in preventive care.
    B. more deficient in several core measures of preventive care.
    C. less likely to see primary care providers.
    D. more likely to receive mandatory immunizations.

13. Which of the following statements is most accurate regarding the use of emergency department (ED) services by Medicaid patients?
    A. The majority of ED visits by Medicaid patients is for nonurgent symptoms.
    B. Those with Medicaid are more than twice as likely to use the ED for nonurgent symptoms compared with those with private insurance.
    C. Medicaid patients use EDs at a similar rate when compared with people with private insurance.
    D. ED visits by Medicaid patients more often involve multiple diagnoses compared with those with private insurance.

▶ Answers

1. B.	6. D.	11. D.
2. D.	7. A.	12. A.
3. C.	8. B.	13. D.
4. B.	9. C.	
5. C.	10. C.	

The Medicaid program was started in 1965 and now covers over 62 million Americans, making it the largest healthcare insurance program in the United States. Medicaid is an entitlement program that was initially established to provide medical assistance to low-income individuals and families receiving public assistance or government welfare benefits. Over time, Congress and the states have expanded Medicaid to reach more uninsured Americans living below or near the poverty line. Medicaid covers a broad population, including pregnant women, children and some parents in both working and jobless families, and children and adults with physical and mental health conditions and disabilities. Additionally, Medicaid provides assistance to low-income Medicare beneficiaries, known as "dual eligible" beneficiaries, providing assistance with Medicare premiums and cost-sharing and covering key services, particularly in long-term care, that Medicare excludes or limits.

Medicaid is the main source of coverage and financing for long-term services and supports (LTSS) since Medicare and private insurance largely does not provide coverage for these services. Of the nearly 10 million Americans that utilize LTSS, about half are elderly and about half are children and working-age adults with disabilities. Medicaid finances 40% of all long-term care spending; more than 60% of nursing home residents are covered by Medicaid.

The cost of Medicaid is shared by the federal government and the states. The federal government matches state Medicaid spending based on a specified formula that varies for each state, but the federal match rate is at least 50% in every state. Though state participation in Medicaid is voluntary, all states participate. The states administer Medicaid within broad federal guidelines. The Centers for Medicare and Medicaid Services (CMS) provides oversight of each state to ensure that the core requirements are met. Beyond these core requirements, each state has flexibility regarding eligibility, benefits, provider payment, delivery systems, and other aspects. Thus, Medicaid programs can vary considerably from state to state.

By design, Medicaid provides coverage for low-income people. States must cover federal core groups of low-income individuals and have flexibility to expand coverage to other groups. Federal core groups include pregnant women, children, parents, elderly individuals, and individuals with disabilities, with income below specified minimum thresholds. Along with the Children's Health Insurance Program (CHIP), Medicaid covers more than a third of all children and more than 50% of all low-income children. Only American citizens and specific categories of lawfully present immigrants can qualify for Medicaid; lawfully present immigrants typically must wait 5 years before enrollment in Medicaid. The Affordable Care Act (ACA) opens Medicaid to a greater number of uninsured adults by creating a new eligibility group of adults younger than 65 years of age with income at or below 138% of the federal poverty line (FPL).

Medicaid provides health and long-term care coverage for people with severe physical and mental disabilities, often in circumstances in which they cannot obtain private insurance or the coverage falls short of meeting their needs. Medicaid currently covers approximately 9.3 million nonelderly people with disabilities, including 1.5 million children. This includes coverage for those with Down syndrome, cerebral palsy, and autism, among others. Medicaid can provide access to a broader range of services needed by the disabled, can help maximize independence, and, if possible, support participation in the workforce.

In addition to the federal core groups to which states must provide coverage in order to receive federal matching funds, states must also cover a set of mandatory services defined by federal law (Table 19–1). These services include benefits typically covered by private insurance but can also include additional services, such as transportation and nursing and community-based long-term care. Services provided by federally-qualified health centers (FQHCs) and rural health clinics (RHCs) are included, reflecting the role of these providers in serving the low-income population. In addition to these services, states have the flexibility to cover optional services, which tend to be vital for individuals with chronic conditions or disabilities and the elderly.

States are allowed to charge premiums and cost-sharing for Medicaid in accordance with federal limitations. Though premiums are prohibited for children and adults with income below 150% FPL, those with higher income can be charged Medicaid premiums. Cost-sharing is largely prohibited from Medicaid-insured children and can vary for adults based on income level. Certain services are exempt from cost-sharing, such as preventive services for children, emergency services, and family planning services. States can terminate Medicaid coverage if premiums are not paid and can permit providers to deny care in certain circumstances if Medicaid patients do not pay their cost-sharing amounts.

Medicaid improves access to healthcare for children. When compared with children with private insurance, children with Medicaid and CHIP demonstrated comparable levels of several core measures of preventive and primary care. However, working-age adults with Medicaid have more difficulty in accessing healthcare compared with adults with private insurance. Medicaid patients use emergency department services at higher rates than those with private insurance. However, only about 10% of Medicaid ED visits are for nonurgent symptoms, compared with 7% for those with private insurers. Adults with Medicaid tend to have higher burden of illness and disability and are more likely to have a secondary diagnosis of a mental disorder; also, a larger share of their visits involve more than one major diagnosis.

DISCUSSION SOURCE

The Kaiser Commission on Medicaid and the Uninsured. Medicaid: A Primer (March 2013). Available at: http://kff.org/medicaid/issue-brief/medicaid-a-primer.

Medicare

14. Medicare is best defined as:
   A. an entitlement program to provide healthcare coverage for low-income elderly persons.
   B. a publicly supported health insurance program for elderly persons and younger persons with permanent disabilities.
   C. a health insurance program for persons ineligible for private insurance.
   D. the nation's insurance program for long-term care coverage in elderly persons.

15. Persons eligible for Medicare include all of the following except:
   A. individuals age 65 and older.
   B. individuals younger than 65 years of age with certain permanent disabilities.
   C. certain individuals concurrently receiving Medicaid.
   D. healthy individuals younger than 65 years with income below 150% of the federal poverty line.

16. to 19. Match the Medicare part with its appropriate benefits.

   16. Part A
   17. Part B
   18. Part C
   19. Part D

   A. allows beneficiaries to enroll in a private plan as an alternative to the traditional fee-for-service plan
   B. covers inpatient and hospital services
   C. provides outpatient prescription drug benefits
   D. helps pay for physician, nurse practitioner, outpatient, home health, and preventive services

---

TABLE 19-1

Mandatory Services Defined by Federal Law for Medicaid

MANDATORY SERVICES

- Physicians' services
- Nurse Practitioners' and Physician Assistants' services
- Hospital services (inpatient and outpatient)
- Laboratory and x-ray services
- Early and periodic screening, diagnostic, and treatment (EPSDT) services for individuals under age of 21
- Federally-qualified health center (FQHC) and rural health clinic (RHC) services

- Family planning services and supplies
- Pediatric and family nurse practitioner services
- Nurse midwife services
- Nursing facility services for individuals 21 y.o. and older
- Home healthcare for persons eligible for nursing facility services
- Transportation services

Source: The Kaiser Commission on Medicaid and the Uninsured. Medicaid: A Primer (March 2013). Available at: http://kff.org/medicaid/issue-brief/medicaid-a-primer.

20. to 22. Indicate (yes or no) if each of the following is eligible for Medicare.

20. A 67-year-old man with multiple comorbidities and high income

21. A 72-year-old permanent legal resident (non-U.S. citizen)

22. A 68-year-old undocumented resident

23. Funding for Medicare include all of the following sources except:
   A. payroll taxes.
   B. monthly premiums from beneficiaries.
   C. sales taxes on alcohol and tobacco products.
   D. taxes from Social Security benefits.

24. All of the following are not typically covered by Medicare except:
   A. long-term care services.
   B. preventive care.
   C. hearing exams and hearing aids.
   D. routine vision care and eyeglasses.

◗ Answers

14. B.	**18.** A.	**22.** No
15. D.	**19.** C.	**23.** C.
16. B.	**20.** Yes	**24.** B.
17. D.	**21.** Yes	

Medicare was initially established in 1965 to provide health insurance for individuals over the age of 65 years regardless of income or medical history. The program has subsequently been expanded to include individuals younger than 65 years with certain medical conditions and disabilities. In 2010, approximately 43 million people received Medicare coverage, including 8 million people under the age of 65 years with disabilities.

Medicare is divided into four parts that each provides different healthcare benefits:

- Part A (Hospital Insurance Program): Covers inpatient hospital services, skilled nursing facilities, home health, and hospice care. This is funded by a tax of 2.9% of earnings paid by employers and workers.
- Part B (Supplemental Medical Insurance Program): Helps pay the outpatient, home health, and preventive services of the healthcare provider. This is funded by general revenues and beneficiary premiums.
- Part C (Medicare Advantage Program): Allows beneficiaries to enroll in a private plan, such as a health maintenance organization, preferred provider organization, or private fee-for-service plan, as an alternative to the traditional fee-for-service plan. These plans receive payments from Medicare to provide Medicare-covered benefits, such as hospital and physician services.
- Part D: Provides prescription drug benefits delivered through private plans that contract with Medicare. A

monthly premium is typically paid by beneficiaries who enroll in these plans.

In addition to funding from payroll taxes and Medicare premiums, other sources of funding include taxation of Social Security benefits, payments from states, and interest.

Individuals aged 65 and over are eligible for Medicare if they are a U.S. citizen or permanent legal resident regardless of prior medical history, comorbidities, income, or assets. Persons younger than 65 years with permanent disabilities are eligible for Medicare after receiving Social Security Disability Income (SSDI) payments for 24 months. Some conditions, such as end-stage renal disease or Lou Gehrig's disease, allow immediate eligibility for Medicare without waiting through 24 months of SSDI payments.

Most beneficiaries of Part A do not pay a monthly premium but may be responsible for a deductible before Medicare coverage begins. Some individuals who are not entitled to Part A coverage (such as those who did not pay enough Medicare taxes during their working years) have the option to pay a monthly premium for Part A benefits. There are also several limitations in Medicare coverage that are commonly needed by the elderly or those with permanent disabilities. These include coverage for custodial long-term care services either at home or in an institution (such as a nursing home or assisted living facility), routine dental care and dentures, routine vision care and eyeglasses, or hearing exams and hearing aids. Medicare also has significant deductibles and cost-sharing requirements for covered benefits.

Medicare Advantage (Part C) allows beneficiaries to enroll in private health plans to receive Medicare-covered benefits. These plans tend to provide all benefits covered under traditional Medicare and can offer additional benefits, including Part D prescription coverage. Medicare contracts with various types of private plans to offer benefits, including HMOs, preferred provider organizations (PPOs), provider-sponsored organizations (PSOs), private fee-for-service (PFFS) plans, high deductible plans linked to medical savings accounts (MSAs), and special needs plans (SNPs) for those eligible for both Medicare and Medicaid, the institutionalized, or those with chronic conditions. Enrollment in Medicare Advantage plans has steadily increased since its inception with approximately one in four Medicare beneficiaries participating in these plans.

DISCUSSION SOURCE

The Henry J. Kaiser Family Foundation. Medicare: A Primer (April 2010). Available at: http://kff.org/medicare/issue-brief/medicare-a-primer.

◗ Malpractice

25. to 28. Match each element of malpractice with its characteristic.

25. Duty of care

26. Breach of the standard of care

27. Injury

28. Proximal cause
  A. failure of a provider to adhere to current practice standards
  B. the existence of damages that flow from an injury such that the legal process can provide redress
  C. results from the establishment of a provider-patient relationship
  D. a causal relationship between a failure to provide standard of care and harm to a patient

29. All of the following establishes a provider-patient relationship except:
  A. professional advice given over the phone to a person who is not officially a patient of the clinic.
  B. observing an accident victim being attended to by paramedics.
  C. helping a neighbor select an OTC cough medicine in the local pharmacy.
  D. covering patients for a colleague who had to leave the clinic for a personal emergency.

30. Which of the following statement about standard of care is true?
  A. Standard of care is rarely argued in court during malpractice claims.
  B. Standard of care generally refers to the care that a reasonable, similarly educated and situated professional would provide to a patient.
  C. Standard of care is constant regardless of geographic area.
  D. Standard of care does not typically apply to NPs.

31. In a malpractice case involving the NP care of a 4-year-old previously well boy with acute otitis media who is seen in a family practice primary care setting, the most appropriate expert the plaintiff may use to establish standard of care would be:
  A. a pediatrician.
  B. a family nurse practitioner.
  C. an infectious disease physician specialist.
  D. an NP specializing in ethical and legal dilemmas.

32. Which of the following examples represents a potential malpractice scenario?
  A. A patient with type 2 diabetes mellitus is prescribed an inappropriate dose of insulin and experiences a severe hypoglycemic episode.
  B. A patient with a known sulfa allergy is prescribed trimethoprim-sulfamethoxazole (TMP-SMX) but no reaction occurs.
  C. A patient with acute bacterial sinusitis does not see any improvement in signs and symptoms 3 days after being given a dose-appropriate prescription for amoxicillin-clavulanate.
  D. Prior to taking a medication, a patient realizes that the wrong drug was dispensed at the pharmacy.

Answers

25. C.	28. D.	31. B.
26. A.	29. B.	32. A.
27. B.	30. B.	

Malpractice is the failure of a person with specialized education and training to act in a reasonable and prudent manner. There are four elements of malpractice, which a plaintiff must prove in order to win a case in court. These include:
- Duty of care
- Breach of the standard of care
- Injury
- Proximal cause (i.e., that the injury was caused by the breach of standard of care)

A duty of care is established when there is a provider-patient relationship. A visit to a nurse practitioner (NP) by a patient establishes an NP's duty to a patient. Duty can also be established outside of an office visit, such as via a telephone conversation. Duty can also be established with an individual who is not officially a patient. If an NP gives professional advice or treatment, in any setting, a duty can be established. If an injured party has reason to believe that there was a provider-patient relationship, there may in fact be such a relationship, even if the provider did not think of the interaction in that manner. For example, a friend of the NP missed an appointment with her primary care provider (PCP) and has now run out of her antihypertensive medications. She asks the NP to renew her prescription as she awaits her next appointment; the NP agrees to provide the antihypertensive prescription but encourages her friend to keep her appointment with her PCP. Although this appears on the surface as a personal favor, in fact the NP's actions have now helped established a provider-patient relationship for healthcare with her friend.

Though the definition of standard of care can differ among jurisdictions, it generally refers to the care that a reasonable, similarly situated professional would have provided for an individual. NPs are duty-bound to use such reasonable, ordinary care, skill, and diligence as NPs in good standing in the same geographical area and in the same general type of practice in similar cases. When an NP is sued for malpractice, the standard of care is argued in court. The attorneys hire expert witnesses, usually other NPs, who will give testimony describing the actions a reasonably prudent NP would have taken in the situation. NPs in a specialty practice will usually not be called as an expert witness in a case that occurred in primary care, nor will a primary care NP be called to comment on a specialty practice situation. The plaintiff's expert's testimony may conflict with the defense's expert's testimony. A judge or jury will accept either the plaintiff or the defendant's expert's explanation of the standard of care and will then decide whether the defendant NP met that standard.

A provider could be negligent, but if there is no injury, there is no malpractice. For example, an NP prescribes penicillin for a patient who has a known allergy to that antibiotic. If the patient takes the penicillin but has no adverse reaction that injures the patient, then there is no malpractice, even though the standard of care has been breached.

For malpractice to have occurred, a breach of the standard of care must have caused an injury to the plaintiff (proximal cause). For example, a patient visits a NP and is diagnosed with otitis media. The NP prescribes amoxicillin, though the patient's chart indicates a penicillin allergy. The patient leaves the clinic with the prescription filled, but before the patient takes any of the potentially problematic medication, the patient falls on the front steps of the clinic, causing a permanent scar on her face. The patient sues the clinic and the NP, claiming the NP had a duty to the patient, the NP breached the standard of care (by prescribing penicillin form for a penicillin-allergic patient), and the patient suffered an injury. All of the above claims are true, but there is no malpractice, because the breach of the standard of care—prescribing amoxicillin to a penicillin allergic patient—did not cause the injury.

Statistics on lawsuits have shown that the top seven conditions that lead to malpractice claims are:

- Breast cancer
- Pregnancy
- Acute myocardial infarction
- Displacement of intervertebral disc
- Cancer of bronchus or lung
- Appendicitis
- Colon and rectal cancer

The following recommendations should be followed to avoid malpractice:

- Comply with the state nurse practice act.
- Maintain effective collaboration, based on state regulations and prudent practice.
- Participate in periodic peer review and comply with protocols and/or guidelines.
- Ensure that collaborating professionals and facilities maintain appropriate insurance.
- Maintain patient records, including an up-to-date problem list and medication list, test results, telephone communications, consultations, and referrals.
- Release information in accordance with the Health Insurance Portability and Accountability Act (HIPAA) regulations and federal rules on human immunodeficiency virus (HIV), substance abuse, and mental health.
- Have systems and policies in place that allow for effective patient follow-up, particularly for high-risk diagnoses.
- Follow up diagnostic tests and referrals.
  - Was it done?
  - Are results on record?
    - If the test results were abnormal, was the condition followed up to a diagnosis or ruled out?
- Revisit an unresolved problem until it is resolved.

DISCUSSION SOURCES

Buppert, C. *The Nurse Practitioner's Business Practice and Legal Guide.* Sudbury, MA: Jones & Bartlett Learning, 2012.

Buppert, C. *The Primary Care Provider's Guide to Compensation and Quality: How to Get Paid and Not Get Sued.* Sudbury, MA: Jones & Bartlett Publishers, 2005.

Buppert, C. *Avoiding Malpractice: 10 rules, 5 systems, 20 cases* (ed 3). Law Office of Carolyn Buppert, 2010. Available at: www.buppert.com/publications.html.

Billing

33. to 37. In order for a NP to be reimbursed by a third-party payer (i.e., Medicare, Medicaid, private insurance), the following questions must be answered "yes":

33. Does the service include a medical evaluation and medical decision making?

34. Does the clinician have legal authority to receive reimbursement for these services?

35. Does the service involve procedures the clinician cannot perform?

36. Is the clinician enrolled with the payer?

37. Is the service covered by the patient's health plan or insurance?

38. In medical coding, the abbreviation CPT stands for:
A. Current Pricing Tier.
B. Current Procedural Terminology.
C. Clinical Practice Terminology.
D. Compendium of Procedures and Therapy.

39. In medical coding, the abbreviation ICD stands for:
A. Insurance Code for Diagnoses.
B. Integrated Clinical Dilemmas.
C. International Classification of Diseases.
D. Initial Classification of the Diagnosis.

40. When billing Medicaid, NPs get the authority to bill for their services from:
A. state law only.
B. federal law only.
C. state and federal law.
D. neither state nor federal law.

41. When billing commercial insurance, NPs get the authority to bill for their services from:
A. state law only.
B. federal law only.
C. state law and/or the commercial payers.
D. federal law and/or commercial payers.

42. All of the following are components of medical decision making according to CPT except:
A. patient history taking.
B. diagnosing.
C. deciding a course of treatment.
D. performing treatments.

43. A fee-for-service system is best defined as:
A. Up-front payments are made prior to any service.
B. A practice gets a set amount each month for all services needed by a patient.
C. Payment for each service is based on a sliding scale according to patient income.
D. For every procedure, there is an associated payment.

44. Which of the following statements is false regarding a capitated system of reimbursement?
    A. The institution or practice gets a set amount per month for all services needed by the patient and covered under a contract between the payer and practice.
    B. Capitated rates are not negotiable.
    C. Capitated rates are based on profit projections and actuarial data.
    D. When payment is capitated, clinics prefer to take care of patients as much as possible through phone calls and mailings rather than seeing a NP or medical doctor (MD).

45. Potential consequences of failing an audit because of upcoding, that is applying an artificially high level code to a visit, include all of the following except:
    A. repaying the money back to the payer.
    B. malpractice lawsuit.
    C. dismissal as a reimbursable provider.
    D. mandated education.

46. All of the following criteria can be used to distinguish a level 3 office visit for an established patient except:
    A. at least six elements of physical examination.
    B. at least one element of history of present illness and at least one positive or negative response to review-of-systems questions.
    C. medical decision making of low complexity.
    D. at least one new prescription or a prescription refill.

47. All of the following criteria can be used to help determine if a level 4 office visit occurred for an established patient except:
    A. at least four elements of physical examination.
    B. at least four elements of history of present illness.
    C. medical decision making of moderate complexity.
    D. positive or negative responses to at least two review-of-systems questions and at least one notation about past history.

48. Services that are an integral, although incidental, part of the physician's personal professional services in the course of diagnosis or treatment of an injury or illness can be classified as:
    A. capitated services.
    B. "incident to" services.
    C. mandatory services.
    D. shared services.

49. Criteria for an "incident to" office visit include all of the following except:
    A. all prescriptions must be written by the physician.
    B. the physician must conduct the initial visit and any visit in which there is a new episode of illness or a change in the plan of care.
    C. the physician, in most instances, must be in the suite of offices, though not in the same room while the NP performs the service.
    D. the physician must remain involved in the care of the patient.

50. "Incident to" billing does not apply to services provided:
    A. in home care.
    B. in a nursing home.
    C. in the physician office.
    D. in a hospital.

Answers

33. Yes	39. C.	45. B.
34. Yes	40. C.	46. D.
35. No	41. C.	47. B.
36. Yes	42. A.	48. B.
37. Yes	43. D.	49. A.
38. B.	44. B.	50. D.

An important part of practice is understanding how the services the NP delivers are reimbursed. Reimbursement follows proper billing. If services of a nurse practitioner (NP) are not billed, or not billed correctly, the practice or employer can miss a significant source of revenue. However, overbilling or "upcoding" (assigning, for billing purposes, a higher than justified billing code) can lead to charges of healthcare fraud. Therefore, NPs must have a thorough understanding of the requirements to receive third-party payments.

NPs seeking reimbursement by third-party payers (Medicare, Medicaid, and commercial health plans and insurers) will require a "yes" response to each of the following questions:

- Is the service historically performed by a physician—that is, does the service include a medical evaluation and medical decision making, or is it a procedure which only a physician (or other authorized provider) is able to perform?
- Does the clinician have the legal authority to perform this level of services?
- Does the clinician have the legal authority to receive reimbursement for these services?
- Is the clinician enrolled with the payer?
- Is the patient's coverage current?
- Is the service covered by the patient's health plan or insurance?
- Is the service medically necessary?
- Is there a CPT code (*Current Procedural Terminology,* a compendium of codes for every medical procedure, published and maintained by the American Medical Association) for the service? Has the appropriate CPT code been submitted on the claim form?
- Is there a diagnosis code (*International Classification of Diseases* or ICD) for the patient's illness or condition? Has the appropriate ICD code been submitted on the claim form?
- If the NP works for or is a specialist, has the primary care provider authorized the visit or procedure?
- Is the service one that is necessary and covered?
- Has a clean claim been submitted—that is, has the practice filled out the claim form fully and appropriately?

- Has the payer's process been followed?
- Have the payers' rules been followed?

Nurse practitioners get the legal authority to bill for their services from various sources, depending on the payer. For Medicare, the authority comes from federal law. For Medicaid, the authority comes from federal and state law. Regarding commercial insurers and health plans, the authority usually comes from state law or may not be mentioned by state law. In the latter case, the commercial payers make their own decisions about whether or not to reimburse nurse practitioners. Whether the payer is Medicare, Medicaid, or a commercial insurer or health plan, there are rules and policies about what can be reimbursed, and these policies can differ significantly from company to company.

Third-party payers reimburse NPs when they are performing these services requiring a high level of clinical skill and decision-making, but not when they are performing nursing services. Nursing services are typically defined as those services that would fall under the practice of the registered nurse. NPs' authority to perform high level services is derived from state law and that legal authority is called "scope of practice." Some state laws are more explicit than others in describing a NP's scope of practice. For example, in select state law, what the NP can do is provided in great detail whereas in other states, the law tends to be more broadly stated.

At minimum, a nurse practitioner would need the scope of practice under state law to bill for "evaluation and management" services. The components of evaluation and management, according to CPT, are taking a history; physical examination; medical (clinical) decision making at the NP, MD, or physician's assistant level; counseling; and coordination of care. Medical (clinical) decision making is defined as diagnosing, deciding upon a course of treatment, and ordering and performing treatments.

The first requirement for reimbursement is having a scope of practice under state law that authorizes the NP to perform services that would historically be considered physician services. States' laws are worded so that there is little question that a nurse practitioner can perform evaluation and management services (taking a history, performing a physical examination, and making medical decisions about further diagnosis and treatment).

Payment for NP services can come in several forms—fee-for-service, capitation, or pursuant to a contract between the practice and another entity. A practice often receives payments under a mixture of fees-for-services, capitation, and contracts.

In the fee-for-service payment system, every procedure performed has an associated payment. A procedure might be a visit for evaluation and management, a consultation, or excising a lesion. Under a fee-for-service payment system, the more services that are billed, the more revenue the practice, agency, or institution will make. As a result, it is important to know which services will be reimbursed and to bill all reimbursable services.

Under a capitated system of reimbursement, the agency, institution, or practice gets a set amount, per month, for all services needed by the patient and covered under a contract between the payer company and the practice company. Capitated rates may be negotiable. The rates are based on profit projections and actuarial data (i.e., data on past utilization of services by males, females, and age cohorts). If a patient's services are reimbursed under a capitated schedule, the practice generates revenue by signing up large numbers of patients, negotiating favorable capitation rates, and keeping expenses to a minimum by providing as few face-to-face visits and services as possible, while providing an acceptable level of care. When payment is capitated, practices want to take care of as much as possible through telephone calls, electronic communication, mailings, or visits with staff other than NPs, MDs, or PAs.

The type of payment system will impact how a NP provides care on a day-to-day basis. If a patient's services are reimbursed under a fee-for-service schedule, a practice receives more revenue with an increasing number of visits and procedures performed. An NP who wants to generate more revenue will see more patients and code comprehensively and at the highest level of service justified by the work performed and the medical necessity of the services. A practice that excels at fee-for-service reimbursement will negotiate favorable fee schedules and be adept at following up unpaid or denied claims.

Under the CPT system, there are five levels of evaluation and management visit performed in an office. For an office visit with an established patient, the most frequently billed visit for Medicare patients is a level 3 visit (CPT 99213). However, many evaluation/management visits with NPs are at level 4 (CPT 99214). Medicare reimbursement for a level 4 visit is significantly greater than for a level 3 visit. As a result, if the NP can meet the requirements for a level 4 visit, he or she will receive additional reimbursement. On the other hand, the NP who bills a level 4 visit but only documents enough work to meet the requirement of a level 3 visit will be in danger of failing an audit, which can result in a demand from the payer for money already paid, fines, mandated education and auditing, and even possible dismissal as a reimbursable provider. If billing errors are frequent, a clinician could be charged with healthcare fraud.

Certain criteria must be met to distinguish between a level 3 and level 4 visit. A level 3 office visit for an established patient requires meeting two of the following three levels of medical work:

- At least one element of history of present illness and at least one positive or negative response to review-of-systems questions.
- At least six elements of physical examination.
- Medical decision making of low complexity.

A level 4 office visit for an established patient requires meeting two of the following three levels of work:

- At least four elements of history of present illness, positive or negative responses to at least two review-of-systems questions, and at least one notation about past history, family history, or social history.
- At least 12 elements of physical examination.
- Medical decision making of moderate complexity.

The difference between the levels is a matter of more extensive history taking, more medical decisions, and higher risk of morbidity and mortality with the higher level code.

Proper coding is essential for the individual and the practice. A clinician who erroneously codes a level higher than is documented could be exposing the individual and the practice to a charge of false claims. However, coding a level lower than the documentation supports is failing to recover full reimbursement to the practice. Documentation and coding need to be appropriate for the specific visit.

Incident-to billing under Medicare is the most misunderstood concept in billing. "Incident-to" services are defined as those which are "an integral, although incidental, part of the physician's personal professional services in the course of diagnosis or treatment of an injury or illness." The purpose of "incident to" billing is to allow a physician to bill for services provided by an assistant or delegate in the office. For example, if a patient being treated by a physician for high blood pressure comes in for a blood pressure check, the physician is able to have a nurse check the blood pressure, and the physician or practice can bill Medicare for CPT 99211 (a level 1 visit). To accomplish this, the physician must be in the office suite at the time of the patient visit, the physician must have documented the plan of care, the physician must employ the nurse (or they both must be employed by the same entity), and the physician must remain involved in the care of the patient. NPs, like physicians, are able to bill the services of an assistant "incident to," if the rules on incident to billing are followed.

Some physicians bill all NP services "incident to" the physician's service. This is legal, if Medicare's rules or the commercial payer's rules are followed. Medicare's rules for a physician billing "incident to" are:

- Services of the NP must be rendered under a physician's "direct personal supervision."
- The NP must be an employee or independent contractor of a physician or physician group.
- Services must be furnished "during a course of treatment where a physician performs an initial service and subsequent services of a frequency which reflect the physician's active participation in and management of a course of treatment."

Medicare administrators have interpreted this last rule as meaning:

- The physician must conduct the initial visit and any visit in which there is a new episode of illness or a change in the plan of care. Note that NPs can evaluate and manage new episodes of illness, but in those cases, the service must be billed under the NP's name.
- The physician must be in the suite of offices, though not in the same room, when the NP performs the service.
- The physician must remain involved in the care of the patient.

"Incident to" billing can only be used for services provided during office visits, with two exceptions. It is permissible to bill "incident to" for a home visit, but both the physician and NP must be present in the home. It is

permissible to bill "incident to" in a nursing home but only if care is provided in an office space rented by the physician, and the physician, NP, and patient all are present. Prudent practice dictates that the NP keeps abreast of current regulations and advisories.

"Incident to" billing does not apply to services provided in a hospital. However, NPs and physicians are able to "share" evaluation and management visits to inpatients, emergency department patients, and outpatients. NP visits for evaluation and management can be billed under a physician employer's number if the physician provides any face-to-face service on the same day. The rules on shared visits are complicated; prior to billing in this fashion, the NP should be well informed on the appropriate regulations.

There are certain monetary advantages for physicians to bill all NP services under the physician's provider number. In this manner, the practice will get 100% of the physician's fee schedule rather than the 85% rate if billing is done under the NP's provider number. However, "incident to" billing cannot be used at all times, such as when the physician is not present in the practice (e.g., out to lunch, visiting hospitalized patients, on vacation, etc.). During these times, visits to patients covered by Medicare and conducted by a NP must be billed under the NP's name.

It is important for NPs to be familiar with when their services can be billed either under the physician's provider number or the NP provider number. A practice can bill some NP services under a physician's number when "incident-to" or "shared visit" rules are followed. Other services can be billed under the nurse practitioner's number, such as when the physician is out of the office, the patient is a new patient, or the patient has a new problem. To optimize reimbursement, NPs must understand the rules on "incident to" and "shared" billing. The NP should preferably bill under the physician's name when the criteria for incident to or shared billing are met and under the NP's name when the criteria are not met.

Medicaid prefers clinicians to bill under their own names. However, each commercial payer (e.g., Blue Cross/Blue Shield and Cigna) develops its own rules and policies, with some following Medicare's incident to rules and some that do not insist on following those rules.

DISCUSSION SOURCES

American Medical Association. *Current Procedural Terminology 2014 Professional Edition.* Chicago: American Medical Association, 2013.

Center for Medicare and Medicaid Services. Documentation Guidelines for Evaluation/Management Services. Available at: www.cms.gov/Outreach-and-Education/Medicare-Learning-Network-MLN/MLNProducts/downloads/eval_mgmt_serv_guide-ICN006764.pdf.

Buppert C. *The Nurse Practitioner's Business Practice and Legal Guide.* Sudbury, MA: Jones & Bartlett Learning, 2012. Available at: www.jblearning.com.

Buppert C. *Billing NP services in specialist's offices, hospitals, nursing facilities, homes and hospice.* Law Office of Carolyn Buppert, 2010. Available at: www.buppert.com.

Buppert C, *Productivity incentive plan for nurse practitioners: How and why.* Law Office of Carolyn Buppert, 2006. Available at: www.buppert.com.

Buppert C. *Safe, Smart Billing and Coding: Evaluation and management:* An educational program on CD. Law Office of Carolyn Buppert, 2012. Available at: www.buppert.com.

Privacy Issues

51. HIPAA stands for:
    A. Health Information Planning and Accessibility Amendment.
    B. Health Information Protection and Accountability Act.
    C. Health Insurance Portability and Accountability Act.
    D. Healthcare Initiative for Patient Access Amendment.

52. A major purpose of the Privacy Rule is to:
    A. define and limit the circumstances in which an individual's protected health information can be used or disclosed by covered entities.
    B. set standards for the distribution and selling of health information to third parties.
    C. define accountability by healthcare providers that can be used in courts when there is suspected breach of information.
    D. protect individuals' health information when access to electronic medical records is illegally obtained.

53. to 56. A covered entity as defined by the Privacy Rule includes (yes or no):

53. Hospitals.

54. Private healthcare insurance companies.

55. Nurse practitioners.

56. Medical assistants

57. Examples of "individually identifiable health information" can include all of the following except:
    A. an individual's past history of schizophrenia.
    B. the type of prescription written for an individual.
    C. a patient's diagnosis of prostate cancer.
    D. the percentage of patients with type 2 diabetes at a clinic.

58. When specific identifiers have been removed from protected health information so that it no longer can be used to identify an individual, the information is said to be:
    A. cleansed.
    B. de-identified.
    C. deprivatized.
    D. HIPAA-certified.

59. Written authorization by the individual is not needed prior to disclosure of protected health information in all of the following circumstances except:
    A. cases of child abuse or neglect.
    B. domestic violence incidents.
    C. when a covered entity believes it is necessary to prevent a serious and imminent threat to the public.
    D. a request of information from a family member.

60. The principle of "minimum necessary" disclosure relates to:
    A. covered entities must provide the requested protected health information in as short a time as possible.
    B. covered entities can only charge a nominal fee for providing requested protected health information.
    C. covered entities must make reasonable efforts to use, disclose, and request only the minimum amount of protected health information needed to accomplish the purpose of the request.
    D. covered entities must make reasonable efforts to provide electronic records, including medical images, of protected health information in as small a file as possible.

61. The penalty for the sale of individually identifiable health information for personal gain is:
    A. $100 fine and up to 1 year probation.
    B. $5000 fine and up to 60 days imprisonment.
    C. $25,000 fine and up to 1 year imprisonment.
    D. $250,000 fine and up to 10 years imprisonment.

Answers

51. C.	55. Yes	59. D.
52. A.	56. Yes	60. C.
53. Yes	57. D.	61. D.
54. Yes	58. B.	

In 1996, the U.S. Department of Health and Human Services (HHS) established for the first time a set of national standards for the protection of certain health information ("Privacy Rule") that implemented the requirement of the Health Insurance Portability and Accountability Act of 1996 (HIPAA). A major goal of the Privacy Rule is to protect an individual's health information but still allow the flow of health information needed to provide and promote high quality healthcare. The Privacy Rule addresses the use of "protected health information" by "covered entities" as well as sets standards for individuals' privacy rights to understand and control how their health information is used. A major purpose of the Privacy Rule is to define and limit the circumstances in which an individual's protected health information may be used or disclosed by covered entities.

A covered entity encompasses every healthcare provider who electronically transmits health information in connection with certain transactions. These transactions can include claims, benefit eligibility inquiries, referral authorization requests, or other transactions identified by HHS under HIPAA. Healthcare providers include any other person or organization that furnishes, bills, or is paid for healthcare. These can include "providers of services" (e.g., institutional providers such as hospitals) or "providers of medical or health services" (e.g., noninstitutional providers such as physicians, dentists, nurse practitioners, or others) as defined by Medicare.

The Privacy Rule protects information held or transmitted by a covered entity or its business associates in any form or media, such as electronic, paper, or oral. "Individually identifiable health information" protected by the Privacy Rule consists of information that identifies the individual or for which there is a reasonable basis to believe the information can be used to identify the individual, including:

- the individual's past, present, or future physical or mental health or condition
- the provision of healthcare to the individual
- the past, present, or future payment for the provision of healthcare to the individual

There are no restrictions on the use of health information that has been de-identified. De-identified health information does not identify an individual nor can it provide a reasonable basis to identify an individual. Information can be de-identified by either 1) having a formal determination made by a qualified statistician, or 2) removing specified identifiers of the individual as well as any relatives, household members, and employers, and is adequate only if the covered entity has no actual knowledge that the remaining information could be used to identify the individual.

A covered entity may not use or disclose protected health information except either 1) as the Privacy Rule permits or requires, or 2) as the individual who is subject of the information authorizes in writing. A covered entity is allowed to disclose protected health information without the individual's authorization under certain circumstances, including:

- to the individual
- treatment, payment, and healthcare operations
- opportunity to agree or object
- incident to an otherwise permitted use and disclosure
- public interest and benefit activities

- limited data set for the purpose of research, public health, or healthcare operations

Covered entities may use and disclose protected health information without individual authorization as required by law in certain situations. This includes disclosure of information to public health authorities authorized by law to collect or receive such information for preventing or controlling disease, injury, or disability and to public health or other government authorities authorized to receive reports of child abuse or neglect. Additionally, covered entities may disclose protected health information to appropriate government authorities regarding victims of abuse, neglect, or domestic violence. Disclosure is also permitted when a covered entity believes it is necessary to prevent or lessen a serious and imminent threat to a person or the public, when the disclosure is made to someone they believe can prevent or lessen the threat. Covered entities can also disclose to law enforcement if the information is needed to identify or apprehend an escapee or violent criminal.

When disclosing information, the covered entity must make reasonable efforts to use, disclose, and request only the minimum amount of protected health information needed to accomplish the intended purpose of the request. This central aspect of the Privacy Rule is called the principle of "minimum necessary" use and disclosure.

Failure to comply with Privacy Rule requirements by a covered entity can result in a fine of $100 per failure. A person who knowingly obtains and discloses individually identifiable health information can face a fine of $50,000 and up to 1 year of imprisonment. The penalty increases to $100,000 and up to 5 years of imprisonment if the wrongful conduct involves false pretenses. If the wrongful conduct involves the sale, transfer, or use of individually identifiable health information for commercial advantage, personal gain, or malicious harm, the penalty increases to $250,000 and up to 10 years of imprisonment.

DISCUSSION SOURCE

U.S. Department of Health and Human Services (HHS). Summary of the HIPAA Privacy Rule. Available at: www.hhs.gov/ocr/privacy/hipaa/understanding/summary/privacysummary.pdf.

ACKNOWLEDGMENT

The contributions of Carolyn Buppert, JD, NP to this chapter are gratefully acknowledged.

Understanding Test Design and Theory

Certification tests can be intimidating to nearly all people taking them because they take place outside of the clinical or classroom setting and usually differ greatly from the assessments that a student encountered in their academic program. As a result, preparing for and taking these standardized tests will usually require a shift in approach and preparation for the exam that is different from the one that saw you through your graduate program.

Consider that standardized tests differ from teacher generated tests in that they tend to be global in focus, rather than limited to a particular course, and rely heavily on the ability to form associations, rather than recall specific details. Moreover, more than 50% of the questions on standardized tests will ask you to apply your knowledge in a manner of context fundamentally different from the one in which you studied.

Despite the major differences between assessment in the context of a graduate program and standardized tests, roughly four of every five test takers who engage in focused, purposeful study pass the exam on their first attempt. Part of effective test preparation involves "demystifying" test design, learning how to "unlock" questions, engaging in preparation that is most effective for your individual learning style, and knowing what to expect on exam day.

Expect that your certification exam will emphasize questions that stress high order thinking skills such as analysis, synthesis, and evaluation of concepts and relationships. Expect few questions that focus on facts, details, and particulars. The testing body is expecting you to think as a competent entry-level nurse practitioner and employ adaptive expertise as you approach your test. NP certification candidates who are expert adaptive experts use conceptual knowledge, including pathophysiology, pharmacology, and principles of assessment and diagnosis, as the basis for thinking but are open to flexibility of thought in relationship to a new context. On the certification exam, this is an important mindset to have, as many questions will present you with a brief context, unlike the one you may experience in clinical practice. Moreover, on test day, you do not have the ability to ask additional questions that might help to bring the "answer" into focus. Therefore, you need to think

as an adaptive expert: Based on the strong conceptual foundation, how do I apply what I know on this new context?

Unlocking the Question

The much maligned multiple-choice question is the bane of many a test taker. In recent years, more and more educators are moving away from the traditional multiple-choice test in favor of questions that encourage students to interact with the test material in a more dynamic way. Nevertheless, the multiple-choice question is the standard instrument of at least part of most high stakes tests.

The multiple-choice question is more easily tackled if you understand how it is designed, what it is attempting to measure, as well as effective strategies for decoding and answering the question. Make frequent practice testing part of your certification exam review.

Multiple-choice questions are made up of multiple parts: a stem (scenario, context), interrogatory (essential question, action), and answer choices. Multiple-choice tests do not lend themselves to plentiful extraneous detail. Stem scenarios or context are there to support, not confuse, you in your analysis. Typical answer choices consist of one best answer, one (obviously) wrong answer, and two partially correct answers. Note: Partially correct answers can cause you to second-guess yourself. Learn to differentiate between partially correct (the "sometimes" or "yes . . . but") and the most common, best answer. On high level tests, the difference between the best answer and the distractor answers will not always be clear; you will be asked to weigh options, interpret data, and arrive at the correct action within the context or scenario of the test question.

There could be many times when you feel that an answer has more than one good choice. In these cases, take another look at the question and then choose the response most specific to the given situation. Sometimes questions that relate to presentation of disease have more than one applicable answer. The response with the most common presentation is likely to be correct. For example, an adult with bacterial meningitis can present with nuchal rigidity and papilledema. Because nuchal rigidity is seen in most adults with this diagnosis, and papilledema is found far less often, nuchal rigidity is a better choice. Childhood development questions often have more than one correct response. A 4-month-old is expected to roll stomach to back and smile. Smiling is a developmental milestone achieved by age 2 months, whereas rolling is typically not seen until an infant is 4 months old. Rolling stomach to back is the best response. Remember: Test questions are designed to have one best, although perhaps not perfect, answer.

Although there are some test items that assess factual knowledge, such as identifying an anatomical landmark, the majority of the test questions are seeking to measure higher order thinking and reasoning skills. These items are testing your clinical judgment and expertise. Most items test your ability to assess or develop a plan of intervention for a clinical situation. You should expect to apply clinical decision-making skills to the test question. Make sure you think through each question. In particular, bear in mind how the pathophysiology of the condition affects the presentation and treatment.

In clinical practice, you would likely gather more information than is given in a scenario in one of the test questions. During the certification examination, you have to decide on the best response given the information in front of you by applying sound clinical judgment. Remember: Multiple choice tests do not lend themselves to plentiful extraneous detail. Decide whether extra information found in a particularly long answer is pertinent to the question and not simply a distractor.

When keeping in mind big information about presenting issues, pharmacology, and best practices, it can be easy to lose sight of important little words—words such as but, however, despite, except, and if. These are common cuing words that tell you that things may not always be as simple as they appear. These words can indicate a shift, a possible contradiction or contraindication, and a conditional situation or scenario. Pay attention to these words. A careful test taker can use these words to construct a strategy for answering the question. For example, in a question that reads "All of the following are symptoms of 'X' except," you can treat this as a mini true/false question. You will be given three or four "true" choices and one "false" choice. That false choice is your answer. On a related note, be wary of options that include extreme words, such as "always," "never," "all," "best," "worst," and "none." Seldom is anything absolute in healthcare.

Sometimes identifying the verb in the question can help you determine the purpose of the question. In addition, look at the information presented and then ask yourself, "Is this question a test of the ability to gather subjective or objective information? Is this question a test of the ability to develop a working diagnosis or to plan a course of intervention?" This thinking helps focus your thought process as you choose the answer. Read each question and all responses thoroughly and carefully so that you mark your option choice only after you are sure you understand the concept being tested in the question. Answering a question quickly might lead to choosing a response that contains correct

information about a given condition but might not be the correct response for that particular question.

Remaining mindful of a conceptual framework that works for you can aid question comprehension and accuracy in your answering. If you are mathematically or visually minded, a good strategy might be to think of the question as a math problem or scientific equation with (patient) + (presentation) + (context) = (best action). Consolidating and storytelling work for people who need to "talk through" answers and thinking to find the best result. Turn the question into a story and predict the ending before you look at the possible answers. When in doubt, process of elimination can be a useful exercise. By eliminating wrong answers, you can narrow down your choices by re-reading the question with remaining possibilities in mind.

With the strategies we have covered here, let's look at the following test item: You see 18-year-old Sam, who was seen approximately 36 hours ago at a local walk-in center for treatment of ear pain. Diagnosed with (L) acute otitis media, amoxicillin was prescribed. Today, Sam states that he has taken five amoxicillin doses since the medication was prescribed but continues to have discomfort in the affected ear. Left tympanic membrane is red and immobile.

This is an action-oriented question, directing you to consider Sam's care and chief complaint. Based on the scenario presented, you can assume:
- Because no chronic health problems are mentioned, implied is that Sam is a young adult who is typically in good health.
- Acute otitis media (AOM) is a common episodic illness usually caused by *S. pneumoniae, H. influenzae, M. catarrhalis,* or respiratory virus.
- A first-line antimicrobial for AOM treatment is amoxicillin. When given in a sufficient dose, this antibiotic is effective against *S. pneumoniae* and both *H. influenzae* and *M. catarrhalis* that do not produce beta-lactamase. Nearly all *M. catarrhalis* and about 30% of *H. influenzae* isolates produce beta-lactamase, rendering amoxicillin ineffective. Clavulanate is a beta-lactamase inhibitor and, when given in conjunction with amoxicillin, is an effective treatment option when AOM fails to respond to amoxicillin alone.
- As inflammation and purulent exudate forms in the middle ear, a small space rich with pain receptors, otalgia is an expected finding in AOM. This usually resolves after 2 to 3 days of antimicrobial therapy.
- Tympanic membrane immobility is a cardinal sign of AOM that, despite antimicrobial therapy, does not resolve for many weeks. A patient report of otalgia is also needed to make the AOM diagnosis.

The following answer choices are given:
A. Advise Sam to discontinue the current antimicrobial and start a course of amoxicillin/clavulanate.
B. Perform tympanocentesis and send a sample of the exudate for culture and sensitivity.
C. Have Sam return in 24 hours for re-evaluation.
D. Recommend that Sam take ibuprofen for the next 2 to 3 days.

Which answer included the best course of action for Sam? Let's review the answers to see which one is correct and why.

A. Advise Sam to discontinue the current antimicrobial and start a course of amoxicillin with clavulanate.

- Choosing this response infers amoxicillin treatment failure. AOM antimicrobial treatment failure is usually defined, however, as persistent otalgia with fever after 72 hours of therapy. Sam has taken fewer than 2 days of therapy, an interval too short to assign continued symptoms to ineffective antimicrobial therapy. In addition, there is no report of Sam's condition worsening in the short time since he was initially seen. Therefore, prescribing an antimicrobial with a broader spectrum activity, such as amoxicillin/clavulanate, is not warranted at this time.

B. Perform tympanocentesis and send a sample of the exudate for culture and sensitivity.

- AOM antimicrobial therapy is based on choosing an agent with activity against the most likely organisms, bearing in mind the most common resistant pathogens. Tympanocentesis is indicated only with treatment failure after 10 to 21 days of antimicrobial therapy with a second-line agent, with the goal of detecting a significantly resistant organism; at that point, culture and sensitivity of middle ear exudate would be appropriate. With fewer than 2 days of treatment, tympanocentesis is not indicated.

C. Have Sam return in 24 hours for re-evaluation.

- If Sam's condition worsens in the next day, re-evaluation is prudent. However, choosing this option ignores Sam's complaint of pain.

D. Recommend that Sam take ibuprofen for the next 2 to 3 days.

- Choosing option D response infers that treating Sam's pain is the most appropriate intervention. This is the best response and the correct answer.

Now consider this question: Which of the following best describes asthma? No clinical scenario is presented; the question simply asks for a definition of a pathological state. When considering the options, the test-taker must recall that asthma is a chronic inflammatory disease of the airways involving an increase in bronchial hyperresponsiveness. This condition leads to a potentially reversible decrease in FEV1-to-FVC ratio. This type of answer lends itself well to becoming a "true/false" question. As you read each answer, ask yourself whether a choice is true or false. You are looking for the "true" answer. If answers seem partially true, or true sometimes, select the one that is mostly true, most of the time.

Here are your answer choices:

A. Intermittent airway inflammation with occasional bronchospasm

B. A disease of bronchospasm leading to airway inflammation

C. Chronic airway inflammation with superimposed bronchospasm

D. Relatively fixed airway obstruction

Let's again look at the choices and reveal the correct answer.

A. Intermittent airway inflammation with occasional bronchospasm

- Because asthma is a chronic, not intermittent, inflammatory airway disease, this option is incorrect.

B. A disease of bronchospasm leading to airway inflammation

- Because asthma is first a chronic inflammatory airway disease that leads to airway hyperresponsiveness, this option is incorrect.

C. Chronic airway inflammation with superimposed bronchospasm

- This option most closely matches the definition of asthma and is the best option.

D. Relatively fixed airway obstruction

- Because the airway obstruction in asthma is largely reversible, this option is incorrect. This answer is more descriptive of chronic obstructive pulmonary disease.

Review That Works for You

With test design in mind, it's time to think about planning an effective study strategy. As you learned in your graduate studies, there are many "right" ways to study. The most important factors to your success, regardless of learning style, depend on an organized and purposeful study plan. This issue of time needed for certification preparation is unique to each exam candidate. That said, one of the major pitfalls in study is the failure to put aside the time to prepare. Map out the demands on your time in the first months after completing your NP program, including work hours, family, personal and professional commitments, as well as time you have perhaps set aside for some well-deserved down time. After doing this, set up a schedule of study time, allotting a greater amount of time to areas of knowledge deficit and less to areas in which you only need to refresh your knowledge base. Make sure you cover all areas listed as possible exam content. Plan your date for certification only after a period of well-planned, systematic, certification-focused study.

Start with reviewing the information on the exam content. Make a list of the areas in which you feel your knowledge base is secure and in which just reviewing material to refresh your memory will likely suffice. Also, make a second list in which you identify areas of weaknesses and areas in which you need to concentrate your review. If you have taken an NP review course, you are likely aware that the content of certain parts of the program were truly review, whereas other sections help to point out areas in which you need to expand on your knowledge base. Knowing on what you need to concentrate your study helps you decide how to allocate your study time.

As you study, please keep in mind that the NP certification examination tests your ability to know the following:

- Why a patient is at risk for a problem.
- How a clinical problem has developed.

- What is the most likely clinical presentation of the condition.
- Why a given intervention is effective.
- How that intervention works.
- What is the most likely clinical outcome.
- Why this clinical problem is of significance to the overall healthcare system.

A poor approach to preparing for the exam and practice is to memorize information so you know what to do but not why you are doing it, in both the exam room and as part of the larger healthcare system. A better approach to preparing for the exam and practice is to understand concepts and apply knowledge so you know what to do and why you are doing it. The Fitzgerald Health Education Associates, Inc. NP Certification Examination Review and Advanced Practice Update prepares you in the why, how, and what of NP practice, as well as helping to prepare you for success on the NP boards.

As you work through practice questions, make a note next to each with words or symbols that indicate how certain you are of your answer. For some, you will be "sure" or "confident" that an answer is correct; for others you may be "mostly" or "somewhat sure"; and for others, you may be offering a best guess. After you score your pretest, examine how your answers match up with your predicted performance. If you marked yourself "confident" on an item you got wrong, start by studying the question and answer choices carefully to glean the possible reasons you might have selected the wrong answer for that particular question. Ask yourself the following: Did I understand the context properly? If so, did I misinterpret or misread the question? Was there unfamiliar content or vocabulary that led me to an incorrect conclusion? What was it about the distractors that distracted me? If you correctly answered a question about which you were not completely certain of the best answer, ask yourself what information in the context, action, or answers helped to lead you in the right direction. Frequent pretesting will not only help you to become more comfortable on test day, it can also help you to be more effective at unlocking a question.

When studying for the NP boards, some people will work best alone, whereas others benefit from collaborating with a study group. Study groups can be helpful and a terrific way to share information and resources. Alternatively, study groups can yield a poor return on time invested if all members are not similarly committed. Study groups can meet in person as well as over technology, such as Skype or Google groups. Here are some guidelines for forming a successful study group.

All group members must treat attendance and participation as they would any other professional commitment, such as work or school. Well in advance, set a schedule, place, and time to meet, as well as a topic for the meeting. Plan a start and end time, with a clear objective for the session. Study groups usually work best when a group member volunteers to research and present information on a subject on a predetermined schedule. The presentation is typically followed with a discussion of the issue and a review of sample exam questions and rationales for the correct response. The leader of a given session should also assume responsibility for keeping the discussion on track, facilitating the efficient use of time and resources.

In order to help avoid the group deteriorating into a chat session, plan for a short period of socialization following high-yield study sessions. Here is an example of a session planned by a highly successful study group with three members, Sarah, Ben, and Helena. "The session will start promptly at 7 p.m. and end at 9 p.m., with the objective of identifying the risk factors, clinical presentation, assessment, and intervention in community-acquired pneumonia in the adult. Sarah is the presenter and also group leader for the evening and is responsible for keeping us on track. A social period from 9 to 9:30 p.m. will follow. We will meet at Helena's apartment. Ben is responsible for refreshments."

Whenever possible, try to create a study situation that will mimic the actual test. Set a timer and be mindful of pacing yourself. During the test, expect to answer about 60 to 70 or more multiple-choice questions per hour. This means you will likely be spending less than a minute, on average, on each question. Some questions take only a few seconds, whereas others require more time for thought. Check yourself at 15- or 20-minute intervals to determine if you are progressing at an acceptable rate, setting a number of questions that you should have answered by a certain time.

Managing Nerves During Review and on Test Day

Everyone who sits for one of the certification examinations is anxious to some degree. This anxiety can be a helpful emotion, focusing the NP certification candidate on the task at hand: studying and successfully sitting for this important examination, a tangible end product of the candidate's graduate or postgraduate education. When excessive, however, anxiety can get in the way of success. Stress yields anxiety, anxiety yields stress; one can be viewed as the product of the other. The stress of preparing for an important examination triggers the sympathetic nervous system to Seyle's three phases of the general adaptation syndrome: alarm, resistance, and exhaustion. In the alarm stage, perhaps triggered by contemplating the preparation needed to achieve certification success, the hypothalamus activates the autonomic nervous system, triggering the pituitary and the body defenses, resulting in a heightened sense of awareness of surroundings, alertness, and focus. At this level of arousal, studying for and taking a test often yields great results. A well-prepared examination candidate is highly focused on what needs to be done to be successful on the examination. Distractions can be filtered out; extraneous information can be discarded in favor of the essentials. During the examination, anxiety and knowledge intersect; information retrieval is facilitated, and examination questions are fluidly processed. Difficult examination items are usually put in perspective, with the test-taker recognizing that most items were answered with relative ease. The NP certification candidate emerges from the test feeling challenged but confident.

Although a moderate amount of anxiety is natural, and even useful, many candidates can find themselves struggling with anxiety that is causing physical or emotional distress. The process of completing a rigorous course of graduate education and study can result in a protracted period of stress. Now, the formerly helpful stress leads to the second stage of the general adaptation syndrome, resistance, in which epinephrine is released to help counteract or escape from the stressor. At that time, the feeling of milder anxiety present in the first stage gives way to a sense of greater nervousness, often accompanied by uncomfortable physical sensations such as dry mouth, tachycardia, and tremor. Studying or test taking becomes difficult; information retrieval is inhibited. This stage is mentally and physically taxing and, if left unchecked, can lead to exhaustion, complicating the challenging task of successfully completing the certification examination. Although the reaction is most severe at the time of the test, most people who have severe test-taking anxiety have a similar, although milder, reaction with the deep study needed to prepare for a critical examination such as NP certification.

The following scenario describes a person with a problematic case of studying-testing anxiety:

The NP certification examination candidate is having a tough day, with a work shift that stretched for 3 unexpected hours and an unusually long commute, all following a poor night's sleep as a result of a noisy neighborhood party. To counteract this, the candidate drank a few extra cups of strong coffee and drank an "energy drink," really nothing more than a can of sugar and caffeine. She also skipped lunch and made a quick trip to a fast food restaurant for some fries as a snack. Studying was part of today's plan, however, so she sits down to prepare for the examination with great intentions of reviewing critical information. Surrounded by great stacks of study material, the NP candidate thinks about what might be on the examination and ponders the wide scope and knowledge base needed to be successful. Now the candidate becomes aware of a dry mouth and tight feeling in the throat. Determined, she sits down and decides to study about antimicrobial therapy. The words on the page seem to blur when the candidate tries to read about the spectrum of activity of an antibiotic; then, having difficulty keeping this information straight, she decides to skip that and focuses on memorizing a few antibiotic dose ranges, information that is unlikely to be on the boards. Even with repeated tries, the NP candidate cannot keep this information at hand and now becomes even more anxious, feeling tension in the back of the neck and a rapidly beating heart. The candidate now tries a few practice examination questions but answers three questions about the appropriate use of antimicrobial therapy in acute otitis media incorrectly. Now, even the thought of sitting for the examination causes the NP candidate to freeze.

In an ideal world, we could all control schedules and set aside vast periods of calm, focused review. Life, however, is complicated. Although developing a study schedule is important, rescheduling study time is likely a good idea when a day has been particularly difficult. Trying to learn when exhausted and stressed by other influences is often counterproductive. Certain scents can be helpful for putting the NP candidate in the right frame of mind to study, particularly under less-than-ideal conditions. These include basil, cinnamon, lemon, and peppermint for mental alertness and chamomile, lavender, and orange for relaxation.

Learning a relaxation technique to use before studying or test taking can help you start your review session with a clear mind and shift focus from whatever events or stress your day may have contained. You can also employ these same techniques on test day to help center yourself if you feel overwhelming anxiety begin to creep in. Start the session by reading or repeating a positive message about being successful on the examination. Avoid excessive amounts of caffeinated beverages prior to studying, which can add to anxious feelings. Eat a light but nourishing meal containing complex carbohydrates, fruit or vegetables, and high-quality protein to feed the body and mind. Avoid refined sugars and excessive fat intake, which can sap energy and derail quality study.

The NP candidate's anxiety started when pondering the wide range of possible topics on the certification examination. Starting the session studying a narrowly focused topic with a specific outcome goal rather than simply studying might have averted this. Setting up a system of study can enhance the success of a study session further. One method is the SQ4R system, in which one surveys the study information to establish goals; formulates questions about the information; and then reads to answer these questions, followed by reciting the responses to the original questions, and reviewing to see if the original goals were met. Study and test-taking anxiety can also be tamed with the help of a learning specialist who can work with the NP candidate to develop the needed skills. Learning specialists can usually be contacted through the academic support centers at universities.

Test Day

You have devoted years of study and months of preparation to this day, and this very thought can be daunting. Approaching test day with an empowered mindset can help alleviate fears and prepare you for what lies ahead. Let's assume you have devoted careful time to a purposeful and organized study regimen, and you are starting to think about the test day itself. Coaches often advise their athletes to avoid anything new on game day. You will be wise to heed this advice as well. This is not the time to change your diet, caffeine intake, medications, or sleep schedule. The test environment will be different from what you are used to, so try to keep your routines as close to "normal" for you as possible.

Visit the website of the certifying body to learn all that you can about test center rules, what you are and are not allowed to bring to the test site, and information about pacing and breaks. On test day, leave yourself plenty of time to arrive at your test center, to park, get settled, and enter the test without feeling rushed. Be sure to have a government-issued photo ID as well as copies of all confirmation numbers and e-mails from the test center or organization. Expect that video surveillance will be used in test centers to limit fraud and ensure security. At many test centers, you will be asked to empty your pockets and place all personal items in a locker provided for your use.

ANCC's test provider, Prometric, offers "test drives" that allow NP certification candidates to practice going through the test day routine ahead of their exam day. More information about test drives can be found on the Prometric Web site, accessible through the ANCC's Web site.

The ANCC examinations consist of 200 questions or test items. Of these, 175 items count toward your score, with the remaining 25 questions serving as sample items that might be used on future examinations but do not contribute to your examination score. The AANP examinations consist of 150 test items, with 15 items as sample questions that do not contribute to your final score. One purpose of adding these items is to evaluate the question's validity and reliability before incorporating the item in the certification examination. These items are integrated throughout the examination, not listed in a separate section. Please check with your certifying body for the most up-to-date information.

As part of your review, you should have some practice pacing yourself as you answer the test questions. Remember, you will have about one minute per test item. Don't get bogged down on a question or questions part of the way through the examination. If you are stumped by a question, move on, with a plan to return to this item at the end of the test. Remind yourself that you have answered many questions with relative ease. Finish all of those questions that you can answer and then come back later to process the problematic questions. The computer-based tests have a mechanism to highlight questions you want to revisit. Expect that the topics you studied will be presented in random order. A question on diabetes mellitus follows one on hypertension and can be preceded by a question on women's health.

Preparing for and taking the NP certification exam takes focus, determination, and courage. You have devoted years of study and months of preparation to this endeavor. Approaching test day with an empowered mindset can help alleviate fears and prepare you for what lies ahead. Emphasize context and adaptive expertise over memorization, become a master at "unlocking" test questions, and be honest with yourself about your learning style and study habits as you prepare to set yourself up for the best outcome. Additionally, consider these clinical practice and certification tips to help you prepare.

Clinical practice and certification tips:

- **Remember that common disease occurs commonly and that the uncommon presentation of a common disease is more common than the common presentation of an**

uncommon disease. *The fundamental tools of NP practice include the ability to procure comprehensively yet succinctly information needed to develop accurate diagnoses. Gathering the needed subjective and objective information in the care of a person with common acute, episodic, and chronic health problems is the most important skill the NP can develop. Develop the skill of taking a thorough yet concise health history that is pertinent to the patient's presenting complaint or health problem. As you proceed through the history, recall the rationale behind each question you ask and how a given response impacts the possible etiology of the patient's health problem. Know how to perform a thorough yet succinct symptom analysis. This process is when the detective work of diagnosis starts. Use the physical examination to confirm the findings of the health history.*

- **Remember that the physical examination is guided by the health history, not the other way around.** *The advanced practice NP role includes the responsibility of arriving at a diagnosis, developing a treatment plan, and providing ongoing evaluation of response to treatment.*

- **Learn to recognize the typical clinical presentation for the 10 most common health problems that present to your practice site, including chief complaint and physical examination findings, needed diagnostics, and intervention.** *Armed with this information, you can focus your study on a thorough knowledge of the assessment and treatment of these conditions. Continue to evaluate the patient's response to therapy.*

  Ask your preceptor to save laboratory results, EKGs, and other diagnostics for you to review at the next session. Do so with a clean eye, as if you were developing a plan of intervention or further diagnosis for the patient. This will help hone your skills. If you prescribed an intervention but will not have the opportunity to see the patient at a follow-up visit, ask your preceptor for an update. Family, cultural, community, developmental, and environmental factors as well as lifestyle and health behaviors influence patient health and the interaction between the NP and the patient. As an advanced practice nurse, the NP provides holistic, wellness-oriented care on an ongoing or episodic basis.

- **Remember to address a patient's primary, secondary, and tertiary healthcare needs at every visit.** *Check for needed immunization, screening tests, and follow-up on previous health problems with every encounter. Think long-term. Envision working with patients during the years ahead and the health problems you may help a person avoid by working together. The healthcare provided by the NP is guided by health and wellness research. The NP is accountable for his or her ongoing learning and professional development and is a lifelong learner. The NP is also knowledgeable in accessing resources to guide evidence-based care.*

- **Ask preceptors and peers what references are most helpful for that particular practice.** *Armed with this information, develop your own reference library that you can* *use with ease. Your investment of time and money to go gather these resources will pay off in your practice.*

REFERENCES

Nugent P, Vitale B. *Test Success: Test-Taking Techniques for Beginning Nursing Students*, ed. 5. Philadelphia: FA Davis, 2008.

Bloom BS (ed). *Developing Talent in Young People.* New York: Ballantine Books, 1985.

Hatano G, Inagaki K. Two Courses of Expertise. In: Stevenson H, Azuma H, Hakuta K (eds). *Child Development and Education in Japan.* New York: Freeman; 1986.

Mastering Tests. http://web.mit.edu/uaap/learning/test/index.html.

Sefcik D. *How to Study for Standardized Tests.* Sudbury, MA: Jones & Bartlett Publishers, 2012.

Taking Multiple Choice Exams. www.uwec.edu/geography/ivogeler/multiple.htm.

Test-taking Strategies. https://casc.byu.edu/testtaking-strategies.

Index

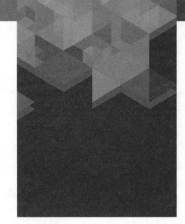

Note: Page numbers followed by f refer to figures, page numbers followed by t refer to tables, and page numbers followed by b refer to boxes.